LIST OF CHAPTERS BY BODY SYSTEM

Common Problems of the Head, Eyes, Ears, Nose, and Throat

14　Earache
19　Hoarseness
22　Nasal Symptoms and Sinus Congestion
27　Red Eye
29　Sore Throat
35　Vision Loss

Common Problems of the Skin

25　Rashes and Skin Lesions

Common Problems of the Cardiovascular System

7　Chest Pain
23　Palpitations
30　Syncope

Common Problems of the Respiratory System

10　Cough
13　Dyspnea

Common Problems of the Abdomen and Gastrointestinal System

2　Abdominal Pain
9　Constipation
11　Diarrhea
26　Rectal Pain, Itching, and Bleeding

Common Problems of the Genitourinary System

17　Genitourinary Problems in Males
24　Penile Discharge

31　Urinary Incontinence
32　Urinary Problems in Females and Children

Common Gynecological Problems

4　Amenorrhea
33　Vaginal Bleeding
34　Vaginal Discharge and Itching

Common Problems of the Breasts

5　Breast Lumps and Nipple Discharge
6　Breast Pain

Common Problems of the Musculoskeletal System

20　Limb Pain
21　Low Back Pain (Acute)

Common Problems of the Neurological System

12　Dizziness
18　Headache

Common Problems in Mental Status

3　Affective Changes
8　Confusion in Older Adults
28　Sleep Problems

Common Systemic Problems

15　Fatigue
16　Fever
36　Weight Loss/Gain (Unintentional)

Advanced Health Assessment *and* Clinical Diagnosis *in* Primary Care

Fourth Edition

Joyce E. Dains, DrPH, JD, RN, FNP-BC, DPNAP
Associate Professor and Advanced Practice Nursing Program Director
Manager, Professional Education for Prevention and Early Detection
The University of Texas MD Anderson Cancer Center
Houston, Texas

Linda Ciofu Baumann, PhD, APRN, BC, FAAN
Professor
University of Wisconsin–Madison
School of Nursing
Madison, Wisconsin

Pamela Scheibel, RN, MSN, CPNP
Clinical Professor
University of Wisconsin–Madison
School of Nursing
Madison, Wisconsin

ELSEVIER
MOSBY

3251 Riverport Lane
St. Louis, Missouri 63043

Notices

Knowledge and best practice in this field are constantly changing. As new research and experience broaden our understanding, changes in research methods, professional practices, or medical treatment may become necessary.

Practitioners and researchers must always rely on their own experience and knowledge in evaluating and using any information, methods, compounds, or experiments described herein. In using such information or methods they should be mindful of their own safety and the safety of others, including parties for whom they have a professional responsibility.

With respect to any drug or pharmaceutical products identified, readers are advised to check the most current information provided (i) on procedures featured or (ii) by the manufacturer of each product to be administered, to verify the recommended dose or formula, the method and duration of administration, and contraindications. It is the responsibility of practitioners, relying on their own experience and knowledge of their patients, to make diagnoses, to determine dosages and the best treatment for each individual patient, and to take all appropriate safety precautions.

To the fullest extent of the law, neither the Publisher nor the authors, contributors, or editors, assume any liability for any injury and/or damage to persons or property as a matter of products liability, negligence or otherwise, or from any use or operation of any methods, products, instructions, or ideas contained in the material herein.

Library of Congress Cataloging-in-Publication Data

Dains, Joyce E.
  Advanced health assessment and clinical diagnosis in primary care / Joyce E. Dains, Linda Ciofu Baumann, Pamela Scheibel.—4th ed.
       p. ; cm.
  Includes bibliographical references and index.
  ISBN 978-0-323-07417-9 (pbk.)
  1. Diagnosis, Differential. 2. Medical logic. 3. Medical history taking. 4. Physical diagnosis. I. Baumann, Linda Ciofu. II. Scheibel, Pamela. III. Title.
  [DNLM: 1. Diagnosis, Differential. 2. Diagnostic Techniques and Procedures. 3. Primary Health Care. WB 141.5]
  RC71.5.D35 2012
  616.07'5—dc22

                                                                          2011002591

Senior Editor: Lee Henderson
Senior Developmental Editor: Rae L. Robertson
Publishing Services Manager: Jeff Patterson
Project Manager: Megan Isenberg
Design Direction: Kim Denando

Printed in the United States of America

Last digit is the print number: 9 8 7 6 5 4 3

REVIEWER FOR THE 4TH EDITION

Kathleen Reeve, DrPH, MSN, ANP-BC, FNP-C
Associate Professor of Clinical Nursing
University of Houston–Victoria
Victoria, Texas

REVIEWERS FOR THE 3RD EDITION

Carin Schofield, RN, ACNP-C
Acute Care Nurse Practitioner
Vallejo Clinic
Tullahoma, Tennessee
Adjunct Faculty
Vanderbilt University School of Nursing
Nashville, Tennessee

Marlene G. S. Sefton, PhD, APN, CNP
Assistant Professor
FNP Option Coordinator
University of Illinois at Chicago
College of Nursing
Department of Public Health, Mental Health
and Administrative Nursing
Chicago, Illinois

ACKNOWLEDGMENTS

No text is ever written as a solitary effort and we have many thanks to offer. We've benefited from the extraordinary support and help of friends, family, and colleagues. We'd like to acknowledge each one. Our thanks are heartfelt; we honor your place in our lives.

To our colleagues at Elsevier who have continued to believe that this text is necessary and who have contributed their time, talent, and expertise—thank you. The remarkable efforts of each member of the publishing team are evident in the final product.

We'd also like to acknowledge the contributors to our first edition. Each is a superb clinician; each shared incredible expertise; and this text is richer because of them:

Katharine E. Hohol, MS, APRN, BC, APNP
Sandra K. Roof, MSN, APRN, BC, APNP
Robert W. Vogler, DSN, RN, CS, FNP
Pam Willson, PhD, RN, CS, FNP

Finally, we want to express our profound appreciation for those faculty, students, and clinicians who have found this book, for those who have shared their enthusiasm with us, and for those who have offered helpful suggestions and comments that have enhanced the content of this text. Thank you.

Joyce E. Dains
Linda C. Baumann
Pamela Scheibel

This text is designed for beginning clinicians and for students who will be using history and physical examination skills in the clinical setting. Its purpose is to take the student to the "next step" of health assessment, that is, beyond basic history and physical examination to using a diagnostic reasoning process. The book is intended to fill the gap between basic physical examination texts and the medical texts that are aimed primarily at disease management. It is not intended as a substitute for a clinical management text nor does it address management of disorders or diseases. Rather, it is designed specifically to focus on the clinical evaluation of common problems that present in primary care settings, using the tools of history and physical examination to engage in the process of clinical diagnosis.

The fourth edition of this text has several changes to further assist the transition to that "next step" of health assessment. Two new chapters have been added that reflect concerns commonly seen in primary care settings: Palpitations (Chapter 23) and Weight Loss/Gain (Unintentional) (Chapter 36). Another new chapter that expands coverage of radiographs, The Abdominal X-ray (Chapter 38), offers a guided approach to reading and interpreting abdominal x-rays. Further, we have expanded content on radiography in Chapter 20, Limb Pain. We have updated chapter content throughout and have increased the number of evidence-based practice guidelines. We continue to provide a list of selected references at the end of each chapter. These references support the information provided and are suggested for further in-depth learning about the problem. New to this edition we have included a list of the *Evidence-Based Practice* boxes on the inside back cover. Another new feature of this edition is arranging chapters alphabetically by chief concern to assist you in locating information.

The focus of *Advanced Health Assessment* is primary care patients. Both adults and children are included, with divergence in questions, examination, or interpretation of findings noted where pertinent. This text does not attempt to address all possible patient concerns but rather seeks to focus on the most common concerns as exemplars of the diagnostic reasoning process.

HOW TO USE THIS BOOK

Each chapter is structured in the context of a commonly occurring chief concern rather than a specific diagnosis or disease entity. Patients generally seek care for relief of symptoms and undiagnosed conditions. The initial challenge for primary care providers is to begin the process of differential diagnosis to determine the cause of a problem, based on history and physical examination and laboratory and other diagnostic tests. However, the steps of the diagnostic reasoning process are seldom articulated in a sequence that reflects the clinician's thought process. Novice clinicians are often left to their own devices, to figure out, for example, which history questions are the most important, which should be asked first and which can be left for later, or to determine which parts of the physical examination must be done as opposed to which will yield little information for a given concern. This text tries to articulate the reasoning process, order the history questions in a meaningful way, and focus the physical examination for a specific chief concern.

The diagnostic or clinical reasoning process is woven into each presenting problem. Each symptom begins with a brief introduction, providing an overview of causative mechanisms and processes. The clinical problem-solving process begins with *Focused History*, which walks through the thinking process involved in obtaining a pertinent, relevant, problem-specific history that will assist with differential diagnosis. The section is designed around questions that experienced clinicians ask themselves to order and organize the questions to be asked of the patient. These "self-questions" are structured according to what information the clinician needs first or most immediately about the presenting complaint, followed by self-questions that help sort through the possible differential diagnoses. The content and order of the self-questions vary, depending on the presenting problem. Sometimes the self-questions are based on what the condition is most likely to be; sometimes they are based on what is too important to miss.

For each of the self-questions there is a list of *Key Questions* to ask of the patient or about the patient if a family member is giving the history. The *Key Questions* are followed by an interpretation or explanation of what the patient responses might signify. For ease of format, the *Key Questions* are written as though the clinician were addressing the patient. Certainly with young children and sometimes with adults, the clinician will be asking questions of another person about the patient. The intent is to convey what questions to ask, rather than to provide every possible format for each question.

Following these two sections is the *Focused Physical Examination* section. It instructs you in what focused physical examination to perform to assist in the diagnostic process. The section is not intended to teach basic physical examination; it assumes you know how, using the techniques of inspection, auscultation, percussion, and palpation. This section, rather, provides focus for the examination, explains how to do more advanced maneuvers, and offers an interpretation of the findings.

Following is the section titled *Laboratory and Diagnostic Studies*. This section provides a brief outline of what kinds of laboratory or diagnostic studies would be appropriate for the chief concern or suspected diagnosis. Because the goal of the text is clinical diagnosis, the laboratory and diagnostic studies included are those that would be a logical starting point, although perhaps not an ending point.

The final section of each presenting concern is the *Differential Diagnosis*. It contains the most common differential diagnoses for the chief concern and summarizes, in a narrative format, the history and physical examination findings, along with the laboratory and diagnostic studies indicated. The section finishes with one or more *Differential Diagnosis* tables, mirroring the narrative summary, which can be used as a quick reference. An index to the *Differential Diagnosis* tables is provided in the text inside the back cover.

A new feature of the 4th edition is ordering the chief concerns alphabetically for easy user access. However, we know that many courses in advanced health assessment use a body systems approach. For ease in translating body systems to the new chapter order, use the quick-reference list found in the text inside the front cover.

The Appendices offer quick reference for often-needed clinical information. Appendices A and B provide height/weight and temperature conversions, and Appendix C provides a Body Mass Index plotting chart.

Perfecting advanced health assessment skills is a lifelong process. It is our hope that this edition continues to assist you in expanding the diagnostic reasoning process.

Joyce E. Dains
Linda C. Baumann
Pamela Scheibel

An Introduction to Clinical Reasoning

Clinical Reasoning, Differential Diagnosis, Evidence-Based Practice, and Symptom Analysis

Basic health assessment involves the application of the practitioner's knowledge and skills to identify and distinguish normal from abnormal findings. Basic assessment often moves from a general survey of a body system to specific observations or tests of function. Such an approach to assessment and clinical decision-making uses a deductive process of reasoning. For example, a specialist, when examining a patient with known hyperthyroidism, would conduct a physical examination to test for deep tendon reflexes. Brisk or hyperreflexic findings would lead the practitioner to conclude that a hyperthyroid state is a likely cause for these findings. This would greatly narrow the choices of diagnostic tests to perform and alterations in treatment to make.

Advanced assessment builds on basic health assessment yet is performed more often using an inductive or inferential process, that is, moving from a specific physical finding or patient concern to a more general diagnosis or possible diagnoses based on history, physical findings, and laboratory and diagnostic tests. The practitioner gathers further evidence and analyzes this evidence to arrive at a hypothesis that will lead to a further narrowing of possibilities. This is known as the process of diagnostic reasoning.

DIAGNOSTIC REASONING

Diagnostic reasoning is a scientific process in which the practitioner suspects the cause of a patient's symptoms and signs based on previous knowledge, gathers relevant information, selects necessary tests, and recommends therapy. The difference between an average and an excellent practitioner is the speed and focus used to arrive at the correct conclusion and initiate the best course of treatment with minimum cost, risk, inconvenience, and delay.

By using diagnostic reasoning, the practitioner accomplishes the following:

- Determines and focuses on what needs to be asked and what needs to be examined
- Performs examinations and diagnostic tests accurately
- Clusters abnormal findings
- Analyzes and interprets the findings
- Develops a list of likely or differential diagnoses

THE DIAGNOSTIC PROCESS
The Primary Care Context

The process of assessment in the primary care setting begins with the patient stating a reason for the visit or a chief concern. Most visits to primary care providers involve concerns or symptoms presented by the patient, such as an earache, vomiting, or fatigue. The initial evidence is collected through a patient history. Demographic information, such as gender, age, occupation, and place of residence, is obtained to place the patient in a risk category that can generally rule out certain diagnoses immediately. In most primary care settings, routine vital signs are obtained, which can include height and weight, temperature, pulse, respiratory rate, blood pressure, last menstrual period, and smoking status. While obtaining the history, the practitioner also makes observations of the patient's appearance, interaction with family members, orientation, and physical condition, and the practitioner notes any unusual findings that could help focus the assessment process.

Symptom Analysis

Presenting symptoms need to be explored with further questions. One useful mnemonic for gathering this information is COLDSPA:

Character—How does it feel, look, smell, sound?
Onset—When did it start?

Location—Be specific. Where is it? Does it radiate?

Duration—How long does it last? Does it recur?

Severity—How do you rate your pain on a scale from 0 (no pain) to 10 (worst pain I've ever had)?

Pattern—What makes it better? What makes it worse? What have you done and did it help?

Associated factors—What other symptoms do you have? How much does it interfere with your usual activities?

Another mnemonic is OLDCARTS: **O**nset; **L**ocation; **D**uration; **C**haracter; **A**ggravating/associated factors; **R**elieving factors; **T**emporal factors; **S**everity.

A final step is to ask about the patient's perception of the meaning of the symptom(s). The practitioner then clusters the information into logical groups based on prior knowledge of symptom clusters associated with specific diagnoses or body systems.

Formulating and Testing a Hypothesis

The practitioner then formulates a hypothesis based on expertise and knowledge of probable processes, such as a pathological, physiological, or psychological process. Further interpretation of evidence refines the hypothesis to a working or probable diagnosis. Hypothesis generation, in fact, probably already began based on the patient's age, gender, race, appearance, and presenting problem. Age is the most significant variable in narrowing the probabilities of a problem. Hypothesis generation forms the context in which further data are collected. This context includes the setting in which care is delivered, such as in a hospital, at an outpatient setting, or at another community-based setting where more than a single individual could be affected. Clinical decision-making can be filled with uncertainty and ambiguity. Because available evidence is almost never complete, hypothesis formation involves some element of subjective judgment.

The hypothesis must then be tested and assessed for the following characteristics:

- Coherence—Are the physiological links, predisposing factors, and complications for this disease present in the patient?
- Adequacy—Does the suspected disease encompass all of the patient's normal and abnormal findings?
- Parsimony—Is it the simplest explanation of the patient's findings? The surest way to make this determination is to ask the patient (or the parents) the reason for seeking care and the current understanding of the problem. This is a crucial step

because patients must find the treatment recommendation acceptable.

- Finally, can a competing hypothesis be eliminated? What other diseases could explain the patient's symptoms?

To confirm the hypothesis, the practitioner establishes a working definition of the problem as a basis for a treatment plan and evaluates the outcome. The goal of a clinical decision is to choose an action that is most likely to result in the health outcomes the patient desires. This step of the decision-making process involves personal preference as to whether the benefits are worth the risks involved, the cost is reasonable, and the most desired outcomes are short or long term.

Clinicians make extensive use of heuristics, or rules of thumb, to guide the inductive or inferential process of diagnostic reasoning. Heuristics are generally accurate and useful rules to make the task of information gathering more manageable and efficient—rules such as familiarity, salience, and resemblance to a patient who has a known disease. On occasion, however, heuristics can be faulty, particularly if the presentation is atypical or the condition is rare. The clinician must always be open to a low probability of a serious diagnosis. Heuristics can have negative effects when stereotypes or biases influence judgment. For example, assuming that a patient is heterosexual can lead to errors in clinical reasoning and differential diagnosis when evaluating the symptoms of rectal pain.

EXPERT VERSUS NOVICE CLINICIANS

Students of advanced assessment have a variety of backgrounds, with many coming from specialized areas of clinical practice. Such students could have difficulty broadening the scope of their observations and clinical possibilities. In any case, whether specialists or not, nonexperts tend to be nonselective in data gathering and in the clinical reasoning strategies they use. Experts, on the other hand, are able to focus on a problem, recognize patterns, and gather only relevant data, with a high probability of a correct diagnosis. The goal for a novice practitioner is to aim for competence and expertise.

The competent practitioner will execute the following steps:

1. Identify the most important cues. These cues are obtained largely through thorough symptom analysis (e.g., COLSDPA), functional assessment, and history to assess the patient's beliefs

and understanding or explanatory model of the illness. Research evidence shows that a person's beliefs or explanatory models of an illness or a symptom include a cause, an opinion about the timeline (acute or chronic), consequences of the condition (minor or life threatening), and some type of verbal label used to identify the cluster of symptoms or sensations (e.g., "the flu," "the blues") (Baumann and Leventhal, 1985; Kleinman et al, 1978). Clinicians need to distinguish between the presence of disease, which has a biological basis, and illness, which is the human experience of being sick that could have little correlation with the objective evidence that is available.

2. Understand and perform advanced examination techniques. These techniques can include special maneuvers and closer observation of fine detail during the physical examination, more in-depth interviews using valid and reliable instruments to assess the patient's risk for a specific diagnosis, and "gold standard" diagnostic tests for the identification of a specific disorder.

3. Test differential or competing diagnoses. A differential diagnosis results from a synthesis of subjective and objective findings, including laboratory and diagnostic tests, with knowledge of known and recognized patterns of signs and symptoms. When using the "rule-out" strategy, the clinician looks for the absence of findings that are frequently seen with a specific condition; the absence of a sensitive finding is strong evidence against the condition being present. When using the "rule-in" strategy, the clinician looks for the presence of a finding with high specificity (low false-positive and high true-negative values); the presence of this finding is strong evidence that the condition is present.

4. See a pattern in the information gathered. A pattern or cluster of findings can emerge from the subjective and objective data. This pattern could be evident during one patient encounter or it could depend on a pattern of signs and symptoms that develops over time. Often the expert clinician can eliminate competing diagnoses only after the initial treatment prescribed is ineffective or after the symptoms either disappear sooner than expected or persist longer than expected.

DEVELOPING CLINICAL JUDGMENT

Brykczynski (1989) studied how advanced practice nurses developed clinical reasoning skills. In her analysis, she observed that didactic content in a lecture or a reference book often discusses the classic presentation of a patient with a specific disorder and does not acknowledge variables that are present in the actual clinical situation. Even the use of case studies has limitations because the data are presented to the reader but in actual clinical practice the practitioner has to be ready to begin the clinical reasoning process by knowing what to ask a patient (Ryan-Wenger and Lee, 1997). Thus theoretical knowledge has limitations in the exercise of expert clinical judgment. Practical knowledge requires actual experience in a situation that is contextual and transactional, and is acquired only through spending time with patients, practicing focused listening, and gaining experience in recognizing subtle cues.

NEGOTIATING GOALS AND EXPECTATIONS OF A PATIENT ENCOUNTER

It is important, especially in an ambulatory care setting, to identify the patient's goals, expectations, and resources to determine what needs to be achieved during an encounter. A patient who seeks care because of a bothersome symptom could be more interested in having the symptom relieved by a particular date than in knowing the cause or diagnostic explanation for the symptom. Other patients could want reassurance that a symptom or sign is not a serious condition and yet do not expect treatment to alleviate the sensations they are experiencing. An explicit discussion between the clinician and patient is necessary to establish what the goals and focus of an encounter will be. Goals can be mutually negotiated to assure clinicians that serious conditions can be "ruled out" and to assure patients that their needs and desires are acknowledged.

EVIDENCE-BASED PRACTICE

Evidence-based practice (EBP) is the integration of clinical judgment with the most current, relevant, and sound research evidence to guide clinical practice decisions. EBP integrates the best research evidence with clinical expertise and the patient's concerns and expectations, and it involves the use of simple rules of logic to apply evidence from research to an individual patient.

EVIDENCE-BASED PRACTICE *Web Sources*

National Guideline Clearinghouse	www.guideline.gov	Evidence-based practice guidelines and best practices
The Cochrane Collaboration	www.cochrane.org	Cochrane Library of systematic literature reviews about treatments and interventions
Cumulative Index to Nursing and Allied Health Literature	www.cinahl.com	CINAHL database on all aspects of nursing, allied health, alternative health, and community medicine
Medscape (from WebMD)	www.medscape.com	MEDLINE database maintained by the National Library of Medicine for biomedical content for dentistry, veterinary medicine, and nursing
Agency for Healthcare Research and Quality	www.ahrq.gov	A resource for information related to improving quality, safety, efficiency, and effectiveness of care
US Preventive Services Task Force	www.ahrq.gov/clinic/uspstfix.htm	Scientific evidence reviews of a broad range of clinical preventive health care services
Clinical Evidence	www.clinicalevidence.org	A compendium of resources for informing treatment and patient care decisions

Some of these rules include evaluating the validity and reliability of the evidence. The levels of evidence range from the "gold standard" of the randomized clinical trial to case studies, correlational studies, and expert opinion. Clinicians and patients increasingly gather evidence from web-based sources, such as the Cochrane Library, which includes databases of systematic reviews of a clinical topic, abstracts of reviews of effectiveness, a controlled trial registry, and review methodology. These databases have gathered the "best evidence" related to clinical problems (Evidence-Based Practice Box). Access to web-based data requires that the practitioner develop skills in health informatics—the application of computer technology to health care delivery. Clinicians need to develop skills in searching for and appraising information for a specific patient in a specific clinical context.

SUMMARY

In the context of primary care practice, the orientation to the patient should be holistic and general and toward the most prevalent or common conditions in a particular population group. This orientation requires that the expert practitioner develop skills in inductive reasoning to arrive at a diagnosis and a treatment plan that are acceptable to the patient. Knowledge of the patient as a person over time greatly enhances the database from which the clinician works to arrive at better clinical judgments. Treatment plans in primary care settings rely on low-level

technology and stress prevention, and encourage self-care behaviors as well as open and effective patient-provider communication. Practitioners need to be able to search for and evaluate the best evidence to guide assessment, treatment, and evaluation of diagnostic efficacy. A practitioner can move from novice to expert and become more efficient in exercising clinical judgment by asking the right questions, seeking pertinent information from the body of scientific evidence, and using clinical reasoning to apply the best evidence to clinical practice.

REFERENCES AND READINGS

Baumann LJ, Leventhal H: I can tell if my blood pressure is up, can't I? *Health Psychol* 4:203, 1985.

Brykczynski KA: An interpretive study describing clinical judgment of nurse practitioners, *Sch Inq Nurs Pract* 3:75, 1989.

Eddy DM: Evidence-based medicine: a unified approach, *Health Aff* 24:9, 2005.

Guyatt GH, Oxman AD, Vist GE, Kunz R, Falck-Ytter Y, Alonso-Coello P, et al: for the GRADE Working Group. GRADE: an emerging consensus on rating quality of evidence and strength of recommendations. *BMJ* 336:924, 2008.

Kleinman A, Benson P: Anthropology in the clinic: The problem of cultural competency and how to fix it, *PLoS Med* 3:e294.

Ryan-Wenger NA, Lee JE: The clinical reasoning case study: a powerful teaching tool, *Nurse Pract* 22:66, 1997.

Straus SE, Richardson WS, Glasziou P, Haynes RB: *Evidence-based medicine: how to practice and teach EBM*, 3rd Ed., London, 2003, BMJ Books.

II

Common Symptoms in Primary Care

2

Abdominal Pain

Abdominal pain is a subjective feeling of discomfort in the abdomen that can be caused by a variety of problems. The goal of initial clinical assessment is to distinguish acute life-threatening conditions from chronic/recurrent or acute mild, self-limiting conditions. Assessment is complicated by the dynamic rather than static nature of acute abdominal pain, which can produce a changing clinical picture, often over a short period of time. In addition, both children and older adults tend to deviate from the usual and anticipated clinical pattern of abdominal pain.

The following three processes can produce abdominal pain: (1) tension in the gastrointestinal (GI) tract wall from muscle contraction or distention; (2) ischemia; and (3) inflammation of the peritoneum. Pain can also be referred from within or outside the abdomen.

Colic is a type of tension pain. It is associated with forceful peristaltic contractions and is the most characteristic type of pain arising from the viscera. Colicky pain can be produced by an irritant substance, from infection with a virus or bacteria, or by the body's attempt to force its luminal contents through an obstruction. Another type of tension pain is caused by acute stretching of the capsule of an organ, such as the liver, spleen, or kidney. The patient with this visceral pain is restless, moves about, and has difficulty getting comfortable.

Ischemia produces an intense, continuous pain. The most common cause of intestinal ischemic pain is strangulation of the bowel from obstruction.

Inflammation of the peritoneum usually begins at the serosa covering the affected and inflamed organ, causing visceral peritonitis. The pain is a poorly localized aching. As the inflammatory process spreads to the adjacent parietal peritoneum, it produces localized parietal peritonitis. The pain of parietal peritonitis is more severe and is perceived in the area of the abdomen corresponding to the inflammation. The patient with parietal pain usually lies still and does not want to move.

Pain can be referred from within the abdomen or from other parts of the body (Box 2-1).

Referral of pain occurs because tissues supplied by the same or adjacent neural segments have the same common pathways inside the central nervous system. Thus stimulation of these neural segments produces the sensation of pain. For example, nerves that supply the appendix are derived from the same source as those that supply the small intestine, resulting in the onset of appendicitis pain in the epigastric area.

Abdominal pain in adults can be classified as acute, chronic, or recurrent. The term acute abdomen refers to any acute condition within the abdomen that requires immediate surgical attention. Not all acute abdominal pain, however, requires surgical intervention. Acute abdominal pain refers to a relatively sudden onset of pain that is severe or increasing in severity and has been present for a short duration. Chronic pain is characterized by its persistent duration or recurrence. Recurrent episodes of pain can be either acute or chronic in nature.

In adults, acute pain requiring surgical intervention is commonly caused by appendicitis, perforated peptic ulcer, intestinal obstruction, peritonitis, perforate diverticulitis, ectopic pregnancy, or dissection of aortic aneurysm. Common causes of acute pain not requiring surgical intervention include cholelithiasis, gastroenteritis, peptic gastroduodenal syndrome, pancreatitis, pelvic inflammatory disease (PID), or urinary tract infection (UTI). Chronic or recurrent pain can be caused by GI disorders, such as irritable bowel syndrome (IBS), diverticulitis, or esophagitis; pelvic disorders, such as dysmenorrhea or uterine fibroids; genitourinary disorders, such as recurrent UTI or chronic prostatitis; or conditions outside the abdomen, such as costochondritis, hip disease, or hernia.

In children, abdominal pain can be classified as acute or recurrent. Common causes of acute pain include appendicitis, food poisoning, UTI, viral gastroenteritis, and bacterial enterocolitis. Recurrent abdominal pain (RAP) is defined as more than three episodes

Box 2-1	Some Causes of Pain Perceived in Anatomical Regions

Right Upper Quadrant
Duodenal ulcer
Hepatitis
Hepatomegaly
Pneumonia
Cholecystitis

Right Lower Quadrant
Appendicitis
Salpingitis
Ovarian cyst
Ruptured ectopic pregnancy
Renal/ureteral stone
Strangulated hernia
Meckel diverticulitis
Regional ileitis
Perforated cecum

Periumbilical
Intestinal obstruction
Acute pancreatitis
Early appendicitis
Mesenteric thrombosis
Aortic aneurysm
Diverticulitis

Left Upper Quadrant
Ruptured spleen
Gastric ulcer
Aortic aneurysm
Perforated colon
Pneumonia

Left Lower Quadrant
Sigmoid diverticulitis
Salpingitis
Ovarian cyst
Ruptured ectopic pregnancy
Renal/ureteral stone
Strangulated hernia
Perforated colon
Regional ileitis
Ulcerative colitis

Modified from Judge R, Zuidema G, Fitzgerald F: *Clinical diagnosis, ed 5,* Boston, 1988, Little Brown.

of pain in 3 months in children older than 3 years. It affects 10% to 15% of children between the ages of 3 and 14; of these children, 90% will not have an organic etiology.

DIAGNOSTIC REASONING: FOCUSED HISTORY

Is this an acute condition?

Key Questions

- How long ago did your pain start?
- Was the onset sudden or gradual?
- How severe is the pain (on a scale of 1 to 10)?
- If a child: What is the child's level of activity?
- Does the pain wake you up from sleep?
- What has been the course of the pain since it started? Is it getting worse or better?
- When was your last bowel movement?
- Have you ever had this pain before?

Onset/Duration

Acute onset of pain that is getting progressively worse could signal a surgical emergency. In general, patients who present with severe pain 6 to 24 hours from the onset probably have an acute surgical condition. Acute abdominal pain can signal a few potentially life-threatening conditions that must be

considered first. The following are possible surgical emergencies that require immediate evaluation and intervention:

- Perforation: look for signs and symptoms of peritonitis (Box 2-2)
- Ectopic pregnancy: in any woman of childbearing age
- Obstruction: in the elderly
- Ruptured abdominal aortic aneurysm: when back pain is present
- Intussusception: in infants
- Malrotation: in infants usually less than 1 month old

Box 2-2	Features of Peritonitis

Pain: front, back, sides, shoulders
Electrolytes fall; shock ensues
Rigidity or rebound of anterior abdominal wall
Immobile abdomen and patient
Tenderness with involuntary guarding
Obstruction
Nausea and vomiting
Increasing pulse rate, decreasing blood pressure
Temperature falls and then rises; tachypnea
Increasing girth of abdomen
Silent abdomen (no bowel sounds)

Modified from Shipman JJ: *Mnemonics and tactics in surgery and medicine, ed 2,* Chicago, 1984, Mosby.

Pain of sudden onset is more likely associated with colic, perforation, or acute ischemia (torsion, volvulus). Slower onset of pain generally is associated with inflammatory conditions, such as appendicitis, pancreatitis, and cholecystitis.

Acute pain that comes and goes can be related to intestinal peristalsis. The onset of pain in relation to food ingestion provides diagnostic clues: pain occurring several hours after a meal suggests a duodenal ulcer (pain with stomach empty), whereas pain immediately after eating occurs with esophagitis.

In children, RAP occurs in attacks usually lasting less than 1 hour and rarely longer than 3 hours and frequently interferes with daily routines. Between episodes, the pain resolves completely. When interviewing a child, remember that the child might not be old enough to have a clear sense of time.

Severity and Progression

Severity is the most difficult symptom to evaluate because of its subjective quality. It is helpful to use a 1-to-10 scale in adults. Children often respond to the use of the pain faces or the Oucher Pain Scale (Figure 2-1).

Determine whether the pain is an acute episode or a chronic or recurrent episode. Acute abdominal pain requires immediate attention, because it can signal an acute surgical condition in the abdomen. Chronic or recurrent episodes of pain can be handled in a more temperate manner.

Pain that is steady, severe, and progressive is worrisome. Pain that causes one to awake from sleep is serious. A sudden pain severe enough to cause fainting suggests perforated ulcer, ruptured aneurysm, or ectopic pregnancy. A severe knifelike pain usually indicates an emergency. Tearing pain is characteristic of an aortic aneurysm. Appendicitis is often described as an ache. Colicky pain that becomes steady can indicate appendicitis or strangulating intestinal obstruction.

Children are poor historians regarding the severity of pain. The caregiver should indicate how severe the child's pain is by a description of the activity level of the child. In general, avoidance of favorite activities or motion indicates an organic problem. Organic disease awakens the child from sleep.

Last Bowel Movement

Obstipation (the absence of stools) occurs with complete obstruction, but diarrhea can be present with partial obstruction. Lack of a bowel movement for 3 days could signal constipation. Children can have sudden onset of constipation that can cause severe abdominal pain.

Previous Pain

Chronic pain could result when a potential surgical event is partially controlled but is not totally resolved. Chronic pain that has been present for longer than 1 year generally is not caused by a neoplasm; consider instead IBS or colorectal, endometrial, or inflammatory causes.

Recurrent attacks of acute pain could be caused by inflammation and exacerbation of a chronic condition, such as functional colonic pain, IBS, cholecystitis, chronic pancreatitis, diverticulitis, or ulcer disease. Acute pain can also be caused by recurrent infection, such as pyelonephritis or cystitis. Urinary tract stones can also cause acute attacks of recurrent pain.

Will the location of pain give me any clues?

Key Questions

- Where is the pain? Can you point to it?
- Does it travel (radiate) anywhere?

Location of the Pain

The viscera is innervated bilaterally so that pain is perceived in the midline. It is often described as a deep, dull, diffuse pain. Visceral pain originates from epigastric, periumbilical, and hypogastric causes; from intraabdominal extraperitoneal organs (pancreas, kidneys, ureters, great vessels, pelvic organs); or from a referred source.

Parietal (also known as peritoneal or somatic) pain is more localized and is described as a sharp pain. Peritoneal pain originates from intraabdominal and intraperitoneal organs.

Inflammation (for example, with appendicitis) can produce either visceral or parietal peritonitis. Initially the inflammation is limited to the serosa covering an inflamed organ. The pain is visceral and is felt diffusely. As the inflammation progresses to the adjacent parietal peritoneum, it produces a more severe localized pain that is perceived in the corresponding area of the abdomen. Children have a poor ability to localize pain and are not helpful in the majority of cases.

The Apley rule states that the further the localization of pain from the umbilicus, the more likely it is that there is an underlying organic disorder.

When blood, pus, or gastric fluid suddenly floods the peritoneal cavity, the pain is frequently reported

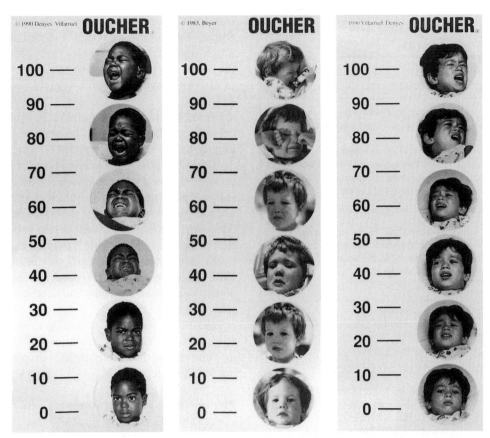

FIGURE 2-1 The Oucher Pain Scale illustrated with African American, Caucasian, and Hispanic children to best fit the child's cultural identity. The African American child version of the Oucher was developed and copyrighted in 1990 by Mary J. Denyes, PhD, RN, FAAN (Wayne State University), and Antonia Villarruel, PhD, RN, FAAN (University of Michigan), at the Children's Hospital of Michigan. Cornelia P. Porter, PhD, RN, and Charlotta Marshall, MSN, RN, contributed to the development of this scale. The Caucasian child version of the Oucher was developed and copyrighted in 1983 by Judith E. Beyer, PhD, RN, currently at the University of Missouri—Kansas City School of Nursing. Photographs were taken by Lynn Julaino, RN, BSN, at Martha Jefferson Hospital in Charlottesville, Va. The Hispanic child version of the Oucher was developed and copyrighted in 1990 by Antonia M. Villarruel, PhD, RN (University of Michigan), and Mary J. Denyes, PhD, RN (Wayne State University). Photographs were taken at Children's Hospital of Michigan in Detroit.

as "all over the abdomen" at first. However, the maximum intensity of pain at the onset is likely to be in the upper abdomen with gastric problems and in the lower abdomen with tubal and appendix rupture. Irritating fluid from a perforated duodenal ulcer produces pain in the right hypochondrium, lumbar, and iliac regions.

Pain arising from the small intestine is always felt in the epigastric and umbilical areas of the abdomen. The ninth and eleventh thoracic nerves supply the small intestine via the common mesentery nerve. Appendicular nerves are derived from the same source

as those that supply the small intestine, resulting in onset of pain in the epigastric area with appendicitis.

Table 2-1 describes the structures involved in specific pain locations.

Radiation of Pain

Radiation of pain can help in diagnosis. Pain that radiates will do so to the area of distribution of the nerves coming from that segment of the spinal cord that supplies the affected area. Biliary colic pain is frequently referred to the region just under the right scapula (eighth dorsal

Table 2-1	Pain Location and Involved Structures
PAIN LOCATION	**INVOLVED STRUCTURES**
Epigastric	Esophagus, stomach, duodenum, liver, gallbladder, pancreas, spleen
Upper abdominal	Esophagus, stomach, duodenum, pancreas, liver, gallbladder, or thorax
Right upper quadrant	Usually esophagus, stomach, duodenum, pancreas, liver, gallbladder, or thorax; often indicates acute cholecystitis
Left upper quadrant	Spleen
Periumbilical	Jejunum, midgut, ileum, appendix, ascending colon; pain caused by inflammation, ischemic spasm, or abnormal distention
Lower abdominal	Colon, sigmoid colon, rectum, and genitourinary structures—bladder, uterus, prostate
Right lower quadrant	Appendix, fallopian tube, ovary
Left lower quadrant	Sigmoid colon, fallopian tube, ovary
Flanks	Kidney(s)
Localized	Occurs from local inflammation of skin or peritoneum, as with appendicitis; lateralized pain occurs in paired organs—kidneys, ureters, fallopian tubes, gonads
Generalized	Produced by diffuse inflammation of gastrointestinal tract, peritoneum, or abdomen wall

segment), whereas renal colic in males is frequently felt in the testicle of the same side. Pain from a ruptured spleen is often referred to the top of the left shoulder.

What do the pain characteristics tell me?

Key Questions

- Can you describe the pain (e.g., burning, sharp, achy, crampy)?
- What makes it worse or better?

Character of Pain

Colicky or cramping pain occurs with obstruction of a hollow viscus that produces distention. Generally there are pain-free intervals when the pain is much

less intense but still present, although it is subtle. During the painful episodes, the patient is exceedingly agitated and restless, and often pale and diaphoretic. The pain from obstruction of the small intestine is rhythmic, peristaltic pain with intermittent cramping. When the obstruction site is in the proximal small intestine rather than in the more distal portion, the paroxysms of cramping occur with greater frequency.

Steady pain is associated with perforation, ischemia, inflammation, and blood in the peritoneal cavity. Burning pain is characteristic of esophagitis. Pain from a duodenal ulcer has been described as burning or "gnawing." Pain of pancreatic origin is steady, epigastric, and prostrating. Pricking, itching, or burning pain comes from superficial causes such as herpes zoster. Dull, aching pain indicates deeper pain. In children, abdominal pain is generally characterized as colicky or inflammatory.

Remember, however, that despite descriptions of characteristic or typical abdominal pain, presentation in children and the elderly is often atypical and might not fit any pattern.

Precipitating or Aggravating Factors

Lying down or bending forward often produces pain from esophagitis. Alcohol can aggravate gastritis or an ulcer.

Pain that is made worse by deep inspiration and is stopped or diminished by a respiratory pause indicates pleuritic origin. If the cause is peritonitis, intraperitoneal abscess, or abdominal distention from intestinal obstruction, pain will increase on deep inspiration. Biliary colic is made worse by forced inspiration. The pain from biliary colic often causes inhibition of movement of the diaphragm.

The patient with visceral pain is restless, moves about, and has difficulty getting comfortable. The patient with parietal pain usually lies still and does not want to move. Children with inflammatory pain secondary to peritoneal irritation usually appear quiet and motionless because movement exacerbates the pain.

Relieving Factors

Food or antacids can relieve pain caused by an ulcer or gastritis. Both colicky pain and inflammatory pain are alleviated significantly with analgesics. However, the pain of a vascular accident will not respond to analgesics.

Are there any precipitating events that will help narrow my diagnosis?

Key Questions

- Is the pain related to any other activity (e.g., eating, lying down)?
- Can you identify any trigger?

Relation to Other Events

Pain that is relieved by defecation, flatus, laxatives, or diet changes implicates the intestine. Pain associated with meals implicates the GI tract.

Pain with sexual activity (dyspareunia) suggests a pelvic origin. Pain that occurs with position changes can be referred from the spine, hips, sacroiliac joint, pelvic bones, or abdominal musculature. Exertional pain can be of cardiac origin.

What does the presence of vomiting or diarrhea tell me?

Key Questions

- Are you vomiting? What does the vomitus look like?
- What do your stools look like?
- How frequent are your stools?

Vomiting

Vomiting that precedes the onset of abdominal pain is unlikely to signal a problem requiring surgery. Vomiting suggests that the pain is visceral in origin. Anorexia is a nonspecific symptom, but its absence makes serious disease less likely.

Vomiting associated with an acute condition of the abdomen may be from one of the following three causes:

- Severe irritation of the nerves of the peritoneum or mesentery. Sudden stimulation of many sympathetic nerves causes vomiting to occur early and to be persistent.
- Obstruction of an involuntary muscular tube. Obstruction of any of the muscular tubes causes peristaltic contraction and consequent stretching of the muscle wall, which results in vomiting. The area behind the obstruction becomes dilated, and, as each peristaltic wave occurs, the tension and stretching of the muscular fibers are temporarily increased; therefore the pain of colic usually occurs in spasms. Vomiting usually occurs at the height of the pain.

- The action of absorbed toxins on the medullary centers. The chemoreceptor trigger zone is stimulated by drugs such as cardiac glycosides, ergot alkaloids, and morphine or by uremia, diabetic ketoacidosis, or general anesthetics. Impulses to the medullary vomiting center then activate the vomiting process.

Pain with Vomiting

In sudden and severe stimulation of the peritoneum or mesentery, vomiting comes soon after the pain. In acute obstruction of the urethra or bile duct, vomiting is early, sudden, and intense. In intestinal obstruction, the timing of the vomiting indicates how high in the gut the obstruction is. If the duodenum is obstructed, vomiting occurs with the onset of pain. Obstruction of the large bowel causes very late or infrequent vomiting.

Vomiting is not usually seen in ectopic pregnancy, gastric or duodenal perforation, or intussusception. Vomiting occurring before pain indicates gastroenteritis. With appendicitis, pain almost always precedes the vomiting.

Vomitus Appearance

Clear vomitus suggests gastric fluid; bile-colored vomitus is from upper GI contents. Feculent vomitus occurs with distal intestinal obstruction. Patients with gastric outlet obstruction vomit fluid that contains food particles if the patient has eaten recently, but later the vomitus becomes clear. Infants with duodenal atresia will vomit bilious fluid, but in pyloric stenosis no bile is seen.

Stool Characteristics

Diarrhea is associated with inflammatory bowel disease, diverticulitis, or early obstruction. The presence of blood in the stool suggests that the pain originates in the intestinal tract. Blood can indicate neoplasm, intussusception, or inflammatory lesions.

Diarrhea can precede perforation of the appendix as a result of irritation of the sigmoid colon, by an inflammatory mass. Some patients will report gas stoppage symptoms: the sensation of fullness that suggests the need for a bowel movement. With appendicitis, the patient often attempts to defecate but without relief.

In children, mild diarrhea associated with the onset of pain suggests acute gastroenteritis but can also occur with early appendicitis. A low-lying appendix, close to the sigmoid colon and rectum, can induce an inflammatory process of the muscle wall of the sigmoid colon. Any distention of the sigmoid by fluid or gas signals the child to pass gas and small amounts of stool. The cycle repeats a few minutes later. In gastroenteritis, typically the child will have large liquid stools. Children can also have abdominal pain from chronic constipation. Constipation that precedes pain suggests disease of the colon or rectum.

Are there any clues to implicate a particular organ system?

If the patient gives a positive response to the following history questions, refer to the topic or chapter indicated for additional discussion. Pain that is not abdominal in origin could be referred to, or perceived to be in, the abdomen. Accompanying symptoms of headache, sore throat, and general aches and pains suggest a viral, flulike cause.

Key Questions

Cardiovascular system (Chapter 7):
- Does the pain occur with exertion or at rest?
- Do you have any chest pain, palpitations, fast heartbeat, or pain that goes to the arm or jaw?

Referred pain from the chest is not uncommon. Pain on exertion signals coronary artery disease (CAD) and angina. Right upper quadrant (RUQ) pain can be caused by congestive heart failure. Myocardial infarction and pericarditis can also cause abdominal pain.

Key Questions

Gastrointestinal system (Chapters 9 and 11):
- Do you have any GI symptoms (e.g., gas, diarrhea, constipation, vomiting, heartburn)?
- Have you had any changes in your bowel habits, stools, or eating pattern?
- Is the pain relieved by defecation or burping?

Gas, bloating, diarrhea, constipation, and rectal bleeding can occur with pain that is intestinal in origin. Heartburn and dysphagia are characteristic of esophagitis. Changes in bowel habits can signal obstruction or neoplasm. Constipation alternating with diarrhea is characteristic of IBS. The patient often also reports distention, bloating, belching, gas, and mucus in the stools.

Pain relieved by defecation or the passage of gas suggests IBS or gas entrapment in the large intestine. Pain relieved by burping suggests distention of the stomach by gas.

Key Questions

Genitourinary system (Chapters 4, 17, 24, and 31 to 34):
- When was your last menstrual period (LMP)? Was it normal for you? Could you be pregnant?
- Do you have any vaginal symptoms or problems, such as unusual discharge, unusual bleeding, or pain with sexual intercourse?
- Do you have any menstrual irregularity or unusual bleeding? (Sexual history could provide information relevant to the possibility of sexually transmitted infections [STIs], PID, and pregnancy.)
- Do you have any urinary symptoms (e.g., frequency, urgency, dysuria, blood in urine, change in urine color)?
- Do you have pain in the back (flank)? Can you point to it?

Menstrual irregularities, vaginal discharge, unusual bleeding, or dyspareunia indicate a pelvic origin of the pain. Sexually active adolescent girls are at the highest risk for contracting PID. Patients with PID may complain of both vaginal discharge and abnormal vaginal bleeding, although pain is often the only presenting symptom. The pain is usually severe and progressive. Pain just before the onset of menses indicates endometriosis. Pain related to ovulation (mittelschmerz) occurs mid-cycle. In women of childbearing age, always consider ectopic pregnancy. Regard women of childbearing age as pregnant until pregnancy is ruled out.

Urinary symptoms (dysuria, hematuria, hesitancy, or frequency) point to a urinary tract cause of the pain. Flank pain is usually associated with renal calculi or pyelonephritis. Upper abdominal pain that radiates to the groin signals ureterolithiasis.

Key Questions

Musculoskeletal system (Chapters 20 and 21):
- Does the pain occur with change in position or movement?
- Do you have any joint pain, heat, swelling, noises, or limitation in range of motion?
- Do you have any difficulty walking?

Pain produced by musculoskeletal problems and referred to the abdomen can be provoked by position changes or walking. Costochondritis can produce pain with vigorous respiration. Symptoms of joint involvement point to either a local cause with referred pain or a systemic cause, such as rheumatoid arthritis.

Key Questions

Respiratory system (Chapters 10 and 13):

- Do you have a cough or difficulty breathing?
- Do you have any shortness of breath?

Pneumonia, especially of a lower lobe, is a common cause of pain perceived in the abdomen, especially in children. Pleurisy can produce pain on deep inspiration. Persistent coughing can produce musculoskeletal soreness that may be referred to the abdomen.

Is the pain psychogenic, organic, or functional?

Key Questions

- Do you feel unhappy, sad, depressed?
- Are you able to eat, sleep, engage in usual activities?
- Have you had recent problems with diarrhea or constipation?
- How is your energy level?
- Have you ever been diagnosed with or treated for a mental health or psychiatric problem?

Abdominal pain can be functional or psychogenic in origin and presents somewhat differently from organic pain (Table 2-2). The presence of vegetative symptoms suggests depression (see Chapter 3).

Table 2-2	Organic Versus Functional Pain	
HISTORY	**ORGANIC PAIN**	**FUNCTIONAL PAIN**
Pain character	Acute, persistent pain increasing in intensity	Less likely to change or get more severe
Pain localization	Sharply localized	Various locations
Pain in relation to sleep	Awakens at night	Does not affect sleep
Pain in relation to umbilicus	Farther away	At umbilicus
Associated symptoms	Fever, anorexia, vomiting, weight loss, anemia, elevated ESR	Headache, dizziness, and multiple system complaints
Psychological stress	None reported	Present

What else do I need to consider?

Key Questions

- What medications are you taking? Why are you taking them?
- Have you had any operations? What were they?
- Have you recently had an involuntary weight loss?
- Have you been camping?
- If a child: Is the child in a day care setting?

Medications

Gastrointestinal distress is a common adverse reaction to many medications. Erythromycin and tetracycline are commonly associated with abdominal pain.

Surgery

Prior surgery can produce adhesions that cause intestinal obstruction. Adhesion of organs to the abdominal wall can also produce pain. Prior appendectomy does not preclude appendicitis; the stump can become inflamed.

Involuntary Weight Loss

Involuntary weight loss raises the index of suspicion for colon cancer. Identify other factors that would lead you to suspect neoplasms, such as a recent change in bowel habits in the middle-age patient, family history of colorectal or gynecological cancer, and the presence of blood in the stool.

Camping or Day Care

Ingestion of untreated water can result in intestinal parasites. Transmission of intestinal parasites is also common in day care settings. Children with intestinal parasites may present with abdominal pain as the only symptom; therefore stools should be evaluated for ova and parasites.

DIAGNOSTIC REASONING: FOCUSED PHYSICAL EXAMINATION
Note General Appearance

Patients with visceral pain are restless, move about, and have difficulty getting comfortable. These are patients with colicky type pain, often indicative of biliary obstruction, ureterolithiasis, obstruction, gastroenteritis, or early peritonitis.

Patients with parietal pain usually lie still and do not want to move. These are patients with localized peritonitis indicative of appendicitis, rupture, or perforation.

In children, note whether the child looks sick (see Chapter 16). Children can react to pain differently than adults. With peritoneal irritation, they are typically quiet and motionless with their knees flexed and drawn up. Children who are septic or have serious diseases, such as perforation or intussusception, generally lie still and look lethargic, withdrawn, and apprehensive. A child with colicky pain frequently writhes in discomfort, occasionally rocking in a rhythmic fashion.

Assess Vital Signs

In patients who are tachycardic and tachypneic, suspect a serious thoracic, intraabdominal, or pelvic disorder that is producing an acute condition in the abdomen. Shallow respirations could indicate pneumonia or pleurisy with referred pain. Orthostatic hypotension, an unusually low blood pressure, or a normal blood pressure in someone who is usually hypertensive can indicate an acute abdominal condition.

The presence of a fever suggests an acute inflammatory condition. A temperature of greater than 39.4° C (102.9° F) is associated more with pulmonary and renal infection than with an abdominal problem and can indicate pneumonia or pyelonephritis.

In adults, look for documented recent involuntary weight loss, which indicates a neoplasm. Weigh a child to determine weight loss and dehydration status.

Observe Abdominal Musculature

A rigid abdomen characterizes peritoneal irritation, whereas a soft abdomen suggests otherwise. A rigid abdomen can signal an acute condition of the abdomen that requires surgical intervention.

Note Coloring of Abdominal Skin

Ecchymosis around the umbilicus (Cullen sign) is associated with hemoperitoneum caused by either pancreatitis or ruptured ectopic pregnancy. Ecchymosis of the flanks (Grey Turner sign) is associated with hemoperitoneum and pancreatitis. Look for skin rashes of viral exanthema.

In children, a rash (palpable purpura) located on the lower extremities, buttocks, and arms indicates Henoch-Schönlein purpura (a syndrome of purpura with urticaria, erythema, arthritis, and GI symptoms).

Note Abdominal Distention

Generalized symmetrical distention can occur as the result of obesity, enlarged organs, fluid, or gas. Distention from the umbilicus to the symphysis can be caused by ovarian tumor, pregnancy, uterine fibroids, carcinoma, pancreatic cyst, or gastric dilation. Asymmetrical distention or protrusion may indicate hernia, tumor, cysts, bowel obstruction, or enlargement of abdominal organs. Remember the Fs of distention: fat, fluid, feces, fetus, flatus, fibroid, full bladder, false pregnancy, fatal tumor.

To determine distention in children, stoop down by the child's side and view across the abdomen. If the skin is tense and taut with a distended abdomen, and if the umbilicus is everted, ascites is often present. Superficial abdominal veins are often distended in children with peritonitis. The healthy child will usually have a flat abdominal profile. A flat abdomen is a straight line from the xiphoid to pelvis with no scaphoiding. A scaphoid abdomen can occur with marked dehydration or high intestinal obstruction.

Auscultate Bowel Sounds

If bowel sounds are absent, suspect peritonitis or ileus. Hyperactive bowel sounds suggest gastroenteritis, early pyloric or intestinal obstruction, or GI bleeding. High-pitched tinkling bowel sounds can indicate obstruction.

In children, use of the stethoscope can be helpful in palpation to determine abdominal pain. Begin listening to the chest; the child accepts this as painless. Then gently move the stethoscope down to the belly, slightly increasing the pressure, watching the child's face and feeling the resistance when painful.

Percuss for Tones and Guarding

In percussion, look for unexpected dullness. Guarding with percussion suggests peritoneal irritation. Tenderness can be elicited with gentle tapping. Tenderness is usually local and only rarely referred.

Palpate the Abdomen

Start with gentle palpation and palpate the area of pain last. Testing for rebound tenderness should be performed gently. Tenderness, guarding, and rebound tenderness suggest peritoneal irritation. The most reliable clinical indicator of parietal peritonitis is involuntary guarding, which must be distinguished from voluntary guarding because of pain or fear of worsening pain as a result of the examination. Guarding is determined with gentle palpation of the abdomen, not by deep palpation of the underlying organs.

You can induce guarding by having the patient place the chin on the chest or cross the arms on the chest and sit up. Palpate the painful area again. Note that intraperitoneal pain is made less severe by induced guarding. If the severity of pain is not decreased by induced guarding, consider other causes such as functional pain or abdominal wall pain.

Palpate for the liver, gallbladder, spleen, kidneys, aorta, and bladder to detect organ tenderness or involvement. Abrupt cessation of inspiration on palpation of the gallbladder (Murphy sign) indicates acute cholecystitis.

Palpate for Masses

Palpation of a mass can indicate neoplasm, obstruction, hernia, or the presence of feces in the colon. Anatomical structures can be mistaken for an abdominal mass. A mass in the upper abdomen that pulsates laterally suggests an abdominal aortic aneurysm.

A sausage-shaped mass can be felt in the upper mid-abdomen in 85% to 95% of infants with intussusception. An olive-shaped mass may be palpable in the RUQ with pyloric stenosis.

Palpate the Groin

The groin must be examined in everyone who has abdominal pain to exclude an incarcerated hernia/ovary or torsion of the ovary or testicle (see Chapter 17).

Palpate for Hernias

Palpate for inguinal, incisional, femoral, and umbilical hernias. Uncomplicated hernias will reduce; strangulated ones will not. Bowel sounds will be present in uncomplicated hernias.

Percuss for Flank Tenderness

The use of direct or indirect percussion over the costovertebral angle (CVA) can elicit tenderness if the kidney is involved. Flank pain, especially with the occurrence of hematuria, can indicate a kidney stone.

Test for Peritoneal Irritation

Several maneuvers can be used to test for peritoneal irritation.

- Obturator muscle test. Perform this test when you suspect a ruptured appendix or pelvic abscess because these conditions can cause irritation of the obturator muscle. Pain in the hypogastric region is a positive sign, indicating obturator muscle irritation. With the patient supine, flex the right leg at the hip and knee to 90 degrees. Hold the leg just above the knee, grasp the ankle, and rotate the leg laterally and medially.
- Iliopsoas muscle test. Perform this test when you suspect appendicitis because an inflamed appendix can cause irritation of the lateral iliopsoas muscle. Pain in the lower quadrant is a positive test. With the patient supine, place your hand over the lower thigh and have the patient raise the leg, flexing at the hip while you push downward against the leg.
- Markle (heel drop) test. Perform this test if you suspect appendicitis. The patient stands with straightened knees, and then raises up on the toes. The patient then relaxes and allows the heels to hit the floor, thus jarring the body. The maneuver will cause abdominal pain if positive.
- Rovsing test. Perform this test if you suspect appendicitis. Press on the left lower quadrant (LLQ). If pain in the right lower quadrant (RLQ) is intensified, the test is positive.

Perform a Pelvic Examination in Women

Perform a pelvic examination in women to rule out STI, PID, ovarian pain, ectopic pregnancy, and uterine fibroids. Vaginal discharge may or may not be present with STI or PID. Bleeding can accompany ectopic pregnancy.

Cervical motion tenderness (CMT) is the hallmark of PID. CMT plus adnexal pain (often bilateral) in the presence of abdominal pain and lower abdominal tenderness are criteria for a presumptive diagnosis of PID.

Adnexal tenderness in the region of pain can signal ectopic pregnancy. An adnexal mass may or may not be palpable, and its presence is not diagnostic. Vague adnexal tenderness can be present with STI. Bilateral, inflammatory ovarian pain and tenderness are usually related to PID, appendicitis, or peritonitis. A functional cyst can produce unilateral tenderness. Uterine fibroids may be palpable as masses in the uterus, or the entire uterus may be enlarged.

Perform Genital and Prostate Examinations in Men

Perform genital and prostate examinations in men to rule out STIs and prostatitis. Look for penile discharge as an indicator of STI and perhaps prostatitis. A tender prostate signals prostatitis. In acute prostatitis, make sure the examination is gentle; vigorous examination or massage of the prostate can cause bacterial release and produce septicemia (see Chapter 17).

Perform Digital Rectal Examination

Look for frank blood and test for occult blood. The presence of blood can indicate an acute process or carcinoma. Palpate for masses, polyps, and lesions. Occasionally patients with a rectocecal appendix and appendicitis can have a tender, localized mass on rectal examination, even though the abdominal examination is normal.

Check Peripheral Pulses

Diminished femoral pulses in the presence of a pulsatile abdominal mass suggest ruptured abdominal aortic aneurysm.

Perform a Generalized Examination as Indicated

Because abdominal pain can be referred from other areas, examine the lungs, cardiovascular system, head and neck structures, and musculoskeletal system. Palpate for regional lymphadenopathy.

LABORATORY AND DIAGNOSTIC STUDIES
Complete Blood Count with Differential

An elevated white blood cell (WBC) count greater than 12,000/microliter indicates an inflammatory or infectious condition. The WBC count is the total number of WBCs in a cubic millimeter of blood. This is an absolute number. The other measure of WBCs is the relative percentage of each of the types. Neutrophils are the body's first defense against bacterial infection and severe stress.

Normally the circulating neutrophils are in a mature form. The mature forms are known as "segs" because the nuclei of the cells are segmented. Immature forms are known as "bands" because the nuclei of the cells are not in segments but are still in a band. An increased need for neutrophils will cause an increase in both the segs (mature cells) and the bands (immature cells). Infection causes both leukocytosis (an increase in the absolute number of WBCs) and an increase in neutrophils, both mature (segs) and immature (bands). This is also called a "shift to the left." When laboratory reports were written by hand, the bands were written first on the left-hand side of the page. Thus a shift to the left means that the bands have increased, which is seen as an increase in the relative percent.

Qualitative Urine/Serum Human Chorionic Gonadotropin Tests

Qualitative urine/serum human chorionic gonadotropin (hCG) tests are monoclonal antibody tests using radioimmunoassay (RIA) to determine or exclude pregnancy. The serum hCG test is more sensitive than the urine hCG test. The serum test can be performed in about 2 hours, and hCG can be detected as early as 6 days after conception. The result is reported as either negative or positive. Because the ß-subunits are measured, it is highly specific and does not cross-react with luteinizing hormone.

Depending on the specific test used, urine testing can detect pregnancy from before a missed period to several days after a missed period. The results are obtained in minutes. A positive test (usually a color change) indicates pregnancy.

Quantitative Serum Human Chorionic Gonadotropin

Quantitative serum hCG is a fluorometric enzyme immunoassay that is highly specific for the ß-receptors of hCG, with almost no cross-reactivity with other hormones. Results are provided as values. The reference ranges for determining an abnormal pregnancy are as follows.

Not significant:	0 to 5.0 mIU/mL
Borderline significance:	5.0 to 25 mIU/mL
Evaluate with serial determinations:	>25 mIU/mL

Use this test if you are concerned about ectopic pregnancy. Ectopic pregnancy causes an increase in hCG levels at the same rate as a normal pregnancy, up to a certain point. In ectopic pregnancy, that point is usually less than 4 to 6 weeks, at which time the hCG levels plateau or begin to fall. Therefore serial determinations are more useful than a single determination.

Erythrocyte Sedimentation Rate

The erythrocyte sedimentation rate (ESR) measures the speed with which red blood cells (RBCs) settle in a tube of anticoagulated blood. The results are expressed as millimeters per hour (mm/hr). A marked increase in ESR during pregnancy is expected because there is an increase in the number of plasma globulins and in the fibrinogen level during pregnancy, causing the cells to stick together and to fall faster than normal. Inflammation or tissue injury also causes an increase in the number of globulins and fibrinogens and causes an increased sedimentation rate. However, the test is nonspecific; although it shows inflammation, it does not show the source. The ESR is often elevated as a result of PID, infectious states, or AIDS.

Cardiac Enzymes

Creatinine kinase MB (CK-MB) isoenzyme, l-lactate dehydrogenase (LDH) levels, and troponin I (Tn-I) are used in diagnosing myocardial infarction (see Chapter 7).

Urinalysis

Evaluation of kidney infection and determination of the presence of a kidney stone, renal failure, or a systemic disease process are done with a urinalysis (U/A). Microscopic hematuria suggests UTI or stone. Glycosuria and ketonuria suggest metabolic disturbances. A positive nitrite test on a U/A dipstick indicates the presence of bacteria, which can be seen on microscopic examination. The finding of 20 or more bacteria per high-powered field (HPF) indicates a UTI. The presence of greater than 0 to 1 RBCs/HPF or greater than 0 to 4 WBCs/HPF on microscopic examination also suggests UTI. RBCs can also be present as a contaminant with vaginal bleeding. The presence of red cell casts suggests kidney disease or renal infarction. White cell casts indicate pyelonephritis.

Urine for Culture and Sensitivity

If you suspect UTI, obtain a urine test for culture and sensitivity (C&S).

Culture for Sexually Transmitted Infection

Perform a culture for STI. Collect a specimen of vaginal or penile discharge on a sterile swab and place in the medium provided for *N. gonorrhoeae, Chlamydia,* or *Mycoplasma.* For penile discharge, use a sterile urethral swab to collect a specimen from the anterior urethra by gentle insertion and scraping of the mucosa (see Chapter 24).

DNA Probe

DNA probes to test for infectious organisms are available for *Chlamydia, Neisseria gonorrhoeae, Trichomonas vaginalis, Gardnerella vaginalis*, and Candida species. Obtain a sample of vaginal or penile discharge with a sterile swab and place it in the medium provided.

This test involves the construction of a nucleic acid sequence (called a probe) that will match a sequence in the DNA or RNA of the target tissue. The results are rapid and sensitive.

Potassium Hydroxide Test

The potassium hydroxide (KOH) test involves direct microscopic examination of material on a slide to determine whether fungus is present. Place a specimen of vaginal or penile discharge on a glass slide, apply a drop of aqueous 10% KOH, and put a coverslip in place. The KOH dissolves epithelial cells and debris and facilitates visualization of the mycelia of a fungus. The presence of fishy odor (the "whiff test") suggests bacterial vaginosis. View under the microscope for the presence of mycelial fragments, hyphae, and budding yeast cells (see Chapter 34).

Saline Wet Prep

In a female with vaginal discharge, this test can demonstrate the presence of *Trichomonas vaginalis* or Gardnerella organisms by microscopic examination. Place a specimen of vaginal discharge on a slide and add a drop of normal saline. Place a coverslip on the slide. The presence of trichomonads indicates *T. vaginalis.* The presence of bacteria-filled epithelial cells (clue cells) indicates bacterial vaginosis (Gardnerella) (see Chapter 34).

Gram Stain

Place a smear of vaginal or cervical discharge on a glass slide for Gram staining. Gram-positive organisms stain purple, whereas gram-negative organisms stain red. *N. gonorrhoeae* is a gram-negative organism.

Fecal Occult Blood Test

Perform the fecal occult blood test (FOBT) to rule out GI bleeding. The test is positive if a stool smear on a prepared card turns color (usually blue or green) when a solution is applied. A three-sample series provides more reliable results.

Fecal Immunochemical Test

Also called immunochemical FOBT (iFOBT), FIT uses antibodies to hemoglobin to detect a specific portion of a human blood protein. FIT does not react with non-human hemoglobin or peroxidase, so food restrictions before the test are not necessary. Immunochemical FOBTs are also more specific for lower gastrointestinal tract bleeding as they target the globin portion of hemoglobin, which does not survive passage through the upper gastrointestinal tract. This test is done essentially the same way as conventional FOBT, but is more specific and reduces the number of false positive results. Vitamins or foods do not affect the fecal immunochemical test, and some forms require only one or two stool specimens.

Electrocardiogram

An electrocardiogram (ECG) can add objective data to the diagnostic process if you suspect the pain is of cardiac origin. ST segment elevation or depression indicates the presence of injured myocardium. T wave inversion will demonstrate the presence of ischemia. The appearance of both strongly supports ischemia but is not diagnostic of CAD. Arterial spasm, pericarditis, and electrolyte imbalance can also cause these variations from normal (Chapter 7).

C-Urea Breath Test

The C-urea breath test is performed in adults and children with epigastric pain for noninvasive testing when *H. pylori* infection is suspected. In the presence of the *H. pylori* organism, urea is converted by the bacterial enzyme urease to carbon dioxide and ammonia. The carbon dioxide is absorbed in the blood and then exhaled in the breath.

Stool Antigen Test

A stool antigen test uses enzyme immunoassay to test for levels of *H. pylori*–specific antigen in a small fecal sample.

Radiography

Abdominal radiographs are of limited value in evaluating abdominal pain. An anteroposterior radiograph of the abdomen shows the kidneys, ureters, and bladder (KUB) and adjacent structures. It can be used to exclude free air (perforation) and obstruction (e.g., renal calculi) or to confirm intestinal obstruction. A chest radiograph can reveal the presence of pneumonia or air under the diaphragm (see Chapters 37 and 38).

Abdominal/Pelvic Ultrasound

Abdominal ultrasound is useful if you are considering ectopic pregnancy, abdominal aortic aneurysm, acute cholecystitis, acute pancreatitis, incarcerated hernia, hernia, or diverticular disease.

Computed Tomography/Magnetic Resonance Imaging

Computed tomography (CT) scanning and/or magnetic resonance imaging (MRI) are appropriate if you suspect retroperitoneal bleeding, pelvic abscess, pancreatitis, obstruction, hernia, incarcerated hernia, or diverticular disease.

Non–Contrast-Enhanced Helical Computed Tomography

This sensitive and specific radiological test is used to definitively diagnose urolithiasis. It is the best imaging study for diagnosing suspected appendicitis.

Colonoscopy or Sigmoidoscopy

If you suspect GI origin of pain, both colonoscopy and sigmoidoscopy are useful in directly visualizing the colon.

Anorectal Manometry

Anorectal manometry is used to evaluate constipation or fecal incontinence. The test measures the pressures of the anal sphincter muscles, the sensation in the rectum, and the neural reflexes that are needed for normal bowel movements. The manometry probe, a thin tube of soft plastic or rigid metal, is inserted into the rectum about 4 inches and then slowly withdrawn halfway. As the probe is withdrawn, the transducer continuously records the pressure at different points. Alternatively, the pressure can be measured with a balloon manometry system, a hollow metal cylinder to which three balloons are attached to measure pressure during anal contraction. A balloon at the tip of the probe is inflated to determine if the patient feels a sensation of rectal fullness and an urge to defecate.

DIFFERENTIAL DIAGNOSIS

When there is no worrisome history or no physical findings, use the specific history questions to point you in the right direction. Then determine whether the clinical findings are consistent. Review the history to see evolution over time, especially of an acute condition.

Identify physical findings that are worrisome as well, such as lower abdominal pain beginning at older age, involuntary weight loss, abnormal bleeding in a perimenopausal or postmenopausal woman, palpable abdominal or pelvic mass, or stool that is positive for occult blood.

Box 2-3	**Indicators of Abdominal Emergencies**

SUBJECTIVE FINDINGS	OBJECTIVE FINDINGS
Progressive intractable vomiting	Involuntary guarding
Lightheadedness on standing	Progressive abdomen distention
Acute onset of pain	Orthostatic hypotension
Pain that progresses in intensity over hours	Fever
	Leukocytosis and granulocytosis
	Decreased urine output

Look initially for surgical problems. Serial abdominal examinations are the best indicator of progression of an abdominal problem. Try to identify what organ seems to be involved and remember that extraabdominal systems can cause abdominal pain (e.g., pneumonia). Try to determine if the pain is organic or functional in origin. Remember that common causes of acute pain differ from common causes of chronic pain. Box 2-3 lists indicators of abdominal emergencies.

ACUTE CONDITIONS THAT CAUSE ABDOMINAL PAIN
Appendicitis

The incidence of appendicitis peaks at age 10 to 20 years, although it can occur at any age. The patient reports sudden onset of colicky pain that progresses to a constant pain. The pain can begin in the epigastrium or periumbilicus and later localize to the RLQ. The pain worsens with movement or coughing. Vomiting after the onset of pain sometimes occurs. On physical examination, the patient will be lying still and will demonstrate involuntary guarding. Classically, tenderness occurs in the RLQ. The other tests for peritoneal irritation will be positive. Rebound tenderness will be present. Variation in presentation is common, particularly with infants, children, and the elderly. Diagnostic testing includes complete blood count (CBC) with differential to confirm or rule out infection and the use of either ultrasonography, CT scan, or laparoscopy (Evidence-Based Practice Box).

Ectopic Pregnancy

Ectopic pregnancy can occur in any sexually active woman of childbearing age, especially those with a history of irregular menses. The patient experiences a sudden onset of spotting and persistent cramping in the lower quadrant that begins shortly after a missed period. On examination the patient shows signs of hemorrhage, shock, and lower abdominal peritoneal irritation that can be lateralized. On pelvic examination, the uterus is enlarged but smaller than anticipated from dates provided. The cervix is tender to motion, and a tender adnexal mass can be palpable. Diagnosis is confirmed by positive hCG test results and ultrasound. Serial quantitative serum hCG levels can be useful. A ruptured ectopic pregnancy is a surgical emergency.

Peptic Ulcer Perforation

The patient reports sudden onset of severe, intense, steady epigastric pain that radiates to the sides, back, or right shoulder. The patient can give a history of burning, gnawing pain that worsens with an empty stomach. The patient lies as still as possible. Epigastric tenderness will be present with palpation or percussion. Rebound tenderness is intense. The abdominal muscles are rigid, and bowel sounds can be absent. Diagnosis is confirmed by upright or lateral decubitus radiographs, showing air under the diaphragm or in the peritoneal cavity. Perforation is a surgical emergency.

 EVIDENCE-BASED PRACTICE *Clinical Diagnosis of Appendicitis*

Historical symptoms that increase the likelihood of appendicitis are RLQ pain, initial periumbilical pain with migration to the RLQ, and the presence of pain before vomiting.

On physical examination, the presence of rigidity, a positive psoas sign, fever, or rebound tenderness increases the likelihood of appendicitis. Conversely, the absence of RLQ pain, the absence of the migration of the pain, and the presence of similar pain previously are historical findings that make appendicitis less likely. On physical examination, the lack of RLQ pain, rigidity, or guarding makes appendicitis less likely. No finding effectively rules out appendicitis.

Although the precision and accuracy of combinations of these findings have not been reported, history and physical examination are at least as accurate as other modalities in diagnosing or excluding appendicitis.

Data from Wagner JM, McKinney WP, Carpenter JL: Does this patient have appendicitis? *JAMA* 276:1589, 1996.

Dissection of Aortic Aneurysm

This condition occurs most frequently in males and persons older than 50 years, especially those with a history of uncontrolled hypertension. The patient experiences the sudden onset of excruciating pain that can be felt in the chest or abdomen and may radiate to the legs and back. Vital signs will reflect impending shock, and there can be a deficit or difference in femoral pulses. Diagnosis can be made by CT or MRI. Additional tests include electrocardiography and cardiac enzymes. This is a surgical emergency with a high death rate.

Myocardial Infarction

In patients older than 50 years, acute MI can present with abdominal pain and gastrointestinal symptoms rather than the classic chest pain. If there is no other explanation for the pain, consider a cardiac origin.

Peritonitis

The most common cause of peritonitis is perforation of the GI tract. It occurs more often in the elderly. The patient experiences the sudden onset of severe pain that is diffuse and worsens with movement or coughing. On examination the patient will be guarding and have rebound tenderness. Bowel sounds will be decreased or absent. Diagnostic tools include CBC with differential and abdominal radiographs.

Acute Pancreatitis

Acute pancreatitis is more common in patients with cholelithiasis or a history of alcohol abuse. The pain is steady and boring in quality and is unrelieved by change of position. It is located in the left upper quadrant (LUQ) and radiates to the back. The patient can also experience nausea, vomiting, and diaphoresis and will appear acutely ill. Abdominal distention, decreased bowel sounds, and diffuse rebound tenderness will be present on physical examination. The upper abdomen can show muscle rigidity. Examination of the lungs can reveal limited diaphragmatic excursion. Diagnostic testing includes CBC with differential, ultrasonography, radiography, and serum amylase and lipase levels.

Mesenteric Adenitis

Adenovirus-induced (commonly *Yersinia*) adenopathy of the mesenteric lymph nodes can result in fever and RLQ abdominal pain that mimics appendicitis. This condition is difficult to diagnose, but the WBC count is elevated and an abdominal radiograph will show abnormalities of the terminal ileus.

Cholecystitis/Lithiasis

Cholecystitis/lithiasis occurs more often in adults than in children and more often in females than in males. The pain is colicky in nature and progresses to a constant pain. The patient reports pain in the RUQ, which can radiate to the right scapular area. The typical pain of cholelithiasis is constant, progressively rising to a plateau and falling gradually. The patient can also experience nausea and vomiting and give a history of dark urine and/or light stools. On physical examination, the patient will be tender to palpation or percussion in the RUQ. The gallbladder is palpable in about half of cases of cholecystitis. Painful splinting of respiration during deep inspiration (Murphy sign) is frequently present with cholecystitis. Diagnostic testing includes CBC with differential, ultrasonography, radiography, and serum amylase and lipase levels.

Ureterolithiasis

The patient reports the sudden onset of excruciating intermittent colicky pain that can progress to a constant pain. The pain is in the lower abdomen and flank and radiates to the groin. The patient can also experience nausea, vomiting, abdominal distention, chills, and fever. There is CVA tenderness on examination along with increased sensitivity in the lumbar and groin areas. Hematuria and increased frequency of urination can be present. U/A should be performed. Urine pH and the presence of crystals can help identify stone composition. Definitive diagnostic testing is via non–contrast-enhanced helical CT.

Urinary Tract Infection/Pyelonephritis

Abdominal pain associated with UTI or pyelonephritis is common in children and could be the only presenting complaint. U/A and C&S are done to confirm the diagnosis.

Pelvic Inflammatory Disease/Salpingitis

PID occurs most commonly in women younger than 35 who are sexually active and have more than one sexual partner. Infection results from organisms transmitted via intercourse, through childbirth, or with abortion. PID is most often caused by *Chlamydia trachomatis* and *Neisseria gonorrhoeae*. Infection begins intravaginally in most cases and then spreads upward, causing salpingitis. The tubal infection produces an exudate, and, as it spreads, peritonitis can result. Onset is usually shortly after menses. Patients have lower abdominal pain that becomes progressively more severe. On examination, abdominal tenderness, CMT, and adnexal tenderness (usually bilateral) are present. With peritonitis, patients can also have guarding and rebound tenderness. Patients can also have a fever, irregular bleeding, vaginal discharge, or vomiting. WBC count and ESR are usually elevated. Cultures and Gram staining can assist with diagnosis.

Obstruction

Obstruction occurs most often in the newborn, the elderly, and those with recent GI surgery. The patient presents with a sudden onset of crampy pain, usually in the umbilical area of the epigastrium. Vomiting occurs early with small intestinal obstruction and late with large bowel obstruction. Obstipation occurs with complete obstruction, but diarrhea can be present with partial obstruction. Hyperactive, high-pitched bowel sounds can be present in small bowel obstruction. A mass can be palpable in lower obstruction. Abdominal distention can be present. The rectum will be empty on digital examination. Diagnosis is confirmed with abdominal radiographs (supine and sitting), MRI, or CT.

Ileus

Ileus is associated with intraperitoneal or retroperitoneal infection, metabolic disturbances, and intraabdominal surgery. The patient experiences abdominal distention, vomiting, obstipation, and cramps. On auscultation, there is minimal or absent peristalsis. Abdominal radiographs show gaseous distention of isolated segments of both the small and large intestines.

Intussusception

Bowel obstruction in children ages 2 months to 2 years usually occurs in the ileocecal region and classically presents with vomiting, colicky abdominal pain with drawing up of the legs, and eventual currant jelly stools. The onset is dramatic. The child is asleep or awake when suddenly he or she cries out with severe pain. The child twists and squirms; nothing gives any relief until, almost suddenly, there is a lull with absence of pain followed by a similar painful episode. The abdomen has a sausage-shaped mass that can be felt in the RUQ. The stool tests positive for blood.

Malrotation/Volvulus

Improper rotation and fixation of the duodenum and colon can cause an artery to obstruct, and the patient experiences ischemic necrosis. This disorder of the embryonic gut is usually seen in the first month of life. The infant presents with bilious emesis followed by abdominal distention and GI bleeding. Shock occurs from progression of the ischemia.

Henoch-Schönlein Purpura

In Henoch-Schönlein purpura, crampy, acute abdominal pain and bleeding are secondary to edema and hemorrhage of the intestinal wall. This disease is an immunoglobulin A (IgA)–mediated vasculitis that affects very small vessels. A urticarial rash occurring on the buttocks and lower extremities progresses to papular purpuric lesions. The laboratory findings show an elevated WBC count but a normal platelet count. A mild increase in ESR, an increase in IgA concentration, and negative antinuclear antibodies (ANA test) are also found.

Incarcerated Hernia

Incarcerated hernia occurs most commonly in the elderly. The patient reports a constant severe pain in the RLQ or LLQ that worsens with coughing or straining. Physical examination reveals a hernia or mass that is nonreducible. Diagnosis is confirmed by MRI or CT. Surgical intervention is indicated.

Pneumonia

Pneumonia is a frequently overlooked cause of abdominal pain in children. The pain is referred from right lower lobe pneumonia because of associated phrenic nerve irritation, which can cause muscular spasm, ileus, and pain referred to the RLQ. The WBC count in pneumonia is typically higher than that in early appendicitis.

CHRONIC CONDITIONS THAT CAUSE LOWER ABDOMINAL PAIN
Irritable Bowel Syndrome

IBS begins in adolescent and young adult years. It produces crampy hypogastric pain that is of variable, infrequent duration. The pain is associated with bowel function, gas, bloating, and distention. Relief is often obtained with the passage of flatus or feces. The patient has a normal abdominal examination and the stool is negative for blood. Consider a proctosigmoidoscopy or barium enema (BE) if onset is at middle age or older, the stool is positive for blood, there is a family history of colorectal cancer or polyps, or the patient fails to improve after 6 to 8 weeks of therapy.

Lactose Intolerance

Lactose intolerance produces crampy pain and diarrhea after the consumption of milk or milk product foods (Chapter 11). It is caused by a deficiency in lactase, an enzyme that decreases in activity with increasing age. It is more common in Asians, Native Americans, and African Americans.

Diverticular Disease

Diverticular disease causes localized abdominal pain and tenderness. The patient will have a fever, elevated ESR, and leukocytosis. Perform a BE or proctoscopy/colonoscopy if there is rectal bleeding.

Simple Constipation

In adults, constipation is associated with infrequency or difficulty passing dry, hard stools and abdominal bloating.

Children with constipation frequently report abdominal pain. The pain is usually colicky in nature but can be dull and steady. The pain varies and is not persistent or progressively worsening. Mild, poorly localized periumbilical tenderness and perhaps guarding are reported. A fecal mass may be palpable.

Habitual Constipation

With habitual constipation, the patient presents with a lifelong history of constipation with onset as a young adult, has a normal physical examination, and does not have occult blood in the stool. Diet, activity, and bowel habits are often causal factors. Consider sigmoidoscopy, anorectal manometry, or colonoscopy if you suspect a metabolic or systemic cause, the stool is heme-positive, or the patient is middle-age or older or fails to respond to treatment.

Dysmenorrhea

Dysmenorrhea, a typically lower abdominal pain or cramping, occurs with menstruation. Dysmenorrhea can be classified as primary (no organic cause) or secondary (pathological cause). In primary dysmenorrhea, the onset is usually soon after menarche and gradually diminishes with age. The woman will have a normal pelvic examination. Secondary dysmenorrhea is associated with specific conditions and disorders such as endometriosis, PID, cervical stenosis, and uterine fibroids. Obtain a gynecological (GYN) consult and/or pelvic ultrasound for secondary dysmenorrhea, dysmenorrhea with increasing severity, or abnormal findings on pelvic examination.

Uterine Fibroids

Fibroids produce pain related to the menstrual cycle and intercourse. The woman can experience dysfunctional uterine bleeding. On examination, palpable myomas are often present. Suspect this cause when there is no suspicion of other pelvic disorder. Order a pelvic ultrasound if ovarian or uterine neoplasm cannot be excluded. Obtain a GYN consult for abnormal bleeding or severe symptoms.

Hernia

A hernia is a loop of intestine that has prolapsed through the inguinal wall or canal or through the abdominal musculature. The patient reports intermittent localized pain that can be exacerbated with exertion or lifting. A physical examination will document the hernia, especially when the patient is instructed in maneuvers or positions to increase intraabdominal pressure. Consider CT or MRI if you suspect strangulation or bowel obstruction.

Ovarian Cysts

Ovarian cysts occur most commonly in young women and produce adnexal pain. The cysts may be palpable, late-cycle (corpus luteum) cysts. A pelvic ultrasound is indicated. Ovarian cysts can become quite large before producing symptoms.

Abdominal Wall Disorder

With abdominal wall disorder, the patient can present with a history of trauma. Ecchymosis or swelling may be visible. The patient may report pain with rectus muscle stress. GI and genitourinary symptoms are absent. A hernia may be palpable. Obtain a CT scan if internal disease cannot be excluded.

CHRONIC CONDITIONS THAT CAUSE UPPER ABDOMINAL PAIN
Esophagitis/Gastroesophageal Reflux Disease

With gastroesophageal reflux disease (GERD), the patient reports a burning, gnawing pain in the mid-epigastrium ("heartburn") that worsens with recumbency.

Regurgitation of gastric contents or water brash (hypersalivation secondary to acid stimulation of the lower esophagus) can also be a complaint. The pain typically occurs after eating or when lying down and may be relieved with antacids. The physical examination is negative. Consider endoscopy if symptoms are severe or the patient does not respond to therapy.

Peptic Ulcer

The patient reports a burning or gnawing pain that occurs most often with an empty stomach, stress, and alcohol intake. The pain is relieved by food intake. Some patients describe the pain as a soreness, empty feeling, or hunger. Typical pain is steady, mild, or severe and located in the epigastrium. Complaints can be atypical in children and minimal in the elderly. There can be epigastric tenderness on palpation. Endoscopy, C-urea breath test and stool antigen test can be used for diagnosis.

Gastritis

Gastritis pain is a constant burning pain in the epigastric area that can be accompanied by nausea, vomiting, diarrhea, or fever. Alcohol, nonsteroidal anti-inflammatory drugs, and salicylates make the pain worse. Physical examination results are negative. No diagnostic testing is necessary if the patient responds to therapy.

Gastroenteritis

Gastroenteritis can occur at any age and produces a diffuse, crampy pain that is accompanied by nausea, vomiting, diarrhea, and fever. Hyperactive bowel sounds will be heard on auscultation. The condition usually resolves on its own, and no diagnostic testing is needed.

Functional Dyspepsia

Functional dyspepsia refers to GI symptoms in which a pathological condition is not present or does not entirely explain the clinical presentation, although altered physiological activity can be present. The patient has vague reports of indigestion, heartburn, gaseousness, or fullness. The patient also reports belching, abdominal distention, and occasionally nausea. The physical examination results are negative. Perform a CBC and fecal testing for occult blood. C-urea breath test and stool antigen test are used for diagnosis of *H. pylori* infection. Consider endoscopy if there is no response to empiric treatment. Consider an upper and lower GI series if the patient also has dysphagia, weight loss, vomiting, or a change in the pattern of the symptoms.

Recurrent Abdominal Pain

Recurrent abdominal pain (RAP) usually presents in children 5 to 10 years of age—rarely after age 14. The patient reports dull, colicky periumbilical pain that is intermittent, occurs daily, and lasts from 1 to 3 hours with complete recovery between episodes. The pain does not awaken the child from sleep but can interfere with the ability to fall asleep. The child can have a low-grade fever, pallor, headache, and constipation. A history of stress associated with school social activities, parental conflicts, or loss is frequently elicited. Physical examination results are essentially negative. Initial laboratory tests are CBC, ESR, U/A, fecal blood testing, and stool for ova and parasites (O & P).

DIFFERENTIAL DIAGNOSIS OF *Common Causes of Acute Abdominal Pain*

CONDITION	HISTORY	PHYSICAL FINDINGS	DIAGNOSTIC STUDIES
Appendicitis	Age 10-20 years, although it can occur at any age; patient reports sudden onset of colicky pain that progresses to constant pain; pain can begin in epigastrium or periumbilicus and then later localizes in RLQ; pain worsens with movement or coughing; vomiting after onset of pain is sometimes present	Patient lying still; involuntary guarding; tenderness in RLQ; other tests for peritoneal irritation positive; rebound tenderness; variation in presentation common, particularly with infants, children, and elderly	CBC with differential, ultrasonography, CT, laparoscopy

Continued

DIFFERENTIAL DIAGNOSIS OF *Common Causes of Acute Abdominal Pain—cont'd*

CONDITION	HISTORY	PHYSICAL FINDINGS	DIAGNOSTIC STUDIES
Ectopic pregnancy	Women of childbearing age; sudden onset of spotting and persistent cramping in lower quadrant that begins shortly after missed period	Signs of hemorrhage, shock, and lower abdominal peritoneal irritation that can be lateralized; enlarged uterus; CMT; tender adnexal mass	Positive hCG, ultrasound; ruptured ectopic pregnancy is surgical emergency
Peptic ulcer perforation	Sudden onset of severe intense, steady epigastric pain that radiates to sides, back, or right shoulder; history of burning, gnawing pain that worsens with empty stomach	Patient lying still; epigastric tenderness; rebound tenderness; abdominal muscles rigid; bowel sounds can be absent	Diagnosis confirmed by upright or lateral decubitus radiograph showing air under diaphragm or in peritoneal cavity; perforation is surgical emergency
Dissection of aortic aneurysm	Most frequent in elderly, especially if hypertensive; sudden onset of excruciating pain that can be felt in chest or abdomen and can radiate to legs and back	Patient appears shocky, vital signs reflect impending shock; deficit or difference in femoral pulses	CT or MRI; additional tests include ECG and cardiac enzymes; surgical emergency
Myocardial infarction	Over age 50; upper or diffuse abdominal pain; can be accompanied by nausea, vomiting, dyspepsia	Hypertension or hypotension, cardiac arrhythmia, paradoxical S2	Serial ECGs, serial cardiac enzymes
Peritonitis	Occurs more often in elderly; sudden onset of severe pain that is diffuse and worsens with movement or coughing	Guarding; rebound tenderness; bowel sounds decreased or absent	CBC with differential, abdominal radiographs
Acute pancreatitis	History of cholelithiasis or alcohol abuse; pain is steady and boring in quality and is unrelieved by change of position; located in LUQ and radiates to back; nausea, vomiting, and diaphoresis	Patient appears acutely ill; abdominal distention, decreased bowel sounds, diffuse rebound tenderness; upper abdomen can show muscle rigidity; can have limited diaphragmatic excursion of lungs	CBC with differential, serum amylase and lipase levels, triglyceride level, calcium level, and liver chemistries; ultrasonography; CT
Mesenteric adenitis	Fever, pain in RLQ, other symptoms suggestive of appendicitis	Pain on palpation in RLQ; there can be pharyngitis, cervical adenopathy	CBC with differential; adenovirus found in tissue of surgical specimen
Cholecystitis/ lithiasis	Appears in adults more than in children, females more than males; colicky pain with progression to constant pain; pain in RUQ that can radiate to right scapular area; pain of cholelithiasis is constant, progressively rising to plateau and falling gradually; nausea, vomiting, history of dark urine and/or light stools	Tender to palpation or percussion in RUQ; gallbladder palpable in about half cases of cholecystitis; positive Murphy sign	CBC with differential, ultrasonography, radiographs, serum amylase and lipase levels
Ureterolithiasis	Sudden onset, excruciating intermittent colicky pain that can progress to constant pain; pain in lower abdomen and flank and radiates to groin; nausea, vomiting, abdominal distention, chills, and fever; increased frequency of urination	CVA tenderness; increased sensitivity in lumbar and groin areas; hematuria	U/A, non–contrast-enhanced helical CT

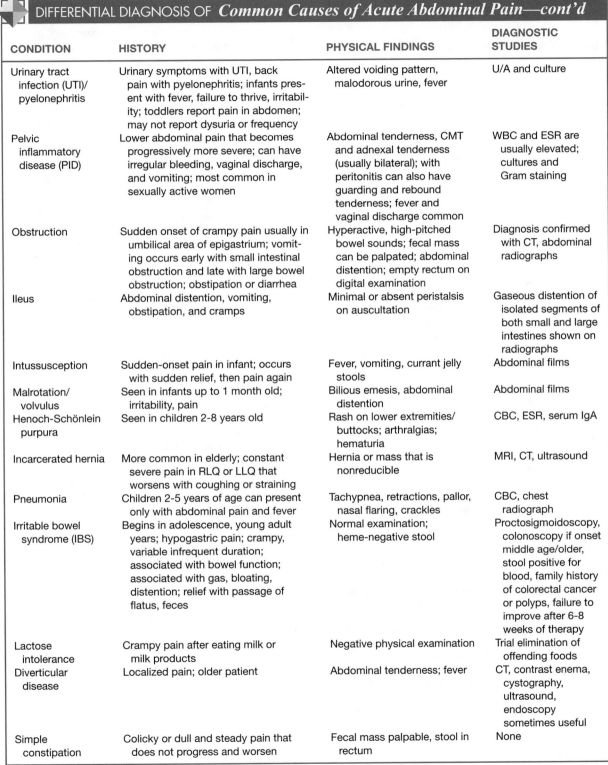

DIFFERENTIAL DIAGNOSIS OF *Common Causes of Acute Abdominal Pain—cont'd*

CONDITION	HISTORY	PHYSICAL FINDINGS	DIAGNOSTIC STUDIES
Urinary tract infection (UTI)/ pyelonephritis	Urinary symptoms with UTI, back pain with pyelonephritis; infants present with fever, failure to thrive, irritability; toddlers report pain in abdomen; may not report dysuria or frequency	Altered voiding pattern, malodorous urine, fever	U/A and culture
Pelvic inflammatory disease (PID)	Lower abdominal pain that becomes progressively more severe; can have irregular bleeding, vaginal discharge, and vomiting; most common in sexually active women	Abdominal tenderness, CMT and adnexal tenderness (usually bilateral); with peritonitis can also have guarding and rebound tenderness; fever and vaginal discharge common	WBC and ESR are usually elevated; cultures and Gram staining
Obstruction	Sudden onset of crampy pain usually in umbilical area of epigastrium; vomiting occurs early with small intestinal obstruction and late with large bowel obstruction; obstipation or diarrhea	Hyperactive, high-pitched bowel sounds; fecal mass can be palpated; abdominal distention; empty rectum on digital examination	Diagnosis confirmed with CT, abdominal radiographs
Ileus	Abdominal distention, vomiting, obstipation, and cramps	Minimal or absent peristalsis on auscultation	Gaseous distention of isolated segments of both small and large intestines shown on radiographs
Intussusception	Sudden-onset pain in infant; occurs with sudden relief, then pain again	Fever, vomiting, currant jelly stools	Abdominal films
Malrotation/ volvulus	Seen in infants up to 1 month old; irritability, pain	Bilious emesis, abdominal distention	Abdominal films
Henoch-Schönlein purpura	Seen in children 2-8 years old	Rash on lower extremities/ buttocks; arthralgias; hematuria	CBC, ESR, serum IgA
Incarcerated hernia	More common in elderly; constant severe pain in RLQ or LLQ that worsens with coughing or straining	Hernia or mass that is nonreducible	MRI, CT, ultrasound
Pneumonia	Children 2-5 years of age can present only with abdominal pain and fever	Tachypnea, retractions, pallor, nasal flaring, crackles	CBC, chest radiograph
Irritable bowel syndrome (IBS)	Begins in adolescence, young adult years; hypogastric pain; crampy, variable infrequent duration; associated with bowel function; associated with gas, bloating, distention; relief with passage of flatus, feces	Normal examination; heme-negative stool	Proctosigmoidoscopy, colonoscopy if onset middle age/older, stool positive for blood, family history of colorectal cancer or polyps, failure to improve after 6-8 weeks of therapy
Lactose intolerance	Crampy pain after eating milk or milk products	Negative physical examination	Trial elimination of offending foods
Diverticular disease	Localized pain; older patient	Abdominal tenderness; fever	CT, contrast enema, cystography, ultrasound, endoscopy sometimes useful
Simple constipation	Colicky or dull and steady pain that does not progress and worsen	Fecal mass palpable, stool in rectum	None

Continued

DIFFERENTIAL DIAGNOSIS OF *Common Causes of Acute Abdominal Pain—cont'd*

CONDITION	HISTORY	PHYSICAL FINDINGS	DIAGNOSTIC STUDIES
Habitual constipation	Lifelong history; younger patient	Normal examination; heme-negative stool	Sigmoidoscopy, anorectal manometry, colonoscopy if alarm symptoms
Dysmenorrhea	Typical premenstrual pain onset soon after menarche, gradually diminishing with age	Normal pelvic examination	GYN consult; pelvic ultrasound if secondary dysmenorrhea, increasing disability, or abnormal pelvic examination
Uterine fibroids	Pain related to menses, intercourse	Palpable myomas; no suspicion of other pelvic disorder	Pelvic ultrasound if ovarian or uterine neoplasm cannot be excluded; GYN consult if abnormal bleeding or severe symptoms
Hernia	Localized pain that increases with exertion or lifting	Physical examination documents hernia	MRI, CT, ultrasound, BE if suspect strangulation or bowel obstruction
Ovarian cyst(s)	Young woman	Adnexal pain and palpable ovarian cysts, especially in late cycle (corpus luteum)	Pelvic ultrasound
Abdominal wall disorder	History of trauma	Visible ecchymosis or swelling; palpable hernia pain with rectus muscle stress; no GI/genitourinary symptoms	CT if internal disease cannot be excluded
Esophagitis/GERD	Burning, gnawing pain in mid-epigastrium that worsens with recumbency; water brash; pain occurs after eating and can be relieved with antacids; in infant: failure to thrive, irritability, postprandial spitting and vomiting	Physical examination negative; in infants: weight loss, in some cases aspiration pneumonia	Endoscopy if symptoms are severe or do not respond to therapy; manometry, pH monitoring
Peptic ulcer	Burning or gnawing pain; soreness, empty feeling, or hunger; occurs most often with empty stomach, stress, and alcohol, and relieved by food intake; pain steady, mild, or severe and located in epigastrium; can be atypical in children and minimal in elderly	Can be epigastric tenderness on palpation	C-UBT, stool antigen test, endoscopy if no response to therapy
Gastritis	Constant burning pain in epigastric area that can be accompanied by nausea, vomiting, diarrhea, or fever; alcohol, NSAIDs, and salicylates make pain worse	Physical examination negative	No diagnostic testing necessary if patient responds to therapy

DIFFERENTIAL DIAGNOSIS OF *Common Causes of Acute Abdominal Pain—cont'd*

CONDITION	HISTORY	PHYSICAL FINDINGS	DIAGNOSTIC STUDIES
Gastroenteritis	Occurs at any age and produces diffuse crampy pain accompanied by nausea, vomiting, diarrhea, and fever; can have history of recent travels, family members ill	Hyperactive bowel sounds will be heard on auscultation; dehydration if severe	No diagnostic testing needed
Functional dyspepsia	Vague reports of indigestion, heartburn, gaseousness, or fullness; belching, abdominal distention, and occasionally nausea	Physical examination negative	C-UBT, stool antigen test, consider endoscopy if no response to empiric treatment; CBC, FOBT, or FIT
Recurrent abdominal pain (RAP)	Children 5-10 years old; history of environmental or psychological stress	Physical examination negative	CBC, U/A, ESR, FOBT or FIT, stool for O & P

CBC, complete blood count; *CMT,* cervical motion tenderness; *CT,* computed tomography; *CVA,* costovertebral angle; *ECG,* electrocardiography; *ESR,* erythrocyte sedimentation rate; *FIT,* fecal immunochemical test; *FOBT,* fecal occult blood test; *GERD,* gastroesophageal reflux disease; *GI,* gastrointestinal; *GYN,* gynecological; *hCG,* human chorionic gonadotropin test; *LLQ,* left lower quadrant; *LUQ,* left upper quadrant; *MRI,* magnetic resonance imaging; *NSAIDs,* nonsteroidal anti-inflammatory drugs; *O & P,* ova and parasites; *RLQ,* right lower quadrant; *RUQ,* right upper quadrant; *WBC,* white blood cell count.

REFERENCES AND READINGS

AGA Institute on "Management of Acute Pancreatitis" Clinical Practice and Economics Committee, AGA Institute Governing Board: AGA Institute medical position statement on acute pancreatitis, *Gastroenterol* 132:2019, 2007.

Aschcraft K: Consultation with the specialist: acute abdominal pain, *Pediatr Rev* 21:363, 2000.

Cartwright SL, Knudson MP: Evaluation of acute abdominal pain in adults, *Am Fam Physician* 77:971, 2008.

Fass R, Longstreth GF, Pimentel M, Fullerton S, Russak SM, Chiou CF, et al: Evidence- and consensus-based practice guidelines for the diagnosis of irritable bowel syndrome, *Arch Intern Med* 161(17):2081, 2001.

Hernia, Corpus Christi, TX, 2008, Work Loss Data Institute.

Kahrilas PJ, Shaheen NJ, Vaezi MF, Hiltz SW, Black E, Modlin IM, et al; American Gastroenterological Association: American Gastroenterological Association medical position statement on the management of gastroesophageal reflux disease, *Gastroenterol* 135:1383, 2008.

Leung A, Sigalet D: Acute abdominal pain in children, *Am Fam Physician* 67:11, 2003.

Levy J: Gastroesophageal reflux and other causes of abdominal pain, *Pediatr Ann* 30:42, 2001.

Lyon C, Clark DC: Diagnosis of acute abdominal pain in older patients, *Am Fam Physician* 74:1537, 2006.

Matthews PJ, Aziz Q: Functional abdominal pain, *Postgrad Med* 81:448, 2005.

McCollough M, Sharieff G: Abdominal surgical emergencies in infants and young children, *Emerg Med Clin North Am* 21:909, 2003.

Rafferty J, Shellito P, Hyman NH, Buie WD, Standards Committee of American Society of Colon and Rectal Surgeons. Practice parameters for sigmoid diverticulitis, *Dis Colon Rectum* 49:939, 2006.

Ros PR, Huprich JE, Bree RL, Foley WD, Gay SB, Glick SN et al: Expert Panel on Gastrointestinal Imaging. Suspected small bowel obstruction. Reston (VA): American College of Radiology (ACR) 2005.

Ross A, LeLeiko N: Acute abdominal pain, *Pediatr Rev* 31:135, 2010.

Rothrock SG, Pagane J: Acute appendicitis in children: emergency department diagnosis and management, *Ann Emerg Med* 36:39, 2001.

Sachs CJ: Abdominal pain: a rational approach, *Consultant* November: 1433, 2005.

Talley NJ; American Gastroenterological Association: American Gastroenterological Association medical position statement: evaluation of dyspepsia, *Gastroenterol* 129:1753, 2005.

Ternent CA, Bastawrous AL, Morin NA, Ellis CN, Hyman NH, Buie WD, Standards Practice Task Force of The American Society of Colon and Rectal Surgeons. Practice parameters for the evaluation and management of constipation, *Dis Colon Rectum* 50:2013, 2007.

Tsipouras S: Nonabdominal causes of abdominal pain—finding your heart in your stomach! *Aust Fam Physician* 37:620, 2008.

Wagner JM, McKinney WP, Carpenter JL: Does this patient have appendicitis? *JAMA* 276:1589, 1996.

Zeiter DK, Hyams JS: Recurrent abdominal pain in children, *Pediatr Clin North Am* 49:53, 2002.

3

Affective Changes

A large percentage of primary care visits have psychological or psychosocial origins. A practitioner must first rule out organic causes for symptoms, mood changes, and behavior changes. Some patients are able to express that their symptoms could be related to situational stress or a psychosocial cause. Others can identify that psychological or emotional difficulties are causing worrisome symptoms or symptoms that interfere with their ability to function. Often the practitioner suspects an underlying psychological or psychosocial disturbance that the patient is not able to articulate. In some cases a parent has concerns about a child's or adolescent's behavior. This chapter focuses on commonly encountered psychological conditions and psychosocial concerns, and provides an approach to elicit more information, determine suicide risk, and evaluate for a diagnosable psychological disorder (Figure 3-1).

Do not assume that an emotional symptom has a psychosocial cause until physical causes have been fully explored. Anxiety and depression are prevalent in the primary care setting. Although they are distinct and separate diagnoses, they often co-occur. Substance use is encountered either as a primary condition or as a comorbid condition and can be a consequence of a psychological or psychosocial condition, or the cause of a psychosocial concern.

DIAGNOSTIC REASONING: FOCUSED HISTORY

Is this a psychosocial problem?

Key Questions (to self)

- Does the presenting concern provide any clues?
- Are behavioral cues present?

Presenting Concern

Fatigue, lack of energy, sleep disturbance, and an inability to concentrate are symptoms that can bring a patient to the primary care setting. These symptoms are common in patients experiencing situational stress, depression, anxiety, or substance use problems. Prolonged somatic symptoms that have not been diagnosed, such as headache, chest pain, abdominal pain, low back pain, or dizziness, can suggest a psychosocial or psychological cause. It is imperative that you consider these clues as you rule out an organic cause. Also see specific chapters that address these symptoms.

A parent could relate that a child's behavior is different from that of other children. On developmental screening the very young child may have deficits in social skills and in preverbal language. Parents of children over the age of 3 years often express concern over absent or delayed speech.

Behavioral Cues

A history of frequent primary care or emergency department visits for unexplained symptoms can point to a psychosocial cause. Sometimes the patient's affect and general appearance do not match the presenting concern. An emotional response that is not consistent with the severity of the presenting problem or situation can point to a psychosocial problem.

Agitation and restlessness are common manifestations of depression, anxiety, and/or substance abuse. Changes in personality or in relationships may be associated with substance abuse, depression, and anxiety.

Language and social skills that seem out of sync with general development are important cues that might indicate a more serious condition.

Could this be a result of a physiological problem?

Key Questions

- Can you describe the symptoms you are having?
- Have you had a major illness recently?
- How long have you had these symptoms?

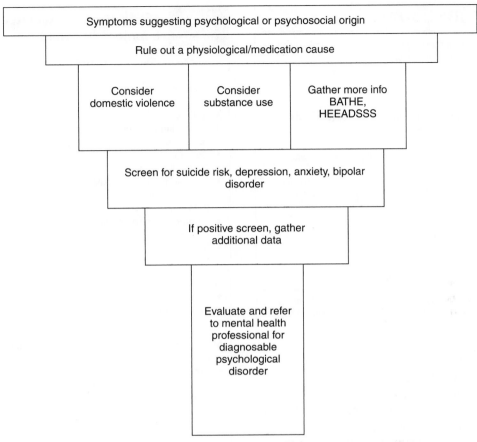

FIGURE 3-1   A suggested approach to the visit. There are areas of overlap.

Symptoms

Physiological problems often present in the patient as abdominal pain (Chapter 2), chest pain (Chapter 7), confusion (especially in the older adult, Chapter 8), dizziness (Chapter 12), fatigue (Chapter 15), headache (Chapter 18), and sleep disturbances (Chapter 28). Refer to the specific chapters that discuss the evaluation of the presenting concern and symptom(s).

Major Illness/Chronic Conditions

Mood disorders can occur secondary to a physiological condition. Patients who have had a major health event, such as a myocardial infarction, stroke, or trauma, or who have chronic symptoms, such as pain, are at risk for the development of depression.

The mnemonic THINC MED is useful when evaluating for underlying organic causes of changes in mood or behavior. Box 3-1 identifies conditions that are commonly associated with anxiety and depression.

Could this be caused by medication?

Key Questions

- What prescribed medications are you currently taking?
- What over-the-counter (OTC) and/or herbal medicines do you take?
- What dietary supplements are you taking?

Medication History

Many medications can cause psychiatric symptoms and mood changes. Box 3-2 lists medications that can produce symptoms of depression, anxiety, and mania.

Box 3-1	**THINC MED**

Major categories of medical conditions that mimic psychological conditions are as follows:

T:	Tumors
H:	Hormones (e.g., thyroid, adrenal, gonads, insulin)
I:	Infections and immune diseases (e.g., AIDS, lupus, syphilis, Lyme disease)
N:	Nutrition
C:	Central nervous system (e.g., head trauma, seizures, multiple sclerosis, Parkinson's disease, dementia)
M:	Miscellaneous (e.g., sleep apnea, anemia, congestive heart failure)
E:	Electrolyte abnormalities and toxins (e.g., hypercalcemia, hypo/hyperphosphatemia, hypo/hypernatremia)
D:	Drugs (including nicotine, caffeine, prescribed medications, illicit drugs, and alcohol)

From Goolsby MJ, Grubbs L: *Advanced assessment: interpreting findings and formulating differential diagnoses,* Philadelphia, 2006, F.A. Davis.

OTC Medications, Herbal Medicines, and Dietary Supplements

Some OTC medications, herbal preparations, and dietary supplements can contribute to psychiatric symptoms. A complete list of all preparations that the patient is taking is a starting point for evaluating side effects and interactions.

Is this a domestic violence situation?

Key Questions

- Have you been hit, kicked, punched, or otherwise hurt by someone within the past year?
- Do you feel safe in your current relationship?
- Is there a partner from a previous relationship who is making you feel unsafe now?

A positive response to any one of these three questions constitutes a positive screen for partner violence (Feldhaus et al, 1997). The first question, which addresses physical violence, has been validated in studies as an accurate measure of 1-year prevalence rates. The latter two questions evaluate the perception of safety and provide estimates of the short-term risk of further violence and the need for counseling, but reliability and validity evaluations have not yet been established. A positive screen

Box 3-2	**Medications Associated with Changes in Mood**

Medications That Can Cause Symptoms of Depression
- Accutane
- Antabuse
- Anticonvulsants
- Antiparkinsonian medications
- Antivirals
- Barbiturates
- Benzodiazepines
- Beta-adrenergic blockers
- Calcium-channel blockers
- Estrogens
- Fluoroquinolone antibiotics
- Interferon alfa
- Narcotics
- Statins

Medications That Can Cause Symptoms of Anxiety
- Albuterol
- Theophylline
- Thyroid hormones

Medications That Can Cause Symptoms of Mania
- Antabuse
- Anticholinergics
- Antiparkinsonian medications
- Capoten
- Cogentin
- Corticosteroids
- Cyclosporine
- Monoamine oxidase inhibitors (MAOIs)
- Opioids
- Tagamet
- Thyroid hormones

requires further assessment and clinical followup, including ascertaining patient safety.

Could this be situational stress or normal grief?

The BATHE model provides a framework for understanding the patient in the context of his/her total life situation (Lieberman, 1997). BATHE is a mnemonic for **B**ackground, **A**ffect, **T**rouble, **H**andling, **E**mpathy.

Key Questions

Background—ascertains the context of the visit
- What is going on in your life?
- What is going on right now?
- Has anything changed recently?

Affect—elicits the emotional response and allows the patient to label the feeling

- How do you feel about that?
- What is your mood?

Trouble—determines the symbolic meaning of the situation for the patient

- What about the situation troubles you most?
- What worries or concerns you?

Handling—helps to assess patient resources and responses to the situation

- How are you handling that?
- How are you coping?

Empathy—reflects an understanding that the patient's response is reasonable under the circumstances

- That must be very difficult for you.
- I can understand that you would feel that way.

BATHE Model

This model provides a patient-centered technique that helps establish a relationship with the patient; serves as a rough screening test for anxiety, depression, or situational stress disorders; and takes minimal time.

Could this be a result of substance abuse?

Key Questions

- In the past year, have you used alcohol or drugs more than you meant to?
- Have you wanted or needed to reduce your drinking or drug use in the past year?

A positive response to one question indicates a substance use concern. When the screen is positive, the CAGE questions can be used to detect alcoholism. Other substances can be substituted for alcohol in the CAGE questionnaire (Box 3-3). Other questionnaires, T-ACE and RAFFT, for alcohol use are also available (Box 3-4 and Box 3-5).

How can I narrow my diagnosis?

Begin with broad screening questions. If the patient's response to the screening question(s) is positive, proceed to elicit more specific symptoms. Although a negative response to a given screening question decreases the likelihood of a disorder, the sensitivity of such screening is not perfect, and answers should be interpreted within the context of the patient's entire history and physical examination.

Box 3-3	**CAGE Questionnaire**

A Framework for Detecting Alcoholism*

C:	Concern, Cut down	Have you ever felt you should cut down on your drinking?
A:	Annoyed	Have people annoyed you by criticizing your drinking?
G:	Guilt	Have you ever felt bad or guilty about your drinking?
E:	Eye-opener	Have you ever had an eye-opener drink first thing in the morning to steady your nerves or get rid of a hangover?

From Ewing JA: Screening for alcoholism using CAGE. Cut down, annoyed, guilty, eye opener, *JAMA* 280:1904, 1998.
*Answering yes to one or more of the four questions raises a high index of suspicion for alcohol abuse and dependence. The CAGE questionnaire has been used and tested extensively in many populations. It is considered to be a reliable method of screening for alcohol abuse in adults. It has reported sensitivities of 43% to 94% and specificities ranging from 70% to 97%.

Box 3-4	**T-ACE Questionnaire**

A Framework for Prenatal Detection of Risk Drinking*

T:	Tolerance	How many drinks does it take to make you feel high? (Positive = more than 2)
A:	Annoyed	Have people annoyed you by criticizing your drinking?
C:	Cut down	Have you felt you ought to cut down on your drinking?
E:	Eye-opener	Have you ever had an eye-opener drink first thing in the morning to steady your nerves or get rid of a hangover?

From Sokol RJ, Martier SS, Ager JW: The T-ACE questions: Practical prenatal detection of risk-drinking, *Am J Obstet Gynecol* 160:863, 1989.
*A positive answer to T alone or to two of A, C, or E can signal a problem with a high degree of probability, and positive answers to all four indicates great certainty of a problem.

Key Questions

- Is there a personal or family history of mental illness?
- Is there a family history of autism?
- Over the past 2 weeks, have you felt down, depressed, or hopeless?
- Over the past 2 weeks, have you had little interest or pleasure in your daily activities?

Box 3-5	**The RAFFT Questionnaire**

A Framework for Detecting Substance Use Disorders in Adolescents

R: Relax — Do you drink or take drugs to relax, feel better about yourself, or fit in?

A: Alone — Do you ever drink or take drugs while you are alone?

F: Friends — Do any of your closest friends drink or use drugs?

F: Family — Does a close family member have a problem with alcohol or drugs?

T: Trouble — Have you ever gotten into trouble from drinking or taking drugs?

From Bastiaens L, Francis G, Lewis K: The RAFFT as a screening tool for adolescent substance use disorders, *Am J Addict* 9:10, 2000.

Box 3-6	**SIG E CAPS**

Neurovegetative Signs In Depression

S: Sleep disorder (either increased or decreased sleep)

I: Interest deficit (anhedonia)

G: Guilt (worthlessness, hopelessness, regret)

E: Energy deficit

C: Concentration deficit

A: Appetite disorder (either decreased or increased)

P: Psychomotor retardation or agitation

S: Suicidality

From Carlat DJ: The psychiatric review of symptoms: a screening tool for family physicians, *Am Fam Physician* 58:1617, 1998.

- Do you tend to be an anxious or nervous person?
- Have you had periods of feeling so happy or energetic that your friends told you were talking too fast or that you were too "hyper"?

Prior Mental Illness, Family History

A personal or family history of prior mental illness increases the likelihood of a current mental illness. Studies support the influence of both behavioral and biological factors in the development of mental health conditions.

Family history of another child with autism increases the risk of autism in a sibling.

Down, Depressed, Hopeless, Loss of Interest or Pleasure

These are cardinal symptoms for depression, and the presence of at least one of these symptoms is required to diagnose clinically significant depression. Research suggests that these two questions (Over the past 2 weeks, have you felt down, depressed, or hopeless? and Over the past 2 weeks, have you felt little interest or pleasure in your daily activities?) are as effective as longer inventories. If screening is positive, confirm with a more thorough assessment of neurovegetative signs (Box 3-6).

Anxious or Nervous

Although there are no validated screening questions for anxiety, asking patients whether they feel anxious or nervous is useful as a general screen. Clinical experts suggest that unexplained somatic symptoms along with reports of agitation and difficulty maintaining concentration suggest anxiety rather than depression.

A positive response to a question about anxiety or nervousness can prompt further screening:

- Do you have anxiety or panic attacks?
- Have you had to limit your activities because of your anxiety?

The first question helps to differentiate anxiety from panic attacks. The second question points toward panic with agoraphobia. If the patient is not certain what you mean by the term "panic attacks," you can provide a simple description to clarify: "A panic attack is a sudden rush of fear and nervousness that makes your heart pound and makes you afraid you're going to die or go crazy" (Carlat, 1998).

Happy, Energetic, Hyper

In the presence of depressive symptoms, a positive response to the last key question is helpful in screening for bipolar disorder. If the screen is positive, the mnemonic DIG FAST can be used to confirm the cardinal symptoms of mania (Box 3-7).

What about special considerations for adolescents?

For adolescents, a psychosocial review of systems can serve as a screen for areas that could be of concern or that have the potential to create problems. The HEEADSSS method of interviewing provides structure and a framework for focusing assessment of the following (Goldenring & Rosen, 2004):

Home environment

Education and employment

Eating

Box 3-7	**DIG FAST**

Cardinal Symptoms of Bipolar Disorder

D: Distractibility
I: Indiscretion (excessive involvement in pleasur-
         able activities)
G: Grandiosity
F: Flight of ideas
A: Activity increase
S: Sleep deficit (decreased need for sleep)
T: Talkativeness (pressured speech)

From Carlat DJ: The psychiatric review of symptoms: a screening tool for family physicians, *Am Fam Physician* 58:1617, 1998.

Activities that are peer-related
Drugs
Sexuality
Suicide/depression
Safety from injury and violence

Key Questions

The HEEADSSS interview progresses from less intimidating questions about home, family members, and the past to more personal and private issues (Table 3-1). Although the HEEADSSS interview is designed to be used in a reasonably short period of time, you often will not have enough time for the adolescent to respond to all questions. Some questions are considered essential; other questions can be asked as time permits or as the situation demands.

Is this patient at risk for suicide?

Key Questions

- Have you been feeling that life is not worth living or that you are better off dead?
- Sometimes when a person feels down or depressed he or she might think about dying. Have you been having thoughts like that?

  If patient answers yes to the preceding questions, then ask the following:
- Do you have a plan?
- What is the plan?
- Do you have the means to carry it out?
- What would cause you to carry out your plan or keep you from carrying it out?
- Have you ever attempted suicide in the past?

Initial Questions

The first set of questions helps determine whether the patient is at risk. Patients rarely volunteer thoughts of suicide, so it is important to ask directly. There is no evidence to suggest that asking about suicide precipitates suicidal thinking or acts.

Follow-Up Questions

The second set of questions helps you evaluate how imminent the risk is. Patients at high risk for suicide should be referred for psychiatric evaluation; those at imminent risk should be admitted for evaluation and treatment. Major risk factors for suicide include hopelessness, substance abuse, and prior suicide attempts.

How do I evaluate for a diagnosable psychological disorder?

All positive screening tests for mental health disorders require a full diagnostic follow-up interview using standard diagnostic criteria, such as those from the *Diagnostic and Statistical Manual of Mental Disorders*, Ed 4, Text Revision (DSM-IV-TR), to determine the presence or absence of specific disorders. The manual describes specific symptom criteria for mental disorders and psychosocial problems. Although primary care providers often diagnose and treat patients with symptoms of depression and anxiety, serious impairment of mental or emotional functioning, psychoses, bipolar disorder, and substance abuse disorders require evaluation, diagnosis, and treatment by qualified mental health specialists. Primary care is not a substitute for psychiatric care. When a patient has been screened and is suspected to be at high risk for a condition, the primary care practitioner has a responsibility to refer the patient to an appropriate resource. See the differential diagnosis table at the end of this chapter for the diagnostic criteria for some common psychological disorders.

DIAGNOSTIC REASONING: FOCUSED PHYSICAL EXAMINATION

Physical examination can yield little additional data that are of diagnostic value. No physical finding is specific for any psychological disorder. The physical examination should be directed at identifying organic-based conditions that mimic psychological disorders. Perform a comprehensive and thorough physical examination if the patient has not had one since the onset

Table 3-1	The HEEADSSS Psychosocial Interview for Adolescents	

ESSENTIAL QUESTIONS	AS TIME PERMITS	FOR MORE IN-DEPTH
Home Who lives with you? Where do you live? Do you have your own room? What are relationships like at home? To whom are you closest at home? With whom can you talk at home? Is there anyone new at home? Has someone left recently? Have you moved recently? Have you ever had to live away from home? (Why?)	Have you ever run away? (Why?) Is there any physical violence at home?	
Education and Employment What are your favorite subjects at school? Your least favorite subjects? How are your grades? Any recent changes? Any dramatic changes in the past? Have you changed schools in the past few years? What are your future education/ employment plans/goals? Are you working? (Where? How much?)	Tell me about your friends at school. Is your school a safe place? (Why?) Have you ever had to repeat a class? Have you ever had to repeat a grade? Have you ever been suspended or expelled? Have you ever considered dropping out? How well do you get along with people at school and work? Have your responsibilities at work increased?	Do you feel connected to your school? Do you feel as if you belong? Are there adults at school you feel you could talk to about something important? (Who?)
Eating What do you like and not like about your body? Have there been any recent changes in your weight? Have you dieted in the last year? (How? How often?) Have you done anything else to try to manage your weight? How much exercise do you get in an average day? Week? What do you think would be a healthy diet? How does that compare to your current eating patterns?	Do you worry about your weight? How often? Do you eat in front of the TV or computer? Does it ever seem as though your eating is out of control? Have you ever made yourself throw up on purpose to control your weight? Have you ever taken diet pills?	What would it be like if you gained (lost) 10 pounds?
Activities What do you and your friends do for fun? (With whom, where, and when?) What do you and your family do for fun? (With whom, where, and when?) Do you participate in any sports or other activities? Do you regularly attend a church group, club, or other organized activity?	Do you have any hobbies? Do you read for fun? (What?) How much TV do you watch in a week? How about video games? What music do you like to listen to?	

Table 3-1 The HEEADSSS Psychosocial Interview for Adolescents—cont'd

ESSENTIAL QUESTIONS	AS TIME PERMITS	FOR MORE IN-DEPTH
Drugs Do any of your friends use tobacco? Alcohol? Other drugs? Does anyone in your family use tobacco? Alcohol? Other drugs? Do you use tobacco? Alcohol? Other drugs? Is there any history of alcohol or drug problems in your family? Does anyone at home use tobacco?	Do you ever drink or use drugs when you are alone? (Assess frequency, intensity, patterns of use or abuse, and how youth obtains or pays for drugs, alcohol, or tobacco.) (Ask the RAFFT questions, Box 3-5.)	
Sexuality Have you ever been in a romantic relationship? Tell me about the people that you've dated. OR Tell me about your sex life. Have any of your relationships ever been sexual relationships? Are your sexual activities enjoyable? What does the term "safer sex" mean to you?	Are you interested in boys? Girls? Both? Have you ever been forced or pressured into doing something sexual that you didn't want to do? Have you ever been touched sexually in a way that you didn't want? Have you ever been raped, on a date or any other time? How many sexual partners have you had? Have you ever been pregnant or worried that you could be pregnant? (females) Have you ever gotten someone pregnant or worried that this could have happened? (males) What are you using for birth control? Are you satisfied with your method of birth control? Do you use condoms every time you have intercourse? Does anything ever get in the way of always using a condom? Have you ever had a sexually transmitted infection (STI) or worried that you had an STI?	
Suicide and Depression Do you feel sad or down more than usual? Do you find yourself crying more than usual? Are you bored all the time? Are you having trouble getting to sleep? Have you thought a lot about hurting yourself or someone else?	Does it seem that you've lost interest in things that you used to really enjoy? Do you find yourself spending less and less time with friends? Would you rather just be by yourself most of the time? Have you ever tried to kill yourself? Have you ever had to hurt yourself (by cutting yourself, for example) to calm down or feel better? Have you started using alcohol or drugs to help you relax, calm down, or feel better?	

Continued

Table 3-1	The HEEADSSS Psychosocial Interview for Adolescents—cont'd		
ESSENTIAL QUESTIONS	**AS TIME PERMITS**		**FOR MORE IN-DEPTH**
Safety (Savagery) Have you ever been seriously injured? (How?) How about anyone else you know? Do you always wear a seatbelt in the car? Have you ever ridden with a driver who was drunk or high? When? How often? Do you use safety equipment for sports and/or other physical activities (for example, helmets for biking or skateboarding)? Is there any violence in your home? Does the violence ever get physical? Is there a lot of violence at your school? In your neighborhood? Among your friends? Have you ever been physically or sexually abused? Have you ever been raped, on a date or at any other time? (If not asked previously.)	Have you ever been in a car or motorcycle accident? (What happened?) Have you ever been picked on or bullied? Is that still a problem? Have you gotten into physical fights in school or your neighborhood? Are you still getting into fights? Have you ever felt that you had to carry a knife, gun, or other weapon to protect yourself? Do you still feel that way?		

From Goldenring J, Rosen D: Getting into adolescent heads: an essential update, *Contemp Pediatr* 21:64, 2004.

of symptoms. This chapter presumes that you have performed the physical evaluation for specific presenting symptoms as part of your process to rule out a physiological cause.

Assess Vital Signs

When substance abuse is suspected, vital signs can quickly confirm the presence of an organic condition related to substance intoxication or withdrawal. Abnormal values for body temperature, blood pressure, heart rate, or respiratory rate indicate a need for a thorough evaluation.

Observe General Appearance

Look for signs of depression or substance abuse, such as an unkempt personal appearance, unusual dress, and general state of poor nutrition (skin condition and appearance of hair and nails). Observe the patient's demeanor and appearance for signs of neglect or a facial expression that might indicate depression. Observe for such behaviors as finger tapping and pacing that indicate anxiety. Methamphetamine users will often have self-induced facial lesions secondary to scratching.

Adolescents who are abusing substances sometimes wear clothing or jewelry that displays drug-oriented graffiti.

Observe the infant or child's engagement. Autistic children make few if any attempts to contact socially with others, prefer to be alone, and ignore attempts to seek attention, affection, or a connection with their surroundings.

Observe Mental Status

Perform a mental status examination. Assess general behavior. Irritability can occur in patients with anxiety. Note body posture, movement, and facial expressions. Assess thought content for suicidality or delusions, which can occur with substance abuse or psychotic disorders. Determine affect for emotional range (broad or restricted), intensity (blunted, flat, or normal), stability, and congruence with the patient's stated mood. Evaluate the patient's cognitive abilities, including attention, concentration, and memory.

Note Speech and Thought Process

Speech tone, quality, and rate reflect mental status. In depression, the speech can be soft and monotonous with little spontaneity. In mania, the speech can be rapid, pressured, and loud, and the speech content consists of a flight of ideas.

Language delay that is not consistent with development should be noted. In some children with autism, language begins to regress instead of increase in skill level.

Examine the Eyes

Substance abusers can have eyes that are injected, jaundiced, puffy, or glassy. Pupils may be dilated or constricted. The patient may have droopy eyelids and a sleepy appearance or a fixed stare. The patient may have difficulty controlling eye movements.

Examine the Ears, Nose, and Mouth

Ears should be examined. If language delay is suspected, hearing loss or deafness should be ruled out.

Substance abusers may have chronic rhinorrhea, frequent nosebleeds, or lesions in the nose or around the nostrils. The patient may have dry lips, halitosis, or an odor of alcohol, marijuana, or tobacco.

Examine the Skin

Look for skin lesions that reflect depression or anxiety, such as neurogenic scratching, nail biting, and hair pulling. Look for evidence of attempted self-injury or suicide. Adolescents may show evidence of cutting scars or superficial cuts on areas of the body. Although typically not suicide attempts, cutting serves as a coping mechanism for unrelieved feelings.

In substance abusers, the skin may be cold and clammy, itching and burning, tight, swollen, or puffy. The person may perspire excessively and have discolored fingers or injection marks along the veins. Tattoos or burn marks, possibly done while under the influence, can disguise injection marks. The patient may have injuries or bruises from falling or fighting.

Assess Balance and Gait

The patient who has a substance abuse problem may have a slow gait or poor balance.

LABORATORY AND DIAGNOSTIC STUDIES

There are no laboratory tests to assist in the diagnosis of most psychological conditions. Base the laboratory and diagnostic studies on the presenting reports (see specific chapters).

Commonly performed tests to help identify underlying conditions include the following: complete blood count (CBC), serum electrolytes, thyroid function, toxicology/blood alcohol levels.

Complete Blood Count with Indices and Differential

The complete blood count (CBC) will provide information about the presence of infection or anemia.

Serum Electrolytes

Hyponatremia or hypernatremia can exacerbate symptoms of depression. Hypercalcemia and hyperphosphatemia can exacerbate depression.

Thyroid Function Tests

An elevated level of thyroid-stimulating hormone (TSH) is related to chronic symptoms of depression. A hyperthyroid state can be associated with anxiety.

Toxicology Screen and Blood Alcohol Level

Urine and blood screening tests can be used to determine alcohol or drug intoxication as a cause of psychological symptoms.

DIFFERENTIAL DIAGNOSIS
Normal Stress

Stress is the nonspecific response of the body to any demand. The perception of a demand as stressful depends on the individual's experience of how much demand for adaptation an event or situation requires. Stressors can be acute or chronic. External stressors include adverse physical conditions (such as pain) or stressful psychological environments (such as poor working conditions, abusive relationships, or major life events). Internal stressors can be physical (such as infections or inflammation) or psychological (such as worry). Daily hassles or situational factors influence the stress load because minor annoyances that happen daily can accumulate. Situational factors can exacerbate a depressive disorder in significant ways. Symptoms of stress include mental, physical, and behavioral symptoms. Common physical symptoms include responses of the autonomic nervous system and musculoskeletal system.

Normal Grief

Grief is a subjective feeling precipitated by the loss of someone or something important to the individual. Normal grief is a process of emotional upheaval, distress, and eventual resolution. Individuals who are grieving often experience both physical and psychological symptoms and can have difficulty functioning. Grief and depression share many of the same characteristics, and normal grief can become clinical depression. An individual with a history of depression is at risk of becoming depressed in times of significant loss. The mood disturbance in depression is typically pervasive and unrelenting. In normal grief, fluctuations in mood are common. Although the pain of grief is intense, the individual is able to experience moments of less intensity or even happiness.

Domestic Violence

Domestic violence is a pattern of assaultive and coercive behaviors that include physical, sexual, psychological, and economic attacks by adults or adolescents against their intimate partners. Individuals who have experienced abuse could present with an injury that is not consistent with the description of how the injury occurred. The individual may be seen frequently for undiagnosed psychosomatic concerns. This patient can appear depressed or show evidence of suicide attempts.

Substance Use Disorders

Substance use disorders are divided into two groups: substance abuse and substance dependence. The categories of substances included are alcohol, amphetamines, cannabis, cocaine, hallucinogens, inhalants, opioids, phencyclidines, sedatives, and hypnotics. Substance abuse occurs when repeated use of alcohol or other drugs leads to significant impairment in functioning and relationships, but does not include compulsive use or addiction, or withdrawal symptoms when stopping the substance. Substance dependence includes a history of substance abuse plus continued use despite related problems, an increase in substance tolerance, and withdrawal symptoms if the substance use is stopped.

Autism Spectrum Disorder

Autism spectrum disorder is a difficult disorder to diagnose because there are no laboratory tests and the clinical signs can be subtle. Infants under the age of 18 months are very difficult to diagnose because the DSM-IV-TR does not have criteria suitable for children this young. Noting a lack of social interaction can be the first sign. After age 3 years the autism diagnostic observation schedule is more useful. Generally children with autism spectrum disorder exhibit mild to severe deficits in social interaction, verbal and nonverbal communication, and have repetitive behaviors or interests. Box 3-8 describes a screening checklist for toddlers.

Adjustment Disorders

There are several adjustment disorder diagnoses. All of the disorders in this category relate to a significantly more difficult adjustment to a life situation than would normally be expected considering the circumstances. The condition is acute if the disturbance lasts less than 6 months and chronic if it lasts for 6 months or longer

---

Box 3-8	**The Five Key Items on The CHAT* Screen**

Ask the Parent:
1. Does your child ever pretend (for example, to make a cup of tea using a toy cup and teapot) or pretend with other things?
2. Does your child ever use an index finger to point, to indicate interest in something?

Health Practitioner Observation:
3. Gain child's attention, then point across the room at an interesting object and say "Oh look! There's a (name of toy)!" Watch child's face. Does the child look across to see what you are pointing at?
4. Gain child's attention, then give child a toy cup and teapot and say "Can you make me a cup of tea?" Does the child pretend to pour out tea, drink it, etc.?
5. Say to the child "Where's the light?" or "Show me the light." Does the child point with an index finger at the light? To record "yes" on this item, the child must have looked up at your face around the time of pointing.

*CHAT = Checklist for Autism in Toddlers.
Reprinted with permission from Baird G, Charman T, Cox A, Baron-Cohen S, Swettenham I, Wheelwright S, et al: Current topic: screening and surveillance for autism and pervasive and developmental disorders, *Arch Dis* 84:471, 2001.

in response to a chronic stressor or one that has enduring consequences.

The disorders in this category can present themselves quite differently. The key to diagnosis is to examine the issue that is causing the adjustment disorder and to determine the primary symptoms associated with the disorder (e.g., anxiety or depression).

Anxiety Disorders

There are several types of anxiety disorders and multiple diagnoses. An anxiety disorder should not be confused with everyday stress and worry. Anxiety disorders are persistent conditions that require careful diagnosis. Anxiety is a group of disorders characterized by a number of both mental and physical symptoms, with no apparent explanation. The primary feature is abnormal or inappropriate anxiety. Apprehension, fear of losing control, fear of going "crazy," fear of impending danger or death, and uneasiness are among the most common psychological symptoms. Common physical symptoms include dizziness, lightheadedness, chest/abdominal pain, nausea, increased heart rate, and diarrhea.

Generalized Anxiety Disorder

Chronic anxiety, also referred to as generalized anxiety disorder, manifests as persistent worries, fears, and negative thoughts lasting a minimum of 6 months. Excessive worry over daily activities and a tendency toward headache and nausea are seen. Typically, generalized anxiety disorder (GAD) develops over a period of time and is not noticed until it is significant enough to cause problems with functioning. Anxiety is persistent, pervasive, and occurs in many different settings.

Panic Disorder

Panic disorder is manifested by sudden attacks of fear accompanied by symptoms that resemble a heart attack (e.g., palpitations, chest pain, dizziness). Often the symptoms develop rapidly and without an identifiable stressor. The individual could have had periods of high anxiety in the past, or could have been involved in a recent stressful situation; however, the underlying cause is typically subtle. Panic attacks subside as abruptly as they begin, typically lasting a few minutes, although they can last several hours. The patient could have thoughts of impending disaster, which can lead to repeated emergency medical presentations. The frequency of these attacks can vary from several times a day to only once or twice a year.

Social Phobia (Social Anxiety Disorder)

Symptoms include extreme anxiety and fear associated with social or performance situations in which the patient is exposed to unfamiliar people or to scrutiny. The patient recognizes that the fear is excessive or unreasonable but avoids the social or performance situations or endures them with intense distress or anxiety.

Mood Disorders

Mood disorders contain several categories, including dysthymia, depression, and bipolar disorder.

The disorders in this category include those in which the primary symptom is a disturbance in mood with inappropriate, exaggerated, or a limited range of affect. The feelings are extreme, pervasive, and unrelenting.

Dysthymia

The patient experiences feelings that are less intense than major depression but still disrupt everyday life. The patient experiences a depressed mood for most of the day and for more days than not, for at least 2 years. During this time, there must be two or more of the following symptoms: undereating or overeating, sleep difficulties, fatigue, low self-esteem, difficulty with concentration or decision making, and feelings of hopelessness.

Major Depressive Disorder

The hallmark symptom of depression is either a depressed mood or a loss of interest or pleasure in usual activities. Major depression can significantly impair a person's ability to function in family, work, and social situations. Patients with depression experience deep, unshakeable sadness and diminished interest in nearly all activities. Crying and feeling depressed or suicidal occur frequently.

Bipolar Disorder

Bipolar disorder has two types. Bipolar I disorder requires the occurrence of at least one manic episode even though other episodes, such as major depressive, hypomanic, or mixed, could have occurred. Bipolar II disorder requires at least one hypomanic episode.

Mania is sometimes referred to as the other extreme of depression. The patient experiences an elevated, expansive, or irritable mood with behaviors and symptoms that reflect a "high." The symptoms are sufficient to interfere with usual social activities and relationships with others.

In bipolar II disorder, there are periods of highs, as described previously, often followed by periods of depression. The high episodes are hypomanic rather than manic. The symptoms are similar but are not severe enough to cause marked impairment in social or occupational functioning and typically do not require hospitalization to ensure the safety of the person.

DIFFERENTIAL DIAGNOSIS OF *Common Causes of Psychological Disorders*

CONDITION	HISTORY	PHYSICAL FINDINGS	DIAGNOSTIC STUDIES
Normal stress	Perceived stress related to external or internal stressors, such as daily life events or situations, psychological environments, relationships Can be acute or chronic Can feel unable to cope or adapt Can have mental, physical, and behavioral symptoms	Could appear unkempt, with unusual dress Could have depressed demeanor Facial expression (e.g., dejected, sad, downcast) Tearing, crying Adolescents could show evidence of cutting	None
Normal grief	Loss of someone or something of importance Can have physical and psychological symptoms Mood fluctuations; feels depressed Can have difficulty functioning	May appear unkempt, with unusual dress, general state of poor nutrition Depressed demeanor Facial expression (e.g., dejected, sad, downcast) Tearing, crying Speech could be soft and monotonous with little spontaneity Adolescents can show evidence of cutting	None
Domestic violence	Reports physical, sexual, psychological, emotional, or economic attacks from family or partners Could seek care frequently for undiagnosed psychosomatic concerns Could report suicide attempts	Can have injuries inconsistent with history Adolescents can show evidence of cutting	None
Substance use disorders*	Reports recurrent substance use that results in failure to fulfill major obligations at work, school, or home and substance-related legal problems Use in situations that are physically hazardous (e.g., driving while intoxicated) Continued use despite significant social or interpersonal problems caused or exacerbated by effects of the substance Report increased tolerance of and need for increased amounts of substance Report withdrawal symptoms Report unsuccessful efforts to cut down or control substance use	Skin can be cold and clammy, itching and burning, tight, swollen, or puffy Excess perspiration Discolored fingers or injection marks along the veins Tattoos or burn marks, injuries or bruises Methamphetamine users can have self-induced facial lesions secondary to scratching Eyes can be injected, jaundiced, puffy, or glassy Pupils can be dilated or constricted Eyelids can be droopy with sleepy appearance or fixed stare Can have difficulty controlling eye movements Can have chronic rhinorrhea, lesions in the nose or around the nostrils Can have dry lips, halitosis, or an odor of alcohol, marijuana, or tobacco	Toxicology screen Blood alcohol level

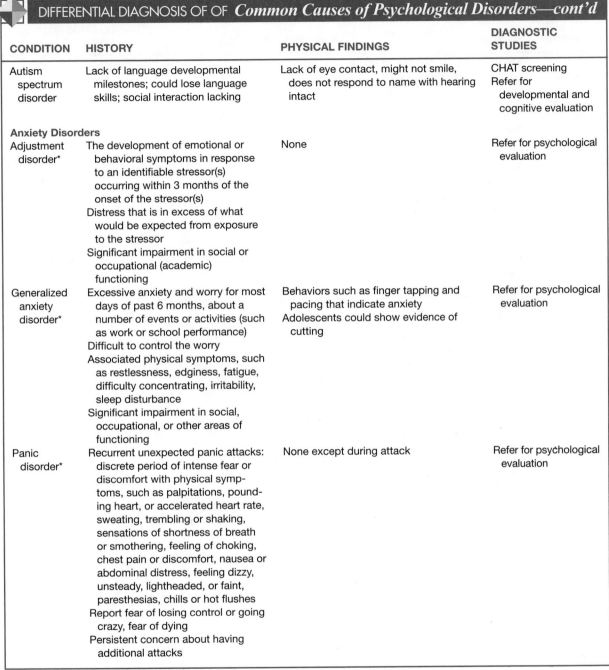

DIFFERENTIAL DIAGNOSIS OF OF *Common Causes of Psychological Disorders—cont'd*

CONDITION	HISTORY	PHYSICAL FINDINGS	DIAGNOSTIC STUDIES
Autism spectrum disorder	Lack of language developmental milestones; could lose language skills; social interaction lacking	Lack of eye contact, might not smile, does not respond to name with hearing intact	CHAT screening Refer for developmental and cognitive evaluation
Anxiety Disorders			
Adjustment disorder*	The development of emotional or behavioral symptoms in response to an identifiable stressor(s) occurring within 3 months of the onset of the stressor(s) Distress that is in excess of what would be expected from exposure to the stressor Significant impairment in social or occupational (academic) functioning	None	Refer for psychological evaluation
Generalized anxiety disorder*	Excessive anxiety and worry for most days of past 6 months, about a number of events or activities (such as work or school performance) Difficult to control the worry Associated physical symptoms, such as restlessness, edginess, fatigue, difficulty concentrating, irritability, sleep disturbance Significant impairment in social, occupational, or other areas of functioning	Behaviors such as finger tapping and pacing that indicate anxiety Adolescents could show evidence of cutting	Refer for psychological evaluation
Panic disorder*	Recurrent unexpected panic attacks: discrete period of intense fear or discomfort with physical symptoms, such as palpitations, pounding heart, or accelerated heart rate, sweating, trembling or shaking, sensations of shortness of breath or smothering, feeling of choking, chest pain or discomfort, nausea or abdominal distress, feeling dizzy, unsteady, lightheaded, or faint, paresthesias, chills or hot flushes Report fear of losing control or going crazy, fear of dying Persistent concern about having additional attacks	None except during attack	Refer for psychological evaluation

Continued

DIFFERENTIAL DIAGNOSIS OF *Common Causes of Psychological Disorders—cont'd*

CONDITION	HISTORY	PHYSICAL FINDINGS	DIAGNOSTIC STUDIES
Social phobia (social anxiety disorder)*	Marked and persistent fear of one or more social or performance situations Anxious about acting in a way that will be humiliating or embarrassing Report panic attack related to exposure to the situation Avoids the situation Avoidance, anxiety, and distress interferes significantly with the person's normal routine, occupational (academic) functioning, or social activities or relationships	None	Refer for psychological evaluation
Mood Disorders			
Dysthymic disorder*	Depressed mood for most of the day, for more days than not, for at least 2 years Reports symptoms of depression such as appetite and sleep disturbance, low energy or fatigue, low self-esteem, poor concentration or difficulty making decisions, feelings of hopelessness	Can appear unkempt, with unusual dress; general state of poor nutrition Depressed demeanor Facial expression (e.g., dejected, sad, downcast) Tearing, crying Speech can be soft and monotonous with little spontaneity Adolescents could show evidence of cutting	Refer for psychological evaluation
Major depressive disorder*	Reports acute symptoms of depressed mood most of the day, nearly every day, or loss of interest or pleasure in all or almost all activities of the day, nearly every day Experiences other symptoms most every day such as appetite disturbance, sleep disturbance, psychomotor agitation or retardation, fatigue or loss of energy, feelings of worthlessness or excessive or inappropriate guilt, diminished ability to think or concentrate, recurrent thoughts of death or suicide	Can appear unkempt, with unusual dress; general state of poor nutrition Depressed demeanor Facial expression (e.g., dejected, sad, downcast) Tearing, crying Speech can be soft and monotonous with little spontaneity Adolescents could show evidence of cutting	Serum electrolytes CBC Thyroid function tests Refer for psychological evaluation

DIFFERENTIAL DIAGNOSIS OF *Common Causes of Psychological Disorders—cont'd*

CONDITION	HISTORY	PHYSICAL FINDINGS	DIAGNOSTIC STUDIES
Bipolar disorder*	History of at least one manic episode or hypomanic episode A distinct period of abnormally and persistently elevated, expansive, or irritable mood, lasting at least 1 week Accompanying symptoms of inflated self-esteem or grandiosity, decreased need for sleep, more talkative than usual or pressure to keep talking, insomnia or hypersomnia nearly every day, psychomotor agitation or retardation, flight of ideas or racing thoughts, easy distractibility, increase in goal-directed activity, excessive involvement in pleasurable activities that have a high potential for painful consequences Report history of one or more major depressive episodes (see above)	In mania, the speech can be rapid, pressured, and loud, and the speech content consists of a flight of ideas	Refer for psychological evaluation

CBC, complete blood cell count; *CHAT,* Checklist for Autism in Toddlers.
*For specific diagnostic criteria, see *Diagnostic and statistical manual of mental disorders,* ed 4, *text revision,* Washington, DC, 2000, American Psychiatric Association.

REFERENCES AND READINGS

Diagnostic and statistical manual of mental disorders, ed 4, text revision, Washington, DC, 2000, American Psychiatric Association.

Baird G, Charman T, Cox A, Baron-Cohen S, Swettenham I, Wheelwright S: Current topic: screening and surveillance for autism and pervasive and developmental disorders, *Arch Dis Child* 84:471, 2001.

Bastiaens L, Francis G, Lewis K: The RAFFT as a screening tool for adolescent substance use disorders, *Am J Addict* 9:10, 2000.

Carlat DJ: The psychiatric review of symptoms: a screening tool for family physicians, *Am Fam Physician* 58:1617, 1998.

Citrome L, Goldberg JF: The many faces of bipolar disorder: how to tell them apart, *Postgrad Med* 117:15, 2005.

Dosreis S, Weiner CL, Johnson L, Newshaffer CJ: Autism spectrum disorder screening and management practices among general pediatric providers, *J Dev Behav Pediatr* 27:88, 2006.

Dunphy LM, Winland-Brown JE: *Primary care: the art and science of advanced practice nursing,* Philadelphia, 2001, FA Davis.

Ewing JA: Screening for alcoholism using CAGE. Cut down, annoyed, guilty, eye opener, *JAMA* 280:1904, 1998.

Feldhaus KM, Koziol-McLain J, Amsbury HL: Accuracy of 3 brief screening questions for detecting partner violence in the emergency department, *JAMA* 277:1357, 1997.

Goldenring J, Rosen D: Getting into adolescent heads: an essential update, *Contemp Pediatr* 21:64, 2004.

Goolsby MJ, Grubbs L: *Advanced assessment: interpreting findings and formulating differential diagnoses,* Philadelphia, 2006, FA Davis.

House A, Stark D: Anxiety in medical patients, BMJ 325, 2002.

Johnson CP: Recognition of autism before age 2 years, *Pediatr Rev* 29:86, 2008.

Lieberman JA III: BATHE: an approach to the interview process in the primary care setting, *J Clin Psychiatry* 58:3, 1997.

Mersy DJ: Recognition of alcohol and substance abuse, *Am Fam Physician* 67:1529, 2003.

Snyderman D, Rovner BW: Mental status examination in primary care: a review, *Am Fam Physician* 80:809, 2009.

Sokol RJ, Martier SS, Ager JW: The T-ACE questions: practical prenatal detection of risk-drinking, *Am J Obstet Gynecol* 160:863, 1989.

Stein M: Attending to anxiety disorders in primary care, *J Clin Psychiatry* 64:35, 2003.

Whooley MA, Avins AL, Miranda J, Browner WS: Case-finding instruments for depression: two questions are as good as many, *J Gen Intern Med* 12:439, 1997.

Williams JW Jr, Noel PH, Cordes JA, Ramirez G, Pignone M: Rational clinical examination. Is this patient clinically depressed? *JAMA* 287:1160, 2002.

Amenorrhea

menorrhea is a lack of menstruation that can be the result of primary or secondary causes. Primary amenorrhea is defined as the absence of menarche by 16 years of age with normal pubertal growth and development, the absence of menarche by 14 years of age with lack of normal pubertal growth and development, or the absence of menarche 2 years after sexual maturation is complete. Primary amenorrhea is a rare condition, with constitutional puberty delay the most common cause. One third of primary amenorrhea cases are genetic in nature, such as Turner syndrome or abnormality of the X chromosome.

Secondary amenorrhea is defined as the absence of menstruation for at least three cycles in women with established normal menstruation or 9 months in females with previous oligomenorrhea (menstrual periods occurring at intervals of greater than 35 days, with only four to nine periods in a year). The most common causes of secondary amenorrhea are the physiological events of pregnancy, lactation, and menopause.

The production of menstrual flow requires an intact outflow tract, a hormonally responsive uterus, and an integrated hypothalamic-pituitary-ovarian (HPO) axis. An important task in the diagnostic evaluation of amenorrhea is to identify the malfunctioning element. The primary care provider begins investigation of etiological reasons for amenorrhea and uses that knowledge to determine the type of amenorrhea. In turn, the suspected cause guides diagnostic tests, treatment, and referrals. This method of classification directs the clinician to evaluate constitutional causes, congenital or chronic disorders, the lower genital tract, and then dysfunction of any component of the HPO axis.

The normal menstrual cycle begins with the pulsatile delivery of gonadotropin-releasing hormone (GnRH) by the medial-basal hypothalamus. In response, the posterior pituitary releases luteinizing hormone (LH) and follicle-stimulating hormone (FSH). These influence the growth and development of a follicle and its release of estradiol, which causes the uterine endometrium to proliferate and initiates the LH surge, which is followed by ovulation and menstruation (Figure 4-1 and Table 4-1).

The hypothalamus is also affected by the central nervous system (CNS) and the thyroid gland, which can determine the amount of GnRH received by the pituitary. Alterations in the pattern of GnRH pulsatile release decreases circulating LH and FSH levels; the consequence is an anovulatory menstrual cycle and amenorrhea.

About 66% of all amenorrheic women are hypoestrogenic because of either hypothalamic-pituitary hypofunction or end-organ failure. Determining whether the patient is hypoestrogenic can expedite finding the reason for her amenorrhea and setting the sequencing of laboratory tests. The progesterone challenge test (PCT) causes withdrawal bleeding if there is estrogen production and an adequate outflow tract. The functional status of the pituitary-ovarian unit is assessed by measuring the gonadotropins (LH and FSH).

DIAGNOSTIC REASONING: FOCUSED HISTORY

Is there a pregnancy?

Key Questions
- Are you sexually active?
- Are you using any birth control methods?
- Are you trying to become pregnant?

Pregnancy

For any female with a uterus, it is important to rule out pregnancy as the first step in determining the cause of amenorrhea. It is rare, but a young girl can become pregnant before the onset of menses. Pregnancy should be ruled out before the administration of androgenic challenge tests. If the woman is pregnant and there is accompanying bleeding, determination of whether the pregnancy is uterine or ectopic is the next priority (see

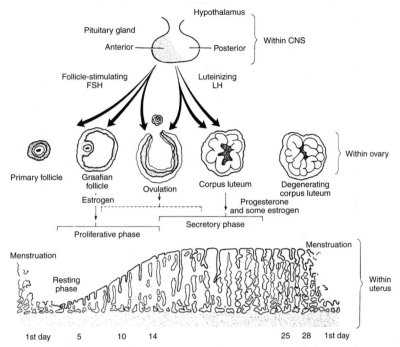

FIGURE 4-1 Interrelationships among cerebral hypothalamic, pituitary, ovarian, and uterine functions throughout the menstrual cycle. (Modified from Lowdermilk DL, Perry SE, Bobak IM: *Maternity & women's health care,* ed 6, St Louis, 1997, Mosby.)

Chapter 33). Be cognizant of domestic violence and sexual abuse, with consequent unintended pregnancy. Ask direct questions in private about being hit, pushed, or slapped or about having nonconsensual sex.

Contraceptive Use

The type and use patterns of contraceptives are important in the search for the cause of amenorrhea. Contraceptive failures can account for an unintended pregnancy. Amenorrhea can occur after discontinuation of oral contraceptives. Measurement of serum gonadotropins is affected by long-acting contraceptives, such as Depo-Provera (medroxyprogesterone acetate [DMPA]), implants, or intrauterine devices (IUDs) containing progestagens; these must be discontinued before testing.

Seeking Pregnancy

Knowing that the patient is seeking pregnancy or, if the patient is pregnant, whether it is intended or unintended allows the interview to be structured appropriately. It also aids in proper counseling and referral. Amenorrheic patients seeking pregnancy who do not

bleed after androgen challenge tests are most successfully treated by an infertility specialist. Young maternal age and early referral to a specialist increase a woman's conception rate.

Is this primary or secondary amenorrhea?

Key Questions

- Have you ever had a menstrual cycle?
- Have you started pubertal development? Can you show me how your breasts and pubic hair (PH) look compared with these pictures? (Use Tanner Sexual Maturity Rating [SMR] scales [Figures 4-2 and 4-3].)
- At what age did you start your periods?
- When was your last normal menstrual period?
- What is the nature of your periods (e.g., frequency, duration, amount of flow)?

Onset of Menstruation

The age range for menarche in the United States is 9 to 17 years. If the woman has had established menses at intervals of every 21 to 38 days, then the

Table 4-1   Correlation of Ovarian and Endometrial Cycles (Ideal 28-Day Cycle)

	MENSTRUAL (1-3 TO 5 DAYS)	EARLY FOLLICULAR (4 TO 6-8 DAYS)	ADVANCED FOLLICULAR (9 TO 12-16 DAYS)	OVULATION (12-16 DAYS)	EARLY LUTEAL (15-19 DAYS)	ADVANCED LUTEAL (20-25 DAYS)	PREMENSTRUAL (26-32 DAYS)
Ovary	Involution of corpus luteum	Growth and maturation of graafian follicle		Ovulation	Active corpus luteum	Active corpus luteum	Involution of corpus luteum
Estrogen	Diminution	Progressive increase		High concentration	Secondary rise	Rising	Decreasing
Progesterone	Absent	Absent	Absent	Appearing	Rising	Rising	Decreasing
Endometrium	Menstrual desquamation and involution	Reorganization and proliferation	Further growth and watery secretion		Active secretion and glandular dilation	Accumulation of secretion and edema	Regressive
Pituitary Secretion							
Follicle-stimulating hormone (FSH)	Fairly constant until just before ovulation			Moderate increase just before	Rapid decrease in previous levels	Rapid decrease in previous levels	
Luteinizing hormone (LH)	Fairly constant until just before ovulation			Marked increase just before	Rapid decrease in previous levels	Rapid decrease in previous levels	

From Thompson JM, McFarland GK, Hirsch JE, Tucker SM: *Mosby's clinical nursing*, ed 4, St Louis, 1997, Mosby.

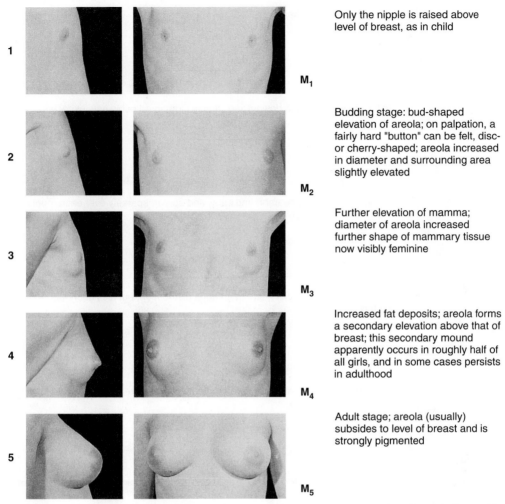

1

M₁ — Only the nipple is raised above level of breast, as in child

2

M₂ — Budding stage: bud-shaped elevation of areola; on palpation, a fairly hard "button" can be felt, disc- or cherry-shaped; areola increased in diameter and surrounding area slightly elevated

3

M₃ — Further elevation of mamma; diameter of areola increased further shape of mammary tissue now visibly feminine

4

M₄ — Increased fat deposits; areola forms a secondary elevation above that of breast; this secondary mound apparently occurs in roughly half of all girls, and in some cases persists in adulthood

5

M₅ — Adult stage; areola (usually) subsides to level of breast and is strongly pigmented

FIGURE 4-2 Five stages of breast development in females. (Photographs from Van Wieringen JC, Wafelbakker F, Verbrugge HP, DeHass JH: *Growth diagrams 1965 Netherlands: Second National Survey on 0-24-year-olds,* Groningen, The Netherlands, 1971, Wolters-Noordhoff; reprinted by permission of Kluwer Academic Publishers.)

classification of secondary amenorrhea would apply. Established menses indicate that there is no outlet flow problem and that the HPO axis and endometrium are functioning.

Pubertal Development

Female pubertal development begins with a growth spurt 1 year before the development of breast buds (thelarche) at around age 11 years. Then there is continued growth for 1 year until the peak height velocity is achieved. PH appears (pubarche), followed by axillary hair and the beginning of menarche. The average age of menarche for U.S. girls is 12 years 4 months. The length of time from thelarche to menarche is 2 to 3 years.

A thorough review of pediatric growth charts is helpful in determining the young girl's norm of growth and development and the centimeters attained by her latest growth spurt. Most adolescent girls have a mean height gain of 29 cm (11.4 inches) and the growth spurt lasts approximately 4 years. Asking adolescents to self-identify their Tanner SMR scales for breast and pubic maturity provides very accurate staging (see Figures 4-2 and 4-3). Additionally, it gives the opportunity for insight into their feelings about their body and self-esteem.

1   No growth of pubic hair

2   Initial, sparse, straight, downy, and slightly pigmented pubic hair, especially along labia

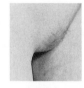

3   Pubic hair is darker, coarser, and curly, and spread sparsely over entire pubis in typical female triangle

4   Pubic hair is denser, curly, and in an adult distribution, but less abundant and restricted to pubic area

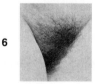

5   Pubic hair is adult in quantity, type, and pattern, with lateral spreading to inner aspect of thighs

6   Further extension laterally, upward, or over the upper thighs (this stage may not occur in all women)

FIGURE 4-3   Tanner sexual maturity development in females. (Photographs from Van Wieringen JC, Wafelbakker F, Verbrugge HP, DeHass JH: *Growth diagrams 1965 Netherlands: Second National Survey on 0-24-year-olds,* Groningen, The Netherlands, 1971, Wolters-Noordhoff; reprinted by permission of Kluwer Academic Publishers.)

Age of Menarche

The lack of menstrual periods and secondary sex characteristics by age 14 or the lack of menses by age 16 in the presence of secondary sex characteristics is considered primary amenorrhea. Fifty-six percent of all adolescents start menses when PH development is at PH stage 4 and 19% at PH stage 3 (see Figure 4-3).

If the adolescent is PH stage 4 but has not had a menses, then primary amenorrhea should be diagnosed. However, if the adolescent does not meet the age and maturation criteria, then suspect she is experiencing delayed puberty or is a so-called "late bloomer." She is likely to have a family history in her mother and sisters of delayed menarche. Almost 80%

of amenorrheic adolescents with intact female genitalia and developed breasts have an inappropriate LH feedback, anovulatory cycles, or high levels of androgenic hormones. They will bleed after a PCT and should be monitored for continued menses to avoid endometrial hyperplasia.

Menstrual History

Absence of a menstrual period for the past 3 months in females with established normal menstruation or 9 months in females with previous oligomenorrhea (menstrual periods occurring at intervals of greater than 35 days, with only four to nine periods in a year) is considered secondary amenorrhea. Sudden cessation of menstruation is more likely to indicate pregnancy or stress as a cause, whereas a gradual cessation suggests polycystic ovarian syndrome (PCOS) or premature ovarian failure.

Are there any constitutional delays causing the amenorrhea?

Key Questions

- Has there been a change in weight, percentage of body fat, or athletic training intensity?
- Are you under unusual stress at school, home, or work?
- Do you or anyone in your family have any congenital disorders or chronic diseases?

Change in Weight, Percentage Body Fat, and Athletic Training Intensity

Underweight persons typically have a low body fat–to–lean muscle ratio. Body fat can be assessed by measuring the body mass index (BMI). The severe stress of anorexia nervosa can produce prolonged amenorrhea. Exercise from various sports—jogging, middle and long distance running, ballet dancing, gymnastics, and track and field events—can lower body fat sufficiently to cause menstrual aberrations. Long distance runners and ballerinas are more apt to be amenorrheic than are swimmers; however, even moderate exercise can cause one or two missed periods a year. The mechanism of action on the HPO axis is unknown but is expressed by delayed puberty, shortened luteal phase, anovulation, and amenorrhea. Obesity can be the cause of amenorrhea or be a sign of PCOS. PCOS causes ovarian dysfunction—elevated androgens, hirsutism, low sex steroid binding globulin (SSBG), and an elevated LH/FSH ratio.

Emotional State

The stress of athletic competition, family situations, school performance, peer relations, and work can disrupt normal cyclic menses. The HPO axis of a teenager is more sensitive to physical and psychological stress than that of an adult female.

Congenital or Chronic Diseases

Turner syndrome stigmata (see the discussion on performing a head and neck examination later in this chapter) or similar physical findings suggest the probability of an abnormality of one or all components (CNS, structural anomalies, or HPO axis) necessary for menstruation. Most structural anomalies that would prevent outflow of the menstrual blood are detectable on physical examination. Chronic diseases, such as anorexia nervosa, diabetes mellitus, Crohn disease, systemic lupus erythematosus, glomerulonephritis, cystic fibrosis, pituitary adenoma, adrenal diseases, and thyroid dysfunction, can cause amenorrhea.

Could this be thyroid dysfunction?

Key Questions

- Have you noticed changes in the texture of your hair or skin?
- Are you bothered by hot or cold temperatures?
- Have you had any changes in your energy level?
- Have you had any changes in your bowel function?

Hair and Skin Changes and Temperature Intolerance

Hypothyroidism and hyperthyroidism are expressed by changes in hair and skin texture. Hyperthyroidism often makes women intolerant of the heat, and this is sometimes confused with menopausal syndrome symptoms. Cold intolerance is frequently exhibited by persons with low-functioning thyroids.

Energy and Bowel Changes

Increased functioning of the thyroid causes restlessness and diarrhea, whereas decreased functioning results in constipation and fatigue. Even mild thyroid dysfunction can cause menstrual irregularities; therefore a thyroid function test is needed to assess the thyroid status.

Could this be caused by hyperprolactinemia?

Key Questions

- Are you able to express a discharge or liquid from your nipples?
- Is there increased stimulation to your nipples?
- Have you had any surgery or disease of the breasts or chest wall?

Galactorrhea

Women notice breast nipple discharge that is not associated with breastfeeding or medications. Offensive medications are listed in Box 4-1 and include primarily the dopamine antagonist agents and estrogens.

Nipple Stimulation and Chest Wall Stimulation

Nipple stimulation from clothing irritation during jogging or nipple manipulation during sexual activity may cause galactorrhea. Surgical interventions, such as lymph node dissection, or disease processes, such as herpes zoster, can also lead to galactorrhea, triggered by peripheral neural stimulation.

Could the hyperprolactinemia be caused by medications?

Key Questions

- What prescription medicines are you taking?
- Have you used any street drugs? What kind of drugs have you used?

Medication History

Some medications, such as phenothiazines or contraceptives, can cause amenorrhea. These drugs increase prolactin levels, induce an estrogenic effect, or are toxic to the ovaries (see Box 4-1). Illicit drugs, such as heroin and methadone, also lead to menstrual abnormalities.

Is a pituitary tumor causing the amenorrhea?

Key Questions

- Have you experienced any visual changes?
- Are you having an increased number of headaches?

Box 4-1	**Drugs That May Cause Amenorrhea**

Prolactin Increase
Antipsychotics: Phenothiazines, haloperidol, pimozide, clozapine
Antidepressants: Tricyclic antidepressants, monoamine oxidase inhibitors
Antihypertensives: Calcium channel blockers, methyldopa, reserpine

Estrogenic Effect
Digitalis, marijuana, flavonoids, oral contraceptives

Ovarian Toxicity
Busulfan, chlorambucil, cisplatin, cyclophosphamide, fluorouracil

Modified from Kiningham RB, Apgar BS, Schwenk TL: Evaluation of amenorrhea, *Am Fam Physician* 53:1186, 1996.

Visual Changes and Headaches

A pituitary tumor could be responsible for the hyperprolactin state. Enlarging pituitary tumors cause headaches. As the tumor grows out of the sella turcica, it compresses the optic chiasm and nerves. The common visual defect is bitemporal hemianopia, although other defects can occur. Changes in visual fields are often self-diagnosed when the patient recognizes vision problems while reading or driving an automobile. Clinical changes in vision warrant a referral to an ophthalmologist and computed tomography (CT) or magnetic resonance imaging (MRI) work-up for a tumor of the sella turcica. A high prolactin level indicates a pituitary adenoma that presents with or without galactorrhea.

Is this a problem of the HPO axis?

Key Questions

- Have you experienced any problems with infertility?
- Do you have excess hair on your face or chest?
- Are you having any menopausal symptoms (e.g., hot flashes, vaginal dryness)?
- Did you hemorrhage during childbirth?

Infertility

Many cases of infertility are caused by failure of ovulation. PCOS affects women between the ages of 15 and 30 years. Basal body temperature charts and endometrial biopsies can reveal anovulatory cycles. Vaginal ultrasound shows enlarged ovaries with multiple small, fluid-filled cysts. Infertility can be caused by low or high estrogen levels. Measurement of gonadotropins, vaginal maturation index (MI), and progesterone levels provide insight into the functioning of the HPO axis.

Androgen Excess
About 50% of women diagnosed with PCOS are hirsute, obese, and have difficulty conceiving. Few other signs of masculinization are present. LH is elevated with PCOS. Truncal obesity, acne, and male pattern baldness can signify androgen excess.

Estrogen Deficiency
Hot flashes or flushes, changes in mood, and difficulty sleeping are common menopausal symptoms that women with low estradiol levels can experience. A dry vagina is often accompanied by dyspareunia and sometimes dysuria. The dysuria can be secondary to the hypoestrogenic state of the urethra and not be the result of a urinary tract infection. Prolonged hypoestrogenic status leads to osteopenia, regardless of age.

Hemorrhage at Childbirth
Amenorrhea can occur subsequent to a pregnancy and delivery if, at the time of delivery, there was severe hemorrhage. Obstetric hemorrhage causes pituitary ischemia and infarction and results in pituitary insufficiency. This pathological process is known as Sheehan syndrome. In this instance, refer the patient to an endocrinologist.

Is this a problem of the uterus?

Key Question
- Have you had a miscarriage or abortion, uterine infection, or any surgery or procedure involving your uterus?

Gynecological Problem
Endometritis, incomplete abortion, or aggressive curettage of the uterus can lead to denuding of the endometrial layer, scarring, and Asherman syndrome. The patient with Asherman syndrome will not bleed after the PCT, nor will she bleed after the uterus is primed with estrogen and challenged with DMPA. The diagnosis can be made by performing weekly serum progesterone tests to determine if any value is within the ovulatory range (>3 ng/mL) yet there are no periods. The diagnosis can also be made by the gynecologist via hysteroscopy, hysterosalpingography, or measuring endometrial thickness by ultrasonography.

What symptoms support a structural outflow problem?

Key Questions
- Do you have cyclic abdominal bloating or cramping?
- Have you been amenorrheic since you had a cervical procedure?

Presence of Premenstrual Symptoms or Dysmenorrhea
Cyclic symptomatology of dysmenorrhea in the absence of menses can be caused by an incomplete outflow tract. Physical examination validates a vaginal opening, imperforate hymen, intact uterus, or congenital imperforate cervical os. If there is no indication of a uterus by examination or lower abdominal ultrasound, a karyotype is needed to determine the congenital disorder. A referral to an endocrinologist or gynecological surgeon could be indicated for removal of any abdominal male gonads, which would be a risk for cancerous degeneration.

Amenorrhea Since Cervical Procedure
Stenosis of the cervical os can occur after gynecological office surgeries, such as cervical biopsies and cryotherapy. However, it is more common after cone biopsies of the cervix, such as the loop electrosurgical excision procedure (LEEP), or carbon dioxide laser treatment.

DIAGNOSTIC REASONING: FOCUSED PHYSICAL EXAMINATION
Note General Appearance
The body morphology of the patient can provide clues to the cause of amenorrhea; often diseases can be diagnosed secondary to short stature, underweight, or overweight. A height less than 5 feet (short stature) in a girl who is 14 years old or older could indicate a congenital chromosomal problem. Assess the woman's general state of health to determine if there are signs of systemic, chronic, or congenital disease.

Assess Nutritional Status and Plot Measurements on Growth Chart in Adolescents

Assess nutritional status, looking for signs of undernutrition or overnutrition. Measure the height, weight, and arm span of the adolescent. Plot on a growth chart if delayed puberty is a consideration. Anorexia nervosa is often found while evaluating an adolescent who has short stature and is underweight.

Assess Sexual Maturity

Use the Tanner SMR scales to assess and rate the stage of breast and PH development. An SMR can be calculated by averaging the girl's stage of PH and breast development. The stage of breast and PH development in the adolescent girl is related to her chronological age, age at menarche, and evidence of growth spurt. The breasts often develop at different rates, so some asymmetry is common. Menarche generally occurs at SMR 4 or breast stage 3 to 4. Plot these physiological events on the growth curve.

Screen for Eating Disorders

If you suspect anorexia nervosa or bulimia, administer a screening instrument to help determine the diagnosis. Refer to the DSM-IV-TR for diagnostic criteria. About half of the females with eating disorders will have short stature.

Calculate the Body Mass Index

Seventeen percent body fat is needed for most females to be menarchal, and about 22% body fat is necessary for ovulation. Calculate the BMI (Box 4-2; also see Appendix C). A BMI of 19 kg/m^2 usually indicates about 17% body fat, which can cause amenorrhea.

Obesity causes amenorrhea secondary to ovarian dysfunction. A BMI of greater than 27 kg/m^2 corresponds to being more than 20% overweight. Adipose cell stroma convert androstenedione to estrogen (estrone) as the body fat increases. Obesity also increases sex hormone binding globulin, thereby increasing free steroid levels. Both processes can cause an imbalance in the HPO axis and lead to amenorrhea.

Examine the Skin and Hair

Observe for signs of thyroid dysfunction or adrenal excess. Features of hypothyroidism include dry, coarse, flaky skin; coarse hair that tends to break; and thick,

---

Box 4-2	**Body Mass Index (BMI)**

BMI is helpful in assessing the nutritional status and total body fat of the patient. You can use the BMI chart, Appendix C, to determine the BMI. You can also calculate the BMI by using the following formula:

Multiply the patient's weight in pounds by 704. Take that number (product) and divide by the height in inches. Once again, divide by the height in inches.

Example: Weight = 75 pounds; height = 4 feet 2 inches or 50 inches

75 × 704	= 52,800
52,800 ÷ 50	= 1056
1056 ÷ 50	= 21.12
BMI	= 21

---

brittle nails. Hyperthyroidism is characterized by fine, warm skin that is hyperpigmented at pressure points. Nails will often separate from the nail plate (onycholysis), and hair will be fine, thin, and limp. Cushingoid features include truncal obesity, striae, and moon face. Observe for other signs of androgen excess, which include hirsutism, acne, and male pattern baldness.

Perform a Head and Neck Examination

During the head and neck examination, note any visual changes, including visual field defects, that might indicate a pituitary tumor. Anosmia might denote a congenital absence of GnRH, resulting in no secretion of LH or FSH from the pituitary. Without LH or FSH production, there is no ovulation; anovulatory cycles are amenorrheic. Also look for Turner syndrome stigmata—webbed neck and low-set ears (other signs are shieldlike chest and short fourth metacarpal).

Palpate the Thyroid Gland and Lymph Nodes

Palpate the thyroid gland for diffuse enlargement, asymmetry, and nodules. Auscultate for thyroid bruits and count the pulse rate. Assess for supraclavicular and infraclavicular lymphadenopathy or carcinogenic masses of the sternal notch and abdomen, which could arise from a tumor of germ cell, adrenal, or pituitary origin.

Perform Clinical Breast Examination

Physical examination verifies sexual maturation level. The growth spurt occurs before breast development (thelarche), which is followed by the appearance of axillary hair. Perform a breast examination and assess breast maturity level using Tanner SMR scales. More than 95% of adolescents are menarchal 1 year after they reach a breast maturity rating of 4. Check for galactorrhea (see Chapter 5).

Perform a Pelvic Examination

Observe for maturation of the female genitalia and secondary sex characteristics. Assign a Tanner SMR scale for PH development. A congenital problem might manifest as vaginal or uterine agenesis and is identified by the absence of a vagina, cervix, or uterus. There could be a small invagination of the perineum below the urinary meatus. It can be explored using a cotton-tipped applicator and otoscope with a large ear speculum or nasal speculum to determine the dimensions of the vault and presence of a cervix. A clitoris larger than 1 cm is suggestive of androgen excess.

Assess for other outlet problems, including an imperforate hymen (painful, bluish bulging of the perineum), stenotic cervix (bulging os or inability to pass a cotton-tipped applicator through the os), or a transverse vaginal septum. The development of hematocolpos, hematometra, or hematoperitoneum from menses behind an obstructed outflow tract needs immediate intervention to prevent inflammatory changes and endometriosis. Needle aspiration is *not* recommended because it might potentiate infection. Refer to a reconstructive gynecological surgeon for MRI and, often, extensive surgery.

If the introitus is small, use a pediatric Pedersen, Huffman-Graves, or Graves' speculum (which measures approximately $1/2$ inch wide and $3^3/4$ inches long), or a Huffman vaginoscope. Vaginal walls that are pale and dry, have few rugations, and are friable are estrogen deficient. Low estrogen levels cause scant cervical mucus. Vaginal cytology reports for women exhibiting such symptoms show an MI lacking or low in estrogen.

The bimanual examination can be performed with only an index finger in the vagina if the vaginal vestibule is small. If the hymen is rigid, a rectal bimanual examination can be completed instead of the usual vaginal bimanual examination. On pelvic bimanual examination, enlarged ovaries are palpated about half the time in patients with PCOS. Assess for position, size, shape, and consistency of the cervix, uterus, and ovaries.

LABORATORY AND DIAGNOSTIC STUDIES
Pregnancy Test

Immunoassay testing for the beta subunit of the human chorionic gonadotropin (ß-hCG) is used to identify or rule out pregnancy and is an essential test on all females presenting with amenorrhea.

Thyroid-Stimulating Hormone

A serum TSH test identifies hypothyroidism. When hormonal supplementation is provided, menses usually resumes for these patients. If the amenorrhea is associated with galactorrhea and hyperprolactinemia, the prolactin level must be measured again after the thyroid function levels become normal.

Prolactin Levels

The prolactin level is most reliable when it is a fasting measurement. When the patient's fasting prolactin level is normal (<50 ng/mL), a PCT is indicated. If the patient's level is high (>50 ng/mL) or if she has galactorrhea, a cone-down view of the sella turcica is taken to rule out a pituitary adenoma. A level >200 ng/mL is highly suggestive of a prolactinoma. A prolactin elevation less than 100 ng/mL but higher than normal is most frequently caused by prescribed or illicit drugs. The hyperprolactinemia usually subsides a few weeks after stopping the offending drug. Microscopic examination of breast discharge will reveal fat globules and no red blood cells (see Chapter 5).

Serum Follicle-Stimulating Hormone Levels

Ovarian failure, which causes a low estradiol secretion, will raise the FSH level higher than 40 mIU/mL. If both the FSH and LH levels are greater than 50 mIU/mL, then primary ovarian failure is established. If the patient is older than 30 years, menopause is diagnosed; if she is younger than 30 years, a karyotype should be done. An FSH measurement of less than 40 mIU/mL denotes a hypothalamic-pituitary dysfunction and secondary ovarian failure.

Serum Luteinizing Hormone Levels

A serum LH level greater than 35 milliunits/mL is frequently seen in patients with PCOS. An LH:FSH ratio higher than 2:1 is suggestive of PCOS, whereas a ratio higher than 3:1 is considered diagnostic of PCOS.

Dehydroepiandrosterone Sulfate

Mildly elevated levels of dehydroepiandrosterone sulfate (DHEA-S) are seen in women with PCOS. Significantly elevated DHEA-S levels (>700 mg dl^{-1}) indicate congenital adrenal hyperplasia.

Central Nervous System Imaging

If both FSH and LH levels are low, indicating a problem of the pituitary, imaging of the CNS is warranted. Either contrast-enhanced CT or MRI of the sella turcica can determine whether there is an abnormality. If the prolactin level is greater than 100 ng/mL or the cone-down view of the sella turcica is abnormal, CT or MRI with contrast enhancement should be obtained.

Pelvic Ultrasound and Vaginal Ultrasound

Pelvic and vaginal ultrasound studies are used to determine the presence of a uterus; the anatomical size and endometrial thickness of a uterus; and whether fibroids or other tumors exist. Ultrasound is used to measure ovarian size, to identify cysts, and to evaluate follicular development. In primary amenorrhea, ultrasound is helpful in assessing müllerian agenesis and gonadal dysgenesis because there could be internal organs and no conduit to the perineum. One third of these patients also have urinary tract abnormalities; therefore an abdominal ultrasound can be obtained at the same time to evaluate that system.

Progesterone Challenge Test

Also called the progesterone withdrawal test, the PCT consists of the administration of oral DMPA 10 mg daily for 7-10 days or parenteral progesterone in oil 200 mg intramuscularly. The patient should respond to the medication within 2 to 7 days. If there is a positive PCT response, the patient bleeds. This demonstrates that there are sufficient endogenous estrogens to prepare the endometrium and confirms that there is a functioning outflow tract. It substantiates an intact HPO axis. Other forms of progesterone can be used: micronized progesterone 400 mg PO daily for 7-10 days or norethindrone 5 mg PO daily for 7-10 days.

Estrogen/Progesterone Challenge Test

The estrogen/progesterone challenge test (E/PCT) consists of the administration of conjugated estrogens 1.25 mg daily or estradiol 2 mg daily for 21 days followed by progesterone as given in the PCT. If there is no menstrual flow, administer the regimen a second time. If there is no flow after both courses of therapy, the cause is either the outflow tract or the uterine endometrium. The E/PCT is positive if there is menstrual flow within 2 to 7 days. A positive test denotes that there is inadequate estrogen production either from inadequate functional ovarian follicles or from inadequate pituitary gonadotropic stimulation.

Chromosome Analysis (Karyotyping)

A buccal smear or vaginal smear of epithelial cells is stained with cresyl violet and examined microscopically. Karyotyping is done to delineate probable chromosomal abnormalities. It is used in the work-up for ambiguous genitalia, primary amenorrhea, oligomenorrhea, delayed puberty, or abnormal development at puberty.

Endometrial Biopsy

Endometrial biopsy can be used to show the hormonal response of the uterine endometrium.

Basal Body Temperature Charting

A woman can take her awakening body temperature each day and chart it to determine if ovulation is occurring. This test is based on the fact that progesterone increases the body temperature by 0.5° F to 0.8° F for 11 days during the luteal phase. If this increase in temperature occurs, ovulation has occurred and a positive estrogen component is inferred. Digital read-out thermometers are quick and easy to use.

Maturation Index

A vaginal cytological smear (Papanicolaou smear) for evaluation of ovarian function can determine the hormonal status of the vagina. The index is read from left to right and refers to the percentage of parabasal, intermediate, and superficial squamous cells appearing on a smear, with the total of all three values equaling 100%. For example, an MI of 0/40/60 represents 0% parabasal cells, 40% intermediate cells, and 60% superficial cells. Lack of estrogen effect is demonstrated by predominance of parabasal cells. Low estrogen effect is demonstrated by predominance of intermediate cells. Increased estrogen effect is demonstrated by predominance of intermediate cells. Both increased and decreased estrogen effects can be reflective of a hormonal imbalance of the HPO axis.

Progesterone Levels

Serum progesterone levels collected at weekly intervals can establish whether ovulation has occurred. A value greater than 3 ng/mL is found with ovulation.

DIFFERENTIAL DIAGNOSIS
Pregnancy

Pregnancy is the most common reason for amenorrhea in women of childbearing age. Determining the pregnancy status of the patient is the first step in the amenorrhea work-up.

Constitutional Problems
Delayed Puberty

A pituitary adenoma must be ruled out for all patients with delayed puberty. Yearly prolactin levels should be performed for those with delayed puberty because of the possibility of occult pituitary adenomas.

Anorexia Nervosa and Bulimia

Anorexia nervosa and bulimia are disorders that are psychiatric in origin. Affected women have such a fear of being fat that they do not eat or they purge after eating. Often these women are overachievers and have low self-esteem. The majority are adolescents, with a mean age of 13 to 14. Amenorrhea is caused by extreme weight loss and/or cachectic state.

Exercise-Induced Amenorrhea

This amenorrhea is common in competitive athletes, but exercise can also cause skipped menses in the casual trainer. Gymnasts, ballerinas, and long distance runners are at high risk, especially if they started their training at a very early age. Body fat of 17% is needed for menarche, whereas 22% body fat is necessary for ovulation. BMI estimates the woman's body fat level.

Congenital or Chronic Disorders
Turner Syndrome

Turner syndrome causes primary amenorrhea because of ovarian agenesis. The typical features are short stature, webbed neck, shieldlike chest, and delayed secondary sex characteristics.

Cushing Syndrome

Cushing syndrome is caused by an excess secretion of adrenocorticotropic hormone (ACTH) from a pituitary or adrenal adenoma. Classically, patients present with a "moon face," acne, hirsutism, kyphosis, purplish striae of the abdomen, and hypertension. CT can reveal pituitary or adrenal adenoma.

Thyroid Dysfunction

Amenorrhea from thyroid dysfunction subsides as soon as serum thyroid levels return to normal. Hypothyroidism frequently causes amenorrhea and is characterized by fatigue, constipation, cold intolerance, and dry skin.

Polycystic Ovary Syndrome

PCOS typically causes infertility in women ages 15 to 30 years. Half of these women exhibit hirsutism and obesity. The ovaries are often large and contain multiple fluid-filled cysts. The diagnosis is established by ultrasonography.

Uterine and Outflow Tract Problems
Imperforate Hymen

The woman with an imperforate hymen could present with a painful, bulging perineum. There is lack of an intact outflow tract, which causes the primary amenorrhea.

Cervical Os Stenosis

Stenosis of the cervical os can be the cause for either primary or secondary amenorrhea. Stenosis is often caused by therapeutic procedures of the cervix such as cryotherapy or cone biopsies. These procedures cause scarring and stenosis of the os, obstructing the outflow tract.

Asherman Syndrome

Asherman syndrome occurs when the uterine endometrial lining is denuded or scarred, usually by infection or curettage. The patient does not respond to either a PCT or an E/PCT.

Hypothalamic-Pituitary-Ovarian Axis Problem
Ovarian Failure

Menopause occurs when the ovaries fail secondary to depletion of ova. The average age of menopause in the United States is 51 years. It is a state of hypoestrogenemia. The gonadotropin levels rise (FSH >40 milliunits/mL), and the estradiol levels fall (<15 pg/mL). Clinical symptoms are hot flashes, night sweats, insomnia, mood changes, and amenorrhea for 12 months. If this occurs before age 40 years, it is considered premature. Common causes of premature ovarian failure include genetic and enzyme disorders, immune disturbances, and chemotherapy.

Sheehan Syndrome

Sheehan syndrome is activated by severe obstetrical hemorrhage, which causes pituitary ischemia and infarction. The pituitary gland becomes dysfunctional.

Medications

Prescription and illicit drugs can increase prolactin levels, which in turn promote galactorrhea. Offending drugs are primarily dopamine antagonist agents, estrogens, and marijuana.

Chest Wall or Nipple Stimulation

Prolactin inhibits the pulsatile secretion of GnRH, unbalancing the HPO axis and possibly causing amenorrhea. The higher the prolactin level, the greater the chance is that the patient will be amenorrheic.

Pituitary Adenoma

Pituitary macroadenomas and microadenomas should be suspected if the prolactin level is greater than 100 ng/mL or if there are any abnormalities of the cone-down view of the sella turcica. Patients with pituitary adenomas should be referred to an endocrinologist. Patients with prolactin levels exceeding 1000 ng/mL probably have an invasive tumor.

DIFFERENTIAL DIAGNOSIS OF *Common Causes of Amenorrhea*

CONDITION	HISTORY	PHYSICAL FINDINGS	DIAGNOSTIC STUDIES
Pregnancy			
Pregnancy	Breast tenderness, morning sickness, urinary frequency	Globular, enlarged uterus; soft, bluish color cervix	β-hCG pregnancy test positive; ultrasonography positive
Constitutional Problems			
Delayed puberty	No menstruation at age beyond 16 years; more than 5 years between initiation of breast growth and menarche	Breast stage 1 persists beyond age 13.4; PH stage 1 persists beyond age 14.1	Prolactin normal; TSH, T_4 normal; CBC, U/A normal; chemistry profile normal; bone age normal; skull radiograph normal
Anorexia nervosa/ bulimia	Mean age 13-14; fear of being fat; low self-esteem; depression; isolation; overachiever; food is parental battleground; preoccupation; hair loss; abdominal bloating, pain, constipation	Amenorrhea before or after weight loss; cachexia; low body fat; short stature; yellow, dry, cold skin; acrocyanosis: increased lanugo hair; hypotension, systolic murmurs, often mitral valve prolapse	TSH normal; prolactin normal; FSH and LH usually low; glucose normal; ECG: bradycardia, low-voltage changes, T wave inversions, and occasional ST segment depression
Exercise-induced amenorrhea	Began athletic training at young age; more common with long distance runners, ballerinas, gymnasts	BMI <17% body fat	TSH normal; prolactin normal

DIFFERENTIAL DIAGNOSIS OF *Common Causes of Amenorrhea—cont'd*

CONDITION	HISTORY	PHYSICAL FINDINGS	DIAGNOSTIC STUDIES
Congenital or Chronic Disorders			
Turner syndrome	Congenital; short stature; infantile sexual development	Characteristics: webbed neck, low-set ears, shield-like chest, short fourth metacarpal	Karyotype (45,X)
Cushing syndrome	Weight gain; weakness; back pain	Moon face, acne, hirsutism, purple striae of abdomen	Cortisol increased; 17-ketosteroids increased; CT adenoma
Thyroid dysfunction	Hypothyroid: delayed growth, weight gain, fatigue, constipation, cold intolerance; hyperthyroid: weight loss, nervousness, heat intolerance	Hypothyroid: dry skin, fine hair, galactorrhea; hyperthyroid: moist skin, hyperpigmentation over bones, thin hair, goiter	Hypothyroid: TSH high; hyperthyroid: TSH low; T_3 high; T_4 high
Polycystic ovary syndrome	Infertility	Hirsutism; obesity; enlarged ovaries	Ultrasonography: enlarged ovaries with multiple fluid-filled cysts; testosterone high; DHEA-S may be elevated
Uterine and Outflow Tract Problems			
Imperforate hymen/stenotic cervical os	Monthly bloating, cramping, and pelvic pressure; no menses; cryotherapy or other procedure to cervix	Fibrotic hymen without patent opening; stenotic cervical os	Clinical diagnosis by history and findings
Asherman syndrome	History of uterine infection; tuberculosis, schistosomiasis; uterine iatrogenic scarring; curettage, irradiation	Pelvic examination normal	PCT negative; E/PCT negative; hysteroscopy adhesions
Hypothalamic-Pituitary-Ovarian Axis Problem			
Ovarian failure	Hot flashes, night sweats, insomnia, mood changes	Pale, dry vaginal mucosa; few rugae	FSH and LH high; estradiol low
Sheehan syndrome	Recent history of postpartum hemorrhage and shock during delivery	Hair loss; depigmentation of skin; mammary and genital atrophy	Pituitary and end-organ hormones low; hemoglobin low
Medications/chest wall or nipple stimulation	Breast nipple discharge; history of dopamine antagonists, estrogens, or illicit drugs; stimulation to nipples: exercise or sexual; history of chest wall surgery or herpes zoster	Nipple discharge: bilateral; multiduct; milky, clear, or yellowish discharge	Wet mount or hemoccult of nipple discharge: negative for RBCs; prolactin high; cone-down view of sella turcica; MRI or CT with contrast
Pituitary adenoma	Delayed puberty; history of visual changes, increasing headaches	Visual field defects; galactorrhea	Prolactin high; cone-down view of sella turcica positive; MRI or CT with contrast positive

BMI, body mass index; *CBC,* complete blood cell count; *CT,* computed tomography; *DHEA-S,* dehydroepiandrosterone sulfate; *ECG,* electrocardiogram; *E/PCT,* estrogen/progesterone challenge test; *FSH,* follicle-stimulating hormone; *LH,* luteinizing hormone; *MRI,* magnetic resonance imaging; *PCT,* progesterone challenge test; *PH,* pubic hair; *RBCs,* red blood cells; T_3, triiodothyronine; T_4, thyroxine; *TSH,* thyroid-stimulating hormone; *U/A,* urinalysis.

REFERENCES AND READINGS

American Academy of Pediatrics, Committee on Sports Medicine and Fitness: Medical concerns in the female athlete, *Pediatrics* 106:610, 2000.

Bielak KS, Harris S: Amenorrhea, *e-Medicine* (website): http://emedicinemedscape.com/article/953850-overview. Updated April 8, 2010. Accessed September 21, 2010.

Deligeoroglou E, Tsimaris P: Menstrual disturbances in puberty, *Best Pract Res Clin Obstet Gynaecol* 24:157, 2010.

Goodman LR, Warren MP: The female athlete and menstrual function, *Curr Opin Obstet Gynecol* 17:466, 2005.

Goswami D, Conway GS: Premature ovarian failure, *Hum Reprod Update* 11:391, 2005.

Heiman D: Amenorrhea, *Prim Care* 36:1, 2009.

Hunter MH, Sterrett JJ: Polycystic ovary syndrome: it's not just infertility, *Am Fam Physician* 62:1079, 2000.

Master-Hunter T, Heiman DL: Amenorrhea: evaluation and treatment, *Am Fam Physician* 73:1374, 2006.

Pletcher JR, Slap GB: Menstrual disorders: amenorrhea, *Pediatr Clin North Am* 46:505, 1999.

Sabatini S: The female athlete triad, *Am J Med Sci* 322:193, 2001.

Wilson GR, Haddad JE, Haddad CJ: Amenorrhea: common causes and evaluation, *Compr Ther* 31:270, 2005.

Breast Lumps and Nipple Discharge

From 80% to 90% of all breast lumps are found by the woman or her partner before diagnosis through clinical breast examination (CBE) or mammography. The three most common breast lumps are fibroadenomas, fibrocystic breast changes, and breast carcinoma. Fibroadenomas are benign solid tumors most frequently seen in women younger than 30 years. Fibrocystic breast changes are a heterogeneous group of nonproliferative changes of stromal and/or glandular elements of the breast tissue that includes benign cysts, diffuse and localized nodularity, nipple discharge, and breast tenderness. Fibrocystic symptoms are seen with great frequency in women ages 30 to 50 years but less often in those who are menopausal.

Breast carcinoma is the most common cancer in women and the second leading cause of cancer-related death. The risk of breast cancer in women rises steadily with age and accelerates rapidly after the age of 50. Although benign conditions that affect the breast are more common, the presence of a lump raises legitimate fears. The goal of the assessment process is to reach a diagnosis that addresses the possibility of breast cancer.

Nipple discharge is a common complaint among postmenarchal female clients. It is often related to pregnancy, recent breastfeeding, or estrogenic medications. In women who are not lactating, nipple discharge is most frequently caused by intraductal papilloma, duct ectasia, or cancer. Nipple discharge is more commonly caused by benign lesions than by cancerous ones. Physiological stimulation (e.g., sucking, pregnancy, mechanical stimulation) of the breasts can produce discharge, as can breast trauma and inflammation (e.g., herpes zoster, mammoplasty), pituitary disorders (e.g., irradiation of pituitary), or tranquilizing drugs (e.g., phenothiazines, methyldopa).

DIAGNOSTIC REASONING: FOCUSED HISTORY FOR BREAST LUMPS

Is this lump likely to be malignant?

Key Questions
- How long has the lump been present?
- Is the lump changing (e.g., getting bigger, worse, or more painful)?
- Is the lump in one breast only or are there lumps in both breasts?
- When was your last menstrual period?
- Is there any discharge from the nipple?
- Have you recently been treated for a breast infection?

Duration and Growth

The primary presenting complaint of a malignant lesion is that of a single, hard, painless lump in the breast that is unchanged by the cyclic hormonal milieu. A change from the patient's normal physical findings is the most persuasive criterion for considering a diagnosis of breast cancer.

Malignant lumps are more likely to be new lumps that show progressive increase in size. The lump grows until there is an alteration in the contour of the breast tissue. An unchanged lump of long duration (years) is almost always benign. Half of all newly appearing benign cysts resolve within two or three menstrual cycles.

Unilateral Versus Bilateral

Breast lumps found bilaterally in identical quadrants of the breast are more likely to be benign. A solitary unilateral lump, although usually a cyst, fibroadenoma, or lipoma (rare), raises more suspicion for malignancy.

Postmenopausal

Cyclic cysts of the breast are less common after menopause and necessitate diagnostic investigation. A postmenopausal woman with unilateral mastalgia (breast pain) has a greater risk for breast cancer. Perimenopausal and postmenopausal women are also at greater statistical risk for breast cancer because of the higher incidence of breast cancer as they age. A new breast lump in a postmenopausal woman warrants a high degree of suspicion for cancer.

Nipple Discharge with a Lump

The occurrence of nipple discharge with the presence of a lump is worrisome because it can represent a ductal cancer. This condition demands further investigation, such as mammogram, ductogram, or biopsy.

Infection

Any residual masses in the breast after antibiotic therapy are suspicious for malignancy and require biopsy.

Does the person have additional risk factors for breast cancer?

Key Questions

- Have you ever had breast cancer?
- Do you have a family history of breast cancer (i.e., first-degree relative)?
- Have you ever had ovarian, endometrial, colon, or thyroid cancer?
- Do you have a family history of ovarian, endometrial, colon, or prostate cancer?
- Have you ever received radiation to the chest or had a malignancy in childhood?

Risk Factors

The presence of risk factors in a woman who has a lump raises the index of suspicion for malignancy. It is important to remember that the absence of such risk factors is not cancer protective. About 70% to 80% of all breast cancer patients have no risk factors for malignancy before their diagnosis. Patients with a personal history of epithelial hyperplasia, ductal carcinoma in situ (DCIS), or lobular carcinoma in situ (LCIS) are usually evaluated every 6 months by a breast specialist because of their increased risk for malignancy. Malignant breast tumors in adolescents are more likely to be metastasis than a primary tumor. Hodgkin lymphoma, rhabdomyosarcoma, or neuroblastoma could be the primary tumor. A history of chest wall irradiation is a risk factor. See Box 5-1 for a summary of characteristics that could increase a woman's risk for breast cancer.

Is this condition more likely to be benign?

Key Questions

- How old are you?
- Do you have a history of cystic breast changes or lumpy breasts?
- Does this lump feel like other lumps you have had?
- Do the lumps change with your periods?
- Have you ever had a mammogram or ultrasound? Why was it done? What were the results?
- Have you ever had a lump drained or biopsied? What was the diagnosis?
- Do you have breast implants?

Box 5-1   **Primary Risk Factors for Breast Cancer**

Female Gender

Age
75% of all cases occur after age 50; no plateau effect with age

Personal History of Breast Cancer or Cancer In Situ
DCIS is a precursor of cancer and increases the risk for invasive breast cancer, usually in the same breast

Previous History of Breast Biopsies for Non-malignant Breast Disease
Biopsy-proved proliferative changes or atypical epithelial hyperplasia; fibrocystic histological findings that indicate increased risk of breast cancer are moderate or severe hyperplasia (1.5-2 times the risk), atypical hyperplasia (5 times the risk), and lobular carcinoma in situ (8-10 times the risk); LCIS is a marker for cancer rather than a precursor; the cancer may occur in either breast

Laboratory Evidence of Specific Genetic Mutation
Increases susceptibility to breast cancer (i.e., mutation in BRCA1 or BRCA2 gene)

Personal History of Cancer
Ovarian, endometrial, colon, or thyroid cancers

Family History of Breast Cancer
In first-degree relatives (mother, sister, or daughter) or in two or more close relatives

Age

Fibrocystic breast changes occur predominantly between the ages of 20 and 30. Fibroadenomas are more frequent in women ages 15 to 39. Intraductal papilloma and ductal ectasia occur in the age range of 35 to 55 years, whereas breast carcinoma is most prevalent in women age 40 to 70 years. Any woman older than 25 years who has a breast lump should be evaluated by CBE, diagnostic mammography, and/or ultrasound. Magnetic resonance imaging (MRI) sometimes can be used in addition to mammography and ultrasound. Additional evaluation with tissue biopsy may be required.

Timing, Consistency, and Duration

The most frequent breast complaint is that of a painful, mobile lump that increases in size and tenderness as the menstrual cycle approaches. The lump commonly has discrete borders that allow for measurement of the length, width, and depth of the lesion by the patient (e.g., size of a pea). The lump remains prominent on breast self-examination, is almost always painful to palpate, and frequently causes pain with changes in position of the arm on the affected side. Fibrocystic breast changes exist on a continuum that corresponds with the menstrual cycle. Tenderness and size variations occur throughout the month.

Previous Mammograms or Biopsies

History or documentation of cyclic changes in lumps or the presence of glandular breast tissue on a mammogram or ultrasound supports a clinical diagnosis of benign disease. More convincing evidence of benign disease occurs when there is a clear fluid aspirate from the cyst with no residual or recurring breast lump, with the caveat that benign disease and malignant disease can occur simultaneously.

Breast Implants

With a ruptured implant, augmented breast tissue is pushed away from the chest wall by the implant.

Could this lump be mastitis related to lactation?

Key Questions
- Have you recently had a baby?
- Are you currently breastfeeding or breast suckling?
- Are your nipples sore or cracked?
- Have you had pierced nipples?
- Is your breast painful or hot? Are there any areas of redness?
- Have you had a fever?

Childbirth

Engorgement or congestive mastitis begins on day 2 or 3 after delivery and affects both breasts. A breast mass in a lactating woman is usually associated with mastitis, an inflammation of breast tissue, and a blocked duct. It occurs most often in primiparous nursing mothers and is usually caused by coagulase-positive *Staphylococcus aureus*. It can also occur during periods of weaning when the flow of milk is disrupted. Inflammatory breast cancer in lactating women is rare but must be considered.

Sore, Cracked, or Pierced Nipples

Cracked or pierced nipples can be a site for the introduction of infection.

Painful or Hot Breast

Mastitis is characterized by a breast that is painful, hot, and red. In lactating women, the most frequent symptom is a painful erythematous lobule in an outer quadrant of the breast. Although mastitis is most common in lactating women, it can also occur in nonlactating women, usually as the result of a generalized dermatitis occurring from insect bites, sunburn, or allergic reactions. However, the most common cause of an inflamed breast in nonlactating women is inflammatory breast cancer. In inflammatory breast cancer, the entire breast is swollen, heavy, and edematous.

Fever

Fever is a sign of infectious mastitis and occurs most often in association with lactation and breastfeeding. High fever does not occur because of simple breast engorgement in the postpartum period. Also, fever does not usually occur in inflammatory breast cancer and is rare in dermatitis reactions.

DIAGNOSTIC REASONING: FOCUSED HISTORY FOR NIPPLE DISCHARGE

A focused history can help sort out the causes of the most frequently presenting cases of nipple discharge. Questioning should address normal lactation, high circulating levels of prolactin, and malignancy.

Is this normal lactation?

Key Questions

- When was your last normal menstrual period? How frequent are your cycles?
- Is it possible that you are pregnant? What are you using for birth control?
- When was your last delivery or miscarriage? How long were you pregnant?
- Did you breastfeed? For how long? When did you stop?
- Is the nipple discharge clear or milky?
- How long have you had the nipple discharge?

Menstrual Cycle

Frequently, fibrocystic breast changes are most marked just before menses and manifest as a spontaneous multiple duct discharge that can be either unilateral or bilateral.

Pregnancy and Lactation

Pregnancy is the most common cause of breast tenderness and clear or milky nipple discharge (galactorrhea). A bloody nipple discharge during pregnancy is usually the result of vascular engorgement and clears within weeks. Recent pregnancy and/or breastfeeding (within 8 weeks) can account for a prolonged clear or milky discharge that is successfully suppressed by decreased breast stimulation or by the administration of dopamine agonist therapy (bromocriptine or pergolide). If the patient has had prolonged lactation, there can be milk formation even though prolactin levels are normal.

Color of Discharge

Normal lactation produces a discharge that is milky and nonpurulent. Mastitis associated with breastfeeding can produce purulent discharge. A subareolar abscess can also produce a purulent discharge. Mastitis and abscesses that produce purulent nipple discharge must be distinguished from inflammatory breast cancer by biopsy or by evoking remission with antibiotic therapy.

Oral contraceptives can cause a clear, serous, or milky discharge from single or multiple ducts. Ductal ectasia and papillomatosis can produce a greenish or brownish nipple discharge. A serous or serosanguineous discharge from a single duct is usually indicative of an intraductal papilloma, but can be from an intraductal cancer. A bloody nipple discharge can occur with benign or cancerous conditions.

Duration of Discharge

Women who breastfeed sometimes experience a milky discharge long after the termination of nursing. New-onset discharge in a woman who is not pregnant or lactating requires further investigation.

Is the discharge related to high prolactin levels?

Key Questions

- What medications are you taking?
- Do you jog or run? If yes: Do you wear a sports bra? Do your nipples rub on your clothing?
- Are your breasts fondled, squeezed, or suckled during sexual activity?
- Do you have a thyroid condition?
- What medical conditions or health problems do you have?
- If a newborn: Has the discharge been present since birth?

Medicines

Patients taking multiple tranquilizing medications are often found to have nipple discharge. Discontinuation of the medication(s) usually eliminates most clear or milky bilateral nipple discharge. However, the condition might not warrant a drug cessation trial. See Box 5-2 for medications that can produce nipple discharge.

Box 5-2	**Drugs that Can Produce Nipple Discharge**

Estrogens or Drugs That Increase Estrogen
Digitalis
Marijuana
Heroin

Dopamine Receptor Blockers
Phenothiazines
Haloperidol
Metoclopramide
Isoniazid

CNS Dopamine Depleters
Tricyclic antidepressants
Reserpine
Methyldopa
Cimetidine
Benzodiazepines

Behavioral Activities

Nipple stimulation (sexual or during jogging) increases prolactin levels, as does the use of marijuana. Only about 13% of men with hyperprolactinemia will develop gynecomastia and galactorrhea. Women with increased prolactin levels commonly experience both galactorrhea and amenorrhea.

Other Causes of Galactorrhea

Certain genetic disorders, medical conditions, and central nervous system (CNS) lesions can be responsible for galactorrhea.

- Genetic disorders: Chiari-Frommel syndrome, Argonzdel Castillo (Forbes-Albright) syndrome
- Medical conditions: chronic renal failure, sarcoidosis, Schüller-Christian disease, Cushing disease, hepatic cirrhosis, hypothyroidism
- CNS lesions: pituitary adenoma, empty sella, hypothalamic tumor, head trauma

Newborn

The breasts of a newborn can be abnormally enlarged secondary to the effects of maternal estrogens. A discharge that is usually white can be present and is commonly referred to as witch's milk.

> ### Can the nipple discharge be a sign of malignancy?

Key Questions

- Is the nipple discharge spontaneous or must it be expressed?
- Does it come from one or both nipples?
- Does it come from one or multiple nipple ducts?
- Do you also have a breast lump?
- Are you postmenopausal?

Spontaneous Versus Expressed Discharge

Spontaneous discharge is more concerning than expressed discharge. Bilateral spontaneous discharge is likely related to lactation or systemic causes (e.g., hyperprolactinemia). Unilateral spontaneous discharge is associated with intraductal papilloma or cancer.

Unilateral Versus Bilateral Discharge

Unilateral discharge is usually associated with an intraductal papilloma or cancer. Bilateral breast findings seldom represent cancer.

Single-Duct Versus Multiple-Duct Discharge

Single-duct involvement is more suspicious for intraductal papilloma or cancer. Multiple-duct discharges usually are caused by hyperprolactinemia or duct ectasia.

Associated Mass

An associated mass could be benign or malignant. Further evaluation is mandatory. Ultrasonography is helpful in differentiating solid from cystic lesions and is often the first step in the evaluation of a cyst or a mass in the woman with firm, dense breast tissue.

Postmenopausal

Postmenopausal women have a higher incidence of breast cancer. Other risky signs for a cancerous cause of nipple discharge are presence of a mass or lump, unilateral nipple discharge, abnormal cytology, and an abnormal mammogram.

Nipple discharge that is spontaneous, unilateral, and from a single duct is suspicious for a cancerous etiology.

DIAGNOSTIC REASONING: FOCUSED PHYSICAL EXAMINATION

Perform a multiposition physical examination of the breasts and nipples. See the Evidence-Based Practice box on the effectiveness of CBE.

Inspect Breasts and Nipples

Inspect the breasts while the patient is sitting with her arms at her sides, arms pushing down on hips (to contract the pectoralis muscles), and arms elevated above head and while the patient is bending forward from the waist (gravity pulling on breast tissue). Look for changes in breast shape or contour, a lump, or dimpling. Contraction of underlying muscles in the different arm positions will accentuate skin findings caused by a fixed adherent lesion, characteristic of cancer. Look for breasts that are notably asymmetrical. The skin over the lesion could then flatten or dimple inward, or the nipple could be directed differently than the nipple of the opposite breast. Normal nipples are everted and point in like directions. Lifelong inversion, either unilateral or bilateral, is also normal, but a new inversion is suspicious. Engorgement (congestive mastitis) involves both breasts, which are enlarged and tense. Infectious mastitis usually involves one lobe or a quadrant of one breast.

EVIDENCE-BASED PRACTICE   *Effectiveness of Clinical Breast Examination in Detecting Breast Cancer*

In a systematic review of the literature, Barton et al. (1999) found that randomized clinical trials demonstrated reduced breast cancer death rates in women screened by both CBE and mammography. Evidence of the effectiveness of CBE alone was less direct. CBE alone detected from 3% to 45% of diagnosed breast cancers that screening mammography missed. The precision of CBE was difficult to determine because of the lack of consistent and standardized examination techniques. The authors estimated CBE sensitivity at 54% and specificity at 94%. The likelihood ratio of a positive CBE result was 10.6 (95% confidence interval [CI], 5.8 to 19.2), whereas the likelihood ratio of a negative test result was 0.47 (95% CI, 0.40 to 0.56). Longer duration of CBE and a higher number of specific techniques used were associated with greater accuracy. The value of inspection was not proved. The authors concluded that indirect evidence supports the effectiveness of CBE in screening for breast cancer. Although the screening clinical examination by itself does not rule out disease, the high specificity of certain abnormal findings greatly increases the probability of breast cancer. The authors' bottom line for the CBE procedure: position the patient properly; use a vertical-strip pattern to cover all breast tissue; make circular motions with the pads of the middle three fingers and examine each breast area with three different pressures; and spend at least 3 minutes per breast.

Data from Barton MB, Harris R, Fletcher SW: Does this patient have breast cancer? The screening clinical breast examination: should it be done? How? *JAMA* 282:1270, 1999.

Observe Skin of Breasts and Nipples

Observe skin color for erythema and unilateral prominent blood vessels, which may be a presentation of breast cancer. Prominent vessels plus a tender cordlike vein suggest thrombophlebitis of the superficial veins of the breast. Both conditions require a CBE and a mammogram to look for a mass. Paget disease begins as a scaling eczematoid area on the nipple and progresses to a deep lump behind the nipple well. Paget disease can produce darkly pigmented lesions that are suspicious for malignant melanoma. An excisional or punch biopsy is recommended to distinguish Paget disease from malignant melanoma or other ulcerative lesions like Bowen disease, eczema, or papillomatosis. Observe the condition of the skin of the nipples for cracks or dried exudate or the presence of nipple flattening or retraction.

Palpate Breasts with Patient Sitting

Place the palm of your right hand at the patient's right clavicle at the sternum. Sweep downward from the clavicle to the nipple, feeling for superficial lumps. Repeat the sweep until you have covered the entire right chest wall. Repeat the procedure using your left hand for the left chest wall.

Perform bimanual digital palpation. Place one hand, palmar surface facing up, under the patient's right breast. Position your hand so that it acts as a flat surface against which to compress the breast tissue. With the fingers of the other hand walk across the breast mound, feeling for lumps as you compress the tissue between your fingers and your flat hand. Repeat the procedure for the other breast.

If the woman has augmentation of breast tissue, small masses, including those from ruptured implants, can best be felt with the patient in the sitting position.

Palpate Lymph Nodes

Palpate the supraclavicular, infraclavicular, and axillary lymph nodes (Figures 5-1 and 5-2). The supraclavicular lymph nodes can be accessed by having the patient shrug her shoulders; then feel deep in the supraclavicular hollow. Feel for lymph nodes, noting their size, shape, consistency, and mobility. The presence of a small (<1 cm), single, rubbery, and mobile lymph node can be a sign of inflammation: rarely is it a sign of early malignancy. On the other hand, finding one or more lymph nodes in the same region that are greater than 1 cm, firm, fixed to the chest wall, or of a matted consistency is highly suggestive of metastatic disease.

Palpate Breasts and Nipples with Patient Supine

With the patient supine, ask her to position one arm above her head. Place a small towel behind the scapula to aid in flattening the breast tissue. Palpate all areas of breast tissue, feeling for lumps or nodules. Remember that the breast tissue extends from the second or third rib to the sixth or seventh rib, and from the sternal margin to the midaxillary line. It is essential to include the tail of Spence in palpation. Recall that the greatest amount of glandular tissue lies in the upper outer quadrant of the breast with tissue extending from this quadrant into the axilla to form the tail of Spence.

Palpate using your finger pads because they are more sensitive than your fingertips. Palpate systematically,

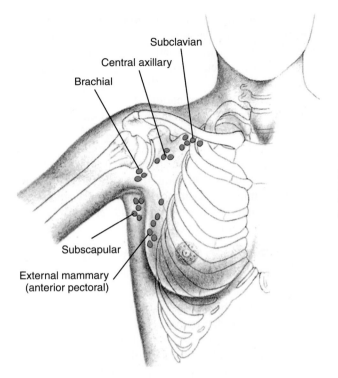

Subclavian

Central axillary

Brachial

Subscapular

External mammary
(anterior pectoral)

FIGURE 5-1 Five groups of lymph nodes accessible to palpation. (From Seidel HM, Ball JE, Dains JE, Flynn JA, Solomon BS, Stewart RW: *Mosby's guide to physical examination,* ed 7, St Louis, 2011, Mosby.)

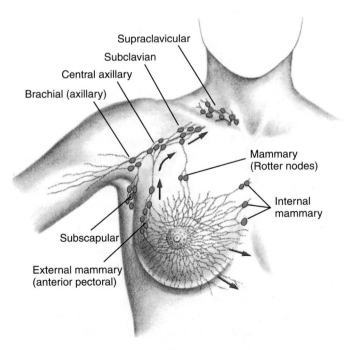

Supraclavicular

Subclavian

Central axillary

Brachial (axillary)

Mammary
(Rotter nodes)

Internal
mammary

Subscapular

External mammary
(anterior pectoral)

FIGURE 5-2 Lymphatic drainage of the breast. (From Seidel HM, Ball JW, Dains JE, Flynn JA, Solomon BS, Stewart RW: *Mosby's guide to physical examination,* ed 7, St Louis, 2011, Mosby.)

pushing gently but firmly, toward the chest with your fingers rotating in a clockwise or counterclockwise pattern. At each point press inward, using three depths of palpation: light, then medium, and finally deep palpation. Strip, concentric circle, or wedge methods are commonly used for ensuring palpation of the entire breast. Any method is acceptable, as long as every part of the breast is palpated. Regardless of the method, glide your fingers from one point to the next. Avoid lifting your fingers off the breast tissue because doing so makes it easy to miss tissue.

Assess Nipple Well

At the completion of the examination return to the nipple and with two fingers gently depress the tissue inward into the well behind the areola. Your fingers and tissue should move easily inward. A normal nipple well is a smooth concave structure. Most lumps in this area are found at the areola border. Repeat with the other breast.

Examine Nipple for Discharge

Palpate for discharge only if the patient presents with a report of nipple discharge. Place the thumb and first finger 1 to 2 cm outside the border of the areolar complex and gently compress, sliding the fingers toward the nipple in a milking fashion. Repeat this maneuver twice, cephalocaudally and laterally. Determine if the discharge is unilateral or bilateral. Look closely to determine if the discharge is from a single duct or multiple ducts. Palpation of a single site on the areola border may reproduce the discharge and reveal the responsible duct. Specimen collection is often easier and of a larger quantity when the patient is sitting.

Inflammatory symptoms and a purulent nipple discharge are suggestive of a breast abscess.

Transilluminate Breast Masses

Transillumination of a breast mass (best performed in a darkened room) sometimes provides diagnostic clues. A fluid-filled cyst will transilluminate whereas a solid mass will not. A solid lump is more frequently a malignant mass, whereas a cystic, fluid-filled lump is more commonly benign.

Characterize Lumps

Accurately measure any lumps by marking the edges with a pen and measuring the width and length with a centimeter ruler. Estimate the depth of the lesion, contour, shape, fluctuation, firmness, and mobility.

Fluctuation can be determined by holding the edges of the mass against the chest wall and pressing the center with finger pads. Fluctuation ("bouncy" consistency) occurs with cysts, lipomas, and abscesses. Cysts are frequently tender, especially premenstrually. Reexamination in 1 or 2 weeks will usually demonstrate cyclic hormonal changes of the tissue, and lump size and tenderness will have changed. In the postmenopausal woman, hormone replacement therapy can stimulate similar symptoms of breast lumps and pain (mastodynia). A single, firm, asymmetrical, immobile mass in a postmenopausal woman will, when biopsied, prove to be cancerous 75% of the time.

LABORATORY AND DIAGNOSTIC STUDIES

The diagnostic accuracy of ultrasound, mammography, and aspiration biopsy ranges from about 70% to 80% and varies with the training and skills of the clinician or technician. Therefore a high degree of suspicion for cancer and excellent patient followup should be sustained for a breast lump or nipple discharge.

Ultrasound

Ultrasound is helpful in differentiating solid from cystic lesions. In women under age 30 years ultrasound is often the first step in the evaluation of a cyst or a mass. The ultrasound finding of a cystic lesion can be followed by aspiration of the cyst, eliminating it to make sure it is not concealing another abnormal breast finding. The ultrasound identification of a solid mass can be followed by tissue biopsy.

Mammography

Screening mammography (conventional film or digital) is used to identify nonpalpable breast lesions. It consists of two views—craniocaudal (CC) and medial lateral oblique (MLO). In the presence of a palpable mass or nipple discharge, a diagnostic mammogram, which involves additional views, spot compression, and magnification views, is necessary.

Diagnostic mammography is used to identify palpable lumps or abnormal screening mammograms. It consists of additional views to clarify the features and location of palpable masses. Additional views could include spot compression, magnification, exaggerated CC to the medial or lateral side, tangential, and 90-degree lateral views. Mammography is of less diagnostic value in women younger than 30 years because of the density of the breast tissue.

Magnetic Resonance Imaging

Magnetic resonance imaging (MRI) is used primarily to evaluate abnormal areas that are seen on a mammogram and to assess breast implants for leaks or ruptures. MRI is sometimes useful in viewing breast abnormalities that can be felt but are not visible with mammography or ultrasound. It also can be used to image dense breast tissue, which is often found in younger women. Contrast is used to enhance the vascularity of malignant lesions. Although MRI is highly sensitive (85% to 100%), it lacks specificity. MRI is inferior to mammography in detecting in situ cancers and cancers smaller than 3 mm.

Fine-Needle Aspiration and Cytological Examination

Fine-needle aspiration (FNA) biopsy uses a small-gauge needle to obtain fluid and cellular material. FNA is a routinely performed office procedure that is both diagnostic and therapeutic. It immediately determines if the lump is a cyst or a solid tumor. The aspirate is sent for cytological evaluation to determine the presence or absence of malignant cells. If the aspirate is negative for cytology and the mass completely goes away and is not present on follow-up examinations, no further treatment is necessary.

Stereotactic or Needle Localization Biopsy

FNA can also be used with ultrasonography or stereotactic imaging to further assess and obtain adequate sampling in poorly defined palpable masses. The lesion is located, marked, and verified by imaging to assist in the identification of the tissue to be sampled.

Core-Needle Biopsy

Core-needle biopsy (CNB) uses a large-gauge needle to obtain several cores of tissue. It produces a larger tissue sample than FNA. It can be used in conjunction with ultrasonography or stereotactic imaging for small or difficult to palpate lesions. Local anesthesia is required.

Excisional Biopsy

Excisional biopsy is the gold standard for evaluating breast masses. It is performed in an operating room using local or general anesthetic, and the entire lesion is removed. Excisional biopsy is indicated if there is a large breast mass or for those lesions in which more conservative biopsy has produced equivocal results. The surgical specimen is evaluated histologically.

Microscopy

Microscopy of nipple discharge can reveal fat cells of galactorrhea, leukocytes of infection, or red blood cells. Care must be taken to prevent the slide from drying out. Place a coverslip on the slide immediately after obtaining the specimen and review the slide shortly after it is prepared.

Cytological Smear

A cytological specimen of discharge is placed directly from the nipple onto the slide, or, if there is only a small amount of discharge, it can easily be collected with a saline-saturated cotton-tipped applicator and spread onto the slide. The slide is then fixed in the same manner as a cervical specimen. This technique can expose cancerous cells. However, a negative smear is not conclusive, and additional work-up is mandated.

Ductography (Ductogram)

A ductogram is useful in evaluating the cause of nipple discharge. Contrast medium is injected by the radiologist into the discharging duct, and a mammogram is taken, which can show a filling defect (commonly an intraductal papilloma), a dilated or cystic appearance (duct ectasia or fibrocystic disease), or an abrupt obstruction (malignancy).

Serum Prolactin Level

Elevated serum prolactin levels can produce nipple discharge. Hyperprolactinemia should be suspected when the prolactin level exceeds 20 to 25 ng/mL. Prolactin elevation secondary to medications is generally less than 100 ng/mL. Prolactinomas are found when the prolactin level exceeds 150 ng/mL.

Thyroid Function Testing

Thyroid-stimulating hormone (TSH) is high in hypothyroidism. About 20% of patients with hyperprolactinemia have hypothyroidism. TSH testing is done to rule out primary hypothyroidism as a cause of the hyperprolactinemia and associated nipple discharge.

DIFFERENTIAL DIAGNOSIS
Single Breast Mass

Cancer

Breast cancer can occur at any time after puberty but it occurs more frequently with increasing age. Classically, breast cancer is a single lump that is hard, nontender, and immobile with borders that are not clearly delineated from the rest of the breast tissue. It occurs most commonly in the upper outer quadrant of the breast. Malignant tumors eventually affix to the skin, ligaments, or chest wall and cause retractions. Cancers infrequently cause pain or tenderness on palpation, but some do. The tumors continually increase in size (although at varying rates) and do not come and go. Other suspicious signs of cancer include nipple inversion, dimpling of the breast, bloody nipple discharge, and axillary lymphadenopathy. Occasionally, breast cancer presents as diffuse swelling, pain, or breast erythema. Unilateral breast pain in a postmenopausal woman is suggestive of cancer. A mammographic finding of a nonpalpable mass or preinvasive lesion associated with macrocalcifications could be the only evidence of a malignant breast mass. Benign lumps are usually smooth, round, and freely movable. However, colloid, medullary, and expansive intraductal cancers can feel like benign tumors.

Fifteen percent of women younger than 40 years who have breast cancer are diagnosed during pregnancy or the postpartum period. Pregnant and postpartum breast cancer patients make up about 2% of total breast cancer patients. The normal physiological changes of the breast tissue during these times necessitate a thorough history and physical examination. A breast lump during pregnancy or lactation is more difficult to sample for a biopsy because of the increased vascularity of the breasts. Additionally, the lactating breast can act as an ideal medium for bacterial infection and is slower to heal.

Cysts

Benign cysts occur with higher frequency than any other type of breast lump. They are typically round or elliptical, soft or fluctuant, and mobile. Cysts are not attached to the surrounding breast, nipple, or chest wall, so there is no dimpling of breast tissue or nipple retraction. There are often multiple cysts, frequently in the upper outer quadrants of each breast. Cysts vary in size throughout the menstrual cycle and are usually at their smallest and least tender stage at the end of menses (end of the secretory phase). Transillumination of a cyst allows light to pass through the lump and supports the clinical diagnosis.

Fibroadenoma

Fibroadenoma usually occurs as a single, nontender, rubbery, firm, ovoid, or lobulated mass that measures 1 to 5 cm in diameter. This lump is freely mobile; thus there is no dimpling or retractions. Fibroadenoma does not vary in size with the menstrual cycle. Fibroadenomas are multiple or bilateral about 25% of the time. They are the most commonly occurring breast mass in adolescence. Only biopsy can distinguish them from dysplasia, cancer, or cystosarcoma phyllodes.

Cystosarcoma phyllodes is a type of fibroadenoma in which the tumor grows rapidly and reaches a large size. Surgical removal of the tumor with a margin of normal breast tissue or simple mastectomy is sometimes necessary to prevent recurrence. The tumor is rarely malignant.

Abscess

Abscesses often follow systemic signs of mastitis. If mastitis is not treated early with antibiotics, it can progress to an abscess. A peripheral abscess is found more than 1 cm away from the areola and is usually caused by *S. aureus* or streptococcal organisms. A subareolar abscess is located in the nipple complex and can be associated with duct ectasia. Anaerobic organisms are the likely cause for subareolar abscesses. A chronic abscess can be encapsulated by fibrous tissue, causing the mass to be an irregularly shaped, firm mass that is nontender. An abscess should be incised and drained, and breastfeeding stopped.

Fat Necrosis

Fat necrosis occurs as the result of thickened and retracted scar tissue from an injury and subsequent hematoma. A biopsy alone can differentiate this single, fixed, often irregular tumor from carcinoma.

Lipoma

A lipoma is a fatty tumor of the breast with borders that are smooth and well-defined. The mass has a fluctuant consistency and is usually nontender and mobile.

Tuberculosis

Tuberculosis is an uncommon breast finding but should be considered, especially in immunocompromised patients. In early stages, tuberculosis can appear as a solitary, firm, irregular, nontender mass.

Ruptured Implant

With a ruptured implant, augmented breast tissue is pushed away from the chest wall by the implant. Masses found in these patients often are best palpated with the patient in the sitting position. The definitive diagnosis is made by mammogram, ultrasound, or magnetic resonance imaging.

Inflammatory Breast Mass
Mastitis and Acute Abscess

An acute abscess typically follows lactational mastitis. It is exquisitely tender on palpation and is very warm to the touch. The breast is erythematous and swollen, and the abscess usually involves only one fourth of the breast. The mass has a fluctuant consistency. Chills and fever can be present. Axillary lymphadenopathy suggests an abscess, but inflammatory breast cancer must be considered.

Inflammatory Breast Cancer

Inflammatory breast cancer presents similarly to acute mastitis but differs from mastitis in that the entire breast is swollen and fever is rarely present. Axillary lymphadenopathy can be present. Inflammatory breast cancer is a rapidly progressing disease; therefore close followup and prompt referral are necessary.

Multiple or Bilateral Breast Lumps
Fibrocystic Breast Changes

Fibrocystic breast changes usually present as multiple, bilateral painful masses, which frequently intensify premenstrually during the luteal phase of the menstrual cycle. The masses often rapidly fluctuate in size, are transient in appearance, and cause cyclic mastodynia (see Chapter 6). They occur most often in women ages 30 to 50 and are rare in postmenopausal women. Fibrocystic histological findings that indicate increased risk of breast cancer are atypical hyperplasia (5 times the risk) and lobular carcinoma in situ (8 to 10 times the risk).

Nipple Discharge
Intraductal Papilloma

Intraductal papillomas are the most common benign lesions to cause a bloody nipple discharge. They usually are unilateral, subareolar lesions occurring in perimenopausal women. Solitary papillomas do not increase breast cancer risk.

Duct Ectasia

Mammary duct ectasia occurs most frequently in menopausal women. The subareolar ducts become blocked with desquamating secretory epithelium, necrotic debris, and chronic inflammatory cells. This condition is frequently bilateral and is characterized by pain, tenderness, periods of inflammation, and a nipple discharge that is spontaneous, sticky, multicolored, and from multiple ducts. Nipple retraction can occur. There is no known association with malignancy.

Neonatal Discharge (Witch's Milk)

Newborns can have breast enlargement and a white nipple discharge secondary to maternal estrogens. This condition disappears within 1 to 2 weeks after birth.

Hyperprolactinemia

Hyperprolactinemia can cause nipple discharge in both men and women. The nipple discharge is usually bilateral, milky, and from multiple ducts. Additional symptoms include amenorrhea, decreased libido, or gynecomastia. Approximately 75% of women presenting with galactorrhea and amenorrhea have hyperprolactinemia. A prolactin-secreting tumor can produce additional symptoms, such as headaches and visual disturbances. Normal serum-fasting prolactin levels are generally less than 30 ng/mL. A prolactinoma is likely if the prolactin level is greater than 250 ng/mL and less likely if the level is less than 100 ng/mL.

Male Breast Disease
Acute Mastitis

Acute mastitis in males occurs from trauma (e.g., nipple chafing from jogging) and presents as previously discussed in the section on mastitis.

Cancer

Male breast cancer is extremely rare and represents about 1% of all breast cancers. It begins as a painless induration, retraction of the nipple, and an attached mass. It progresses to include lymphadenopathy and skin and chest wall lesions.

DIFFERENTIAL DIAGNOSIS OF *Common Causes of Breast Lumps and Nipple Discharge*

CONDITION	HISTORY	PHYSICAL FINDINGS	DIAGNOSTIC STUDIES
Single Breast Mass			
Cancer	Usually older than 35; unilateral new lump	Single, hard, nontender, fixed lump; borders irregular or not discrete; can be erythema dimpling, increased vessel patterns; can have nipple discharge	Diagnostic mammogram; ultrasound; tissue biopsy
Cysts	Younger age, often younger than 35; often multiple	Round or elliptical; soft or fluctuant; mobile	Clinical examination; FNA: clear aspirate; mammogram; ultrasound: cyst(s)
Fibroadenoma	Common in adolescence	Single, sharply circumscribed, mobile lump	Diagnostic mammogram; ultrasound; biopsy
Abscess	History of mastitis	Single mass; irregular shape; chronic abscess can be nontender	Biopsy
Fat necrosis	Can have history of injury at site	Single, fixed, and often irregular tumor	Biopsy
Lipoma	Can have others on arms, trunk, buttocks, or back; usually nontender	Single tumors; smooth, well-defined; fluctuant consistency	Biopsy
Tuberculosis	History of tuberculosis, positive PPD, or chest radiography; immunocompromised patient status	Single; irregular shape; nontender	Biopsy
Ruptured implant	History of augmentation; change in size or shape of breast	Nodule palpated best when patient is sitting	Diagnostic mammogram; ultrasound; MRI
Inflammatory Breast Mass			
Mastitis and acute abscess	Primigravidas more often than multigravidas; >1 wk after delivery; breastfeeding; tender nipples	Red, warm, tender; usually unilateral, one fourth of breast, or one lobule; breast engorgement; fever; nipple discharge: pus	Culture positive for *S. aureus, Escherichia coli, Streptococcus;* elevated WBC
Inflammatory breast cancer	History of mastitis or inflammatory process of breast	Entire breast swollen; fever rarely present; axillary lymphadenopathy	Biopsy
Multiple or Bilateral Breast Lumps			
Fibrocystic breast changes	Multiple breast lumps of both breasts; cyclic changes that worsen at time of menses	Bilateral nodularity, dominant lumps; tender, mobile	FNA; ultrasound; mammogram
Nipple Discharge			
Intraductal papilloma	Bloody nipple discharge; usual age is 40-50 yr	Unilateral, subareolar	Diagnostic mammogram; ultrasound; ductogram
Fibrocystic breast changes	Milky nipple discharge; cyclic changes that worsen at time of menses	Spontaneous, clear or milky, bilateral, multiduct nipple discharge; multiple breast lumps of both breasts	Diagnostic mammogram; ultrasound; ductogram

DIFFERENTIAL DIAGNOSIS OF *Common Causes of Breast Lumps and Nipple Discharge—cont'd*

CONDITION	HISTORY	PHYSICAL FINDINGS	DIAGNOSTIC STUDIES
Duct ectasia	Green nipple discharge	Greenish or brownish nipple discharge	Diagnostic mammogram; ductogram
Neonatal discharge (witch's milk)	Milky discharge 1-2 wk after birth	Enlarged breast tissue, milky discharge lasting 1-2 wk after birth	None
Hyperprolactinemia	Milky or clear nipple discharge; amenorrhea; history of medications: estrogenic, dopamine blockers, or dopamine depleters; hypothyroidism; pregnancy; postabortion; nipple stimulators; visual changes	Spontaneous, unilateral or bilateral, multiduct; clear or milky nipple discharge	Serum prolactin levels; TSH; MRI if indicated
Male Breast Disease Acute mastitis	History of clothing rubbing nipple (e.g., jogging); swelling or lump of chest wall; tenderness of site	Red, warm, tender; usually unilateral, one fourth of breast, or one lobule; breast engorgement; fever; nipple discharge/pus	Culture: positive for *S. aureus, E. coli, Streptococcus*; elevated WBC
Cancer	Family history of male breast cancer; painless lump of chest wall	Induration, retraction of nipple or mass in nipple well; fixed, nontender; lymphadenopathy	Mammogram; FNA; tissue biopsy

FNA, fine needle aspiration; *MRI,* magnetic resonance imaging; *PPD,* purified protein derivative (tuberculin), *TSH,* thyroid-stimulating hormone; *WBC,* white blood cell count.

REFERENCES AND READINGS

Apantaku LM: Breast cancer diagnosis and screening, *Am Fam Physician* 62:596, 2000.

Arca MJ, Caniano DA: Breast disorders in the adolescent patient, *Adolesc Med Clin* 15:473, 2004.

Ballesio L, Maggi C, Savelli S, Angeletti M, De Felice C, Meggiorini ML: Role of breast Magnetic Resonance Imaging (MRI) in patients with unilateral nipple discharge: preliminary study, *Radiol Med* 113:249, 2008.

Barton MB, Harris R, Fletcher SW: Does this patient have breast cancer? The screening clinical breast examination: should it be done? How? *JAMA* 282:1270, 1999.

Fallat M, Ignacio Jr R: Breast disorders in children and adolescents, *J Pediatr Adolesc Gynecol* 21:311, 2008.

Kerlikowske K, Smith-Bindman R, Ljung BM, Grady D: Evaluation of abnormal mammography results and palpable breast abnormalities, *Ann Intern Med* 139:274, 2003.

Klein S: Evaluation of palpable breast masses, *Am Fam Physician* 71:1731, 2005.

Parikh JCR: Appropriateness criteria® on palpable breast masses, *J Am Coll Radiol* 4:285, 2007.

Pena KS, Rosenfeld JA: Evaluation and treatment of galactorrhea, *Am Fam Physician* 63:1763, 2001.

Pruthi S: Detection and evaluation of a palpable breast mass, *Mayo Clin Proc* 76:641, 2001.

Santen R, Mansel R: Benign breast disorders, *N Engl J Med* 353:275, 2005.

Sickles E: Galactography and other imaging investigations of nipple discharge, *Lancet* 356:1622, 2000.

Templeman C, Hertweck SP: Breast disorders in the pediatric and adolescent patient, *Obstet Gynecol Clin North Am* 27:19, 2000.

Breast Pain

Nearly 70% of women experience breast pain (clinically known as mastalgia) during their lives; it is the most common breast-related complaint among women. Although a common problem in menstruating women, breast pain is less common in postmenopausal women. The pain can be mildly annoying or severe, and it can be periodic or nearly constant. Breast pain can occur in one or both breasts or in the underarm (axilla) region of the body.

Because of awareness about breast cancer, many women worry that breast pain indicates malignancy. The cause of breast pain is not known. Its relationship to the menstrual cycle and its occurrence in premenopausal women suggest a hormonal etiology. Breast pain is rarely associated with breast cancer and is usually related to fibrocystic changes in premenopausal women.

Breast pain associated with gynecomastia is seen in some young males. An abnormal ratio of estrogen to androgen causes the breast tissue to grow and become tender. It is also seen with Klinefelter syndrome, a sex chromosomal disorder (XXY) that occurs in males.

DIAGNOSTIC REASONING: FOCUSED HISTORY

Could age help explain the cause?

Key Question

- How old are you?

Breast tissue changes with age. Women under the age of 25 years have more stromal and lobular breast characteristics, and fibroadenomas are more frequently seen in this kind of tissue. Women ages 25 to 40 years are more likely to have cyclic mastalgia and nodularity. After age 40, women's breasts begin to involute and they are more likely to have cysts and duct ectasia. Women over the age of 50 years have an increased risk of breast cancer.

In adolescent males, an abnormal ratio of estrogen to androgens can occur, causing breast tissue to grow and become tender.

Is this cyclic or noncyclic mastalgia?

Key Questions

- Are you still menstruating?
- What is the relationship of the pain to your menstrual cycle?
- What is the pattern and severity of the pain?

Pre- or Postmenopausal
Cyclic mastalgia occurs premenopausally and is associated with the menstrual cycle. Postmenopausal pain is not cyclic.

Relationship to Menstrual Cycle/Severity
Cyclic mastalgia occurs in relation to the menstrual cycle. Typically it is most severe before the menses and goes away spontaneously with or after the menses. Premenstrual water retention in the breasts has also been proposed as a cause of breast pain.

What other characteristics of the pain will help me with a diagnosis?

Key Questions

- Can you describe the pain?
- Is the pain in one breast or both?
- Where in the breast(s) is it?
- Does the pain radiate?

Pain Description
Cyclic mastalgia is usually described as a heaviness most likely caused by hormonal changes that affect the breast tissue, resulting in edema and increased nodularity. Noncyclic mastalgia is described as sharp and burning.

Location and Radiation

Cyclic mastalgia is usually bilateral and poorly localized. Women often describe it as radiating to the axillae and arms. Noncyclic mastalgia is often unilateral and well localized.

Is the pain associated with a lump or discharge?

Key Questions

- Have you felt a lump?
- Do you have a history of cystic breast changes or lumpy breasts?
- Do the lumps come and go or change with your periods?
- Have you ever had a mammogram or ultrasound? Why was it done? What were the results?
- Have you ever had a lump drained or biopsied? What was the diagnosis?
- Do you have any nipple discharge?

Lumps

Noncyclic mastalgia is occasionally secondary to the presence of a fibroadenoma or cyst. Cysts that increase in size and tenderness as the menstrual cycle approaches can contribute to breast pain. Cyclic cysts of the breast are less common after menopause and necessitate diagnostic investigation. A postmenopausal woman with unilateral breast pain has a greater risk of a diagnosis of breast cancer.

Previous Mammograms or Biopsies

History or documentation of cyclic changes in lumps or the presence of cystic or glandular breast tissue on a mammogram or ultrasound supports a clinical diagnosis of benign disease.

What else could be causing the pain?

Key Questions

- When was your last period?
- Have you missed any periods?
- Could you be pregnant?
- Is your breast hot or red?
- Does the pain get worse with deep inspiration?
- What medications are you taking?
- Have you had any trauma to your chest?
- Have you had chicken pox?

Missed Periods/Pregnancy

Pregnancy is the most common cause of breast tenderness.

Hot or Red Breast

Mastitis is characterized by a breast that is painful, hot, and red. In lactating women, the most frequent symptom is a painful erythematous lobule in an outer quadrant of the breast. Although mastitis is most common in lactating women, it can also occur in nonlactating women, usually as the result of generalized dermatitis occurring from insect bites, sunburn, or allergic reactions. However, the most common cause of an inflamed breast in nonlactating women is inflammatory breast cancer. In inflammatory breast cancer, the entire breast can be swollen, heavy, and edematous.

Pain with Deep Inspiration

Pain with deep inspiration suggests a musculoskeletal etiology. Costochondritis especially affects the second and third ribs.

Medications

In postmenopausal women, hormone therapy can stimulate symptoms of breast lumps and pain. Many herbal products, especially ginseng and dong quai, can also cause some women to experience an onset of breast pain, as do soybean products or tofu. Women on liquid diet supplements that have a soy base can experience breast changes and discomfort.

Gynecomastia can occur as a result of such medications as corticosteroids, hormonal medications, diazepam, and illicit drugs.

Trauma to Chest

Chest trauma, whether by accident or from abuse, can cause breast pain. In female adolescents, breast pain has been linked to sexual abuse.

Chicken Pox

Persons who have had varicella infection are susceptible to reactivation of latent varicella-zoster virus (VZV) infection in dorsal root ganglia or cranial nerve ganglia.

Could the pain be related to another system?

Key Questions

- Have you ever had chest pain or shortness of breath?
- Have you had abdominal pain with this breast pain?

Chest Pain or Shortness of Breath

See Chapter 7 for a discussion of chest pain. It is important to rule out cardiac disease when assessing any type of chest pain, including breast pain. The most common cause of death in North American women is heart disease with atypical presenting symptoms.

Abdominal Pain

See Chapter 2 for a discussion of abdominal pain. Gallbladder disease and hiatal hernia can also refer pain to the breast region. These conditions must be ruled out when evaluating breast pain.

DIAGNOSTIC REASONING: FOCUSED PHYSICAL EXAMINATION
Perform a Breast Examination

Perform a multiposition physical examination of the breasts, nipples, and regional lymph nodes as described in Chapter 5. In the vast majority of women with breast pain, the physical examination is negative. In children, assess for breast development using the Tanner Sexual Maturity Rating (SMR) scale of breast development (see Chapter 4).

Characterize Lumps

If you find a mass on physical examination, determine its size, depth, contour, shape, fluctuation, firmness, and mobility. Fluctuation can be determined by holding the edges of the mass against the chest wall and pressing the center with finger pads. Fluctuation ("boucy" consistency) occurs with cysts, lipomas, and abscesses. Cysts are frequently tender, especially premenstrually. Reexamination in 1 or 2 weeks usually demonstrates cyclic hormonal changes of the tissue and change in lump size and tenderness.

Examine the Chest Wall

Palpate the intercostal spaces for costochondral margin tenderness and swelling. Palpation that reproduces the pain, especially affecting the second and third ribs, suggests costochondritis.

Skin

Look for the vesicular eruption along a single dermatome. Unilateral pain precedes the eruption of herpes zoster by 3-5 days (see Chapter 25).

Examine the Genital Area in the Male

Sexual maturation should be assessed by using the Tanner SMR scale (Figure 6-1). Boys with Klinefelter syndrome have sparse or absent pubic hair and small testes and penis. Testicular palpation should be performed to estimate the size of the testicles.

LABORATORY AND DIAGNOSTIC STUDIES
Urine for Human Chorionic Gonadotropin

Test the urine for human chorionic gonadotropin (β-hCG) to rule out pregnancy.

Mammography

In the absence of a mass on physical examination, women 40 years of age and older should have a screening mammogram unless one was obtained in the previous 10 to 12 months. The purpose of the mammogram is to look for concurrent breast pathology in women whose age places them at risk for breast cancer. Screening mammography (conventional film or digital) is used to identify nonpalpable breast lesions. It consists of two views: craniocaudal (CC) and medial lateral oblique (MLO). When the physical examination is normal, mammograms are not indicated in women younger than 30 years. In the vast majority of women with breast pain, mammography shows no evidence of breast pathology. If a mass is found on a screening mammogram, additional views and imaging can be ordered.

Ultrasound

If a mass is found on mammography, ultrasound is helpful in differentiating solid from cystic lesions. In women under age 30 years, ultrasound is often the first step in the evaluation of a cyst or a mass. The ultrasound finding of a cystic lesion can then be followed by aspiration of the cyst, eliminating it to make sure it is not concealing another abnormal breast finding. The ultrasound identification of a solid mass should be followed by tissue biopsy.

Fine-Needle Aspiration and Cytological Examination

Fine-needle aspiration (FNA) biopsy uses a small-gauge needle to obtain fluid and cellular material if a mass is present. It immediately determines if the lump

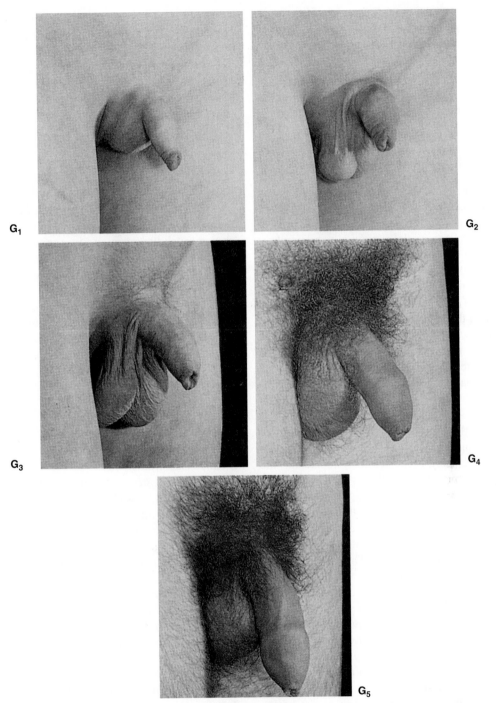

FIGURE 6-1 Tanner stages of penis, testes, and scrotal development in boys. (Photographs from Van Wieringen JC, Wafelbakker F, Verbrugge HP, DeHaas JH: *Growth diagrams 1965 Netherlands: Second National Survey on 0-24-year-olds,* Groningen, The Netherlands, 1971, Wolters-Noordhoff; reprinted with permission of Kluwer Academic Publishers.)

is a cyst or a solid tumor. The aspirate is sent for cytological evaluation to determine the presence or absence of malignant cells.

Karyotyping

Chromosomal testing determines the presence of the XXY chromosomal disorder or related chromosomal variants.

DIFFERENTIAL DIAGNOSIS
Cyclic Mastalgia

Cyclic mastalgia—pain that corresponds to changes in the menstrual cycle—is the most common type of breast pain and accounts for as much as two thirds of breast pain. Cyclic mastalgia is usually bilateral; is often greatest in the upper outer breast quadrant; and is described as dull, heavy, and aching, often radiating to the axilla and arm. The pain has a variable duration and is often relieved after the menses. Typically for several days preceding the menstrual flow, the breasts of these women enlarge, become lumpy and tender to touch, and produce a generalized aching. The nipples can become extremely sensitive and very uncomfortable. Cyclic mastalgia is usually bilateral and poorly localized. Compared with noncyclic mastalgia, cyclic mastalgia occurs more often in younger women.

Cyclic mastalgia is attributed to the fluctuations of hormones during the menstrual cycle. As the breasts prepare for pregnancy each month by increasing the number of milk-producing cells, as much as 15 to 30 mL of fluid can be stored in each breast. This fluid can cause breast enlargement and the possibility of tenderness and pain. Additional factors that contribute to cyclic mastalgia include caffeine intake, high-sodium diets, and high-fat diets. Thyroid conditions have also been shown to cause cyclic mastalgia.

Noncyclic Mastalgia

Noncyclic mastalgia is most common in women 40 to 50 years of age. It accounts for about one fourth of breast pain cases. The duration of symptoms tends to be shorter than that of cyclic mastalgia, and noncyclic mastalgia resolves spontaneously in 50% of cases. The pain is localized to a specific area in the breast and is described as sharp, stabbing, burning, and throbbing. Noncyclic mastalgia is occasionally secondary to the presence of a fibroadenoma or cyst, and the pain can be relieved by treatment of the underlying breast lesion.

Noncyclic mastalgia has no relationship to the menstrual cycle. It can be constant or intermittent with irregular exacerbations, and increased nodularity is often noted on physical examination. Cysts, fibroadenomas, duct ectasia, mastitis, breast injury, and breast abscesses have been associated with noncyclic mastalgia. Additional causes include referred pain from infected teeth, medication-induced pain, and musculoskeletal pain.

Mastitis/Abscess

Mastitis is inflammation and infection of the breast tissue characterized by sudden onset of swelling, tenderness, erythema, and heat, which is usually accompanied by chills, fever, and increased pulse rate. Most infections are staphylococcal, often *Staphylococcus aureus*. Mastitis is most common in lactating women after milk is established, usually the second to third week after delivery; however, it can occur at any time. Mastitis is not an indication to discontinue breastfeeding unless an abscess forms. An abscess presents as a large, hardened mass with a discharge of pus (suppuration) and an area of fluctuation, erythema, and heat. The underlying pus-filled abscess can impart a bluish tinge to the skin.

Mammary Duct Ectasia

Mammary duct ectasia occurs most frequently in menopausal women. The subareolar ducts become blocked with desquamating secretory epithelium, necrotic debris, and chronic inflammatory cells. This condition is frequently bilateral and is characterized by pain, tenderness, periods of inflammation, and a nipple discharge. Nipple retraction can occur. There is no known association with malignancy. Mammogram and ultrasound can show ectasia.

Pregnancy

Pregnancy is the most common cause of breast tenderness. Test the urine for ß-hCG to rule out pregnancy.

Costochondritis

A common musculoskeletal cause of breast pain is Tietze syndrome or costochondritis, which is inflammation of the cartilage of the ribs. This pain, which originates in the area of the sternum and the ribs, is localized close to the sternum and causes tenderness on palpation when moving the rib cage or when taking a deep breath.

Herpes Zoster (Shingles)

Herpes zoster is caused by reactivation of the VZV from a dorsal root ganglion to a cutaneous nerve and the adjacent skin. Herpes zoster eruption can occur in the chest area, producing breast pain. An area of erythema and pain can precede the development of grouped vesicles.

Klinefelter Syndrome

This sex chromosomal disorder (XXY) occurs in males and is characterized by gynecomastia and prepubertal testes. In some adolescent boys, the first sign of Klinefelter syndrome is breast pain and gynecomastia. Patients may lack secondary sexual characteristics because of a decrease in androgen production. This results in sparse facial, body, pubic, and axillary hair; a high-pitched voice; a female type of fat distribution, and small testes and penis. See Fig. 6-1 for Tanner SMR scale. By late puberty, 30% to 50% of boys with Klinefelter syndrome manifest gynecomastia, which is secondary to elevated estradiol levels and increased estradiol/testosterone ratio. The risk of developing breast carcinoma is at least 20 times higher than normal.

Breast Lumps/Nipple Discharge Associated with Breast Pain

See Chapter 5 for a discussion of breast lumps and nipple discharge.

DIFFERENTIAL DIAGNOSIS OF *Common Causes of Breast Pain*

CONDITION	HISTORY	PHYSICAL FINDINGS	DIAGNOSTIC STUDIES
Cyclic mastalgia	Corresponds to changes in menstrual cycle Bilateral; pain often greatest in upper, outer breast quadrant Dull, heavy, and aching pain; radiates to axilla and arm; varying duration	Often no physical findings; breasts can be tender	None; history and clinical examination
Noncyclic mastalgia	Women 40-50 years No relationship to menses Pain localized to specific area in breast; described as sharp, stabbing, burning, throbbing	Often no physical findings; breast can be more nodular; lump can be present	Mammogram; ultrasound
Mastitis/abscess	Sudden onset of swelling, tenderness, erythema, and heat, which is usually accompanied by chills, fever, and increased pulse rate Lactating women after milk is established, usually second to third week after delivery	Swelling, redness, tenderness Possible abscess formation with hardened mass, area of fluctuation, erythema, and heat Underlying pus-filled abscess can impart bluish tinge to skin	None; clinical examination
Mammary duct ectasia	Menopausal women Bilateral or unilateral pain, tenderness; periods of inflammation; nipple discharge	Often no physical findings Nipple retraction can occur; lump may be present	Mammogram; ultrasound
Pregnancy	Missed period; contraceptive use failure	Breast tenderness and swelling	Urine for β-hCG
Costochondritis	Pain in area of sternum and ribs; pain with deep inspiration	Tenderness on palpation, when moving rib cage, or when taking a deep breath	None; trial of NSAIDs
Herpes zoster	Pain; history of chicken pox	Vesicular eruption along a cutaneous dermatome	None

Continued

DIFFERENTIAL DIAGNOSIS OF *Common Causes of Breast Pain—cont'd*

CONDITION	HISTORY	PHYSICAL FINDINGS	DIAGNOSTIC STUDIES
Klinefelter syndrome	Adolescent boy with breast tenderness and enlargement	Testes prepubertal, gynecomastia, decreased body hair	Karyotyping
Breast lumps associated with breast pain	See Chapter 5 for discussion on breast lumps and nipple discharge.		

β-hCG, human chorionic gonadotropin; *NSAIDs,* nonsteroidal anti-inflammatory drugs.

REFERENCES AND READINGS

Amory JK, Anawalt BD, Paulsen CA, Bremner WJ: Klinefelter's syndrome, *Lancet* 356:333, 2000.

Duijm LE, Guit GL, Hendriks JH, Zaat JO, Mali WP: Value of breast imaging in women with painful breasts: observational follow up study, *BMJ* 317:1492, 1998.

Hamed H, Fentiman IS: Benign breast disease, *Int J Clin Pract* 55:461, 2001.

Johnson C: Benign breast disease, *Nurse Pract Forum* 10:137, 1999.

Morrow M: The evaluation of common breast problems, *Am Fam Physician* 61:2371, 2000.

Neinstein LS: Breast disease in adolescents and young women, *Pediatr Clin North Am* 46:607, 1999.

Padden DL: Mastalgia: evaluation and management, *Nurse Pract Forum* 11:213, 2000.

Santen R, Mansel R: Benign breast disorders, *N Engl J Med* 353:275, 2005.

Smith RL, Pruthi S, Fitzpatrick LA: Evaluation and management of breast pain, *Mayo Clin Proc* 79:353, 2004.

Templeman C, Hertweck SP: Breast disorders in the pediatric and adolescent patient, *Obstet Gynecol Clin North Am* 27:19, 2000.

Wright WL: Diagnosis and treatment of herpes zoster: role of the nurse practitioner, *J Am Acad Nurse Pract* 15:10, 2003.

7

Chest Pain

The first task in the evaluation of a patient with chest pain is to determine whether the pain is a life-threatening condition, such as ischemic heart disease, aortic dissection, or pulmonary embolism (PE). Myocardial ischemia and myocardial infarction (MI) are life-threatening causes of chest pain and must be assessed rapidly so emergent treatment can be initiated. Aortic dissection is a rare but equally catastrophic cardiovascular cause of chest pain that also must be diagnosed quickly. PE, which is also a life-threatening cause of acute chest pain, is accompanied by the sudden onset of dyspnea.

If acute ischemic heart disease is an unlikely cause, other causes of acute chest pain should be considered, such as pulmonary, gastrointestinal (GI), psychological, musculoskeletal, or other conditions (such as pericarditis). A significant proportion of patients whose presenting symptoms include acute chest pain have esophageal spasm or gastroesophageal reflux disease (GERD); however, harmless conditions can mimic more serious disease. Pericarditis and valvular diseases, such as aortic stenosis and mitral valve prolapse, are less emergent causes of cardiac pain.

Clue: A quick diagnosis of acute MI greatly increases the patient's chances of survival.

Pain in any organ or system can be the result of inflammation, obstruction/restriction, or distention/dilation. All pain arising from the GI, musculoskeletal, respiratory, cardiac, and pulmonary systems transmits to the same spinal cord segments—T1 through T5—and makes identification of the specific origin of discomfort difficult. Many causes of noncardiac chest pain relate to chest anatomy, specifically skin, muscles, ribs, cartilage, pleura, lungs, esophagus, mediastinum, and thoracic vertebrae.

In children, chest pain is rarely associated with serious organic disease. The most common causes of chest pain in children are costochondritis; trauma and muscle strain to the chest wall; and respiratory conditions associated with cough. Chest pain from cardiac disease is relatively rare in children. However, patients and families often associate chest pain with heart disease and can be anxious about the condition because of reports of sudden death in young athletes.

DIAGNOSTIC REASONING: FOCUSED HISTORY

The identification of potentially acute life-threatening situations must be made immediately. After you have determined that there is no immediate risk of severe oxygen deprivation to vital organs (e.g., MI, aortic dissection, and PE), proceed with a focused history (Table 7-1).

First, is this a life-threatening condition?

Key Questions
- Can you describe the pain? What does it feel like? (Dull, sore, stabbing, burning, squeezing?)
- When did it start?
- What were you doing when it started?
- How long have you had the pain?
- What other symptoms have you noticed?

Characteristics of Pain

Typical anginal pain is described as substernal heaviness, pressure, or a squeezing sensation that is provoked by exertion and relieved with rest or nitroglycerin. The substernal pain or discomfort radiates to the left shoulder and down the left arm and can extend to the neck and lower jaw. An abrupt tearing pain, located in the anterior or posterior chest, characterizes aortic dissection. It can migrate to the arms, abdomen, back, or legs. Patients with Marfan syndrome are at risk for aortic dissection.

Pneumonia, PE, and pneumothorax present with chest pain. The patient with PE is able to point to the area of pain over the affected lung and usually describes a gripping, stabbing pain that is moderate to severe in intensity. The pain can radiate to the neck or

Table 7-1	Differentiating Ischemic from Nonischemic Chest Pain	
FACTORS	**ISCHEMIC ORIGIN**	**NONISCHEMIC ORIGIN**
Character of pain	Constricting, squeezing, burning, heavy feeling	Dull or sharp pain
Location of pain	Substernal, midthoracic; radiates to arms, shoulders, neck, teeth, forearms, fingers; interscapular	Left submammary and hemothorax areas
Precipitating factors	With exercise, excitement, stress, after meals	Pain after exercise; provoked by specific body movements or deep breaths

Modified from Selzer A: *Principles and practices of clinical cardiology,* ed 2, Philadelphia, 1983, Saunders.

shoulders. Patients experiencing a pneumothorax most frequently report mild to severe chest pain of sudden onset located in the lateral thorax and radiating to the ipsilateral shoulder. The quality of pain is described as sharp or tearing. Chest pain of pneumonia is located over the area of infiltration and does not radiate. It frequently has a burning or stabbing quality and is associated with cough (see Chapter 10).

Remember that chest pain is subjective and that prior experience, personal attitudes, and cultural values form the patient's perception of pain. The severity of the chest pain is not an indication of the severity of the condition. Assessment of the severity of the pain is often made easier by the use of rating scales that use 1 to 10 or happy to sad faces (see Figure 2-1).

Onset of Pain

Onset. Determine if the onset of pain was sudden or gradual and what the patient's activity was at the time of onset. The typical onset of angina occurs during exercise, exertion, or emotional stress. It is relieved by rest or nitroglycerin. Chest pain of MI can occur at any time and is not relieved by rest or nitroglycerin. Sudden onset of chest pain and dyspnea is common with PE. In a pneumothorax, the patient usually reports that severe coughing, exertion, or straining suddenly precipitated the chest pain. Chest pain caused by pneumonia occurs gradually over several hours or days. Chest pain in adolescents that occurs after activity can indicate organic cardiac disease.

Most MIs occur in the morning hours, with a peak on Mondays. Patients might also report acute chest pain hours after heavy exertion, such as snow shoveling, sexual intercourse, or other physical activity.

In children, ask about recent choking episodes or swallowing a foreign body when the pain increases with attempts to swallow. Pain that usually occurs when lying down after eating is associated with GERD. Trauma to the chest wall from a fall or strenuous activity can cause rib fractures or chest contusions.

Duration. The most life-threatening conditions produce an acute onset of chest pain. The more chronic the pain, the less likely it is that a specific cause will be found. Intermittent chest pain that occurs frequently probably indicates a more serious problem, such as angina, than one episode of brief, mild pain.

Associated Symptoms

The person experiencing an acute MI frequently reports nausea, vomiting, diaphoresis, shortness of breath, and syncope. PE is often associated with shortness of breath, apprehension, hemoptysis, and chest pain that increases with deep breathing. Fever, cough, and thick sputum production usually accompany chest pain caused by pneumonia.

Does the patient have risk factors for coronary artery disease?

Key Questions

- How old are you?
- Do you smoke?
- Do you have high blood pressure, diabetes, or heart disease?
- Do you have a history of myocardial infarction?
- Has anyone in your family had a heart attack or stroke before the age of 60?

Risk Factors

According to the report of the U.S. Preventive Services Task Force, clinically significant coronary artery disease (CAD) is uncommon in men under 40 and premenopausal women, but risk increases with advancing age. The presence of risk factors, such as smoking, hypertension, diabetes, high cholesterol level, obesity, and family history of heart disease increases the risk of CAD. The National Cholesterol Education Program (2001) identifies the following major risk factors for CAD: cigarette smoking, hypertension, low high-density lipoprotein (HDL) cholesterol level (<40 mg/dL), a family history of premature coronary heart disease, and age (men 45 years and older; women 55 years and older). In addition, a lipoprotein panel after fasting should be obtained that includes low-density lipoprotein (LDL) (<100 mg/dL is optimal) and total cholesterol values (<200 mg/dL is desirable).

If this is not a life-threatening condition, what does a description of the pain tell me?

Key Questions

- Is the pain acute or chronic?
- What were you doing when the pain first occurred?
- Point to where the pain is located. Does it spread to any other part of your body?
- What seems to trigger the pain?
- Does the pain awaken you from sleep?

Acute or Chronic

After life-threatening causes of acute chest pain are ruled out, sudden-onset pain can be associated with trauma, musculoskeletal injury, or inflammation. Chronic, gradual-onset chest pain is rarely an emergent situation. Chest pain can be the sequelae to an upper respiratory tract infection. Pain from GERD often occurs at night or after a large meal.

Location and Character of Pain

Pain arising from the thoracic skin and other superficial tissues, such as that associated with furuncles, contusions, and abrasions, is sharply localized.

Irritation of the intercostal nerves can result in a neuritis that produces sudden onset of a stabbing, burning pain, and tenderness. The pain is easy to locate at the intercostal spaces and along inflamed nerves with three maximal pain points: adjacent to the vertebrae, in the axillary lines, and along the parasternal lines. Pain can be severe when the patient breathes deeply, coughs, or moves suddenly.

Dorsal root irritation associated with herpes zoster can present with intense burning or knifelike pain along the spine to the lateral thoracic wall and the anterior midline. This pain can restrict movement of the trunk and respirations. Generally this pain is continuous and increases in severity.

Nerve root pain is caused by mechanical irritation or edema of the nerve root. This pain can be felt at the point of irritation but is frequently referred to points along the peripheral course of the nerve. Thoracic spinal segment root pain is often referred to the lateral and anterior chest wall and is seen with spinal diseases and thoracic deformities.

Costal cartilage that loosens from the fibrous attachment most often causes localized dulling, aching pain and tenderness over the eighth, ninth, and tenth ribs on either side; however, the pain can be acute, paroxysmal, or stabbing.

Musculoskeletal pain is produced by irritation of tissues and transmitted through the sensory nerves. The stimulus travels through the nerve to the dorsal ganglion up the spinal afferent pathway to the central nervous system.

Bone pain results from irritation of sensory nerve endings in the periosteum and is intense and well localized. Chronic diseases affecting the bone marrow can cause a poorly localized pain of varying severity. Ribs are common sites for metastatic malignant deposits, probably because of their rich vascularity. When metastasis expands to the rib and involves the periosteum, pain results. Referred pain from a nerve dermatome is described as intense, aching, and boring.

When tumors involve the mediastinum, chronic aching or dull substernal chest pain is produced by pressure of the tumor against the spine or ribs.

Lung pain is caused by the involvement of adjacent structures. The trachea and large bronchus are innervated by the vagus nerve (cranial nerve X). The finer bronchi and lung parenchyma are free of pain innervation, and therefore extensive disease can occur in the periphery of the lungs without pain until the process extends to the parietal pleura. Pleural pain, or pleuritis, results from the loss of normal lubricating function and irritation of the serous membranes of the pleural surfaces. It is a constant, localized, cutting sensation that is accentuated with respiratory movement. Diaphragmatic pleural pain can be referred to the base of the neck or abdomen. Children often report chest pain from tachyarrhythmia because they are unable to differentiate between true pain and the unusual sensation of the arrhythmia. Cardiac causes of chest pain in children are usually associated with congenital anomalies or acquired diseases of the coronary artery, such as Kawasaki disease.

Sleep

Distinguish between awakening with pain and awakening from pain. Awakening because of pain signals a more serious problem of organic origin, such as cardiac ischemia. Psychogenic chest pain in adolescents commonly accompanies sleep disturbances.

What do associated symptoms tell me?

Key Questions

- Do you have a cough or a change in your usual cough?
- Do you bring up sputum? If so, how much and what color?
- Do you have a fever?
- Are you lightheaded or dizzy?
- Do you feel like your heart is racing?

Cough and Sputum Production

Chest pain associated with cough and colored sputum production is usually caused by an acute infection, such as pneumonia. Pain results from a pleural effusion or the collection of fluid in the pleural space. Sputum associated with pneumonia can be dark green, rust color, or red. Frequent lower respiratory tract infections can be caused by congenital heart disease with large left-to-right shunts and an increase in pulmonary blood flow. Children and older adults with persistent cough can experience chest pain related to the musculoskeletal strain associated with coughing. Asthmatic persons can develop chest pain from straining of the chest wall muscles caused by tachypnea, coughing, or retraction.

Fever

Fever can indicate pneumonia, myocarditis, or PE. It is possible that elderly and immunosuppressed persons will not have fever, even with bacterial infections.

Lightheadedness, Dizziness, or Fainting

Arrhythmias caused by hypoxia, trauma, or electrical shock can cause insufficient coronary blood flow and chest pain. Premature atrial tachycardia (PAT) can cause lightheadedness. Diastole is shortened in PAT, and thus cardiac output is decreased. Most cases of syncope in adults are caused by cardiac problems, such as structural heart disease, arrhythmias, and coronary insufficiency. Most cases of syncope in children are benign and are the result of breath holding, orthostatic syncope, hyperventilation, or vasosyncopal episodes.

Palpitations

Caffeine, stress, and hormonal changes can cause the sensation of a rapid or forceful heartbeat. Mitral valve prolapse can present with a history of palpitations.

Theophylline and ß-adrenergic agents can cause such arrhythmias as supraventricular tachycardia, which can be perceived as palpitations.

Is the pattern of pain related to activity and position change?

Key Questions

- Can you describe your recent physical activities?
- Have you had any injury to the chest?
- Does chest movement or position make the pain better or worse?

Recent Activities

Recent strenuous exercise (especially weight lifting) or horseplay can strain the pectoral, trapezius, latissimus dorsi, serratus anterior, and shoulder muscles. Rib fractures and musculoskeletal strains and contusions can cause significant chest pain, especially with movement. Musculoskeletal disorders are the most common cause of chest pain in children and younger adults.

Decreased exercise tolerance can result from significant heart disease, such as shunts, arrhythmias, or CAD. In children, congenital coronary anomalies can arise abnormally (as from the pulmonary artery), take an abnormal course, or have fistula connections to other structures, and thus result in exertional chest pain. Any episode of moderate to severe chest pain during or after exercise should be investigated as cardiac in origin.

History of Chest Trauma

A careful history of preceding activities should be obtained to detect any recent muscle strain. Posttraumatic pericardial effusion can develop 1 to 3 months after chest trauma. Blunt injury can cause hemothorax, pneumothorax, soft tissue injury, and rib fracture. A ruptured spleen can cause irritation of the phrenic nerve, producing shoulder pain.

Pain with Movement

Pain of cardiac origin, except for pericarditis, is not affected by respiration. Pain on inspiration suggests pleural etiology. A sharp, pleuritic pain relieved by sitting upright and leaning forward suggests pericarditis. Pain that is aggravated by chest wall movement, especially along the sternal border, is most frequently costochondritis; adults and children can experience this inflammatory condition of the costal cartilage. Lying flat, consuming alcohol, taking aspirin, eating spicy meals, and wearing tight clothing often precipitate the pain of esophagitis. Frequently, patients report that this pain occurs after lying down following eating a meal.

Is there a gastrointestinal origin for the patient's chest pain?

Key Questions

- Does the pain get better or worse from eating?
- Do you have blood in your stools?
- Have you vomited any blood?

Food Association

Differentiating between esophageal and cardiac origin of chest pain can present a challenge because the character and location of the pain can be very similar. Nitroglycerin can relieve both the pain of angina and the pain of esophagitis. In these instances, an electrocardiogram is indicated.

Esophagitis is the most frequent GI cause of chest pain. Patients describe this pain as "heartburn," or a dull, burning sensation in the epigastric and retrosternal area. The esophagus is more pain sensitive in its proximal portion. Therefore chest pain that is temporally related to eating meals or particular foods should suggest esophagitis.

Sometimes associated symptoms of a sour taste in the mouth and mild nausea are associated with esophagitis. An esophageal tear or spasm causes more acute, severe chest pain, described as a "tearing" or "crushing" sensation. Frequently the patient experiencing pain of GI origin reports mild to moderate chest pain occurring intermittently over days to months.

Peptic ulcer and cholecystitis can cause chest pain intermittently. Hematemesis (blood in the emesis) or hematochezia (blood in the stool) frequently accompanies peptic ulceration. Cholecystitis is frequently reported as right anterior chest pain that radiates to the shoulder or upper back.

Acute pancreatitis should be considered if the chest pain is excruciating and constant and is reported in the left upper quadrant of the abdomen radiating to the chest, shoulder, and arm. Pancreatitis is often accompanied by hypotension. Physical examination and diagnostic tests are necessary to differentiate it from chest pain of cardiovascular origin.

Could this pain be from a systemic cause?

Key Questions

- Do you have any skin problems?
- Do you have any chronic health problems?

Skin Symptoms

If the patient reports persistent unilateral chest pain of pruritic, burning, or stabbing quality, consider herpes zoster. This pain will follow the distribution of a cervical or thoracic nerve root. A vesicular rash in the area of pain is characteristic; this rash occurs several days after the occurrence of chest pain.

Systemic Conditions

Chest muscle pain can be caused by localized inflammation of the muscles in collagen diseases, such as polymyositis, fibromyalgia, or systemic lupus erythematosus. Arthritic inflammatory changes of the cervical and thoracic spine and shoulders can produce upper chest pain. This pain is aggravated by range of motion of the affected joints.

Sickle cell disease (SCD) can cause chest pain. In sickle cell anemia, the erythrocytes become rigid and "sickle," leading to capillary occlusion and sickle cell crisis. The heart increases the stroke volume to compensate for the anemia. The heart gradually dilates and heart failure ensues. Chest pain in a patient with SCD can also originate from acute coronary syndrome (ACS). In this condition, chest pain, fever, dyspnea, and cough are caused by infarction of lung tissue or an infectious agent.

Marfan syndrome is a hereditary connective tissue disease. Cardiovascular involvement occurs in more than 50% of persons by age 21. Mitral valve involvement is common, with auscultatory findings of mitral regurgitation and mitral valve prolapse. Marfan syndrome is associated with an increased risk of aortic dissection.

Kawasaki disease often has a long-term complication of CAD, coronary occlusion, or MI.

What does the family history tell me?

Key Questions

- Has anyone in your family had heart disease, chest pain, or sudden death from cardiac arrest?
- Was anyone in your family born with heart problems?
- Does anyone in your family have high cholesterol?

Family History

History of congenital heart disease in close relatives increases the chances of its occurrence in a child. When one child has the condition, the risk of siblings having the condition increases by one third. Essential hypertension and CAD show a strong family pattern. Hypertrophic cardiomyopathy has a positive family history with autosomal dominant transmission in one third of patients.

Children who have a homogenous family history of hypercholesterolemia can present with CAD before the age of 20.

What is the emotional state of the patient?

Key Questions

- In the past 6 months, have you had a spell or an attack in which you suddenly felt frightened, anxious, or very uneasy?
- In the past 6 months, have you had a spell or an attack in which for no apparent reason your heart suddenly began to race, you felt faint, or you could not catch your breath?

Panic Disorder

The two preceding questions can be a highly sensitive screen for panic disorder. A "yes" answer to either of these questions is a positive screen for panic disorder. Patients with anxiety or depression often describe feelings of chest heaviness or tightness that can last for days, unrelated to exertion or rest. Patients can also report difficulty taking a deep breath.

DIAGNOSTIC REASONING: FOCUSED PHYSICAL EXAMINATION

A focused physical examination of the patient experiencing chest pain will provide objective data for the assessment. A thorough examination of the cardiovascular, pulmonary, upper GI, and upper body musculoskeletal systems is essential.

Clue: The electrocardiogram (ECG) greatly improves the accuracy of the diagnosis of acute chest pain and should be obtained early in the assessment if cardiac causes are suspected.

Observe General Appearance

Initial observation of the patient will provide clues to the severity of the problem. Observe the patient for grimacing, diaphoresis, pallor, cyanosis, tachypnea, use of accessory muscles for breathing, splinting of chest wall, and unequal chest wall excursion. Persons experiencing an MI can be diaphoretic, pale, and anxious. Patients manifesting PE appear diaphoretic and anxious; respirations are rapid; splinting of the chest is common; and peripheral cyanosis can be present. Persons with fractured ribs or significant chest wall contusions splint their chest wall and take shallow breaths to avoid aggravating pain with respiratory expansion.

Observe the height and weight of a child. Abnormal findings for age can indicate chronic disease.

Measure Vital Signs and Respiratory Patterns

Vital signs for persons experiencing angina can be within normal ranges. Frequently, however, with acute MI, blood pressure is elevated and cardiac arrhythmias are present. If cardiogenic shock ensues, hypotension will occur.

The patient with aortic dissection can be hypotensive with unequal peripheral pulses. Pericarditis can be accompanied by fever, rapid and shallow respirations, and hypertension. Myocarditis can present with fever, respiratory distress, and paradoxical pulse.

In heart failure, decreased stroke volume reduces the systolic blood pressure and compensatory vasoconstriction maintains a constant diastolic pressure. This can result in a decreased pulse pressure.

Pneumothorax is manifested by tachypnea and unequal chest wall excursion. The patient with pneumonia can also be tachypneic, with signs of infection that include fever and a productive cough.

In children, chest pain with tachycardia and hypotension is generally caused by hypovolemia secondary to a hemothorax, hemopneumothorax, or vascular injury. Pain can also be caused by rhythm disturbance.

The rate, rhythm, and depth of respirations in patients experiencing costochondritis, GI disease, or herpes zoster are not usually altered.

Hyperventilation can cause chest pain as a result of hypercapnic alkalosis or coronary artery vasoconstriction. Most hyperventilation is associated with a stressful event or emotional upset; however, aspirin overdose, severe pain, and diabetic ketoacidosis can be organic causes.

Inspect the Skin

Cool, pale, moist skin can accompany an acute MI, PE, or aortic dissection. Observe the skin overlying the area of chest pain for signs of a vesicular rash of herpes zoster. Petechial rash on the face and shoulders can be a sign of protracted coughing as a result of pneumonia, asthma, or upper respiratory tract infection. Bruises can indicate trauma or abuse.

Sweat on the forehead of an infant can indicate congenital heart disease (CHD). A decrease in cardiac output causes a compensatory sympathetic overactivity, resulting in a cold sweat on the forehead. Examine the color of the mucous membranes, conjunctivae, soft palate, lips, and tongue for central cyanosis.

Palpate Trachea and Chest

Tracheal shift can occur with pneumothorax and, in children, with atelectasis involving a significant portion of one lung. To assess the trachea for lateral displacement, position your index finger first on the right side of the suprasternal notch and then the left. If the trachea has shifted to the side, you will feel the wall on one side but only soft tissue on the other. In a pneumothorax, the trachea is deviated to the opposite side during exhalation and toward the side of the pneumothorax during inspiration. The trachea is displaced toward a lung that is atelectatic, with the displacement exaggerated during inspiration.

Palpate the entire chest wall for tenderness, depressions, or bulges. Fractured ribs and contusions will result in tenderness to palpation and possible deformity. Palpate each costochondral and chondrosternal junction. Costochondritis will be manifested by pain with palpation over the cartilage between the sternum and the ribs. Palpation and range of joint motion can elicit arthritic pain in the shoulder or cervical spine. Musculoskeletal chest pain is usually reproduced with palpation or by moving the arms and chest through a variety of positions. Subcutaneous emphysema may be palpable at the neck or upper chest wall. Rib pain on palpation in children without a reported history of trauma can indicate child abuse.

To check the chest wall for symmetry, first test for diaphragmatic excursion of both the anterior and the posterior thorax between the eighth and tenth ribs. As the patient takes a deep breath, each hand should move the same distance from the spine. Pneumothorax, pneumonia, and fractured ribs can alter this finding.

Percuss the Chest

Percussion in the area of pneumothorax will result in a hyperresonant sound of an air-filled cavity. Areas of infiltration, as in pneumonia, will produce a dull or flat sound.

Auscultate Breath Sounds

Instruct the patient to breathe through the mouth slowly and deeply. Auscultate systematically from the lung apexes to the lower lobes anteriorly, posteriorly, and laterally (Table 7-2).

Auscultation of bronchial or bronchovesicular breath sounds over the peripheral lungs can indicate consolidation. If breath sounds are diminished over all lung fields, suspect chronic obstructive pulmonary disease (COPD). Obese patients can have breath sounds that are difficult to auscultate. Breath sounds will be inaudible in areas of pneumothorax.

Auscultate for Adventitious Sounds

Adventitious lung sounds are superimposed on normal sounds and can be auscultated over any area of the lung field during inspiration or expiration. Documentation of abnormal lung sounds should include the type of sound heard, location, and changes during both inspiration and expiration phases of respiration.

Crackles or rales are discontinuous popping sounds heard most often during inspiration. Any disease process that increases peripheral airway resistance, obstructs the peripheral airway, or causes a loss of elastic recoil will produce crackles. These indicate the presence of fluid, mucus, or pus in the smaller airways. Fine crackles are soft and high pitched. Medium crackles are louder and lower pitched. Crackles might be heard over the site of a PE.

Wheezing is frequently described as a whistling sound and can be heard during inspiration, expiration, or both. The sound is high pitched and musical. Wheezing indicates that there is fluid in the large airways, such as in severe heart failure; more often it is associated with bronchospasm, as seen in asthma. Wheezing occurs on exhalation because that is when

Table 7-2   Normal Breath Sounds

BREATH SOUND	LOCATION	QUALITY	INSPIRATION/EXPIRATION RATIO
Bronchial	Heard on chest over sternum and on back between scapulae	Loud, high pitched	Expiration longer than inspiration
Bronchovesicular	Heard over bronchi at first and second intercostal spaces anteriorly and between scapulae posteriorly	Loud, medium pitched	Equal inspiratory and expiratory phases
Vesicular	Heard over most of peripheral lung fields	Soft, low pitched	Inspiration longer than expiration

small airways collapse. During inhalation, the negative pressure in the chest tends to hold open the airways. However, during exhalation, positive pressure in the alveoli is conducted from the outside of the small airways and tends to collapse them. The sound is usually polyphonic; this means that multiple slightly different high-pitched sounds are heard at the same time. Most of the causes of wheezing affect many small airways at the same time; each one collapses at a slightly different time, creating a slightly different tone. The presence of a single-tone wheeze suggests a single area of blockage, such as with a foreign body. A prolonged expiratory phase of respiration is produced by intrathoracic airway obstruction associated with lower respiratory tract involvement.

Rhonchi are continuous, deep-pitched, coarse breath sounds usually heard during expiration. They are generated by turbulent air passing through secretions in large airways. Rhonchi can be present when the patient has pneumonia.

Pleural friction rub is a grating or squeaking sound heard in the lateral lung fields during inspiration and expiration. It indicates that inflamed parietal and visceral pleural linings are rubbing together.

If abnormal lung sounds are detected, additional auscultation for bronchophony, egophony, and whispered pectoriloquy are indicated (see Chapter 13).

Auscultate Heart Sounds

Auscultate for normal heart sounds in all positions, identifying S_1, S_2, rate, and rhythm. Identification of myocardial ischemia cannot be reliably performed by physical examination alone. An ECG must be obtained to assess electrical conduction and the condition of myocardial function. Abnormal sounds, such as paradoxical S_2 during pain, are a sign of coronary ischemia. A transient, paradoxical S_2 could indicate a transient left ventricular dysfunction, congestive heart failure, or left bundle-branch block. A transient S_3 (ventricular gallop) or mitral regurgitation murmur at the apex can occur occasionally with myocardial ischemia or congestive heart failure. An S_4 (atrial gallop) typically indicates a stressed heart, which can be the result of hypertension, MI, or CAD causing heart failure. A summation gallop is the result of an S_3, S_4, and rapid rate; this can also occur with heart failure. Abnormal rhythms, including tachycardia, bradycardia, and irregular rhythms, are often heard during MI. ECGs are necessary to identify the specific rhythm.

Also note any murmurs and their location, grade, and radiation. Incompetent heart valves produce murmurs and can be the cause of heart failure. In children, a loud murmur, best audible at the upper right sternal border or upper left sternal border with a thrill, can indicate a congenital heart defect.

Aortic diastolic murmur can be present with a dissecting aorta. In aortic valve stenosis, a harsh ejection systolic murmur with radiation to the neck is heard on auscultation.

Midsystolic click/late systolic murmur (honk) is heard with mitral valve prolapse. The patient must be examined in both the supine and upright positions to elicit the characteristic sounds.

Observe the Spine for Evidence of Scoliosis

Persons with scoliosis are at increased risk for pulmonary problems because of structural variations that can cause compression of intrathoracic contents.

Examine the Abdomen

Auscultate for bowel sounds. Palpate the abdomen for tenderness and masses. Epigastric pain with palpation can occur with esophagitis or peptic ulcer disease. Cholelithiasis or cholecystitis can be manifested by pain on palpation in the right upper quadrant. Pancreatitis can produce left upper quadrant tenderness.

Examine the Extremities

Clubbing of the fingers can be an indication of chronic hypoxia resulting from CHD in children or COPD in adults. Peripheral cyanosis indicates hypoxia if accompanied by central cyanosis. Consider exposure to a cold environment or anxiety if peripheral cyanosis is observed. Lower extremity edema is a sign of heart failure or venous stasis. Note the progression of the edema or whether there is pitting edema up the leg.

Absent peripheral pulse(s) can be a sign of atherosclerotic vessel disease or dissecting aortic aneurysm. Compare the quality of the pulses bilaterally.

LABORATORY AND DIAGNOSTIC STUDIES

Diagnostic tests are usually indicated when cardiovascular, pulmonary, or GI pathology is the suspected cause of chest pain. Musculoskeletal and neurological causes of pain usually do not require diagnostic tests.

Electrocardiogram

An ECG can add objective data to the diagnostic process in evaluating chest pain. ECGs are most valuable when there is a previous ECG with which to compare the findings or when serial ECGs are obtained. ST segment elevation or depression indicates the presence of injured myocardium. T wave inversion demonstrates the presence of ischemia. The appearance of both strongly supports ischemia but is not diagnostic of CAD. Arterial spasm, pericarditis, and electrolyte imbalance can also cause these variations from normal. Q waves are indicative of myocardial muscle loss but are not diagnostic of CAD.

Evidence of ischemia is not always obvious on an ECG even when the patient is reporting anginal pain.

Stress Testing

Persons experiencing intermittent chest pain who have a normal ECG and are not taking digoxin should have an exercise stress ECG for diagnostic and prognostic purposes. Treadmill exercise testing uses a standardized protocol of increasing workload with continuous ECG recording. Stress tests provide information on myocardial function determined by blood flow. An important objective of stress testing is to identify patients who have a high risk of severe (left main or three-vessel) CAD. The sensitivity of the test ranges from 65% to 70%.

Exercise Myocardial Perfusion Imaging

This imaging has greater accuracy than the standard treadmill test when the resting ECG is abnormal. Because of its higher sensitivity, the test is able to localize and characterize the extent of myocardial ischemia and to provide direct measurement of left ventricular function. This test is more costly than a treadmill test.

Cardiac Enzymes

Levels of creatinine kinase-MB (CK-MB) isoenzyme rise above normal within 4 hours after an MI and will peak at around 24 hours. The patient who has had an MI will have a CK-MB result that is five or more times the normal value. Cardiac troponins T and I are sensitive and specific markers of myocardial injury and are more predictive of future coronary events. Levels of cardiac troponins T and I are affected less than those of CK-MB in the first 12 hours following an acute MI, but the troponin levels remain elevated for 7 to 10 days after the cardiac event.

Echocardiography

An echocardiogram is a noninvasive test for examining the heart that provides information about the position, size, and movements of the valves and chambers as well as the velocity of blood flow by means of reflected ultrasound. This test is used to determine biological and prosthetic valve dysfunction and pericardial effusion, to evaluate velocity and direction of blood flow, to furnish direction for further diagnostic study, and to monitor patients with cardiac disease over an extended period.

Ventilation/Perfusion Lung Scan

With PE, the blood supply distal to the embolus is restricted. Imaging will show poor or no visualization of the affected area. The ventilation scan demonstrates movement or lack of movement of air in the lungs. The perfusion scan demonstrates blood supply to the affected area of the lungs. The ventilation/perfusion scan is reported as one of three categories: normal, high probability, and nondiagnostic. A normal scan is characterized by even distribution of the radiotracer throughout both lungs and rules out significant pulmonary emboli; no additional diagnostic tests are required. A high-probability scan is represented by multiple segmental or larger defects with normal ventilation in at least one area of abnormal perfusion. This is also known as a ventilation/perfusion mismatch. When a scan does not fit into either the normal or the high-probability category, the study is considered to be nondiagnostic and further investigation is required.

Pulmonary Angiography

A pulmonary angiogram (arteriogram) is necessary if an embolectomy is considered. Radiographic contrast medium is injected into the pulmonary arteries, and the vasculature is visualized. This test can detect emboli as small as 3 mm in diameter. The test sensitivity is 98%, and the specificity is 96%. This test is the gold standard for diagnosing PE, but it is expensive and carries a small risk of cardiac arrhythmias, anaphylaxis, and death.

Arterial Blood Gases

Arterial blood gases (ABGs) are obtained to detect respiratory alkalosis resulting from hyperventilation, decreased carbon dioxide pressure (Pco_2), and sometimes decreased oxygen pressure (Po_2) (hypoxemia). Hypoxemia often correlates with the extent of the lung area occluded in a PE.

Radiography

Pneumothorax and pneumonia can be identified by chest radiography. Pneumothorax reveals evidence of pleural air, whereas pneumonia is seen on radiographs as a parenchymal infiltrate. Chest radiography with suspected PE is usually nonspecific; it can be normal or an elevated hemidiaphragm or pulmonary infiltrate can be present. Rib radiographs will confirm rib fracture.

Cervical and thoracic spine and shoulder radiographs can show degenerative joint changes.

Computed Tomography Scanning

Computed tomography (CT) scans produce cross-sectional images of anatomical structures without superimposing tissues on each other. They show the different characteristics of tissue structures within solid organs. Aortic dissections and tumors of the lung and pancreas can be detected with CT scans.

Magnetic Resonance Imaging

Magnetic resonance imaging (MRI) is a noninvasive technique that produces cross-sectional images of the body through exposure to magnetic energy sources. It does not involve radiation and is used to differentiate healthy and diseased body tissues. It is useful in detecting tumors, infection sites, and diseased vessels.

Activated Partial Thromboplastin Time and Prothrombin Time

Activated partial thromboplastin time (aPTT) is a clotting test that screens for coagulation disorders and is used to monitor the effectiveness of heparin therapy. Prothrombin time (PT) measures a potential defect in stage II of the clotting mechanism through analysis of the clotting ability of five plasma coagulation factors. PTs are commonly ordered to measure the effects of oral anticoagulant therapies. Ineffective anticoagulation therapy places the patient at risk for PE. These tests can also be ordered to search for the cause of PE.

Serum Amylase and Lipase

Amylase is an enzyme that helps convert starch to sugar; it is produced in the pancreas, liver, salivary glands, and fallopian tubes. If there is inflammation of the pancreas or salivary glands, increased levels of amylase enter the bloodstream. Lipase is the enzyme responsible for the breakdown of fats to fatty acids and glycerol. The pancreas is the main source of lipase. Pancreatic damage results in elevated serum lipase levels. Therefore, determining the levels of serum amylase and lipase is useful in the diagnosis of pancreatitis. Amylase levels return to normal before lipase levels.

Abdominal Ultrasound

Abdominal ultrasound is a noninvasive procedure to visualize solid organs. It is useful in detecting masses, fluid collections, and infection. Pancreatitis and gallbladder disease can be detected with ultrasound.

Bronchoscopy

Bronchoscopy permits visualization of the trachea, bronchi, and select bronchioles. It is useful to diagnose tumors, hemorrhage, and trauma; to obtain brushings for cytological examinations; and to remove foreign bodies from the lower respiratory tract.

Complete Blood Count

A complete blood count (CBC) is obtained to detect an elevated white blood cell count that occurs with infection. Hemoglobin and hematocrit levels are useful if anemia is suspected as an underlying cause of chest pain.

Esophageal pH

When GERD is suspected, 24-hour esophageal pH monitoring is performed to document pathological acid reflux.

Endoscopy

Upper endoscopy with biopsy is necessary to document the type and extent of tissue damage in GERD. A normal endoscopy, however, does not rule out mild gastric reflux disease.

Erythrocyte Sedimentation Rate

The erythrocyte sedimentation rate value will be elevated with inflammation, such as in arthritis and pericarditis. The test is not specific for a particular disease.

DIFFERENTIAL DIAGNOSIS
Common Causes of Emergent Chest Pain
Acute Myocardial Infarction

Assessment of the patient experiencing acute chest pain must first focus on the potential diagnosis of myocardial infarction (MI) to facilitate prompt initiation of treatment to limit infarct size. The patient with an acute MI generally describes a sudden onset of pain at rest. It is a persistent, often severe, deep, central chest pain and can radiate, as does angina, to the throat or neck, across both sides of the chest to the shoulder, and/or down the medial aspect of either or both arms. Rest or nitroglycerin does not relieve the pain. The chest pain is often associated with shortness of breath, nausea, vomiting, and diaphoresis.

The quality of the pain or discomfort is generally more intense than any previously experienced anginal symptoms. Patients can also express a sense of impending doom. Quick review for positive risk factors (men age 45 years and older; women age 55 years and older; cigarette smoker; hyperlipidemia; hypertension; diabetes; obesity; history of CAD; family history of CAD) is useful. Objective evidence of an MI can include skin pallor, cool

diaphoretic skin, and transient paradoxical S_2. The patient can be hypertensive or hypotensive.

The patient with severe chest pain or a suspected MI should be placed on a cardiac monitor as soon as possible. Observe for premature ventricular contractions and classic electrocardiographic changes that indicate MI, including ST segment elevations, T wave inversions, and Q waves. Performing a 12-lead ECG and determining levels of cardiac isozymes will help confirm or rule out an MI.

Aortic Dissection

The patient often is in a great deal of distress, describing the unrelenting chest pain as ripping and tearing and radiating to the interscapular region, jaw, neck, or lower back. Physical examination reveals severe hypertension and unequal or absent peripheral pulses. Chest radiography demonstrates a wide mediastinum with extension of the aortic wall beyond the calcific border. A CT scan or MRI can be ordered, but aortography remains the gold standard. Patients with suspect aortic dissection should be referred for emergent care.

Acute Coronary Insufficiency

Acute coronary insufficiency refers to those situations in which chest pain is caused by lack of oxygen to the myocardium but there is no evidence of infarct. The patient reports severe, oppressive, constricting, retrosternal discomfort lasting longer than 30 minutes. The patient may report prior history of MI or angina. The ECG can show intermittent ischemic changes or be normal. Cardiac isozymes are normal.

Pulmonary Embolus

Patients presenting with PE usually report sudden onset of severe sharp, crushing, nonradiating chest pain if there is an embolus impacted in a major artery. Infarction of the pulmonary parenchyma closer to the pleural surface will cause pleuritic chest pain often accompanied by the sudden onset of dyspnea and hemoptysis. Patients frequently express feelings of impending doom.

A review of risk factors will likely reveal one or more of the following: older age, prior venous thromboembolism, prolonged immobility or paralysis, cancer, heart failure, other chronic disease, pelvic or lower extremity surgery, recent pregnancy or delivery, obesity, oral contraceptive use, or varicose veins. Physical findings include restlessness, tachycardia, tachypnea, fever, diminished breath sounds, crackles and/or wheezes, and possible pleural friction rub. There can be signs of thrombophlebitis of the extremities. Initial diagnostic tests should include chest radiograph and ECG; these can both be normal but if clinical signs still point to PE, referral for consultation and further tests, including ABGs, venous Doppler studies, ventilation/perfusion scans, and pulmonary angiography, are indicated.

Pneumothorax

Pneumothorax can be a life-threatening event, especially if the patient has underlying COPD or asthma. The patient reports sharp or tearing chest pain that can radiate to the ipsilateral shoulder. Sudden onset of shortness of breath is also associated with spontaneous pneumothorax. Objective findings include decreased or absent breath sounds on the affected side, tachycardia, tachypnea, and possible deviated trachea. A chest radiograph is needed to evaluate the possible complete or partial collapse of the lung.

Arrhythmias

Patients report palpitations and/or forceful heartbeats. These arrhythmias can be the result of myocardial ischemia, cocaine abuse, or such conditions as prolapsed mitral valve or anxiety. Syncope associated with palpitations indicates a more serious cardiac arrhythmia.

Congenital Coronary Anomalies

The coronary arteries can arise abnormally, take an abnormal course, or have fistulous connections to other structures, resulting in exertional chest pain that can lead to sudden death in the young athlete. The child or adolescent can have a history of moderate to severe chest pain during or after exercise. Risk factors include the following: family history of sudden death at an early age, heart disease, or seizures; history of light-headedness or loss of consciousness during exercise; and tall and lanky body type with double-jointedness. Referral to a pediatric cardiologist is warranted.

Common Causes of Nonemergent Chest Pain
Stable Angina

Stable angina refers to chest pain typically described as substernal chest pressure or heaviness, radiating to the left shoulder and arm, neck, or jaw. The pain onset is usually gradual, brought on and exacerbated by exercise and stress; it is associated with nausea, diaphoresis, and shortness of breath and is alleviated with rest and/or nitroglycerin. Pain typically lasts 2 to 10 minutes. Physical examination is usually normal. An S_4 gallop can be transiently present during an episode of pain. Tests for angina include performing an ECG during an episode of pain, which can show ST segment depression and T wave inversions, or the findings can be normal.

Myocarditis

Myocarditis is an inflammation of the myocardium and is commonly caused by viruses. The heart is unable to contract properly because the inflammatory process interferes with the contractile function of the myocardial cells and eventually leads to cell death. It is frequently accompanied by pericarditis. The chest pain is caused by ischemia or arrhythmia. Patients have fever and dyspnea and can have evidence of heart failure. Heart murmurs and friction rubs can be heard. Chest radiographs show cardiomegaly.

Pericarditis

The pain associated with pericarditis is described as sharp, located in the center of the chest, short-lived, episodic, and radiating to the back in the trapezial area. The pain is worse when the patient is supine and sitting, whereas leaning forward often reduces the intensity of the pain. Shallow breathing can be an associated symptom in an effort to avoid pain. Dyspnea can be present with compression of the bronchial tree by a large pericardial effusion. Risk factors for pericarditis include recent viral or bacterial infection, recent MI, uremia, myxedema, and history of autoimmune disease. Objective signs include fever before the onset of pain, tachycardia, and pericardial friction rub. The rub is pathognomonic for pericarditis but is found in only 60% to 70% of patients with pericarditis. Diagnostic tests show elevated white blood cells and erythrocyte sedimentation rate and diffuse ST segment elevation in the early stages. Chest radiography can be normal or show effusion with an increase in cardiac shadow.

Aortic Stenosis

Aortic stenosis can cause exertional chest pain. Associated symptoms include fatigue, palpitation, dyspnea on exertion (DOE), dizziness, and syncope. Physical examination will reveal a loud, harsh crescendo-decrescendo murmur best heard at the second right intercostal space with the patient leaning forward. The murmur can radiate to the neck and is often associated with a thrill. An echocardiogram will provide diagnostic evidence of aortic stenosis.

Mitral Regurgitation

Symptoms of mitral regurgitation are similar to those of aortic stenosis: they include exertional substernal chest pain, fatigue, palpitation, dizziness, DOE, and syncope. The murmur associated with mitral regurgitation is holosystolic and blowing and often is heard best at the apex in the left lateral position. The murmur decreases with inspiration and can radiate to the left axilla and occasionally to the back. Again, echocardiography will provide evidence of mitral regurgitation.

Pneumonia

Signs and symptoms of pneumonia include pleuritic chest pain; a productive, moist cough with dark sputum; shortness of breath; and fever and chills. Risk factors include ineffective cough reflex, inability to swallow, advanced age, or very young age. Auscultation of the lungs reveals diminished breath sounds over affected areas, and crackles and wheezes can be heard. Rales and rhonchi are frequently heard on auscultation of the lungs. Dullness with percussion is heard over areas of consolidation. Vocal fremitus is positive. In addition, physical findings can include tachycardia, tachypnea, bronchophony, and egophony. Chest radiography, sputum culture, and ABGs will further support the diagnosis of pneumonia. Follow-up chest radiographs are indicated after pneumonia because lung tumors can be hidden by pneumonia. The very young and very old are most often hospitalized for observation and treatment of pneumonia. Healthy adults are usually managed on an outpatient basis.

Mitral Valve Prolapse

Patients with chest pain from mitral valve prolapse report a range of symptoms, including arrhythmias, palpitations, and anxiety. Physical examination can be normal, or a midsystolic click can be heard over the apex while the patient is sitting or squatting. An echocardiogram will provide evidence of mitral valve prolapse.

Pleuritis

Pleuritic chest pain occurs suddenly and is worsened by deep breathing, coughing, and sneezing. Pleuritic chest pain can be a manifestation of pneumonia or can represent pleural inflammation, especially following a viral upper respiratory tract infection. Physical examination of the chest can be normal, or a pleural friction rub can be heard over the area of inflammation. The patient's respiration rate is normal, but respirations are often shallow or guarded. Unless pneumonia is suspected, no diagnostic tests are indicated because the cause of pleuritic chest pain is likely of viral etiology.

Esophagitis

Esophagitis or esophageal spasm symptoms often mimic angina. In fact, sublingual nitroglycerin can also relieve the symptoms, but usually relief takes longer than the 3 to 5 minutes for angina to be relieved. Patients frequently report that the pain is worse after eating spicy foods or large meals or if they lie down after eating. They sometimes report a sour taste in their mouth. Physical examination is normal except for possible epigastric tenderness with palpation. The most reliable way to detect reflux as the cause of chest pain is to correlate episodes of chest pain with results of 24-hour esophageal pH monitoring.

Chest Trauma

Rib fractures usually follow trauma. Pain is made worse by deep breathing. The patient's respirations are shallow, and pain is exacerbated by palpation in the area of the fracture. Chest or rib radiographs will confirm suspected rib fractures.

Costochondritis and Tietze Syndrome

Costochondritis and Tietze syndrome are both identified by severe pain with palpation along the anterior cartilage where the ribs meet the sternum. Deep breathing and movement of the chest wall intensify the pain. In Tietze syndrome, swelling also occurs along this border.

Herpes Zoster

Herpes zoster is manifested by unilateral chest pain that follows a dermatome. The pain is usually described as burning, stabbing, or pruritic. Early in the course of the disease, no objective manifestations are present. As the course of herpes zoster progresses, a vesicular rash appears in the area of pain (see Chapter 25).

Peptic Ulcer Disease

Subjective manifestations of peptic ulcer disease include episodes of pain 1 to 3 hours after eating. The pain can awaken the patient at night and is frequently relieved by antacids or eating. The patient can report hematemesis and/or melena. A CBC can show iron-deficiency anemia. Personal or family history of ulcer disease can be a risk factor, as well as cigarette smoking and alcohol abuse. Upper GI radiography and endoscopy are diagnostic tests that can confirm peptic ulcer disease.

Cholecystitis

Cholecystitis is reported as colicky, intermittent epigastric or right upper quadrant pain that often follows a high-fat meal. Nausea and vomiting can accompany the pain, which often radiates to the right infrascapular area. Physical examination can show a positive Murphy sign, as indicated by tenderness in the region of the gallbladder. The gallbladder can be distended and palpable. Gallbladder ultrasonography is the most important diagnostic test in the evaluation of this problem.

Acute Pancreatitis

Acute pancreatitis occurs as the sudden onset of severe, steady upper epigastric or left upper quadrant abdominal pain, which frequently radiates to the left anterior chest, shoulders, or back. The pain is worse in the supine position. The patient appears restless, and pain can be associated with nausea and severe vomiting, hypotension, and unexplained shock. Left upper quadrant abdominal pain with palpation is present. Determination of serum amylase and lipase levels confirms the diagnosis. A rise in amylase level is seen 2 to 12 hours after the onset of symptoms. The lipase level returns to normal slower than the amylase level and thus is more useful in diagnosing pancreatitis later in its course. Pancreas ultrasonography and CT are necessary to show positive evidence of pancreatitis.

Lung and Mediastinal Tumors

Lung and mediastinal tumors can be manifested by chest pain. Associated symptoms include shortness of breath, cough, and hemoptysis. Pneumonia is often the initial diagnosis, and persistence of symptoms after treatment can lead to further investigation for tumors. Risk factors include a smoking history and family history of cancer. Physical examination can be normal or reveal diminished breath sounds in the area of the tumor. Dull sounds on percussion of the chest can be an objective manifestation of a chest mass. Chest radiography and CT of the chest are diagnostic tools to identify these lesions. Bronchoscopy is performed to obtain a biopsy.

Cocaine Use

Cocaine increases the metabolic requirement of the heart for oxygen and decreases the supply of oxygen, producing myocardial ischemia and chest pain. Cocaine causes adrenergic stimulation, thus increasing heart rate, blood pressure, and left ventricular contractility. Concomitantly, myocardial oxygen supply declines because of cocaine-induced vasoconstriction of the coronary arteries. ECGs, serial cardiac enzymes, and urine drug screens are useful diagnostic tools.

Psychogenic Origin

Adults and adolescents with a history of a recent stressful situation can present with chest pain. Physical examination is negative.

Pleurodynia

Group B coxsackieviruses can cause pleurodynia. Presentation is usually a sudden, severe onset of stabbing, paroxysmal pleuritic pain over the lower rib cage and substernal area. Deep breathing aggravates the pain. Fever, headache, malaise, and unproductive cough are usually present. The chest examination is negative except for pleuritic friction rub in 25% of cases. The condition lasts from 1 to 14 days.

Precordial Catch Syndrome

Recurrent brief episodes of sudden, sharp, but not distressing pain occurring at rest or during mild exercise can indicate precordial catch syndrome. It is localized near the apex of the heart and along the left sternal border or beneath the left breast. It is seen in adolescents and is benign in nature.

DIFFERENTIAL DIAGNOSIS OF *Common Causes of Emergent Chest Pain*

CONDITION	HISTORY	PHYSICAL FINDINGS	DIAGNOSTIC STUDIES
Acute myocardial infarction	Severe, oppressive, constricting retrosternal discomfort, radiating to left or right arm, neck, and/or jaw, lasting >30 min; diaphoresis, dyspnea, nausea; history of CAD, cigarette smoker, positive family history of CAD, history of elevated lipids	Hypertension or hypotension, cardiac arrhythmia, paradoxical S_2	Serial ECGs, serial cardiac enzymes, nuclear scan, troponin, T & I, chest radiograph, echocardiogram, angiography
Aortic dissection	Sudden, tearing pain in anterior or posterior chest; migrates to arms, abdomen, and legs	Pulse deficits, hypertension; possible neurological changes in legs; aortic diastolic murmur	Echocardiogram, angiography, CT scan/MRI, emergency referral, chest radiograph
Acute coronary artery insufficiency	Severe, constricting retrosternal chest pain lasting >30 min; anxiety, diaphoresis, dyspnea; prior history of angina or MI	Restlessness, cool and clammy skin, tachycardia	ECG, isoenzymes
Pulmonary embolus	Acute onset; sense of doom; pleuritic pain, restlessness; mild to severe pain; hemoptysis; history of DVT, recent trauma to lower extremity, surgery; oral contraceptives	Fever, dyspnea, cough, tachycardia, tachypnea, diminished breath sounds; crackles, wheezing	PT/aPTT, ABGs, chest radiograph, ventilation/perfusion scans, CT, pulmonary angiography
Pneumothorax	Sharp or tearing pain, can radiate to ipsilateral shoulder; dyspnea; children with asthma, CF, or Marfan syndrome at risk	Tachycardia; diminished breath sounds; crackles, wheezing	Chest radiograph, ABGs
Arrhythmias	Palpitations, dizziness, forceful heartbeats; history of CHD, fever, and medications (sympathomimetics and β-adrenergic agents); history of cocaine abuse	SVT = tachycardia of 150-250 beats/min, sinus or ventricular tachycardia, irregular pulse	ECG during episode, Holter 24-hour ECG
Congenital coronary anomalies	In children and adolescents, history of moderate to severe chest pain during or following exercise; family history of early sudden death	Can have murmurs, clicks, decreased lower extremity pulses, irregular pulse, BP	ECG, referral to pediatric cardiologist

ABG, arterial blood gas; *aPTT,* activated partial thromboplastin time; *BP,* blood pressure; *CAD,* coronary artery disease; *CF,* cystic fibrosis; *CHD,* coronary heart disease; *CT,* computed tomography; *DVT,* deep venous thrombosis; *ECG,* electrocardiogram; *MI,* myocardial infarction; *MRI,* magnetic resonance imaging; *PT,* prothrombin time; *SVT,* supraventricular tachycardia.

DIFFERENTIAL DIAGNOSIS OF *Common Causes of Nonemergent Chest Pain*

CONDITION	HISTORY	PHYSICAL FINDINGS	DIAGNOSTIC STUDIES
Stable angina	Substernal chest pressure following exercise or stress and relieved by rest or nitroglycerin; nausea, SOB, diaphoresis, sternal chest pressure	Normal examination; possible transient S_4	ECG during episode of chest pain
Myocarditis	Chest pain; history of fever, dyspnea	Heart murmur, friction rub, fever	ECG, chest radiograph

Continued

CONDITION	HISTORY	PHYSICAL FINDINGS	DIAGNOSTIC STUDIES
Pericarditis	Sharp, stabbing pain referred to left shoulder or trapezius ridge, usually worse during coughing or deep breathing; can be relieved by sitting forward; history of viral or bacterial infection, autoimmune disease	Fever before onset of pain, tachycardia, pericardial friction rub	WBC, ESR, ECG, chest radiograph
Aortic stenosis	Chest pain on exertion, substernal and anginal in quality; fatigue, palpitations, DOE, dizziness, syncope	Radial pulse diminished; narrow pulse pressure; loud, harsh, crescendo-decrescendo murmur heard best at second right ICS with patient leaning forward; thrill	Echocardiogram, ECG, chest radiograph
Mitral regurgitation	Exertional chest pain, fatigue, palpitations, dizziness, DOE, syncope	Holosystolic, blowing, often loud murmur heard best at apex in left lateral position and decreases with inspiration; murmur can radiate to axilla and possibly back	Chest radiograph, ECG, echocardiogram
Pneumonia	Productive cough of yellow or green or rust sputum, dyspnea, pleuritic pain	Fever; tachycardia, tachypnea; inspiratory crackles; vocal fremitus; percussion dull or flat over area of consolidation; bronchophony; egophony	Chest radiograph, sputum cultures, ABGs
Mitral valve prolapse	Chest pain, varies in location and intensity; palpitations; anxiety; nonexertional pain of short duration; history of Marfan syndrome	Arrhythmias, possible midsystolic click heard over apex; heard best while patient is in sitting or squatting position; thoracoskeletal deformity common in children	ECG, echocardiogram
Pleuritis	Mild, localized chest pain, worse with deep breathing; recent URI	Shallow respirations, local tenderness, pleural friction rub	None initially
Esophagitis	Substernal pain worse after eating and lying down; sour taste in mouth	Epigastric pain with palpitation	Esophageal pH
Chest trauma (rib fracture)	History of injury or trauma; pain with deep breaths; splinting of chest wall	Shallow respirations; chest wall pain on palpitation	Chest radiograph
Costochondritis	Pain along sternal border, increases with deep breaths; history of exercise, URI, or physical activity	Pain with palpitation over costochondral joints; normal breath sounds	None
Herpes zoster	Unilateral chest pain; painful rash	Normal breath sounds; vesicular rash along dermatome	None
Peptic ulcer disease	Epigastric pain 1 to 2 hours after eating, can be relieved by antacids; hematemesis and melena; risk factors include smoking and alcohol overuse	Tenderness to palpitation in epigastric area; signs of hypovolemia	Upper GI radiograph, upper endoscopy, CBC
Cholecystitis	Right upper quadrant abdominal pain radiating to right chest, often after eating high-fat meal; nausea and vomiting	Positive Murphy sign; palpable gallbladder	Gallbladder ultrasound

DIFFERENTIAL DIAGNOSIS OF *Common Causes of Nonemergent Chest Pain—cont'd*

CONDITION	HISTORY	PHYSICAL FINDINGS	DIAGNOSTIC STUDIES
Acute pancreatitis	Severe left upper quadrant abdominal pain radiating into left chest; pain worse in supine position; nausea, vomiting, fever	Left upper abdominal pain with palpation; hypotension	Serum analysis, pancreas ultrasound or CT scan
Lung tumors	Chest pain, SOB, cough, hemoptysis, history of cigarette smoking; history of pneumonia	Normal exam or diminished breath sounds over tumor and dull percussion sound over tumor	Chest radiograph, CT scan of chest, bronchoscopy
Cocaine use	Chest pain, SOB, diaphoresis, nausea; can relate to substance use	Tachycardia, hypertension	ECG, serial cardiac enzymes, drug screen
Psychogenic origin	Precordial chest pain, history of stressful situations	Normal exam	ECG, chest radiograph
Pleurodynia	Severe, acute onset, stabbing, paroxysmal, pleuritic pain over lower rib cage and substernal edge; headache, malaise, nonproductive cough	Pleural friction rub 25% of time; chest examination normal; fever usually present	None
Precordial catch syndrome	Sudden, sharp, nondistressing pain near apex of heart; seen in adolescents	Normal examination	None

CBC, complete blood cell count; *CT,* computed tomography; *DOE,* dizziness on exertion; *ECG,* electrocardiogram; *ESR,* erythrocyte sedimentation rate; *GI,* gastrointestinal; *ICS,* intercostal space; *SOB,* shortness of breath; *URI,* upper respiratory tract infection; *WBC,* white blood cell count.

REFERENCES AND READINGS

Bettmann MA, Lyders EM, Yucel EK, Khan A, Haramati LB, Ho VB, Expert Panel on Cardiac Imaging. Acute chest pain—suspected pulmonary embolism [online publication]. Reston (VA): American College of Radiology (ACR); 2006.

Canadian Cardiovascular Society, American Academy of Family Physicians, American College of Cardiology, American Heart Association, Antman EM, Hand M, Armstrong PW, Bates ER, Green LA, Halasyamani LK, et al: 2007 focused update of the ACC/AHA 2004 guidelines for the management of patients with ST-elevation myocardial infarction: a report of the American College of Cardiology/American Heart Association Task Force on Practice Guidelines, *J Am Coll Cardiol* 51:210, 2008.

Cava J, Saygor P: Chest pain in children and adolescents, *Pediatr Clin North Am* 51:1553, 2004.

Cayley WE: Diagnosing the cause of chest pain, *Am Fam Physician* 72:2012, 2005.

DeVon HA, Ryan CJ: Chest pain and associated symptoms of acute coronary syndromes, *J Cardiovasc Nurs* 20:232, 2005.

Eslick GD, Coulshed DS, Talley NJ: Diagnosis and treatment of noncardiac chest pain, *Natl Clin Pract Gastroenterol Hepatol* 2:10, 2005.

Expert Panel on Detection, Evaluation, and Treatment of High Blood Cholesterol in Adults: Executive summary of the third report of the National Cholesterol Education Program (NCEP) Expert Panel on Detection, Evaluation, and Treatment of High Blood Cholesterol in Adults (Adult Treatment Panel III), *JAMA* 285:2486, 2001.

Grundy SM, Cleeman JI, Merz CN, Brewer HB Jr, Clark LT, Hunninghake DB: Implications of recent clinical trials for the National Cholesterol Education Program Adult Treatment Panel III Guidelines, *Circulation* 110:227, 2004.

Imazio M, Cecchi E, Demichelis B, Chinaglia A, Ierna S, Demarie D: Myopericarditis versus viral or idiopathic acute pericarditis, *Heart* 94:498, 2008.

Kruip MJ, Leclercq MG, van der Heul C, Prins MH, Büller HR: Diagnostic strategies for excluding pulmonary embolism in clinical outcome studies: a systematic review, *Ann Intern Med* 138:941, 2003.

Lane JR, Ben-Shachar G: Myocardial infarct in healthy adolescents, *Pediatrics* 120:1, 2007.

Lange RA, Hill LD: Acute pericarditis, *N Engl J Med* 351:2195, 2004.

Lee TH, Goldman L: Evaluation of the patient with acute chest pain, *N Engl J Med* 342:1187, 2000.

Reddy S, Singh H: Chest pain in children and adolescents, *Pediatr Review* 31:929, 2010.

Swap CJ, Nagurney JT: Value and limitations of chest pain history in the evaluation of patients with suspected acute coronary syndromes, *JAMA* 294:20, 2005.

Confusion in Older Adults

Confusion is a symptom rather than a disease state. It is the inability to think quickly or coherently. A confused patient is disoriented to time, person, or place and can demonstrate impaired cognitive function. Older adults are far more likely to experience an acute confusional state as a result of hospitalization or surgery, systemic or electrolyte imbalance, organ failure, excessive medication, nutritional deficiency, systemic infection, or cerebral insufficiency, such as stroke or transient ischemic attacks. When an older patient presents with confusion, the differential diagnosis includes delirium, dementia, or depression.

Delirium, caused by alteration in brain metabolism, is characterized by abrupt onset, reduced level of acute consciousness, and sleep/wake cycle disturbance. **Delirium is a medical emergency** and can occur as a result of medications, alcohol use or alcohol withdrawal, narcotic reaction or narcotic withdrawal, Wernicke-Korsakoff syndrome (vitamin B_{12} deficiency), hepatic encephalopathy, acute illness, chronic illness, interacting diseases, or trauma (e.g., head injury).

Dementia, a chronic generalized impairment of brain function, affects thinking but not level of consciousness. A common early complaint in dementia is forgetfulness, with loss of concentration and loss of memory. Causes of dementia can be classified as reversible (or partially reversible), modifiable, or irreversible (Box 8-1).

Depression as a cause of confusion, especially in the elderly, is considered a reversible cause of dementia. When anxiety symptoms are also present, depression can manifest as mild delirium (see Chapter 3).

DIAGNOSTIC REASONING: FOCUSED HISTORY

Obtaining an appropriate history from a confused patient involves the use of another person as the historian. Preferably that person is someone who has had consistent contact with the patient and can report about usual behavioral patterns and the conditions involved with this episode.

Is this a condition that requires immediate intervention?

Key Questions

- How suddenly did the confusion start?
- Is the patient alert and aware of time, person, and place?
- Has the patient expressed thoughts of suicide (in words or actions)?
- Does the patient use alcohol or other drugs?

Confusion that is acute in onset and persistent can indicate delirium, a cerebrovascular event, cerebral infection, subdural hematoma, or neoplasm. A history of altered level of consciousness and the patient's current state indicate a medical condition that requires immediate intervention. Acute-onset confusion can produce paranoia and aggression. Suicidal ideation can accompany depression and is an indication for immediate intervention and further evaluation. If the patient has been abusing alcohol or other chemical substances, acute withdrawal can require immediate medical intervention.

If the onset is gradual and the patient is not seriously ill, consider depression or dementia. Remember that depression and dementia can coexist. Unless the patient is suicidal or seriously ill, both depression and dementia can be handled in a more temperate manner.

What distinguishing characteristics of confusion does this patient exhibit?

Key Questions

- Was the onset of the confusion abrupt (i.e., over a period of minutes or hours) or gradual (i.e., a few days, weeks, or months)?
- Does the confusion change within a 24-hour period (stable or fluctuating)?

<table>
<tr><td colspan="2">

Box 8-1   **Causes of Dementia**

Reversible Causes of Dementia

D	Drugs/medications
E	Emotional illness/depression
M	Metabolic/endocrine disorders
E	Eye/ear involvement/environmental
N	Nutritional/neurological
T	Tumors/trauma
I	Infection
A	Alcoholism/anemia/atherosclerosis

Modifiable Causes of Dementia
- Normal pressure hydrocephalus
- Hepatic encephalopathy
- HIV encephalopathy (AIDS dementia complex)

Irreversible Causes of Dementia
- Alzheimer disease
- Multi-infarct dementia
- Huntington chorea

</td></tr>
</table>

- Is there a change in the sleep pattern?
- Is the patient alert and aware?
- Has the patient experienced seeing, hearing, or feeling things that are not there?
- Is there any history of head trauma?

Onset and Duration

Confusion that is abrupt in onset but short-lived can indicate a transient ischemic attack (TIA). Sudden onset, usually over a period of hours, is characteristic of delirium. In delirium, the condition is persistent but has been present for no longer than 1 month. In an acute confusional episode, the symptoms are less severe than with delirium with a less sudden onset. The onset in depression is usually gradual, over a period of weeks, and is persistent over time. In dementia, the onset is insidious and gradual; the condition has often been present for many weeks or months.

Fluctuation in Symptoms

With delirium, the symptoms can fluctuate over the course of a day and frequently are worse at night and with fatigue. The course is more stable with both depression and dementia, with little variation over a 24-hour period.

Disturbance in Sleep/Wake Cycle

The sleep/wake cycle in delirium is always impaired. Either the wakefulness is abnormally increased and the patient gets little or no sleep, or the patient has night

insomnia and is drowsy and tired during the day. Thus the sleep/wake cycle is usually fragmented, and the patient tends to be restless and agitated and has hallucinations while awake during the night.

Level of Consciousness

In both dementia and depression, the individual is likely to be both alert and aware, although the mood can be depressed. With delirium, the patient will have a decreased level of consciousness, be less alert and aware, and can be difficult to arouse. With an acute confusional state, the person will demonstrate impaired concentration and make errors in thinking.

Hallucinations

Visual, tactile, and auditory hallucinations are common with delirium, especially at night when changes in environment or activity occur. Hallucinations are uncommon in both depression and dementia, although hallucinations can occur in late-stage dementia.

Head Trauma

Head trauma can produce confusion and disorientation. In older adults, common causes of head trauma include motor vehicle crashes, physical abuse, and falls.

Are there any associated symptoms that will point me in the right direction?

Key Questions

- Has the patient shown any tremor, especially at rest?
- Has the patient had any trouble walking?
- Has the patient reported severe headache and/or nausea?
- Has the patient had a fever?
- Has the patient gained or lost weight?
- Does the patient engage in his/her usual activities?

Tremor and Gait Disturbance

Tremors are associated with parkinsonism, human immunodeficiency virus (HIV) encephalopathy, and liver disease. Gait disorder is associated with parkinsonism, medication reactions, and head trauma.

Headache, Nausea, and Fever

Headache and nausea are associated with head trauma, stroke, and tumor. Fever is usually present with HIV infection, other systemic infections, or acute alcohol withdrawal.

Change in Weight and Usual Activities

Patients with depression can exhibit vegetative symptoms (e.g., cessation of talking, eating, dressing, and toileting; insomnia; weight loss or gain; diminished interest in most activities or former pleasures) and feelings of worthlessness.

What does the pattern of cognitive losses tell me?

Key Questions

- What specific problems with mental abilities or thinking have you noticed?
- What behavioral changes or personality changes have you noticed?

Changes in Mental Abilities and Behaviors

Patients with delirium have global cognitive losses that involve memory, thinking, perception, and judgment. These patients can become completely disoriented, irritable, and fearful. They can be difficult to arouse or conversely have insomnia. Families sometimes note visual hallucinations.

Patients in an acute confusional state can be disoriented—especially for time, less for place, and almost never for self. They show impaired concentration, experience sensory misperceptions, and make errors in thinking.

Dementia, particularly early in the disorder, presents with more selective cognitive losses. Family members report that patients cannot remember recent events, are disoriented, are irritable or depressed, have poor hygiene, show poor judgment, make financial errors, are socially withdrawn, have difficulty finding or saying the right words, are clumsy or fall, have urinary incontinence, have deteriorating interpersonal relationships, and show personality changes.

Fewer cognitive losses occur with depression. These persons can exhibit cognitive losses consistent with confusion—apathy and drowsiness, impaired concentration, and errors in thinking. The most common cognitive symptoms are severe negative thinking, guilt, and remorse.

Is the confusion caused by a concurrent health problem?

Key Questions

- Does the patient have any chronic health conditions?
- Has the patient been hospitalized recently, and if so, for what reason?

- Has the patient been acutely ill recently?
- Is there a history of mental illness or similar thought disturbance?

Current and Past Health Status

Obtain past medical records to make a complete medical history. Most likely you will have to use a relative or close friend to determine current and past health status. Many systemic conditions and disorders can produce alteration in mental status, particularly in older patients (Box 8-2). Chronic health problems (such as alcoholism, renal failure, liver disease, severe anemia, chronic obstructive pulmonary disease [COPD], severe cardiovascular disease, and HIV) predispose individuals, especially the elderly, to the development of confusion. Patients with multiple chronic health problems are particularly at risk.

Could the confusion be caused by medication?

Key Questions

- What medications is the patient taking?
- Is the patient taking the medications correctly?

Medications

Drugs that can produce altered mental status include the following:

- Alcohol
- Antibiotics (e.g., isoniazid, aminoglycosides)
- Anticholinergic agents
- Anticonvulsants
- Antidepressants
- Antihypertensive agents (e.g., reserpine, ß-blockers, methyldopa, clonidine, hydralazine)
- Antiparkinsonian agents
- Cardiac drugs (e.g., digitalis, lidocaine, ß-blockers, vasodilators, diuretics)
- Chemotherapeutic agents (e.g., methotrexate)
- Gastrointestinal drugs (e.g., H_2 blockers, metoclopramide)
- Illicit drugs (e.g., amphetamines, cocaine, opiates)
- Narcotics
- Over-the-counter cold/allergy preparations
- Sedatives
- Tranquilizers

Taking Medication Correctly

Combinations of these medications increase the probability of medication-induced confusion. People who are confused may be taking medications improperly,

Box 8-2	**Systemic Conditions Associated with Confusional States**

Endocrine
- Hypo/hyperthyroidism

Metabolic
- Anemia (severe)
- Hypo/hypercalcemia
- Hypo/hypercortisolism
- Hypo/hyperglycemia
- Hypomagnesemia
- Hypo/hypernatremia
- Wilson disease (copper disorder)
- Porphyria

Infectious
- AIDS
- Cerebral amebiasis
- Cerebral cysticercosis
- Cerebral toxoplasmosis
- Cerebral malaria
- Fungal meningitis
- Lyme disease
- Neurosyphilis
- TB meningitis

Cardiovascular
- Congestive heart failure
- Hyperviscosity

Cerebrovascular
- Cerebral insufficiency (TIA, CVA)
- Postanoxic encephalopathy

Pulmonary
- COPD
- Hypercapnia
- Hypoxemia

Renal
- Renal failure
- Uremia

Neurological
- Hepatic encephalopathy
- Hypertensive encephalopathy
- Limbic encephalitis
- Head trauma

Other
- Alcoholism
- Anemia (severe)
- Leukoencephalopathy
- Metastatic cancer to brain
- Sarcoidosis
- Sleep apnea
- Vasculitis (e.g., SLE)
- Vitamin deficiencies (B_{12}, folate, niacin, thiamine)
- Whipple disease

which compounds the problem. Further, older adults may need lower doses or a gradual increase in dosages of medications used to treat both acute and chronic conditions.

What risk factors do I need to consider?

Key Questions
- How old is the patient?
- How many medications is the patient taking?
- Is the patient HIV positive?
- Has the patient experienced recent life losses?

Age

Older adults are at risk for the development of confusion, delirium, dementia, and depression. Factors that place them at risk include the use of multiple medications, the existence of multiple medical conditions, and the physiological changes associated with aging. Dementia occurs in approximately 5% to 10% of adults 65 to 80 years of age, 20% of those older than 80 years, and almost half of those older than 85 years.

Polypharmacy

Older adults who are taking multiple medications are at risk for medication interactions and resulting confusion (see also the preceding list of medications that can produce altered mental status).

Human Immunodeficiency Virus

Patients with HIV infection or those who are immunocompromised are at increased risk for the development of HIV encephalopathy (AIDS dementia complex) or dementia caused by central nervous system (CNS) opportunistic infections.

Recent Bereavement

Recent loss and the lack of a social network place an individual at risk for depression. Both cause profound biopsychosocial stress that can easily exceed the person's resources and skills. Extreme mourning or isolation can be physically and emotionally draining.

DIAGNOSTIC REASONING: FOCUSED PHYSICAL EXAMINATION
Take Vital Signs

The presence of a fever can indicate infection or alcohol withdrawal. A diastolic blood pressure greater than 120 mm Hg suggests hypertensive encephalopathy, whereas a systolic blood pressure less than 90 mm Hg can indicate impaired cerebral perfusion.

Note Level of Consciousness

In both dementia and depression, the individual is likely to be alert and aware, although the mood can be depressed. With delirium, the patient will have a decreased level of consciousness, be less alert and aware, and can be difficult to arouse. With an acute confusional state, the patient will demonstrate impaired concentration and have difficulty thinking.

Perform a Mental Status Examination

A thorough mental status examination is essential. Mental status assessment is used to determine cognitive function. A number of assessment instruments are available, including the Mini Mental State Examination (MMSE) (see Figure 8-1 for sample items from the MMSE). Patients with delirium may be unable to cooperate or answer questions. Patients with dementia are cooperative and willing to try but make mistakes and give incorrect or "near miss" answers. Patients with depression are less cooperative and are more likely to give "don't know" answers, refuse to answer questions, or be less willing to try.

Global cognitive loss is consistent with delirium. Losses occur in the following areas: memory, thinking, perception, information acquisition, information retention, information processing, information retrieval, and information use. Thus the MMSE score will be very low with inability to perform most or all of the items.

Dementia, particularly early in the disorder, presents with selective cognitive losses that can occur in one or more of the following areas. Specific losses include the following:

- Apraxia (i.e., cannot draw simple geometric figures)
- Visuospatial problems (e.g., cannot draw intersecting pentagons)
- Cannot perform commands
- Selective cognitive loss
- Loss of abstract reasoning
- Problems with orientation
- Problems with recent memory
- Problems with number retention

Fewer cognitive losses occur with depression than with dementia. Loss of concentration is an important symptom of depression. The individual is aware of losses and can highlight disabilities, especially memory loss. Along with loss of memory, impaired concentration and errors in judgment are common.

Orientation to Time
    "What is the date?"

Registration
    "Listen carefully, I am going to say three words. You say them back after I stop. Ready? Here they are. . .
    HOUSE (pause), CAR (pause), LAKE (pause). Now repeat those words back to me."
    [Repeat up to 5 times, but score only the first trial.]

Naming
    "What is this?" [Point to a pencil or pen.]

Reading
    "Please read this and do what it says." [Show examinee the words on the stimulus form.]

CLOSE YOUR EYES

FIGURE 8-1   Sample items from the MMSE. For a full copy of the MMSE, administration instructions, and scoring guidelines, contact Psychological Assessment Resources. (Reproduced special permission of the Publisher, Psychological Assessment Resources, Inc., 16204 North Florida Avenue, Lutz, FL 33549, from the Mini Mental State Examination, by Marshal Folstein and Susan Folstein, Copyright 1975, 1988, 2001 by Mini Mental LLC, Inc. Published 2001 by Psychological Assessment Resources, Inc. Further reproduction is prohibited without permission of PAR, Inc. The MMSE can be purchased from PAR, Inc., by calling (800) 331-8378 or (813) 449-4065.)

In older persons, also administer the Geriatric Depression Scale (Figure 8-2). The test is positive for depression if the score is above 5.

The Confusion Assessment Method (CAM) can be used to assess delirium. The CAM instrument assesses the presence, severity, and fluctuation of nine delirium features: acute onset, inattention, disorganized thinking, altered level of consciousness, disorientation, memory impairment, perceptual disturbances, psychomotor agitation or retardation, and altered sleep–wake cycle. The CAM diagnostic algorithm is based on four cardinal features of delirium: (1) acute onset and fluctuating course, (2) inattention, (3) disorganized thinking, and (4) altered level of consciousness. Permission to use the CAM and the training manual for it can be obtained through ElderLife@hrca.harvard.edu.

Perform a Complete Neurological Examination

Normal neurological findings are typical of early dementia and depression. Abnormal findings suggest other organic involvement.

Geriatric Depression Scale (short form)

Choose the best answer for how you felt over the past week.

1. Are you basically satisfied with your life? yes/no
2. Have you dropped many of your activities and interests? yes/no
3. Do you feel that your life is empty? yes/no
4. Do you often get bored? yes/no
5. Are you in good spirits most of the time? yes/no
6. Are you afraid that something bad is going to happen to you? yes/no
7. Do you feel happy most of the time? yes/no
8. Do you often feel helpless? yes/no
9. Do you prefer to stay at home, rather than going out and doing new things? yes/no
10. Do you feel you have more problems with memory than most? yes/no
11. Do you think it is wonderful to be alive now? yes/no
12. Do you feel pretty worthless the way you are now? yes/no
13. Do you feel full of energy? yes/no
14. Do you feel that your situation is hopeless? yes/no
15. Do you think that most people are better off than you are? yes/no

This is the scoring for the scale. One point for each of these answers. Cut-off: normal (0-5), above 5 suggests depression.

1. no	6. yes	11. no
2. yes	7. no	12. yes
3. yes	8. yes	13. no
4. yes	9. yes	14. yes
5. no	10. yes	15. yes

FIGURE 8-2 Geriatric Depression Scale (short form). (From Sheikh JI, Yesavage JA: Geriatric Depression Scale: recent evidence and development of a shorter version, *Clin Gerontol* 5:165, 1986.)

Cranial Nerves

Check vision, hearing, and sensory impairment as contributing factors in confusion. Dilated pupils suggest alcohol withdrawal; pinpoint pupils can indicate narcotic excess or use of eye drops. Changes in pupil size can also indicate neurological changes, such as those that occur with stroke or neoplasm. The sense of smell is often impaired in dementia. Patients with parkinsonism can exhibit a typical facial presentation: masked facial expression, poor blink reflex, and drooling. Speech is slowed, slurred, and monotonous.

Proprioception and Cerebellar Function

Test coordination through rapid alternating movements (RAMs), accuracy of movement, balance (Romberg test), and gait. Slowed RAMs are characteristic of early HIV encephalopathy. Tremor and restlessness are associated with alcohol intoxication or withdrawal. Tremor (especially resting), rigidity, and bradykinesia indicate parkinsonism. Asterixis, sometimes referred to as liver flap or liver tremor, is an involuntary tremor of the hands, tongue, and feet that is characteristic of hepatic or metabolic encephalopathy. Postural tremor is present with HIV encephalopathy. Writhing movements (chorea) typify Huntington disease.

Gait abnormalities are found with multi-infarct dementia, normal pressure hydrocephalus, and HIV encephalopathy.

Sensation (Primary and Cortical)

Agnosia (failure to identify or recognize objects despite intact sensory function) is present with dementia.

Deep Tendon Reflexes

Test deep tendon reflexes (DTRs) and the superficial plantar reflexes. Hyperreflexia and primitive reflexes are present in late dementia. Hyperreflexia is also present in multi-infarct dementia, HIV encephalopathy, and costovertebral angle (CVA).

A positive Babinski sign on testing the plantar reflex is present in multi-infarct dementia, CVA, and head injury. Cogwheeling (resistance to a passively stretched hypertonic muscle resulting in a rhythmical jerk similar to a ratchet) suggests parkinsonism.

Motor Tone and Function

Apraxia (impaired ability to carry out motor activities despite intact motor function) indicates dementia. Motor weakness, especially of the legs, loss of coordination, and impaired handwriting are consistent with early HIV encephalopathy.

Language

Aphasia (language disturbance) is often present in dementia and can occur with CVA and head injury.

Localizing and Lateralizing Signs in CNS

Focal neurological signs (i.e., exaggerated DTRs, positive Babinski sign, gait abnormalities, and hemiparesis) are consistent with multi-infarct dementia. Focal deficits also occur with cerebrovascular injury.

Patients with late HIV encephalopathy demonstrate weakness that is greater in the legs than in the arms; ataxia; spasticity and hyperreflexia; positive Babinski sign; myoclonus; and bladder and bowel incontinence.

Psychomotor agitation or retardation is consistent with depression. An agitated confusional state without focal signs can occur with head trauma.

Perform a Respiratory Examination

Monitor the rate and effort of respirations. Auscultate the lung fields. Tachypnea suggests hypoxia. Bibasilar crackles indicate congestive heart failure (CHF) with hypoxia. Asymmetrical crackles suggest pneumonia with hypoxia. Patients with dementia or depression in the absence of concomitant lung disease will have normal findings.

Evaluate the Cardiovascular System

Perform a careful cardiovascular examination. Tachycardia suggests sepsis, hyperthyroidism, hypoglycemia, agitation, anxiety, or alcohol withdrawal. Be alert for indicators of cardiovascular problems that can produce hypoxia, such as CHF or myocardial infarction (MI).

Examine the Abdomen

Examine the abdomen and percuss for CVA tenderness. Specific findings can indicate a local or systemic cause for the confusion. For example, urinary retention suggests urinary tract infection, CVA tenderness points to pyelonephritis, and an enlarged liver can indicate hepatic encephalopathy.

LABORATORY AND DIAGNOSTIC STUDIES

Diagnostic testing is aimed at detecting or confirming a metabolic/organic cause of the confusion. If dementia seems likely, these same tests can rule in or rule out reversible or modifiable causes of the dementia. Most tests will be normal when the diagnosis is depression.

Complete Blood Count

Leukocytosis suggests infection. Anemia as a cause of confusion in chronic illness can also be detected.

Blood Chemistry

High or low potassium or sodium levels, dehydration, and acidosis can all produce confusion. Elevated or depressed magnesium and calcium levels, hypoglycemia, and hyperglycemia can also cause confusion. Elevated blood urea nitrogen (BUN) and creatinine levels or an elevated BUN/creatinine ratio can indicate renal failure. Elevation in liver enzymes suggests liver dysfunction.

Thyroid Function Tests

Abnormal levels of thyroid-stimulating hormone (TSH) can indicate thyroid dysfunction, either thyroid toxicosis or a hypothyroid state. An elevated TSH level is related to chronic symptoms of depression.

Serum B$_{12}$ and Folate

Deficiencies of vitamin B$_{12}$ and folate are reversible causes of dementia.

Serology for Syphilis

A positive test can indicate neurosyphilis as the cause of confusion.

Arterial Blood Gases

Arterial blood gases (ABGs) are used to determine the presence or degree of hypoxia.

Toxicology Screen and Blood Alcohol Level

These tests can be used to determine alcohol or drug intoxication as a cause of confusion.

Urinalysis

Urinalysis is used to detect infection and can point to renal indicators of systemic disease. See Chapter 32 for a complete discussion of urinalysis.

Chest Radiograph

A chest radiograph is used to detect infection, CHF, COPD, pneumonia, or other respiratory-associated causes of hypoxia.

Lumbar Puncture

Lumbar puncture is used to rule out bacterial, fungal, or tumor meningitis (see Chapter 18).

Electrocardiography

Electrocardiography (ECG) is used to rule out certain cardiovascular causes of hypoxia, such as MI or dysrhythmias.

Electroencephalography

Electroencephalography (EEG) can be used to identify a seizure disorder as a cause of or a contributing factor to confusion.

Computed Tomography or Magnetic Resonance Imaging

Computed tomography (CT) or magnetic resonance imaging (MRI) is used to diagnose cerebrovascular bleeding, injury, abscess, or tumor or whether focal neurological signs are present. These imaging tests usually do not yield useful information related to the diagnosis of dementia.

Positron Emission Tomography Scan

Positron emission tomography (PET) is useful in confirming the diagnosis of Alzheimer disease. PET images demonstrate the metabolic activity of organs and other tissues. A radiopharmaceutical, which includes both sugar (glucose) and a radionuclide (a radioactive element) that releases signals, is injected into the patient and its emissions are measured by a PET scanner. Using the gamma ray signals discharged by the injected radionuclide, PET measures the amount of metabolic activity at a site in the body and a computer reassembles the signals into images. PET highlights areas with increased, diminished, or no metabolic activity, thereby pinpointing problems. A distinctive image appears in the area of the brain affected by Alzheimer disease. It can be seen in early disease. PET also is useful in differentiating Alzheimer disease from other forms of dementia, such as vascular dementia, and from other memory disorders, such as clinical depression.

DIFFERENTIAL DIAGNOSIS
Delirium

The incidence of delirium increases progressively after the fourth decade of life. Because delirium is associated with an increased risk of death, it should always be considered first in patients who exhibit cognitive impairment or behavioral changes.

Delirium is characterized by reduced ability to maintain attention to external stimuli, disorganized thinking, decreased level of consciousness (LOC), perceptual disturbances, disturbed sleep/wake cycle, disorientation, and memory impairment. The patient will evidence a decreased LOC and impaired arousal, increased or decreased psychomotor activity, and irritability. The onset is rapid, and the condition can last from hours to weeks. Fluctuations over the course of the day are common, with lucid intervals during the day and worse symptoms at night. The thought process is disorganized, and the patient is usually disoriented, most commonly to time. There is a tendency for the patient to mistake the unfamiliar for familiar places and people. Hallucinations, usually visual, are common. Physical examination findings depend on the underlying cause of the delirium. The patient often exhibits asterixis or tremor. Speech is incoherent, hesitant, slow, or rapid. Table 8-1 shows the distinguishing characteristics of delirium.

Confusion

Confusion is less abrupt and less severe than delirium, with less severe disorientation and more subtle motor signs. The diurnal variation is less severe than in delirium. The person can be apathetic and drowsy and will show disorientation—especially for time, less for place, and almost never for self. Concentration is impaired, and the person lacks direction and selectivity and is easily distracted. Errors in thinking are common. The person may exhibit tremor and difficulty in motor relaxation.

Table 8-1	Distinguishing Characteristics of Delirium, Dementia, and Depression		
CHARACTERISTIC	**DELIRIUM**	**DEMENTIA**	**DEPRESSION**
Onset	Sudden	Insidious, relentless	Sudden or insidious
Duration	Hours, days	Persistent	For longer than 2 weeks
Time of day	Increases and decreases during the day	Stable, no change	Throughout the greater part of the day
Consciousness	Altered	Not impaired except in severe cases	Not impaired
Cognition	Impairment of memory, attentiveness, consciousness, numerous errors in assessment tasks	Minimal cognitive impairment initially, progresses to impaired abstract thinking, judgment, memory, thought patterns, calculations, agnosia	Impaired concentration, reduced attention span, indecisiveness, slower thought processes, impaired short-term and long-term memory
Activity	Increased or decreased, can fluctuate	Unchanged from usual behavior	Insomnia or excessive sleeping, fatigue, restlessness, anxiety, increased or decreased appetite
Speech/language	Rambling and irrelevant conversation, illogical flow of ideas, incoherent	Disordered, rambling, incoherent; struggles to find words	Slower speech
Mood and affect	Rapid mood swings; fearful, suspicious	Depressed, apathetic, uninterested	Sad, hopeless, feels worthless, loss of interest or pleasure
Delusions/ hallucinations	Misperceptions, illusions, hallucinations, and delusions	Misperceptions usually absent, delusions, no hallucinations	No delusions or hallucinations
Reversibility	Potential	No, progressive	Can be treated, can recur
Pathophysiology	Associated with infections, medications, electrolyte and metabolic disorders, major organ failure, brain insults, and acute alcohol withdrawal	Usually related to structural diseases of the brain	Associated with grief, a stressful life event, reaction to medical or neurologic diseases, or a change in lifestyle

Dementia

Dementia is characterized by acquired persistent and progressive impairment of intellectual function, with compromise in at least two of the following areas:

- Language (aphasia)
- Memory
- Visuospatial skills (apraxia, agnosia)
- Emotional behavior or personality
- Cognition (e.g., calculation, abstraction, judgment)

Refer to Table 8-1 for the distinguishing characteristics of dementia.

The onset of symptoms is insidious, with the course stable through the day and night. The condition can be present for months or years, with progressive deterioration. Recent and remote memory is impaired. The patient is alert and attention is relatively unaffected, although orientation is usually impaired. Hallucinations are usually absent until late in the course of the disease. Speech is usually unimpaired although the person has difficulty finding words. Sleep is often fragmented. On mental status examination, the patient tries hard and provides "near miss" answers. Physical findings are often absent. The olfactory sense can be impaired. Box 8-3 lists common presentations of dementia, Box 8-4 lists phases of Alzheimer-type dementia, and Box 8-5 describes a staging system for Alzheimer disease.

Alzheimer-type dementia can sometimes be distinguished from vascular or multi-infarct dementia (MID) by obtaining a cardiovascular history, determining the progression of symptoms, and detecting the presence or absence of focal neurological signs and symptoms (Table 8-2).

Depression

Depression can produce confusion, especially in the elderly. The onset of the confusion is often abrupt, with some diurnal variation. Generally, depression is more consistent over time than delirium. The confusion is of short duration compared with dementia. A past history of psychiatric problems, including undiagnosed depressive episodes, is common. During mental status examination, the patient tends to highlight disabilities, especially memory loss. The memory loss is equal for recent and remote events. The cognitive losses, however, are fluctuating rather than stable over time. The patient manifests a depressed or anxious mood, including sleep and appetite disturbance. Hallucinations are usually absent,

| Box 8-3 | Common Presentations of Dementia |

Memory loss	Language difficulty
Depression	Social withdrawal
Irritability	Behavioral change
Poor hygiene	Urinary incontinence
Insomnia	Hallucinations (late)
Paranoia	Anxiety
Weight loss	Failure to thrive
Poor work performance	Falls, clumsiness
Financial errors	Deteriorating interpersonal
Poor judgment	relationships
Delirium	Personality changes

| Box 8-4 | Phases of Alzheimer-Type Dementia |

Progression of symptoms corresponds with the progression of underlying nerve cell degeneration. Damage typically begins with cells involved in learning and memory and gradually spreads to cells that control thinking, judgment, and behavior. The damage eventually affects cells that control and coordinate movement.

Limbic
- 2 to 3 years after onset
- Olfactory system involved
- Memory loss
- Can perform tasks

Parietal
- 3 to 6 years after onset
- Loss of comprehension of spoken language
- Cannot name common objects
- Apraxia: cannot perform motor skills although motor system intact
- Agnosia: failure to identify or recognize objects despite intact sensory function
- Misinterprets visual and auditory stimuli
- Delusions

Late Frontal
- 6 to 8 years after onset
- Motor disturbances: walking, swallowing, moving
- Primitive reflexes
- Seizures
- Sensation remains intact

although the patient may have suicidal thoughts. Depression as a cause of confusion can be easy to miss because it is often associated with anger, anxiety, and unclear thinking as well as denial (see Chapter 3). Table 8-1 presents distinguishing characteristics of depression.

Box 8-5　Stages of Alzheimer's Disease

Staging systems for Alzheimer's disease vary. The Alzheimer's Association uses seven stages to describe the progression of Alzheimer's disease.

Stage 1: No impairment (normal function)

Stage 2: Very mild cognitive decline (may be age-related changes or earliest signs of Alzheimer's disease)

- Memory lapses, especially in forgetting familiar words or names or the location of everyday objects.
- Symptoms not evident during a medical examination or apparent to friends, family, or co-workers.

Stage 3: Mild cognitive decline

- Problems with memory or concentration; may be measurable in clinical testing or apparent during a detailed medical interview.
- Friends, family, or co-workers begin to notice deficiencies.
- Common difficulties include:
  1. Word- or name-finding problems noticeable to family or close associates
  2. Decreased ability to remember names when introduced to new people
  3. Performance issues in social or work settings
  4. Reading a passage and retaining little material
  5. Losing or misplacing a valuable object
  6. Decline in ability to plan or organize

Stage 4: Moderate cognitive decline (Mild or early-stage Alzheimer's disease)

- The affected individual may seem subdued and withdrawn, especially in socially or mentally challenging situations.
- Clear-cut deficiencies in the following areas:
  1. Decreased knowledge of recent occasions or current events
  2. Impaired ability to perform challenging mental arithmetic (e.g., counting backward from 100 by 7s)
  3. Decreased capacity to perform complex tasks, such as marketing, planning dinner for guests, or paying bills and managing finances
  4. Reduced memory of personal history

Stage 5: Moderately severe cognitive decline (Moderate or mid-stage Alzheimer's disease)

- Major gaps in memory and deficits in cognitive function emerge. Some assistance with day-to-day activities becomes essential.
- Individuals may:
  1. Be unable during a medical interview to recall such important details as their current address, their telephone number, or the name of the college or high school from which they graduated
  2. Become confused about where they are or about the date, day of the week, or season

  3. Have trouble with less challenging mental arithmetic (e.g., counting backward from 40 by 4s or from 20 by 2s)
  4. Need help choosing proper clothing for the season or the occasion
  5. Usually retain substantial knowledge about themselves and know their own name and the names of their spouse or children
  6. Usually require no assistance with eating or using the toilet

Stage 6: Severe cognitive decline (Moderately severe or mid-stage Alzheimer's disease)

- Memory difficulties continue to worsen, significant personality changes may emerge, and affected individuals need extensive help with customary daily activities.
- Individuals may:
  1. Lose most awareness of recent experiences and events as well as of their surroundings
  2. Recollect their personal history imperfectly, although generally able to recall their own name
  3. Occasionally forget the name of their spouse or primary caregiver but generally can distinguish familiar from unfamiliar faces
  4. Need help getting dressed properly; without supervision, may make such errors as putting pajamas over daytime clothes or shoes on wrong feet
  5. Experience disruption of their normal sleep/wake cycle
  6. Need help with handling details of toileting (flushing toilet, wiping, and disposing of tissue properly)
  7. Have increasing episodes of urinary or fecal incontinence
  8. Experience significant personality changes and behavioral symptoms, including suspiciousness and delusions, hallucinations, or compulsive, repetitive behaviors
  9. Tend to wander and become lost

Stage 7: Very severe cognitive decline (Severe or late-stage Alzheimer's disease)

- This is the final stage of the disease when individuals lose the ability to respond to their environment, the ability to speak, and, ultimately, the ability to control movement.
  1. Lose capacity for recognizable speech, although words or phrases may occasionally be uttered
  2. Need help with eating and toileting and there is general incontinence of urine
  3. Lose the ability to walk without assistance, and then the ability to sit without support, the ability to smile, and the ability to hold their head up
  4. Reflexes become abnormal and muscles grow rigid; swallowing is impaired

From Reisberg B, Ferris SH, de Leon MJ, Crook T: The global deterioration scale for assessment of primary degenerative dementia, *Am J Psychiatry* 139:1136, 1982. Copyright © 1983 by Barry Reisberg, MD. Reproduced with permission.

Table 8-2 | Multi-Infarct Versus Alzheimer-Type Dementia

FACTORS SUGGESTING DEMENTIA	HACHINSKI ISCHEMIA POINT SCORE*
Abrupt onset	2
Stepwise deterioration	1
Fluctuating course	2
Emotional lability	1
Relative preservation of personality	1
Depression	1
Somatic complaints	1
History of hypertension	1
History of strokes	2
Evidence of associated arteriosclerosis	1
Focal neurological symptoms[†]	2
Focal neurological signs[†]	2

*A score of 4 or more is indicative of Alzheimer-type dementia. A score of 7 or more is indicative of multi-infarct dementia.
[†]Focal neurological signs/symptoms: exaggerated DTRs, positive Babinski sign, gait abnormalities, hemiparesis.
From Siu AL: Screening for dementia and investigating its causes, *Ann Intern Med* 115:122, 1991.

DIFFERENTIAL DIAGNOSIS OF *Common Causes of Delirium, Confusion, Dementia, and Depression*

CONDITION	HISTORY	PHYSICAL FINDINGS	DIAGNOSTIC STUDIES
Delirium	Onset abrupt; fluctuations over course of day common with lucid intervals during day and worst symptoms at night; lasts hours to weeks; unable to maintain attention to external stimuli; disorganized thinking, perceptual disturbances, disturbed sleep/wake cycle; hallucinations, usually visual, common	Decreased LOC, impaired arousal, decreased psychomotor activity; disoriented, most commonly to time; physical examination findings depend on underlying cause of delirium; patient often exhibits asterixis, tremor, and difficulty in motor relaxation; speech incoherent, hesitant, slow, or rapid	CBC, electrolytes, glucose, BUN, creatinine, LFTs, TFTs, serum B_{12}, folate, serology for syphilis, ABGs, toxicology screen, blood alcohol level, U/A, ECG, EEG, chest radiograph, lumbar puncture, CT or MRI (when CVA or injury suspected)
Confusion	Less abrupt, less severe than delirium; diurnal variation less severe than delirium; concentration impaired, easily distracted; errors in thinking common	Apathetic, drowsy; disoriented especially for time, but less for place, almost never for self; less severe disorientation, more subtle motor signs than in delirium	CBC, electrolytes, glucose, BUN, creatinine, LFTs, TFTs, serum B_{12}, folate, serology for syphilis, ABGs, toxicology screen, blood alcohol level, U/A, ECG, EEG, chest radiograph, lumbar puncture, CT or MRI (when CVA or injury is suspected)

Continued

DIFFERENTIAL DIAGNOSIS OF *Common Causes of Delirium, Confusion, Dementia, and Depression—cont'd*			
CONDITION	**HISTORY**	**PHYSICAL FINDINGS**	**DIAGNOSTIC STUDIES**
Dementia	Onset insidious, course stable through day and night; present for months or years, with progressive deterioration; recent and remote memory impaired; hallucinations usually absent until late in course of disease; sleep often fragmented	Alert, attentive; orientation usually impaired; on mental status examination, patient tries hard, provides "near miss" answers; demonstrates one or more of following cognitive disturbances: aphasia (language disturbance); apraxia (impaired ability to carry out motor activities despite intact motor function); agnosia (failure to identify or recognize objects despite intact sensory function); disturbance in executive functioning (planning, organizing, sequencing, abstracting); physical findings often absent in Alzheimer type; olfactory sense can be impaired; speech usually unimpaired although difficulty with finding words; findings in multi-infarct dementia include focal neurological signs/symptoms: exaggerated DTRs, positive Babinski sign, gait abnormalities, hemiparesis	CBC, electrolytes, glucose, BUN, creatinine, LFTs, TFTs, serum B_{12}, folate, serology for syphilis, ABGs, toxicology screen, blood alcohol level, U/A, ECG, EEG, chest radiograph, lumbar puncture, CT or MRI (when CVA or injury suspected; does not yield useful information for dementia); PET scan
Depression	Onset of confusion often abrupt, with some diurnal variation, generally more consistent over time than delirium; confusion of short duration compared to dementia; past history of psychiatric problems common, including undiagnosed depressive episodes; cognitive losses fluctuating rather than stable over time; sleep/appetite disturbance; hallucinations usually absent although person can have suicidal thoughts	Depressed or anxious mood; tends to highlight disabilities, especially memory loss; memory loss equal for recent and remote events; physical examination often normal	Geriatric Depression Scale in elderly; CBC, electrolytes, glucose, BUN, creatinine, LFTs, TFTs, serum B_{12}, folate, serology for syphilis, ABGs, toxicology screen, blood alcohol level, U/A, ECG, EEG, chest radiograph, lumbar puncture, CT or MRI (when CVA or injury suspected)

ABGs, arterial blood gases; *BUN,* blood urea nitrogen; *CBC,* complete blood count; *CT,* computed tomography; *CVA,* costovertebral angle; *DTRs,* deep tendon reflexes; *ECG,* electrocardiography; *EEG,* electroencephalography; *LFTs,* liver function tests; *LOC,* level of consciousness; *MRI,* magnetic resonance imaging; *PET,* positron emission tomography; *TFTs,* thyroid function tests; *U/A,* urinalysis.

REFERENCES AND READINGS

Adelman AM, Daly MP: Initial evaluation of the patient with suspected dementia, *Am Fam Physician* 71:745, 2005.

Alistair Burns A, Iliffe S: Dementia, *BMJ* 338:405, 2009.

American Psychiatric Association: *Diagnostic and statistical manual of mental disorders*, ed 4, text revision: DSM-IV-TR, Washington, DC, 2000, American Psychiatric Association.

Bostwick JM: The many faces of confusion: timing and collateral history often hold the key to diagnosis, *Postgrad Med* 108:60, 2000.

Espino DV, Jules-Bradley AC, Johnston CL, Mouton CP: Diagnostic approach to the confused elderly patient, *Am Fam Physician* 57:1358, 1998.

Galvin JE, Roe CM, Powlishta KK, Coats MA, Muich SJ, Grant E et al: The AD8: a brief informant interview to detect dementia, *Neurology* 65:559, 2005.

Gleason OC: Delirium, *Am Fam Physician* 67:1027, 2003.

McCusker J, Cole MG, Dendukuri N, Belzile E: The Delirium Index: a measure of the severity of delirium: new findings on reliability, validity, and responsiveness, *J Am Geriatr Soc* 52:1744, 2004.

Sendelbach S, Guthrie PF: Evidence-based practice guideline: acute confusion/delirium. Iowa City (IA): University of Iowa Gerontological Nursing Interventions Research Center, Research Translation and Dissemination Core; 2009 Mar. 66 p. National Guideline Clearinghouse 7:14340, Dec 2009. Available online at http://www.guideline.gov/content.aspx?doc_id=14340. Accessed September 24, 2010.

Snyderman D, Rovner B: Mental status exam in primary care: a review, *Am Fam Physician* 80:809, 2009.

Thibault JM, Steiner RW: Efficient identification of adults with depression and dementia, *Am Fam Physician* 70:1101, 2004.

Wei LA, Fearing MA, Sternberg EJ, Inouye SK: The Confusion Assessment Method: A systematic review of current usage, *J Am Ger Soc* 56:823, 2008.

Young J, Sharon K, Inouye SK: Delirium in older people, *BMJ* 334:842, 2007.

Constipation

Constipation is a common symptom and is a subjective interpretation of a disturbance of bowel function. There is lack of general agreement on the norms for stool frequency, size, or consistency, with considerable uncertainty on how much deviation is required to warrant the label of constipation. Generally, constipation refers to a failure to completely evacuate the lower colon. This is associated with difficulty in defecating, infrequent bowel movements, straining, abdominal pain, and pain on defecating. It can also refer to hardness of stool or a feeling of incomplete evacuation. Obstipation refers to intractable constipation or the regular passage of hard stools at 3- to 5-day intervals.

There are five areas in the defecation process where interference can cause a disturbance in motility and lead to clinical problems: (1) the peristaltic reflex, (2) the spinal arc, (3) relaxation of the anal sphincter, (4) contraction of the voluntary muscle associated with defecation, and (5) the autonomic and cortical control of defecation. Both functional and organic disturbances can cause constipation.

Acute constipation refers to a sudden change for that individual, suggesting an organic cause, such as mechanical obstruction, adynamic ileus, or traumatic interruption of the nervous system from medications or following anesthesia. Persistent constipation occurs when the condition lasts for weeks or occurs intermittently with increasing frequency or severity. Partial obstruction or local anorectal conditions could be the cause.

Chronic constipation occurs as the result of disruption of the storage, transport, and evacuation mechanisms of the colon. Functional causes are the most common and include poor bowel habits; inadequate intake of dietary fiber, bulk, and fluids; and anal fissure pain. Genetic predisposition to constipation seems to exist.

DIAGNOSTIC REASONING: FOCUSED HISTORY

Is this really constipation?

Key Questions

- How many stools are there per day?
- What is the consistency of the stool?

Frequency of Stool

Stool frequency is the easiest parameter to quantify. In the general adult population, the "normal" frequency of bowel movements ranges from 3 to 12 per week. Having fewer than three bowel movements per week is considered constipation.

Infants and children have decreasing stool frequency with age, from more than 4 stools per day during the first week of life to 1.2 per day at age 4. Infants who have a fewer number of stools than average are at greater risk of developing constipation.

Alternating episodes of constipation and diarrhea are characteristic of irritable bowel syndrome (IBS). Patients describe their constipation stools as hard, round balls.

Stool Consistency

Dry, hard stools suggest a lack of sufficient dietary fluids or fiber. Stools that are marginally frequent but are soft and moist do not indicate constipation, whereas this same number of stools that are hard and dry would indicate constipation. Liquid stool and fecal incontinence, particularly in children and the elderly, can represent stool impaction and overflow.

What red flags do I need to consider?

Key Questions

- Is there any rectal bleeding or blood in the stool?
- Have you had an unintentional weight loss >10 lb?

- Have you had inflammatory bowel disease (IBD)?
- Have you or your family members had colorectal cancer?

Bleeding

Black stools can indicate bleeding from a site in the upper gastrointestinal (GI) tract because blood mixed with gastric acid makes the stools appear black. Bright red blood indicates bleeding from the lower GI tract and can indicate a mass. Hemorrhoids and anal/rectal fissures can also produce bleeding. Brisk bleeding is uncommon with hemorrhoids and requires immediate investigation.

Unintentional Weight Loss

An unintended weight loss of greater than 10 pounds can signal an underlying cancer (see Chapter 36).

History of IBD/Colorectal Cancer

The patient with a history of IBD (Crohn disease or ulcerative colitis) or with a personal or family history of colorectal cancer is at increased risk for colorectal cancer. A change in bowel habits can signal an intestinal tumor.

Is the constipation acute or chronic?

Key Questions

- When did the constipation start?
- How long have you been constipated?
- Is this an individual episode or is it chronic?
- At what age did the constipation first begin?

Onset and Duration

Recent onset usually reflects changes in lifestyle or physical health, such as dietary changes, activity changes, new medications, partially obstructing lesions, or recent illness. Chronic constipation or constipation of long duration is usually associated either with functional causes, such as lack of dietary fiber and bulk, or with concurrent systemic disorders, such as diabetes mellitus (DM) or hypothyroidism.

Age of Onset

New-onset constipation in adults older than age 40 is suspicious for colon lesions. Constipation in the newborn is likely to have an anatomical cause. In infants, the cause is likely inadequate fluid and fiber in the diet. In children, the cause is likely to be diet as well as developmental and psychological factors. In adults, the cause is usually related to dietary and bowel habits.

If the constipation is acute, what conditions should I consider?

Key Questions

- Have you been ill recently?
- Have you had a fever?
- Do you have any chronic health problems?

Recent Illness

Dehydration and fever cause hardening of the stools by diminishing intestinal secretions and increasing water absorption from the colon. A transient period of constipation is common during an acute febrile illness. Also, reflex ileus is sometimes seen with pneumonia.

Chronic Illness

Hardened stools are found in patients with renal acidosis and diabetes insipidus. Infants and children with hypotonia of the abdominal and intestinal musculature from neurological conditions are predisposed to constipation.

Neurological gut dysfunction, myopathies, endocrine disorders, and electrolyte abnormalities can cause constipation. Constipation in infants can be an early symptom of congenital hypothyroidism.

If the constipation is chronic or recurrent, what should I consider?

Key Questions

- What do you usually eat in a day?
- How many glasses of liquid do you drink each day?
- Do you eat breakfast?
- What are your usual bowel habits?
- How active are you?
- What medications are you taking?
- Do you use laxatives? How often do you take laxatives? How long have you used laxatives?

Dietary Pattern

A 3-day dietary history is more accurate than a 24-hour recall, although a 24-hour recall can provide a reasonable picture of the patient's dietary habits. Diets that lack roughage result in lack of fecal bulk, causing an inadequate stimulus for peristaltic movement. Diets that are high in protein result in complete digestion of the protein, leaving little residue to stimulate movement. Diets high in calcium content lead to the formation of calcium caseinate in the stools, which does not stimulate peristalsis. Teenagers often drink several quarts of milk per day, causing constipation. Inadequate fluid intake (less than six 8-ounce glasses per day) contributes to dry, hard, and infrequent stools.

Breakfast
Colonic motility is greatest following breakfast. Skipping this meal decreases the postprandial effect associated with food intake.

Bowel Habits
Postponing a bowel movement because of time constraints or other reasons suppresses the normal gastrocolic reflex and can produce constipation.

Activity Level
Constipation is a common problem in individuals with a sedentary lifestyle. The lack of physical activity reduces the peristaltic reflex. Over-activity can also cause constipation due to the lack of adequate fluid replacement.

Medications
Medications that commonly cause or contribute to constipation include narcotics, imipramine, diuretics, calcium channel blockers, anticholinergics, psychotropic agents, antacids, decongestants, anticonvulsants, iron, bismuth, and lead.

Use of Enemas, Laxatives, and Suppositories
Use of stimulants to empty the colon removes the peristalsis stimulus for 2 to 3 days. Diarrhea is usually followed by infrequent stools for several days. Chronic use of stimulants can produce chronic atonic constipation.

How can I further narrow the causes?

Key Questions
- What does your stool look like?
- Is the stool size large or small?
- What is the general shape of the stool (e.g., small, round, ribbonlike)?
- Is the stool formed or liquid?

- Have you had any involuntary loss of stool?
- Does the constipation alternate with periods of diarrhea?

Size or Caliber of Stool
Infrequent passage of small, hard stools can indicate congenital aganglionic megacolon. Very large stools can indicate functional constipation, with the size of the stools a function of the size of the colon. Ribbonlike stools suggest a motility disorder, such as IBS. They can also be caused by narrowing of the distal or sigmoid colon from an organic lesion. A progressive decrease in the caliber of stool suggests an organic lesion. Stools with a toothpaste-like caliber suggest fecal impaction. Constipation can also be the result of dietary habits and can be seen in teenagers who drink several quarts of milk per day.

Consistency of Stool/Fecal Incontinence
Dry, hard stools suggest a lack of sufficient dietary fluids or fiber. Liquid stool and fecal incontinence, particularly in the elderly, can represent stool impaction and overflow. Overflow incontinence in children can indicate constipation from a fecal impaction.

Alternating Constipation and Diarrhea
Alternating episodes are characteristic of IBS. Patients often describe the stool during the constipation episodes as hard and pellet-like.

What else do I need to consider?

Key Questions
- Do you have the urge to defecate?
- Do you have any urinary tract symptoms?
- Do you have any nausea or vomiting?
- Is there any pain with defecation?
- Is there any bleeding with defecation? How much?
- What color are your stools? Are the stools very dark colored or black?

Urge to Defecate
Children with Hirschsprung disease (aganglionic megacolon) do not have an urge to defecate because the stool accumulates proximal to the lower portion of the rectum where the proprioceptors for defecation are located. Evidence of stiffening, squeezing, and crying indicates stool is being propelled to the rectum. Adults

who overuse laxatives or other stimulants also cannot experience the urge to defecate.

Associated Urinary Tract Problems

Voiding problems can indicate an abdominal mass. Day and night enuresis is seen in some children with encopresis (fecal soiling). Rarely does a neurological lesion produce fecal incontinence without a disturbance in bladder control.

Vomiting

Bilious vomiting can indicate intestinal obstruction in the newborn. Vomiting associated with pain in adults can indicate obstruction.

Pain

Chronic recurrent abdominal pain is commonly present in constipation. Pain is intermittent and can be localized to the periumbilical region. Crampy lower abdominal pain is usually caused by bowel distention, which can result from IBS, intermittent obstruction, or adhesions. Noncrampy dull pain in the left abdomen is associated with diverticulosis. Pain on defecation can indicate an anal or a rectal lesion, such as hemorrhoids or anal fissures.

Bleeding

Bright red blood in the stool indicates hemorrhoids, fissure, or possible rectal mass. Black stools can indicate bleeding from a site in the upper GI tract because blood mixed with gastric acid makes the stools appear black. Brisk bleeding is uncommon with hemorrhoids and requires immediate thorough investigation.

Color

Red stools can be the result of using laxatives of vegetable origin or ingestion of foods, such as red beets. A black or very dark brown color can be caused by drugs, such as iron and bismuth, both of which contribute to constipation.

If this is a child, is there anything else I need to consider?

Key Questions

- Is there fecal soiling of underpants?
- Is there crying with defecation?
- If an infant: Is there a history of delayed passage of meconium stool?

- Has the child begun to drink milk?
- Has the child recently started toilet training?
- Does the child have urinary frequency?

Crying with Defecation

Small children with constipation will cry with movement when a fissure is present. With large hard stools, the child will not want to defecate because of the pain and will do stool-holding mannerisms, such as sitting and standing still.

Fecal Soiling of Underpants

Repeated fecal soiling from involuntary passage of small amounts of feces into the underpants of children older than age 4 is consistent with encopresis from functional megacolon secondary to chronic constipation. The constipation is usually secondary to painful defecation, with a resultant anal fissure. Coercive bowel training, fear of the toilet, or reactive voluntary withholding of bowel movements can also cause this condition.

History of Delayed Passage of Meconium Stool

Such a history can indicate congenital aganglionic megacolon (Hirschsprung disease).

Change in Diet

Cow's milk is a common cause of constipation in young children who have been on breast milk or formula.

Toilet Training

Some children develop stool withholding when toilet training is initiated.

History of Urinary Frequency

Urinary frequency, enuresis, and urinary tract infections can be the result of constipation. Fecal soiling can cause urinary tract infection by the ascending of the fecal flora. Further, an enlarged dilated rectum can push on the bladder, causing frequent need to urinate.

Is there a family history or genetic predisposition?

Key Question

- Is there a family history of constipation or IBS?

Genetic predisposition to constipation seems to exist. It is common for more than one family member to have a history of chronic constipation or IBS.

DIAGNOSTIC REASONING: FOCUSED PHYSICAL EXAMINATION
Plot Growth Curve in Children

Slow growth can indicate congenital aganglionic megacolon. Also incorrect formula mixing, underfeeding, starvation, and anorexia nervosa can first be recognized by a complaint of constipation.

Perform Abdominal Examination

Observe abdominal contour, looking for distention. Abdominal distention is frequently not marked in patients with functional constipation but can be present with other causes. Auscultate for bowel sounds. Silent or abnormal bowel sounds can also indicate an organic cause, such as obstruction. On palpation, stool can be felt as mobile, nontender masses in the left lower quadrant (LLQ). Firm, rubbery masses of stool palpable in the right lower quadrant (RLQ) in newborns can indicate meconium ileus. Palpable abdominal masses or organomegaly point to an organic cause. Note tenderness, which can indicate an organic cause, although a tender bowel can be palpable in IBS. Inspect the sacral region of the back. The presence of dimpling could indicate a spinal deformity contributing to the constipation.

Look for hernias. Large abdominal wall hernias can interfere with the ability to generate the intraabdominal pressure that is required to initiate defecation.

Perform Digital Rectal Examination

On perianal inspection, look for skin excoriation, skin tags, fissures, strictures, tears, or hemorrhoids, any of which can cause painful defecation. Early fissures have the appearance of superficial erosions. More advanced lesions are linear or elliptical breaks in the skin. Long-standing fissures are deep and indurated. Internal fissures are seen when the anal sphincter relaxes as the examining finger is withdrawn. To examine for a fissure in a child, place the infant/child in the knee-chest position and spread the buttocks to reveal the mucocutaneous junction of the anus.

Look for rectal prolapse and feel for a rectocele, which might interfere with defecation. A normal anal sphincter with an empty rectal ampulla can indicate Hirschsprung disease. In functional constipation, expect to find a large dilated rectum full of stool. Sphincter tone is increased in functional problems and strictures but is decreased in neurological diseases. The presence of a mass in the rectum indicates an impaction or obstructive lesion. A pilonidal dimple is seen with spinal bifida occulta.

Perform a Focused Neurological Examination

Test relevant deep tendon and superficial reflexes. Interruption of T12-S3 nerves causes loss of voluntary control of defecation (Table 9-1).

LABORATORY AND DIAGNOSTIC STUDIES
Fecal Occult Blood Test

A positive fecal occult blood test (FOBT) indicates blood in the stool, which can be the result of ulcerative or malignant lesions. The sensitivity of this test in detecting colorectal cancers and adenomas ranges from 50% to 90%. It is an inexpensive and noninvasive method to screen for bleeding lesions. A stool sample is placed on filter paper, and an activating solution is applied. A positive test is indicated by the appearance of a color (usually blue or green). Serial testing (3 days) is done using stool cards at home that are returned by mail for analysis. Annual FOBT, beginning at age 50 years, is one of the recommended screening tests for colon cancer. The Evidence-Based Practice box describes the current recommendations.

Table 9-1	Superficial and Deep Tendon Reflexes and Spinal Level Tested
REFLEX	**SPINAL LEVEL TESTED**
Superficial	
Upper abdominal	T7, T8, T9
Lower abdominal	T10, T11
Cremasteric	T12, L1, L2
Deep	
Biceps	C5, C6
Brachioradial	C5, C6
Triceps	C6, C7, C8
Patellar	L2, L3, L4
Achilles	S1, S2

◎   EVIDENCE-BASED PRACTICE   *Screening for Colon Cancer*

The preferred screening for asymptomatic persons at average risk is cancer prevention testing. Patients who decline cancer prevention testing should be offered cancer detection tests. Average risk patients are those who are age ≥50 years and who have:

- No personal history adenoma or colorectal cancer (CRC)
- No personal history of IBD
- Negative family history (no first-degree relative or two second-degree relatives with CRC)

Cancer Prevention Tests

- Cancer prevention tests should be offered first. The preferred CRC prevention test is colonoscopy every 10 years, beginning at age 50 years (Grade 1 B). Screening should begin at age 45 years in African Americans (Grade 2 C).

Alternative CRC Prevention Tests

- Flexible sigmoidoscopy every 5-10 years (Grade 2 B)
- CT colonography every 5 years (Grade 1 C)

Cancer Detection Tests

- The preferred cancer detection test is annual FIT for blood (Grade 1 B).

Alternative Cancer Detection Tests

- Annual Hemoccult Sensa (Grade 1 B)
- Fecal DNA testing every 3 years (Grade 2 B)

Grade of Recommendation/Description

- 1A/Strong recommendation, high-quality evidence
- 1B/Strong recommendation, moderate-quality evidence
- 1C/Strong recommendation, low-quality or very low-quality evidence
- 2A/Weak recommendation, high-quality evidence
- 2B/Weak recommendation, moderate-quality evidence
- 2C/Weak recommendation, low-quality or very low-quality evidence

Data from Rex DK, Johnson DA, Anderson JC, Schoenfeld PS, Burke CA, Inadomi JM: American College of Gastroenterology guidelines for colorectal cancer screening 2008, *Am J Gastroenterol* 104:739, 2009.

Fecal Immunochemical Test

Also called immunochemical FOBT (iFOBT), fecal immunochemical test (FIT) can be used as an alternative to FOBT. FIT uses antibodies to human globin to detect a specific portion of a human blood protein. FIT does not react with non–human hemoglobin or peroxidase, so food restrictions before the test are not necessary. Immunochemical FOBTs are also more specific for lower GI tract bleeding because they target the globin portion of hemoglobin, which does not survive passage through the upper GI tract. This test is done essentially the same way as conventional FOBT, but is more specific and reduces the number of false positive results. Vitamins or foods do not affect the FIT, and some forms require only one or two stool specimens.

Fecal/Stool DNA

Cells from precancerous polyps and cancerous tumors are shed in the stool and contain recognizable DNA markers. A stool DNA test can identify several of these markers, indicating the presence of precancerous polyps or colon cancer.

Complete Blood Count

Obtain a complete blood count (CBC) when you suspect bleeding. Hematocrit and hemoglobin levels will be below the expected reference range with a bleeding lesion.

Serum Electrolytes

Severely ill patients can develop hypokalemia and hypercalcemia, which are causes of constipation. Patients on thiazide diuretics can develop hypokalemia and subsequent constipation.

Serum Thyroid-Stimulating Hormone

An elevated thyroid-stimulating hormone (TSH) level can suggest hypothyroidism, which can be a cause of constipation. Screen for elevated TSH levels in persons with other symptoms suggestive of hypothyroidism, such as sparse, coarse, dry hair; hirsutism; dry skin; or hoarse speech.

Urinalysis

A urinalysis and culture should be done if a child has an associated rectosigmoid impaction because of encopresis.

Anoscopy

Anoscopy is indicated if digital rectal examination detects hemorrhoids, fissures, strictures, or masses in the anus or rectum. It enables a view of the immediate internal anal canal that is not possible on manual digital rectal examination. A hand-held anoscope is warmed, lubricated, and slowly eased into the anus while the patient bears down to relax the external sphincter muscle. A light source is necessary; a head lamp is preferable. Anoscopy may not be possible initially with a fissure or abscess because of the pain. However, it should be performed on a follow-up visit to detect IBD or rectal cancer.

Flexible Sigmoidoscopy and Colonoscopy

These tests are indicated for patients in whom conservative treatment fails; for persons older than age 50 years or with new-onset constipation; and for persons with anemia or fecal occult blood. Colonoscopy is indicated for the patient with rectal bleeding.

Barium Enema

This contrast technique can be used to detect diverticula, polyps, and masses. It is also used to determine the extent of dilated bowel in megacolon. The barium enema in children is reserved to rule out Hirschsprung disease. A barium enema is contraindicated if enterocolitis is suspected.

Colon Transit Studies

Colon transit studies are useful for patients with severe chronic constipation that responds poorly to treatment.

Anorectal Manometry

This test measures the pressure of the anal sphincter muscles, the sensation in the rectum, and the neural reflexes that are needed for normal bowel movements. The manometry probe, a thin tube of soft plastic or rigid metal, is inserted into the rectum about 4 inches and then slowly withdrawn halfway. As the probe is withdrawn, the transducer continuously records the pressure at different points. Alternatively, the pressure can be measured with a balloon manometry system, a hollow metal cylinder to which three balloons are attached to measure pressure during anal contraction. A balloon at the tip of the probe is inflated to determine whether the patient feels a sensation of rectal fullness and an urge to defecate.

DIFFERENTIAL DIAGNOSIS

Despite the high prevalence of constipation, only a small number of adults or children with constipation have a significant abnormality. In otherwise healthy individuals, first consider functional causes, particularly dietary, fluid, bowel, and laxative habits. In adults, depression can be associated with constipation.

Simple Constipation

Typically individuals with simple constipation report a diet low in fiber and bulk and/or inadequate fluid intake. A sedentary lifestyle is common. They also often report pain before and with bowel movements because of the hard, dry nature of the stools. Patients can also complain of loss of appetite. The physical examination of the abdomen and rectum is normal. It may be possible to feel fecal masses in the colon and rectum. No diagnostic workup is needed unless the patient does not respond to therapy.

Functional Constipation

Functional constipation is seen in children who have large, hard stools that become difficult or painful to pass. The resulting fecal retention sets up a cycle in which the sensitivity of the defecation reflex and the effectiveness of peristalsis lessen. Watery stool from the proximal colon soils the underwear. On physical examination, stool is present in the LLQ and the rectum is dilated and filled with packed stool. The external sphincter is intact.

Irritable Bowel Syndrome

IBS is common in adults, with onset usually in young adulthood. The presenting complaint can be either diarrhea or constipation. Alternating episodes of each is characteristic of IBS. Mucus in the stools is common. Abdominal pain often occurs, usually in the LLQ, and the bowel may be tender to palpation. A tender bowel may be palpable (see Chapter 11).

Fecal Impaction

Fecal impaction is common in older adults and in those who are confined to bed. The passage of hard stools at 3- to 5-day intervals can occur. Some persons with impaction have continuous diarrhea-like passage of stools and can experience incontinence. Stools can be of small caliber, sometimes described as toothpaste-like. On rectal examination, large quantities of hard feces will be palpable in the rectal ampulla. On abdominal examination, feces-filled bowel may be palpable.

Idiopathic Slow Transit

This condition is most common in older persons, especially those who are less active and have inadequate dietary fiber and fluid intake. These patients experience decreased stool frequency; stools are typically dry and hard.

Hirschsprung Disease (Congenital Aganglionic Megacolon)

Hirschsprung disease is present from birth and is usually detected in young children. Delayed passage of meconium stool can indicate Hirschsprung disease in infants. Children with Hirschsprung disease do not have an urge to defecate because the stools accumulate proximal to the lower portion of the rectum where the proprioceptors for defecation are located. Evidence of stiffening, squeezing, and crying indicates stool is being propelled to the rectum. On examination the rectal ampulla is empty.

Secondary Constipation from Anorectal Lesion

Because defecation is painful with an anorectal lesion, the patient suppresses it. With the eventual passage of hard stools, the patient can report blood on the surface of the stool, on the toilet paper, or in the toilet. On digital rectal examination, look for hemorrhoids (very rare in children), fissures, tears, or abrasions.

Drug-Induced Constipation

Drug-induced constipation is consistent with a history of chronic laxative use or taking those medications that can produce constipation. It occurs most often in older persons. Abdominal and rectal examinations are usually normal.

Tumors

Tumors are uncommon in children, and the frequency increases in the population over the age of 40. Colicky abdominal pain and distention can occur in persons with bowel tumors. Persons with rectosigmoid tumors may report rectal discomfort, stool leakage, urgency, and tenesmus. The patient may report rectal bleeding or blood in the stool. Stool may test positive for occult blood. An abdominal mass may be palpable. Elderly patients who present with constipation, anemia, anorexia, and weight loss are at high suspicion for colorectal cancer. Constipation occurs in less than one third of persons with colon cancer; diarrhea is more common. Onset is recent, and there can be progressive narrowing of stool caliber.

DIFFERENTIAL DIAGNOSIS OF *Common Causes of Constipation*

CONDITION	HISTORY	PHYSICAL FINDINGS	DIAGNOSTIC STUDIES
Simple constipation	Low dietary fiber and bulk; inadequate fluid intake; physical inactivity; pain before and with bowel movements; anorexia	Normal abdominal and rectal examination; can feel fecal masses in colon and rectum	None if resolved; consider colonoscopy/ sigmoidoscopy, anorectal manometry, colon transit studies if not resolved
Functional constipation	Preschool and school-age children; history of abdominal pain and stool soiling	Palpable stool in LLQ; large dilated rectum with packed stool; external sphincter intact	Abdominal radiography, unprepped barium radiography
Irritable bowel syndrome (IBS)	Onset in young adulthood; alternating diarrhea and constipation; mucus in stools	Can have tender, palpable colon	Colonoscopy/ sigmoidoscopy if indicated
Obstipation/ impaction	Passage of hard stool at 3- to 5-day intervals; diarrhea, small caliber stools; common in those confined to bed	Hard feces in rectal ampulla; can have palpable feces-filled bowel	Colonoscopy/ sigmoidoscopy if indicated
Slow transit	Common in older adults; physical inactivity; decreased stool frequency; stool dry and hard	Normal abdominal and rectal examination	Colonoscopy/FOBT or FIT to rule out tumors; consider anorectal manometry, colon transit studies
Hirschsprung disease	Delayed passage of meconium at birth; no urge to defecate	Empty rectal ampulla on examination	Colonoscopy

DIFFERENTIAL DIAGNOSIS OF *Common Causes of Constipation—cont'd*

CONDITION	HISTORY	PHYSICAL FINDINGS	DIAGNOSTIC STUDIES
Anorectal lesions	Rectal pain on defecation; history of hemorrhoids; blood on stool, on toilet tissue, or in toilet	On rectal examination: hemorrhoids, fissures, tears, abrasions; increased sphincter tone	Anoscopy
Drug induced	History of chronic laxative use; history of taking medications that produce constipation	Normal rectal and abdominal examinations	None if resolved; consider colonoscopy/ sigmoidoscopy, barium enema if not resolved
Colorectal cancer	Recent onset: pain and abdominal distention, stool leakage, urgency; late onset: weight loss, anorexia; rectal bleeding; increased incidence over age 40; uncommon in children	Can have palpable abdominal mass or organomegaly	CBC, FOBT, FIT, fecal/stool DNA; colonoscopy

CBC, complete blood count; *FIT,* fecal immunochemical test; *FOBT,* fecal occult blood test; *LLQ,* left lower quadrant.

REFERENCES AND READINGS

American Gastroenterological Association (AGA): American Gastroenterological Association Medical Position Statement: Guidelines on Constipation, *Gastroenterology* 119:1761, 2000.

Arce DA, Ermocilla CA, Costa H: Evaluation of constipation, *Am Fam Physician* 65:2284, 2002.

Basson MD: Constipation, *eMedicine*, last updated Jan 28, 2009; available at http://www.emedicine.medscape.com/article/184704-overview. Accessed on September 24, 2010.

Bleser SD: Chronic constipation: let symptom type and severity direct treatment, *J Fam Pract* 55:587, 2009.

Borum ML: Constipation: evaluation and management, *Prim Care* 28:577, 2001.

Coughlin E: Assessment and management of pediatric constipation in primary care, *Pediatr Nurs* 29:296, 2004.

Dosh SA: Evaluation and treatment of constipation, *J Fam Pract* June:555, 2002.

Hsieh C: Treatment of constipation in older adults, *Am Fam Physician* 72:2277, 2005.

McCallum I, Ong S, Mercer-Jones MM: Chronic constipation in adults, *BMJ* 338:763, 2009.

Rao SS, Ozturk R, Laine L: Clinical utility of diagnostic tests for constipation in adults: a systematic review, *Am J Gastroenterol* 100:1605, 2005.

Rao SS: Constipation: evaluation and treatment, *Gastroenterol Clin North Am* 32:659, 2003.

Tobias N: Management principles of organic causes of childhood constipation, *J Pediatr Health Care* 22:12, 2008.

Wald A: Constipation, *Med Clin North Am* 84:1231, 2000.

Walia R: Recent advances in chronic constipation, *Current Opinion Pediatr* 21:645, 2009.

Youssef NN, Di Lorenzo C: Childhood constipation: evaluation and treatment, *J Clin Gastroenterol* 33:199, 2001.

Youssef NN: Adolescent constipation: evaluation and management, *Adolesc Med Clin* 15:37, 2004.

Cough

Cough is one of the most common symptoms for which patients seek health care. Cough occurs when inspiration is followed by an explosive expiration. Coughing promotes clearance of secretions and foreign bodies from the airways. Cough is usually the result of a reflex initiated by stimulation of the sensory nerve endings beneath and between the epithelium of the larynx and tracheobronchial tree. A cough arises from the stimulation of the cough reflex in the upper respiratory tract by postnasal drip, clearing of the throat, or both. The reflex stimulation follows the vagus nerve to the "cough center," which is located in the medulla oblongata of the brainstem. However, other anatomical locations can be stimulated and initiate the cough reflex, including the pleura, pericardium, ear canals, esophagus, and stomach. The cough reflex is absent in very young infants. Effective coughing can also be impossible in emaciated persons, in persons whose respiratory musculature is weak or paralyzed, and in those with massive ascites.

Although most coughs are a symptom of minor upper respiratory infections (URIs), such as the common cold, a persistent cough can greatly affect a patient's quality of life and ability to sleep. Keep in mind, however, that a cough in a patient in acute distress can signal a life-threatening problem (such as foreign body aspiration with occlusion of airway), severe asthma, escalating heart failure, or pneumonia.

DIAGNOSTIC REASONING: FOCUSED HISTORY

What type of cough is this?

Key Question

- How long have you had a cough?

Duration
Cough can be characterized by the following three categories of duration: (1) acute, less than 3 weeks; (2) subacute, lasting 3 to 8 weeks; and (3) chronic,

lasting more than 8 weeks. A cough of recent onset is most often the result of viral or bacterial infection in the respiratory system. Allergies can also precipitate acute onset of cough in both children and adults. Coughs of longer duration (>3 weeks) are more likely caused by chronic lung or heart disease, such as chronic obstructive pulmonary disease (COPD), cystic fibrosis, chronic bronchitis, asthma, postnasal drainage, heart failure, pertussis, and chronic sinusitis. Gastroesophageal reflux disease (GERD) and a foreign body in the ear canal should also be considered in both adults and children.

Is this cough related to a life-threatening condition?

Key Questions

- Are you short of breath?
- Do you have a history of heart failure?
- Do you have a history of asthma?
- If a child: Have you noticed the child putting small objects in his or her mouth?

Shortness of Breath
Cough associated with shortness of breath (SOB) usually suggests a physical obstruction of the airway caused by a foreign body or the effects of acute asthma. Persons with heart failure report orthopnea, paroxysmal nocturnal dyspnea (PND), cough with possible frothy sputum, possible weight gain with swollen feet and ankles, and often a history of heart disease. Cardiac failure of any kind results in decreased lung compliance and cough.

History of Asthma
Acute exacerbation of asthma is characterized by an irritating nonproductive cough that can progress to tachypnea, dyspnea, wheezing, grunting, cyanosis, fatigue, and finally respiratory and cardiac failure. Viral infection, especially respiratory syncytial virus

(RSV), parainfluenza viruses, and rhinoviruses, are the most important triggers of asthma in children.

Foreign Body

Consider a foreign body aspiration in any child. A child who has aspirated a foreign body can have a varied presentation; generally, the onset of cough is sudden and unexpected. A brief period of severe coughing, gagging, and choking occurs; then a quiet period ensues of no coughing. This can last for hours, days, or even months. A foreign body in the lower airway can produce either emphysema caused by a ball-valve phenomenon or complete distal atelectasis because of absorption of the trapped gas. A mobile foreign body in the lower airway can also produce a paroxysmal cough, with cyanotic episodes and stridor as a result of proximal migration and subglottic impaction.

A foreign body in the esophagus can also produce airway obstruction and cough as well as dysphasia to solid foods because the posterior trachea is compliant and adjacent to the anterior esophagus. Coins are the most frequently found foreign bodies.

What do I need to know if the cough is acute (<3 weeks' duration)?

Key Questions

- Do you have nasal congestion or a sore throat?
- Do you have or have you had a fever? Do you have chills?
- Do you have a headache?

Nasal Congestion

Nasal congestion occurs as a result of a cascade of events. First, the offending organism invades the epithelial cells of the upper respiratory tract. Inflammatory mediators are released, resulting in altered vascular permeability, edema, and nasal stuffiness. Stimulation of cholinergic nerves in the nose and upper respiratory tract leads to increased mucus production (rhinorrhea) and occasionally to bronchoconstriction, which causes cough. It is hypothesized that cellular damage to the nasopharynx is probably what causes the sore and scratchy throat.

Runny nose with cough and mild fever followed by a persistent cough for more than 1 week with clear to off-white mucus greater in the morning suggests bronchitis.

Nasal congestion or a sensation of postnasal discharge, especially associated with facial pain or pressure, suggests sinusitis. A history of bloody nasal discharge can also be present.

Infants with nasal congestion 3 days to 8 weeks after birth who have a cough but are afebrile could have *Chlamydia trachomatis*, contracted from the mother during childbirth. Older children, adolescents, and adults with a sore throat, fever, headache, and malaise progressing to a cough could have mycoplasmal pneumonia.

Fever

In adults, a temperature that is less than 38.3° C (101° F), small amounts of clear to yellow sputum production, nasal congestion, sore throat, and generalized malaise most frequently accompany acute cough with a viral etiology. Acute cough of a more serious nature (e.g., bacterial pneumonia) is usually accompanied by a temperature of greater than 38.3° C (101° F), chest pain, SOB, and purulent or dark sputum. Acute cough resulting from noninfectious processes (heart failure or pulmonary embolism) lacks the signs of infectious disease, such as fever, chills, and purulent sputum.

Viral infection is the most common cause of a low-grade fever in a child who has nasal congestion and little interruption of appetite and activity. An acute cough associated with a persistent fever, loss of appetite, and ill appearance indicates a more serious illness, such as bacterial pneumonia.

Headache

Headache pain can signal sinusitis as the cause of the cough (see Chapter 14).

What does the nature of the sputum tell me?

Key Questions

- Do you cough up sputum?
- Does it have an odor?
- How much have you coughed up?
- What color is the sputum?

Malodorous sputum suggests anaerobic infection of the lungs and sinuses. Very thick, tenacious, dark sputum is characteristic of bronchiectasis. Cloudy, thick sputum suggests lower respiratory tract infection but can also reflect an increase in the number of eosinophils from an asthmatic process. Viral bronchitis rarely causes more than 2 tablespoons of mucopurulent sputum per day. Bacterial bronchitis, however, is frequently associated with purulent sputum, often more than 2 tablespoons per day. Clear, mucoid sputum indicates allergic disorder. Hemoptysis, uncommon in children, usually indicates a more serious disease, such as bacterial pneumonia, an acute inflammatory bronchitis, cystic fibrosis, tumor, or a foreign body.

Children tend to swallow rather than expectorate sputum. Occasionally emesis will have mucus in it and can be used to identify the sputum. A child with a persistent cough and purulent sputum is likely to have an infectious lung disease.

What does the nature of the cough tell me?

Key Questions

- Is the cough getting worse or more frequent?
- What time of day is the cough most bothersome?
- If a child: Did the child have an episode of severe cough, gagging, and choking a few weeks ago?
- What type of work do you do?
- What does the cough sound like?

Severity and Progression of Cough

A cough in children or adults that becomes progressively worse can indicate pertussis. Pertussis has three stages. The first stage presents with a mild cough, rhinorrhea, conjunctivitis, and low-grade fever for 1 to 2 weeks. In the next stage, the cough becomes severe and comes in short paroxysms. There is a "whoop" on the inspiration effort at the end of the paroxysm. In the convalescent stage, the coughing and paroxysmal whooping decrease, but the cough can persist in a milder form for 3 months.

Young infants and older adults with pertussis do not "whoop."

A cough in children that begins with a history of mild URI followed in 2 to 3 days with a cough that is brassy in sound can indicate croup. The cough is usually worse at night. Symptoms escalate as compromise of the upper airway continues from the viral agent (usually parainfluenza). Obstruction increases, stridor becomes continuous, and there is nasal flaring and suprasternal, infrasternal, and intracostal retraction. The child is agitated and sits up. In most children recovery occurs within a few hours. However, any intensification of symptoms of respiratory obstruction requires hospitalization.

Persistent paroxysmal coughing is often associated with asthma.

Timing of Cough

Coughs that awaken persons at night are frequently associated with respiratory problems in which bronchial irritation is a factor, such as asthma or chronic bronchitis, or with nonrespiratory conditions, such as GERD or heart failure. A hallmark of asthma is coughing at night, usually between midnight and 2:00 AM. This is because of the low level of glucocorticol in the body at this time. A severe cough in the early morning indicates postnasal drip, cystic fibrosis, or bronchiectasis. Secretions accumulate through the night, and fits of coughing are followed by bronchorrhea. Cough that is worse at night indicates croup, postnasal drip, lower respiratory tract infection, and allergic reaction. A cough that disappears with sleep is a habit cough.

History of Choking Episode

Consider foreign body aspiration in any child with a cough lasting longer than 3 weeks. Frequently the caregivers report an episode of severe coughing and choking occurring 1 to 3 weeks before with a period of absence of cough (because the level of obstruction is in a lobar or segmental bronchus) and then sudden recurrence of coughing. This period of absence can last for hours, days, or even months. The cough can reappear when irritation of the foreign body or reaction to the foreign body occurs.

Occupation

An occupational and hobby review is warranted. Asbestos or coal dust exposure increases a person's risk of lung disease, including lung cancer. Aerosol sprays, insecticides, chemical exposures, and sawdust can cause cough.

Nature of the Cough

A throat-clearing cough is indicative of postnasal drip caused by irritation of the cough receptors in the pharynx, which are sensitive to mechanical stimulation, such as secretions. A dry, brassy cough indicates pharyngeal or tracheal irritation, allergy, or habit. A loose or moist cough can indicate lung disease, such as cystic fibrosis or asthma.

A paroxysmal cough is seen with asthma, pertussis, and cystic fibrosis and occasionally after inhalation of a foreign body. A barking, croupy cough indicates an irritation in the glottic and subglottic area. A sudden short burst of a cough in infants, called a staccato cough, is indicative of *Chlamydia trachomatis*. A harsh, dry cough caused by airway compression from enlarged nodes in the perihilar or paratracheal region seems to occur with tuberculosis (TB) or fungal infection.

A loud, bizarre cough that seems to be attention seeking can have a psychogenic origin. The cough usually is vibrating, throaty, and dry. The severity can range from occasional clearing of the throat to spells lasting several minutes. The cough usually follows a respiratory tract infection. The cough disappears with sleep or when the child is distracted. School absences are common.

Is the cough related to any event that would help me narrow down the cause?

Key Questions
- Does eating affect your cough?
- Does your cough get worse during certain times of the year?
- Does exercise affect your cough?

Eating
Inhalation into the tracheobronchial tree can occur as a result of lack of esophageal motility, GERD with regurgitation into the pharynx, or central nervous system and neuromuscular disorders. Difficulty with sucking and swallowing or coughing and choking during eating are highly suggestive of an underlying disorder, such as congenital malformations, congenital heart disease, or pneumonia.

In the adult, GERD probably causes cough through direct stimulation of cough receptors with acid or through inflammation from aspiration of stomach contents into the airway.

Season
Chronic cough during winter months suggests viral infections. Exacerbation of cough during spring, summer, and fall is suggestive of allergic disease with increased pollen counts. Croup occurs most commonly in the fall from the parainfluenza virus type 1. Smaller peaks of croup are seen with influenza B outbreaks in the winter months. RSV is common in infants during the winter months. In the warmer months, parainfluenza type 3 is the agent frequently isolated.

Exercise
The hyperpnea of exercise causes bronchospasm because of heat loss from the airway surface and is more pronounced in cold dry air. Asthma attacks are frequently exercise related, as is cough resulting from heart disease or airway compression.

Is this something that is going around?

Key Questions
- Is anyone else at home ill?
- Is anyone else ill in day care, school, or the workplace?

Exposure to respiratory viruses is very common in day care, school, and the workplace. Viruses that cause the common cold are shed in nasal secretions. Contacts acquire the virus by being sneezed on or by touching a sneezed-on object and then touching their own nose or conjunctivae. The incubation period is 2 to 5 days. *Mycoplasma pneumoniae* tends to spread through school/households slowly as the incubation period is 21 days.

Is there anything that would lead me to suspect allergies or reactive airway disease?

Key Questions
- Does anyone in your family have allergies or asthma?
- Is there anything you do or take that stops the cough?
- Do you have pets?

Family History
Allergy-prone individuals are at increased risk for coughs associated with postnasal drip and asthma. Allergy-prone adults and children are those persons with personal or family history of atopic dermatitis, asthma, and allergic rhinitis. Pets residing in the household are frequently the source of the allergen, especially cats and dogs.

Environmental Exposure
Frequently persons notice that the cough occurs after exposure to certain environmental irritants, such as smoke, pollen, dust, or animals. The cough can resolve spontaneously with withdrawal from these irritants.

Ingestion of antihistamines or inhalation of bronchodilators can relieve a cough associated with allergies or asthma.

Smoke Exposure

Chronic cough is not uncommon in persons who smoke. Smoke exposure can trigger cough in persons with allergies or asthma.

Getting Better or Worse

A change in the chronic cough of a smoker can indicate the development of a new and serious underlying problem, such as pneumonia or lung cancer.

> **Does the patient have any risk factors for systemic disease that could present with cough?**

Key Questions

- Do you have any chronic health problems?
- Do you have human immunodeficiency virus (HIV) infection, heart disease, or high blood pressure?
- Are you receiving treatment for cancer?
- Have you ever been exposed to TB?

Chronic Health Problems

Chronic lung and heart disease can present with cough, indicating an exacerbation and/or complication of the disease. In addition, information about chronic health problems can indicate which medications patients take, placing them at risk for cough. Angiotensin-converting enzyme (ACE) inhibitors can be given to treat hypertension or heart failure. Consider exacerbation of heart failure or consider an ACE inhibitor–induced dry, hacking cough, which can be eliminated by stopping the medication. In addition, a medication history can reveal use of drugs that treat or cause immunocompromise.

Immunocompromise

Cancer therapy, HIV, and administration of steroids should raise suspicion of immunocompromise. Adults and children who are immunocompromised are at high risk for infectious lung problems.

Tuberculosis

Inquiry should be made about potential exposure to TB. Family history of TB, incarceration, international travel, and inner city habitation put persons at risk for TB.

DIAGNOSTIC REASONING: FOCUSED PHYSICAL EXAMINATION
Note General Appearance

When a patient appears to be in acute distress with manifestations of oxygen deprivation, dehydration, and fever, think first of bacterial pneumonia. If a patient has significant oxygen deprivation that is not accompanied by fever, consider foreign body aspiration, acute heart failure, or pulmonary embolism.

The setting in which the patient is encountered will influence your response to the situation of acute distress. In most instances, oxygen is started immediately. If obstruction by a foreign body is strongly suspected, emergency personnel should be summoned for removal of the object if you are unable to accomplish this. Emergency chest radiographs could be needed to look for pulmonary infiltrates, and pulse oximetry can be ordered to assess oxygen saturation. Adults and children in acute respiratory distress require specialized care by health care professionals, and their assistance should be requested immediately.

Persons with viral respiratory tract infections or chronic cough from postnasal drainage, GERD, and chronic bronchitis appear less acutely ill and are able to participate in the interview process without difficulty. Those whose cough is caused by bronchospasm can exhibit varying degrees of distress.

Assess Mental Status

Diminished level of consciousness, confusion, and restlessness are likely manifestations of hypoxia in the patient experiencing respiratory problems. Frequently the patient with a pulmonary embolus expresses a sense of impending doom.

Restlessness and agitation in the child can indicate hypoxemia. A lethargic and somnolent child can have CO_2 retention.

Take Vital Signs

An elevated pulse rate and temperature can signal bacterial or viral infection.

Respiratory rate is the best indicator of pulmonary function in young infants. The respiratory rate and tidal volume together produce adequate alveolar ventilation. For any given level of alveolar ventilation, there is an optimum respiratory rate at which the muscular work of breathing is at a minimum. Airway resistance increases at higher flow rates. In children with decreased compliance (e.g., pneumonia, pulmonary edema), respirations are very rapid and shallow. Children with increased airway resistance (e.g., asthma) have respirations that are relatively slow and deep to minimize the high-resistance work. The most reliable and reproducible respiratory rate is the sleeping respiratory rate.

Weigh the Patient

Children with a cough from a chronic disease can present with failure to thrive.

Examine the Head and Neck

Erythema of upper respiratory tract mucous membranes, accompanied by enlarged anterior cervical nodes, is a common finding in a URI.

Observe the neck for jugular venous distention; this can be a sign of heart failure.

The ororespiratory reflex is mediated by the Arnold nerve, the auricular branch of cranial nerve X, and is a rare cause of chronic cough. Careful examination of the ears with removal of cerumen and any hairs in contact with the tympanic membrane (TM) or the opposite wall of the external auditory canal should be done.

A cobblestone appearance of the posterior pharynx is caused by lymphoid hyperplasia secondary to chronic stimulation by postnasal drip.

Inspect the Chest for Shape, Symmetry, and Use of Accessory Muscles

To inspect the chest, have the patient assume a sitting position. Note if the patient has to lean forward or sit up to breathe comfortably. Also observe the patient in a supine position to note if cough or respiratory symptoms change with position. Some respiratory abnormalities are unilateral or localized, such as pulmonary embolus. Compare findings on one side of the body with those on the other. Also compare front to back.

Upper airway obstruction causes suprasternal and supraclavicular retractions. Intercostal retractions and subcostal retractions occur with lower airway obstructive disease. Severe obstruction of either upper or lower airways causes retractions of all the accessory muscles. Retractions occur when an increase in the work of breathing requires an increase in the negative pressure within the chest. Remember that the pediatric airway is much smaller in diameter than that of the adult, and because resistance to flow is related inversely to the fourth power of the radius, decreased diameter of this airway causes enormous increases in resistance. The chest wall is pliable and the softest parts of the thorax are pulled inward on inspiration, causing retractions of the intracostal, suprasternal, and infrasternal spaces. The degree of retraction is proportional to the negative pressure generated within the thorax and therefore correlates with the severity of the problem.

Normally, the anteroposterior (AP) diameter is approximately one third to one half of the lateral diameter. If the AP diameter is equal to the lateral diameter, the condition known as barrel chest is evident and indicates probable COPD. Children with chronic cough because of cystic fibrosis or severe asthma can have an increase in the AP diameter. In children up to 6 months of age, the head circumference is larger than the chest circumference. After 6 months of age, the chest circumference is larger than the head circumference (see Chapter 13).

Observe Respirations

Next, observe the rate, rhythm, and depth of the patient's breathing. The normal respiratory rate in adults is 12 to 20 breaths per minute; in the elderly, it is 16 to 25 breaths per minute. Children younger than 12 years can have respiratory rates up to 30 to 40 breaths per minute. The only way the infant or child can increase oxygen uptake is to increase the ventilation rate. The depth and pattern of respiration change: the infant has more shallow and more frequent breaths.

Exhalation normally lasts about twice as long as inhalation, but in patients with COPD it can take up to four times longer. Note any abnormal breathing patterns (see Box 13-1).

Listen to the Cough

Note whether the cough is dry or moist. Listen also for the quality of the cough, such as whooping or honking.

Palpate the Chest

Palpate the entire chest for tenderness, depressions, bulges, and crepitus. Assess for chest symmetry by measuring diaphragmatic expansion and chest excursion. As the patient takes a deep breath, each hand should move the same distance out from the spine. With COPD, less movement will be seen. Pneumonia and partial paralysis of the diaphragm will result in a reduction in expansion of one side of the chest wall.

Assess for vocal fremitus (the vibrations transmitted to the chest wall during speech) by placing the ball of the hand lightly on the chest and asking the patient to repeat the words "ninety-nine." Evaluate the intensity of the vibration over all lung fields, comparing side to side. Dense tissue conducts sound better than does air; thus such conditions as pneumonia, heart failure, and tumors can increase fremitus. Fremitus is diminished in pneumothorax, asthma, and emphysema.

Percuss the Chest

Percuss systematically at 3- to 5-cm intervals, starting just above the scapulae and moving downward from side to side. Note any differences in volume and pitch. Resonance is a long, low-pitched sound that can normally be heard over most lung fields. Hyperresonance is an abnormally long, low-pitched sound that can signal emphysema or pneumothorax. Dullness or flatness can be heard with pleural effusion, pneumonia, or large tumors.

Auscultate Breath Sounds

Instruct the patient to breathe through the mouth slowly and deeply. Determine the presence, type, and location of both normal and abnormal breath sounds (see Chapter 13).

Most children know what a stethoscope is, and you should use this to your advantage. Infants see the shiny parts; have older children listen to their own chests. Some clinicians begin by listening to the child's leg or hand first. Ensure that the stethoscope is warm before you place it on the chest. Infants are in good position when supine, toddlers should be on the parent's lap, and older children should be sitting or standing.

Auscultate Heart Sounds

Note the location of normal and abnormal heart sounds, the location of their greatest intensity, and the heart rate and rhythm. Also note any murmurs and their location, grade, and radiation. Incompetent heart valves could be the cause of heart failure. In COPD, lung hyperinflation can muffle heart sounds. Poor tissue oxygenation or fever can result in tachycardia.

Examine the Skin and Extremities

Note the presence of cyanosis of the oral cavity (central cyanosis). It is associated with low arterial saturation and can result from inadequate gas exchange in the lungs or from cardiac shunting. Mucous membranes in dark-skinned patients can appear gray with central cyanosis. This can also be seen in persons with COPD. Bluish color of the extremities (peripheral cyanosis) can be observed in Caucasians and is associated with low venous saturation, resulting in vasoconstriction, vascular occlusion, or reduced cardiac output.

Clubbing is a loss of the angle between the skin and nail bed. This is a manifestation of chronic tissue hypoxia, which occurs with chronic lung disease. Edema of the lower extremities can be a sign of increased right-heart filling pressure, caused by primary lung disease or left ventricular failure.

Examine the Abdomen

Epigastric tenderness to palpation can be elicited in the patient with GERD, or the abdominal examination can be entirely normal. In addition, if heart failure is the cause of cough, ascites or hepatojugular reflex can be present. To test for hepatojugular reflex, position the patient so that the jugular pulsation is evident in the neck. Exert firm and sustained pressure with the hand over the patient's right upper quadrant for 30 to 60 seconds. An increase in the jugular venous pressure of more than 1 cm during this maneuver is abnormal.

LABORATORY AND DIAGNOSTIC STUDIES

Some authorities suggest all patients with a cough lasting longer than 3 weeks have a chest radiograph. If the radiograph is abnormal and consistent with infectious or noninfectious inflammatory disease or malignancy, the health care provider should order expectorated sputum studies, computed tomography (CT) scan of the lungs, or bronchoscopy. If the history, physical examination, and radiography suggest heart failure, an ECG, echocardiogram, or both are indicated (see Chapter 7).

If the patient's history and physical examination strongly suggest a specific etiology (i.e., postnasal drip, asthma, GERD), proceed to those treatments initially. Keep in mind that there can be more than one cause for the cough. For those patients whose history and physical examination suggest chronic symptoms, sinus radiography or CT scan of the sinuses can be indicated. Also consider allergy testing for those individuals whose history indicates allergens precipitated the syndrome.

In those situations in which investigation of signs and symptoms leads to probable asthma or if no likely cause is identified, a spirometry test (see Chapter 13) should be performed. If the test is normal but asthma is still suspected, a methacholine challenge test can be done. This test is performed in the laboratory and involves administering methacholine chloride by nebulizer and then repeating the spirometry test. If the patient's cough is related to reactive airways disease, the patient exhibits a 20% decrease in FEV_1.

Complete Blood Count

A complete blood cell count can provide evidence of acute infection with an elevated white blood cell count. Eosinophilia indicates atopy.

Esophageal Probe

GERD is best diagnosed with 24-hour esophageal pH probe monitoring. A barium swallow is less sensitive, and a gastroscopy will verify ulcerative disease but not mild reflux.

Sputum Culture

Sputum culture is important for the diagnosis of a specific infectious agent in the pulmonary system. A sputum specimen must originate from deep within the bronchi. Coughing usually enables the patient to produce a satisfactory specimen. Examination includes macroscopic appearance, cellular composition, and bacterial count.

Sweat Test

A result of >60 mEq/L of chloride is considered diagnostic of cystic fibrosis.

Tuberculin Skin Testing

The Mantoux test is used to detect TB. A Mantoux test result is considered positive at three different levels (≥5, ≥10, and ≥15 mm) of induration (diameter transverse to the long axis of the arm measured and recorded), depending on the individual's degree of risk for TB. In adults, a diameter of less than 5 mm is considered negative, a 5- to 9-mm diameter is considered a weak positive, a 10- to 14-mm diameter is considered an intermediate positive, and a ≥15-mm diameter is considered a strong positive. In a child who has no known risk factors for TB, only a large reaction (≥15 mm) is considered to be positive. If a child is very young (<4 years old), has other medical risk factors, or has some environmental exposure to TB, then an intermediate reaction (≥10 mm) is considered to be positive. If a child is at high risk (e.g., a child who

lives in a household with someone who has TB), then a small reaction (≥5 mm) is considered to be positive.

Nasal Swab for Pertussis

Nasopharyngeal secretions for culture should be obtained using a calcium alginate or Dacron-tipped swab. The swab is inserted into the posterior nasopharynx and gently rotated for a minimum of 15 seconds and optimally for 1 minute. Throat swabs are not acceptable for the diagnosis of pertussis.

Rapid Influenza Testing

Rapid influenza testing is used to detect a virus in nasal or throat secretions. It can help differentiate influenza from other viral and bacterial infections with similar symptoms. Rapid influenza tests are best used within the first 48 hours of the onset of symptoms. The positive and negative predictive values vary considerably depending upon the prevalence of influenza in the community. Testing is most effective when flu prevalence is high.

Chest X-Ray

A chest x-ray is suggested in patients whose cough with accompanying fever persists longer than 3 days, or presents with an unusual clinical course. If a foreign body is suspected, an expiratory film can identify the object (see Chapter 37).

DIFFERENTIAL DIAGNOSIS

Life-threatening causes of cough must be initially considered when arriving at a differential diagnosis. Conditions that present with cough as a symptom are discussed in Chapters 7 and 13 and include pulmonary embolus, heart failure, bacterial tracheitis, foreign body aspiration, and asthma. Review those conditions associated with cough.

Common Cold (Nasopharyngitis)

The common cold is a self-limiting viral infection of the upper respiratory tract that is generally caused by a rhinovirus. The virus invades the mucous membranes of the upper respiratory tract and causes swelling and hypersecretion of mucus. Associated symptoms include a low-grade fever, mild sore throat, and rhinorrhea of clear to yellow mucus. Hypersecretion of mucus causes coughing, especially at night when secretions pool in the nasopharyngeal cavity. Physical examination findings can include red and swollen nasal mucosa with secretions present, mild pharyngeal erythema, and enlarged cervical lymph nodes. Other physical examination findings are negative. The patient is advised to return if the cough persists for more than 3 weeks or if additional symptoms develop, such as temperature of more than 38.3° C (101° F), chest pain, or SOB.

Chronic Obstructive Pulmonary Disease Exacerbation

COPD is a condition primarily consisting of emphysema and chronic bronchitis. It is almost always a condition of heavy smokers. Acute exacerbations of COPD include three clinical findings: worsening dyspnea, increase in sputum purulence, and increase in sputum volume. Patients will have a chronic cough, associated with barrel chest, tachypnea, and distant breath sounds on physical examination. Chest radiography will show hyperexpansion of the lungs, and spirometry will indicate airflow obstruction when emphysema is present. Acute COPD exacerbations can also be associated with a URI, fever without a known cause, increased wheezing or cough, and a 20% increase in respiratory rate and heart rate above baseline.

Bordetella pertussis Infection

Pertussis (whooping cough) is an acute infection of the respiratory tract caused by *Bordetella pertussis*. It is a condition primarily seen in children under the age of 2 and in persons who have not had adequate diphtheria and tetanus toxoids and pertussis (DTP) vaccination. Pertussis infection has occurred among adolescents who become susceptible approximately 6 to 10 years after childhood vaccination. It begins with a prodromal stage of malaise, cough, coryza, and anorexia. The cough then becomes more severe and ends in a high-pitched inspiratory "whoop." Vomiting and cyanosis can also be present. Physical examination can be within normal limits. Pertussis is associated with extremely high white blood cell counts.

Bacterial Pneumonia

Pneumonia is usually associated with dyspnea, pleuritic chest pain, cough with greenish or rusty-colored sputum, fever, and chills. Infants and young children will not produce sputum. Anorexia, malaise, and post-tussive vomiting are seen. Objective manifestations of pneumonia include fever, tachycardia and tachypnea, inspiratory crackles, asynchronous breathing and vocal

fremitus, dull percussion sound over area of consolidation, and bronchophony. Pneumonia can be confirmed by chest radiography, complete blood cell count, and sputum and nasal bacteria cultures.

Fever is frequently absent in the elderly with pneumonia, and thus a new onset of cough, especially when accompanied by either tachypnea or altered mental status, should suggest pneumonia.

The majority of pediatric pulmonary infections are viral and usually caused by RSV, parainfluenza viruses, or influenza viruses. In the infant and young child, acute nonbacterial pneumonia presents after a 1- to 2-day history of coryza, decreased appetite, and low-grade fever. Increasing fretfulness, respiratory congestion, vomiting, cough, and fever can occur. Objective manifestations include tachypnea, tachycardia, nasal flaring, and retractions.

Viral Upper Respiratory Infection

Viral agents include a vast number of serotypes. Cough, nasal congestion, sore throat, fever, chills, and myalgias are the most common symptoms. Most symptoms of URIs, including local swelling, erythema, edema, secretions, and fever, result from the inflammatory response of the immune system to invading pathogens and from toxins produced by pathogens. An initial nasopharyngeal infection can spread to adjacent structures resulting in sinusitis, otitis media, epiglottitis, laryngitis, tracheobronchitis, and pneumonia. Influenza (flu) caused by the family of influenza viruses typically causes more severe symptoms and has more serious sequelae. Fever is usually higher, and stuffy nose and sneezing can be absent. Because flu cannot be distinguished from other URIs on symptoms alone, rapid flu testing can be useful during flu outbreaks.

Mycoplasma Pneumoniae

Mycoplasma pneumoniae is the most common cause of infection of the lower respiratory tract in children and young adults. There is a slow onset of symptoms with fever (39° C or 102.2° F), a cough that is usually dry at the onset, headache, malaise, and sore throat. The child does not look particularly ill, but on auscultation rales and rhonchi are frequently present. The white blood cell count is usually normal, and cold agglutinin titer can be elevated during the acute presentation in more than half of patients with this infection. A titer of 1:32 or higher supports the diagnosis.

Chlamydial Pneumonia

Chlamydial pneumonia is a pulmonary disease caused by *C. trachomatis* transmitted during delivery. It also occurs in young adults. In infants 3 to 11 weeks of age, it is one of the most common causes of interstitial pneumonitis and presents with tachypnea and a characteristic staccato cough in an afebrile child. In adults, infection is associated with upper respiratory tract symptoms followed by fever and a nonproductive cough. Fine rales, usually without wheezes, are heard on auscultation. Chest radiographs show hyperinflated lungs with diffuse interstitial or alveolar infiltrates.

Bronchiolitis

RSV is mainly responsible for bronchiolitis in children less than 2 years old. The infection is associated with 1 to 2 days of fever, rhinorrhea, and cough, followed by wheezing, tachypnea, tachycardia, and respiratory distress. Nasal flaring and retractions with accessory muscle use are seen, along with shallow, rapid respirations. Cough increases as inflammation increases. The infant appears lethargic and has circumoral cyanosis. Wheezes are predominant, with a long expiratory phase. Crackles and rhonchi can also be heard diffusely throughout the lung fields. The chest radiograph shows hyperinflation with mild interstitial infiltrates. Viral isolates from sputum, throat swabs, or nasal washings are used for diagnosis.

Acute Bronchitis

Inflammation of the large airways causes bronchitis that begins with a dry, nonproductive cough usually seen in winter. Continued cough and nasal congestion produce a productive cough and fever. Chest pain can accompany the cough. Lung auscultation reveals diffuse rhonchi on expiration. White blood cell count is normal or mildly elevated.

Croup (Acute Laryngotracheobronchitis)

Inflammation or edema of the subglottic area causes obstruction of the airways of the larynx, trachea, or bronchi. Parainfluenza virus causes most inflammation. Generally the onset occurs after a few days of a URI. Hoarseness, inspiratory stridor, and a characteristic barking cough are heard and are usually worse at night. A low-grade fever can be present. Inspiratory stridor, suprasternal and intercostal retractions, and an increased respiratory rate are seen. Lateral neck radiographs in croup show a normal epiglottis, subglottic narrowing, and ballooning of the hypopharynx. The posteroanterior neck view shows a steeple sign (narrowing of the air column at the top).

Subacute and Chronic Cough
Postnasal Drainage Syndrome

Postnasal drainage syndrome is the most common cause of chronic cough. The cough results from stimulation of the afferent limb of the cough reflex in the upper respiratory tract. Causes of postnasal drip include allergic response, secondary infection after an upper respiratory tract illness, environmental irritants, vasomotor rhinitis, or sinusitis. Both children and adults report dry cough, throat clearing, sensation of something in the back of the throat, and nasal congestion. Physical examination can reveal mucus in the posterior pharynx or a cobblestone appearance of the posterior pharynx. Sinus radiographs, CT scan of the sinuses, and allergy testing can be indicated if this syndrome is suspected to be the cause of cough.

Asthma

Asthma is the most common cause of chronic cough in children. It initially produces a dry cough, commonly worse at night, characteristically exercise related, and often triggered by respiratory tract infections. Physical examination findings depend on the severity of the disease. Prolonged expiratory phase of respiration can be heard. Lungs can have crackles that clear with coughing, and overt or latent wheeze can be produced with forced expiration. Use of neck muscles to facilitate inspiration (called tracheal tugging or chin lag) can be seen. A chest radiograph can show hyperinflation during acute attacks. Pulmonary function testing with and without an aerosolized sympathomimetic bronchodilator is positive.

Gastroesophageal Reflux Disease

GERD should be considered when patients report heartburn, a sour taste in the mouth, or a history of esophagitis. Often persons with GERD are cigarette smokers, overuse alcohol, and are overweight. Microaspiration into the airways or reflux of acid into the esophagus occurs. Young infants can also experience reflux with their cough, usually worsening after feeding, which could be the only symptom. A recurrent, effortless vomiting with failure to gain weight and irritability can also occur. The physical examination of persons with GERD is most often normal. The diagnostic test of most significance is esophageal pH monitoring; values outside the normal physiological range indicate reflux.

Chronic Bronchitis

Chronic bronchitis should be considered when the patient expectorates sputum on most days during a period spanning at least 3 consecutive months and such periods have occurred for more than 2 successive years. In addition, exposure to smoke, irritating dust, or fumes is highly likely. Cigarette smoking as well as fumes and dust stimulate the afferent limb of the cough reflex as irritants, inducing inflammatory changes in the mucosa of the respiratory tract, causing hypersecretion of mucus and slowing of mucociliary clearance. Persons with chronic bronchitis exhibit a rasping, hacking cough, possible rhonchi that clear with coughing, resonant to dull chest, possible barrel chest, prolonged expiration, and possible wheezing. Chest radiography and pulmonary function tests are indicated.

Angiotensin-Converting Enzyme Inhibitor–Induced Cough

This cough occurs hours to months after beginning an ACE inhibitor. Persons report a nonproductive cough associated with an irritating, tickling, or scratching sensation in the throat. Physical examination is normal. The cough resolves within days to weeks after the drug is discontinued.

Bronchogenic Carcinoma

Hemoptysis reported by a cigarette smoker as well as weight loss and/or shortness of breath are frequent health concerns reported by a patient with bronchogenic cancer. Physical findings can include enlarged supraclavicular nodes, dull chest percussion over the tumor, and increased breath sounds distal to the tumor. Hemoptysis should be evaluated with a chest radiograph and a CT scan if indicated.

Cystic Fibrosis

A chronic cough is associated with cystic fibrosis. The cough is productive, and the child has signs of failure to thrive with poor weight gain. The child could have a family history of the disease. The cough is initially dry and hacking but eventually becomes loose and productive of purulent material. Physical examination often shows an increased AP diameter of the chest. Scattered or localized coarse rales and rhonchi are audible. Digital clubbing is often present. Sweat chloride test is positive.

Foreign Body Aspiration

Foreign body aspiration occurs most frequently in children and the elderly. A child or adult who aspirates a foreign body can have a varied presentation. Generally the onset of cough is sudden and unexpected. A brief period of severe coughing, gagging, and choking occurs. If the foreign body does not completely obstruct the airway, an asymptomatic period ensues. This period can last for hours, days, or even months. A foreign body in the lower airway can present with emphysema because of the ball-valve phenomenon or can occur as a complete distal atelectasis created by absorption of the trapped gas. A mobile foreign body in the lower airway can also produce a paroxysmal cough, with cyanotic episodes and stridor because of proximal migration and subglottic impaction. A foreign body in the esophagus can also cause airway obstruction and cough as well as dysphagia for solid foods because the posterior trachea is compliant and opposed to the anterior esophagus. Coins are the most frequent culprit.

Allergic Rhinitis

Upper airway allergy and vasomotor rhinitis can cause a reflex cough secondary to postnasal drip and irritation of the cough receptors. Such a cough is generally seasonal in nature, with a history of sneezing. Allergic shiners, allergic salute, and eczema can be present. Rhinorrhea with clear, watery drainage is seen. Skin testing for allergies is positive.

Chronic Sinusitis

Chronic sinusitis produces a recurrent cough that is especially worse at night because of trickling of infected mucus from the nasopharynx down the posterior pharyngeal wall. Involvement is usually in the maxillary sinuses. History reveals cold-like symptoms that become persistent or recurrent. Noisy breathing and snoring with sleep can also be present. Physical examination reveals clear to mucopurulent secretions in the posterior throat. Purulent rhinorrhea can be present. Sinus tenderness is less frequently present than in acute sinusitis. A radiograph using the Waters view of the head is positive.

Tuberculosis

Brassy cough is the most common symptom of TB but is often ascribed to smoking, a recent cold, or a bout of influenza several weeks before. At first, it is minimally productive of yellow or green mucus, usually on arising in the morning. As the disease progresses, the cough becomes more productive. In adults, a multi-nodular infiltrate above or behind the clavicle (the most characteristic location) suggests recurrence of an old TB infection. In younger persons in whom recent infection is more common, infiltration can be found in any part of the lung, and unilateral pleural effusion is often seen. In sputum examination, the finding of acid-fast bacilli (AFB) in a sputum smear is strong presumptive evidence of TB. A definitive diagnosis is made only on results of a culture.

Smoking

Smoking is most prevalent in female adolescents, and many smoke in closed rooms, increasing their respiratory irritation. History of a mildly productive hacking cough can be indicative of smoking. Infants exposed to passive cigarette smoke inhalation have increased bronchial reactivity. Physical examination can reveal yellow stains on the fingers, teeth, or tongue. Mild chronic conjunctivitis can also be present. Chest radiography can be positive with interstitial markings.

Psychogenic Origin

Psychogenic or habit cough is a rare cause of cough and can be misdiagnosed in a patient with postnasal drip syndrome. School-age children or adolescents with a history of a loud, brassy, disturbing cough that is nonproductive and explosive can indicate a psychogenic etiology. The child usually has missed many school days. The cough is not heard while sleeping, and the child is afebrile with no weight loss. The physical examination is negative.

DIFFERENTIAL DIAGNOSIS OF *Common Causes of Recent Onset of Cough*

CONDITION	HISTORY	PHYSICAL FINDINGS	DIAGNOSTIC STUDIES
Nasopharyngitis	Acute-onset, low-grade fever, rhinorrhea, cough especially at night	Nasal mucosa red and swollen, pharynx mildly red; otherwise negative	None
COPD exacerbation	Worsening dyspnea, increased wheezing or coughing, smoker	Purulent sputum, fever, and increased respiratory and heart rates	Chest radiograph, spirometry
Pertussis	Persistent hacking cough; can have inspiratory whoop, vomiting	Fever absent, coryza	Nasopharyngeal aspirate positive, chest radiograph to rule out pneumonia
Pneumonia*	Noisy cough, dyspnea, pleuritic chest pain, sputum production (yellow, green, red color), chills; in children also see poor feeding and irritability	Fever, tachycardia, tachypnea, inspiratory crackles, asynchronous breathing, vocal fremitus, percussion dull or flat over area of consolidation, bronchophony, egophony	Chest radiograph, CBC, sputum and nasal cultures, O_2 saturation, blood cultures
Viral URI	Cough, nasal congestion, sore throat, fever, chills, myalgias	Fever, pharyngitis, enlarged anterior cervical lymph nodes, normal TMs, nasal mucosa erythema, normal chest examination	None. Rapid influenza testing during outbreaks
Mycoplasmal pneumonia	Child or young adult: dry cough, headache, malaise, sore throat	Fever, rales and rhonchi on auscultation	Cold agglutinin, chest radiograph
Chlamydial pneumonia	Paroxysmal staccato cough in infant 4-12 weeks	Afebrile, conjunctivitis in 50% of infants, tachypnea of 40-80 breaths/min, crackles, no wheezing	Radiograph shows hyperexpansion of lungs with diffuse interstitial infiltrates
Bronchiolitis (RSV)*	Grunting, sneezing, cough, anoxia, exposure to passive smoke	Fever, wheezing on auscultation, prolonged expiratory phase, tachypnea of 60-80 breaths/min, tachycardia >200 beats/min	WBC 5000-24,000/mm³ with increased PMNs; chest radiograph shows hyperinflation; infants less than 2 months, refer; progressive respiratory distress, refer

Continued

DIFFERENTIAL DIAGNOSIS OF *Common Causes of Recent Onset of Cough—cont'd*

CONDITION	HISTORY	PHYSICAL FINDINGS	DIAGNOSTIC STUDIES
Acute bronchitis	Duration <3 months, winter months, URI for 3-4 days; loose, hacking cough that becomes productive, afebrile	Coarse, fine crackles on auscultation; low-grade fever or afebrile	Chest radiograph negative
Croup (acute laryngo-tracheobronchitis)*	History of URI; brassy, barking cough usually at night	Low-grade fever, inspiratory stridor, flaring of nares, prolonged expiratory phase, can see retraction of accessory muscles, breath sounds diminished	None

*Because of the possible rapid changes in condition in infants and children, nonemergent causes of cough can become emergent.
COPD, Chronic obstructive pulmonary disease; *PMNs,* polymorphonuclear neutrophils; *RSV,* respiratory syncytial virus; *TM,* tympanic membrane; *URI,* upper respiratory infection.

DIFFERENTIAL DIAGNOSIS OF *Common Causes of Chronic Cough*

CONDITION	HISTORY	PHYSICAL FINDINGS	DIAGNOSTIC STUDIES
Postnasal drainage	Cough, sore throat	Mucoid secretions in posterior pharynx, cobblestone appearance of posterior pharynx, tenderness to palpation of sinuses, normal chest examination	Sinus radiographs, sinus CT scan, allergy testing
Asthma	Dry, hacking cough, especially at night, and with feeding and laughter	End-expiratory wheeze, prolonged expiratory phase	Pulmonary function testing, chest x-ray, O_2 saturation, bronchoprovocation, allergy testing
GERD	Cough worse at night, sour taste in mouth, heartburn, history of esophagitis, cigarette smoker, alcohol abuse, overweight; in children 0-18 months: failure to thrive, dysphagia, cough after eating and lying down, vomiting	Normal chest examination, normal upper respiratory tract examination, possible epigastric pain with palpation or normal abdominal examination	Esophageal pH monitoring, blood count for anemia, radiograph for aspiration pneumonia; endoscopy if no response to therapy; manometry
Chronic bronchitis	Cough, mild dyspnea, history of COPD, history of cigarette smoking, yellow sputum	Hacking, rasping cough; normal breath sounds or rhonchi that clear with coughing; resonant to dull chest, possible barrel chest, prolonged expiration, possible wheezing	Chest radiograph, pulmonary function tests
ACEI-induced cough	Begins hours to months after starting ACEI; nonproductive, dry cough; scratching sensation in throat	Normal examination	Trial off ACEI
Bronchogenic carcinoma	Cough with hemoptysis; history of cigarette smoking, weight loss, shortness of breath	Enlarged supraclavicular nodes, dull chest percussion over tumor, increased breath sounds distal to tumor	Chest radiograph, CT scan of chest
Cystic fibrosis	Failure to thrive, chronic cough, bulky stools, family history	Nasal polyps, clubbing of fingernails, sputum	Sweat test positive

DIFFERENTIAL DIAGNOSIS OF *Common Causes of Chronic Cough—cont'd*

CONDITION	HISTORY	PHYSICAL FINDINGS	DIAGNOSTIC STUDIES
Foreign body in ear canal	Cough	Cerumen in ears, hairs in contact with TM or opposite wall of external auditory canal	None
Foreign body aspiration	History of environmental hazard, choking episode	Asymmetrical physical findings of decreased breath sounds, wheezing	Asymmetrical radiograph with forced expiratory view
Allergic rhinitis	History of sneezing, cough	Allergic shiners, allergic salute, rhinorrhea clear and watery	Chest radiograph negative, allergy testing positive
Chronic sinusitis	Rhinorrhea >7-10 days	Mucopurulent rhinorrhea	Waters radiograph
Mycoplasmal pneumonia	School-age child, gradual onset, headache, malaise, sore throat, hacking cough	Reddened pharynx, slightly enlarged lymph nodes, rales often fine and crackling	Radiograph shows interstitial pneumonia; cold agglutinins positive, ESR elevated, CBC, O_2 saturation, sputum cultures, blood cultures
Tuberculosis	History of exposure, high-risk group, weakness, malaise, weight loss	Brassy cough, weight loss, can have fever, night sweats	Mantoux test, chest radiograph shows abnormalities in apical and hyaline, sputum culture positive for *M. tuberculosis*
Smoking (passive/active)	History of smoking or being around a smoker	Yellow teeth, fingers; odor of smoke, productive sputum	Radiograph can be positive with interstitial markings
Psychogenic origin	School age or adolescent; dry, hacking cough present only during waking hours	None	As indicated to rule out other causes

ACEI, Angiotensin-converting enzyme inhibitor; *CBC,* complete blood cell count; *COPD,* chronic obstructive pulmonary disease; *CT,* computed tomography; *ESR,* erythrocyte sedimentation rate; *GERD,* gastroesophageal reflux disease.

REFERENCES AND READINGS

Asilsoy S, Bayram E, Agin H, Apa H, Can D, Gulle S et al: Evaluation of chronic cough in children, *Chest* 134:1122, 2008.

Centers for Disease Control and Prevention: Seasonal influenza. Available online at http://www.cdc.gov/flu/index.htm, Accessed May 25, 2010.

Chang AB, Asher MI: A review of cough in children, *J Asthma* 38:299, 2001.

de Jongste JC, Shields MD: Cough 2: chronic cough in children, *Thorax* 58:998, 2003.

Irwin RS, Madison JM: The diagnosis and treatment of cough, *N Engl J Med* 342:1715, 2000.

Kahrilas PJ, Shaheen NJ, Vaezi MF, Hiltz SW, Black E, Modlin IM et al., American Gastroenterological Association: American Gastroenterological Association Medical Position Statement on the management of gastroesophageal reflux disease, *Gastroenterology* 35:1383, 2008.

Malhotra A: Influenza and respiratory syncytial virus. Update on infection, management and prevention, *Pediatr Clin North Am* 47: 353, vi, 2000.

Mandell LA, Wunderink RG, Anzueto A, Bartlett JG, Campbell GD, Dean NC, et al: Infectious Diseases Society of America/American Thoracic Society consensus guidelines on the management of community-acquired pneumonia in adults, *Clin Infect Dis* 44:S27, 2007.

Morton RL, Sheikh S, Corbett ML, Eid NS: Evaluation of the wheezy infant, *Ann Allergy Asthma Immunol* 86:251, 2001.

National Asthma Education and Prevention Program (NAEPP): Expert panel report 3: guidelines for the diagnosis and management of asthma, *J Allergy Clin Immunol* 120:S94, 2007.

Shields MD, Bush A, Everard ML, McKenzie S, Primhak R: British Thoracic Society guidelines: Recommendations for the assessment and management of cough in children. *Thorax.* 63: Suppl 3:iii1, 2008.

Snow V, Lascher S, Mottur-Pilson C: Evidence base for management of acute exacerbations of chronic obstructive pulmonary disease, *Ann Intern Med* 134:595, 2001.

Tierney LM, McPhee SJ, Papadakis MA: *Current medical diagnosis and treatment,* ed 44, New York, 2005, McGraw-Hill.

Valente J: Diagnosing persistent childhood cough, *Practitioner* 245:337, 2001.

CHAPTER 11

Diarrhea

Next to respiratory disease, acute gastroenteritis is the most common illness in families in the United States. Most cases are of viral origin and are self-limiting. In children, 50% are of viral origin, approximately 25% are of bacterial origin, and approximately 25% are of undetermined cause. Diarrhea can be classified according to its pathophysiological pattern (osmotic, secretory, exudative, or motile), its cause (infectious or noninfectious), or its duration (acute or chronic).

Osmotic or malabsorptive diarrhea occurs when nonabsorbable water-soluble solutes remain in the bowel and retain water. This can occur through damage to the intestinal microvillus membrane. The result is malabsorption of luminal solutes with osmotic loss of free water into the gut lumen. This is the most common cause of chronic diarrhea in children. Lactose intolerance is an example of this kind of diarrhea. Ingestion of large amounts of sugar substitutes in diet foods, drinks, candies, and chewing gum can cause osmotic diarrhea through a combination of slow absorption and rapid small bowel motility.

Secretory diarrhea occurs when the balance between fluid secretion and absorption across the intestinal mucosa is altered. When there is a change in this balance produced by physiological causes, diarrhea occurs. The loss of water and electrolytes can be rapid and massive. Traveler's diarrhea and diarrhea caused by *Vibrio cholerae* are examples.

Exudative diarrhea occurs in the presence of mucosal inflammation or ulceration, which results in an outpouring of plasma, serum proteins, blood, and mucus. The consequence is an increase in fecal bulk and fluidity. Many mucosal diseases, such as regional enteritis, ulcerative colitis, and carcinoma, can cause this exudative enteropathy.

Diarrhea from abnormal intestinal motility (either increased or decreased) results in an alteration in contact between the luminal contents and the mucosal surface. Examples include irritable bowel syndrome (IBS) and laxative use.

Infectious bacteria can be caused by viral, bacterial, or parasitic agents.

DIAGNOSTIC REASONING: FOCUSED HISTORY

What does this patient mean by "diarrhea"?

Key Questions
- How frequent are the stools?
- What is the volume of stools?
- Are the stools formed or liquid?
- At what intervals does the diarrhea occur?

Frequency of Stools
In the United States, typical bowel frequency ranges from 1 to 3 times a day to 2 or 3 times per week and varies considerably from person to person. Changes in stool frequency, consistency, or volume can indicate disease.

Stool Volume and Consistency
Processes involving the small bowel tend to produce large-volume watery stools that are relatively infrequent. Large bowel involvement, usually resulting from a bacterially induced inflammatory process, tends to produce more frequent and less watery stools.

Intervals
A history of acute diarrhea followed by continuous or intermittent episodes of loose stools suggests malabsorption commonly caused by lactase deficiency exacerbated by the ingestion of lactose in milk or milk products. Intermittent diarrhea alternating with constipation suggests IBS.

Proximal Colon Symptoms
Proximal colon symptoms include large-volume, less-frequent, more-homogeneous stools, without urgency or tenesmus (painful defecation), and

suggest food intolerance or infectious or inflammatory disease.

Distal Colon Symptoms

Symptoms of small volume, frequency, urgency, tenesmus, incontinence, and mucus suggest proctocolitis, colon cancer, diverticular disease, or IBS.

If this is an infant, is there a risk of dehydration?

Key Questions

- How many wet diapers has the infant produced in the past 24 hours?
- Does the infant seem thirsty?
- Does the infant have tears when crying?

Wet Diapers

Dehydration in infants and young children can occur quickly and with fatal consequences, especially in infants. Diagnosis and treatment must be done in a timely manner. A general rule of thumb to determine signs of dehydration in infants is fewer than six wet diapers per 24 hours or a period of longer than 4 hours without urination.

Thirst

Infants demonstrate their thirst with irritability, crying, and eagerness to drink fluid that is offered to them. Test for thirst by offering fluids either in a bottle or on a spoon. The child with mild dehydration will exhibit increased thirst; the moderately dehydrated child will be very thirsty; and, with severe dehydration, the child will continue to be very thirsty. If left untreated, a child can become stuporous and unresponsive and therefore unable to manifest thirst.

Tears

In mild dehydration, tears are present; in moderate dehydration, tears are or are not present; and in severe dehydration, no tears are present.

If this is an adult, is there risk for dehydration?

Key Questions

- How many times have you urinated in the past 24 hours?
- Are you thirsty?
- Do you have a dry mouth or dry eyes?

Dehydration

Symptoms of dehydration in an adult are more related to the rate of fluid loss than to the absolute degree of fluid loss. The degree of dehydration can be estimated by symptoms of thirst, dry mouth, or dry eyes, and by frequency and volume of urination. Patients can also experience weakness.

Is this an acute or chronic problem?

Key Questions

- How long have you had diarrhea?
- Have you had this problem before?

Acute Diarrhea in Adults

An acute onset of diarrhea in a previously healthy patient without signs or symptoms of other organ involvement suggests an infectious cause. Acute diarrhea in adults is commonly viral in origin. The viral illnesses are self-limited, and an aggressive diagnostic workup is not indicated. Acute diarrhea in adults usually has an abrupt onset and lasts less than 2 weeks. Most of the disorders cause some combination of abdominal pain, diarrhea, nausea, vomiting, fever, and tenesmus.

Acute Diarrhea in Children

Acute diarrhea in children is characterized by loose or liquid stools. A large quantity of fluid and electrolytes that become pooled in the intestinal lumen is lost as stool is expelled. The number of stools is usually increased, but this is not an essential manifestation. Severe or protracted diarrhea can lead to metabolic acidosis, dehydration, azotemia, and oliguria. Diarrhea in the neonate and young infant is considered more serious than that in the older child because of lower tolerance to associated fluid shifts and the greater likelihood of associated infection or congenital anomaly.

Chronic Diarrhea in Adults

Diarrhea is chronic when it lasts more than 2 weeks. Unless the diarrhea is bloody or the patient has a systemic illness, the most common causes of chronic diarrhea are parasites, medications, IBS, lactose intolerance, and inflammatory bowel disease.

Chronic Diarrhea in Children

Chronic diarrhea in children is defined as diarrhea for longer than 3 weeks. The major causes of diarrhea change with age. In the infant, formula protein intolerance is the most common cause. Toddler's diarrhea (irritable colon of infancy), protracted enteritis following a viral infection, and *Giardia* are the common causes in the toddler. In children and adolescents, malabsorption disorders are the most common causes. The diarrhea is the result of the ingestion of solutes that cannot be digested or absorbed, such as lactose products or excessive intake of sorbitol. Another cause of diarrhea in this age-group is inflammatory bowel disease (ulcerative colitis and Crohn disease).

Does the presence or absence of blood help me narrow the cause?

Key Questions

- Is there any noticeable blood in the stool or tissue? How much?
- What color is the blood?
- What color are the stools?

Blood in the Stools

Bright red blood limited to small spots on the toilet tissue suggests that the source of bleeding is from hemorrhoids and not from a diarrheal process higher in the gastrointestinal (GI) tract. Because diarrhea and repeated cleansing of the rectum produce local irritation, minor bleeding from hemorrhoids is not uncommon and must be distinguished from true blood in the stool. Reports of blood in the stool in acute diarrhea are suggestive of a bacterial pathogen, notably *Shigella*. The blood is red.

In infants and children, blood in the stool is most commonly caused by cow's milk intolerance or anal fissures. In the newborn, blood in stools can be a result of hemorrhagic disease of the newborn, thought to be caused by a lack of vitamin K. Premature infants or infants who are of low birth weight are at risk for necrotizing enterocolitis presenting with red or maroon stools (hematochezia) as well as vomiting and abdominal distention.

In adults and children, chronic bloody diarrhea can indicate inflammatory bowel disease, dysentery, colitis, or an invasive organism. Blood that is red usually indicates lower GI tract bleeding, whereas dark or black, tarry stools (melena) typically indicate upper GI tract bleeding. However, bleeding from the small bowel or right colon can also produce melena.

Color of Stools

Some patients believe they have blood in their stool based on stool color. Sources of black stools are blood, iron, charcoal, bismuth, licorice, huckleberries, and lead. Sources of red or pink stools include blood, food (beets, cranberries, tomatoes, peppers), food coloring (breakfast cereals, Jell-O), and drugs (anticoagulants, salicylates, rifampin, pyridium pamoate, diazepam syrup, phenolphthalein in alkaline stool). Green-black stools can be caused by grape-flavored drinks and iron. Dark gray stools occur with cocoa and chocolate ingestion. Pale gray or white stools can be caused by cholestasis, obstructive jaundice, malabsorption, excessive milk ingestion, and antacid ingestion. Green stools are produced by bile salts and chlorophyll-containing vegetables, such as spinach.

What does the presence or absence of pain tell me?

Key Questions

- Are you having any pain or gas with the diarrhea?
- Where is the pain?
- What does the pain feel like?
- Is the pain constant or does it come and go?
- Does the pain awaken you at night?
- Does the pain interfere with your activities (e.g., working, sleeping, eating)?

Occurrence of Pain

Diarrhea with abdominal pain and flatulent stools is characteristic of a malabsorptive process. Most self-limiting viral diarrheas cause some combination of abdominal pain, diarrhea, nausea, vomiting, fever, and tenesmus.

Abdominal pain is common when diarrhea is caused by infective bacteria in the colon, such as ingestion associated with food poisoning. *Giardia lamblia*, introduced through the ingestion of contaminated water or by the orofecal route, produces crampy abdominal pain and is frequently seen in children and diapered infants in day care where handwashing is not done between diapering.

Location of Pain

Generalized abdominal pain is produced by diffuse inflammation of the GI tract as occurs with inflammatory bowel disease or abdominal cramping from infective diarrhea. The pain from ulcerative colitis can be perceived over the entire abdomen or localized to the lower quadrants. The pain associated with IBS is usually confined to the lower quadrants or over the sigmoid colon. Large intestine pain is felt in the lower abdominal quadrants, whereas small intestine pain is felt in the epigastric and umbilical areas.

Severity of Pain
Self-limited diarrhea usually presents with cramping but not severe abdominal pain. Other causes of abdominal pain should be investigated (see Chapter 2).

Sleep-Related Pain
Persistent diarrhea that awakens the patient from sleep usually indicates a serious organic disease, such as diabetes enteropathy or human immunodeficiency virus (HIV) enteropathy. The symptoms associated with IBS occur during the waking hours.

What do associated symptoms tell me?

Key Questions
- Do you have any fever? Did you take your temperature?
- Do you have any vomiting?
- What occurred first: the diarrhea or the vomiting?

Fever
Patients often report having a "fever" when they have such symptoms as facial flushing, shaking chills, headache, malaise or muscle aches, or a sensation of warmth. These symptoms are usually not validated by measuring body temperature with a thermometer. Fever is a cardinal manifestation of disease. GI tract and respiratory tract infections are responsible for 80% of febrile illnesses.

Vomiting
Vomiting is often present early in the course of viral gastroenteritis (especially the Norwalk virus), food poisoning, and food-borne bacterial infection. Vomiting is one of the main causes of dehydration in acute diarrhea. Also, small bowel processes commonly associated with viral agents cause delayed gastric emptying and luminal distention, which often induces vomiting before the onset of diarrhea.

Occurrence of Vomiting and Diarrhea
When diarrhea occurs before the vomiting, suspect a bacterial etiology.

Could this be caused by exposure to others or to contaminated food?

Key Questions
- If a child: Does the child attend day care?
- If a child: Are any of the other children in day care ill?
- Have you been around others who have similar symptoms?

Day Care Attendance
Children who attend day care are at greater risk of acquiring many bacterial infections transmitted through orofecal contamination and diapering.

Others with Similar Symptoms
It is common for food-borne infections to be acquired at social gatherings in which food is served; in this case, others at the gathering can become ill with similar symptoms. However, patients do not always know if others became ill, especially when the onset of diarrhea occurs 1 to 2 hours after food ingestion.

Could this be the result of exposure to animals?

Key Questions
- What pets do you have?
- Have you had contact with or have you handled dogs, cats, or turtles?

Exposure to Infectious Agents Through Animal Contact
Campylobacter jejuni infection can be acquired from infected dogs or cats. Infected turtles are a source of *Salmonella*.

Could this be caused by exposure to contaminated water?

Key Question
- Have you traveled recently? Where?

Recent Travel
Travel outside of the United States carries the potential to acquire enterotoxigenic *Escherichia coli* or, less commonly, *G. lamblia, Salmonella, Shigella, C. jejuni,*

or *Entamoeba histolytica*. Camping exposes individuals to *Giardia* and *Campylobacter* through untreated water. Outbreaks of diarrhea caused by *Cryptosporidium* have been linked to contaminated water in urban areas of the U.S.

Could sexual activities explain the diarrhea?

Key Question

■ Do your sexual practices include anal sex?

Suspect *Shigella* infection in patients who engage in anal sex, particularly homosexual males. Accompanying pain, tenesmus, and the passage of mucus suggest the presence of proctitis.

Could this be the result of an immune problem?

Key Questions

■ Have you been diagnosed with an immune system problem?
■ Do you have frequent colds or other illnesses?
■ Are you receiving chemotherapy?

Immunocompromised Host
Immunoglobulin A (IgA) and immunoglobulin G (IgG) deficiencies are frequent causes of chronic diarrhea in children. Patients with a compromised immune system from acquired immunodeficiency syndrome (AIDS) or chemotherapy often develop enteropathy.

Could this be caused by medications?

Key Questions

■ Have you taken any antibiotics recently? Which one(s)?
■ What prescription medications are you taking?
■ What over-the-counter medications/preparations are you currently using?

Recent Treatment with Antibiotics
Pseudomembranous enterocolitis caused by *Clostridium difficile* has been reported in persons who have been recently treated with antibiotics, most commonly ampicillin, clindamycin, or cephalosporins. Pseudomembranous enterocolitis is a very serious disorder that can lead to paralytic ileus. More often, antibiotics disturb the normal flora of the gut, leading to diarrhea.

Medications
Diarrhea can be caused by antacids that contain magnesium, antibiotics, methyldopa, digitalis, ß-blockers, systemic anti-inflammatory agents, colchicine, quinidine, phenothiazine, high-dose salicylates, and laxatives.

Could this be related to a surgical procedure?

Key Question

■ Have you had surgery recently?

Recent Gastrointestinal Surgery
GI surgery can result in dumping syndrome after the ingestion of meals. Inadequate mixing and digestion take place in the stomach, resulting in rapid transit and diarrhea. Anatomical derangement from surgery can also cause stagnant loops of bowel. This stagnation leads to bacterial overgrowth and results in diarrhea. Extensive bowel resection can produce short bowel syndrome, which results in diarrhea from malabsorption.

Is this diet-related?

Key Questions

■ How much fruit juice or soda do you drink in a day?
■ Do you drink milk or eat milk products?
■ Do you eat wheat products?
■ What have you eaten in the past 3 days?

Excessive Intake of High-Carbohydrate Fluids
The ingestion of large amounts of apple juice or nonabsorbable fillers, such as sorbitol, can lead to malabsorptive diarrhea. Bacterial contamination of nonpasteurized apple juice can cause diarrhea.

Lactose Intolerance
The ingestion of specific disaccharides, such as lactose, produces a malabsorptive osmotic diarrhea in persons with lactose intolerance.

Cow's Milk Protein/Soy Protein Hypersensitivity
Diarrhea, vomiting, colic, occult or grossly bloody stools, and white blood cells within the stools that begin within 2 to 3 weeks after starting either cow's milk or soy formulas can be caused by protein hypersensitivity.

Celiac Sprue (Gluten Enteropathy)

Gluten enteropathy is manifested by increasing frequency, looseness, paleness, and bulkiness of stool within 3 to 6 months of dietary intake of wheat, rye, barley, or oat products. Patients have a hypersensitivity reaction to the protein in these grains.

Starvation Stools

The history of this condition includes diarrhea that persists for 2 to 3 weeks. Stools are loose because the liquid low-fiber diet used to ease the symptoms of acute diarrhea is continued for too long. Health care providers can neglect to tell patients or parents to resume a regular diet when acute diarrhea begins to resolve. New guidelines recommend feeding soon after rehydration has been achieved.

Could this be caused by food preparation problems?

Key Questions

- Have you recently eaten raw or undercooked poultry, shellfish, or beef?
- Have you recently ingested unpasteurized milk?
- Do you prepare poultry and/or beef on the same surface as other foods?
- Is anyone else you know ill with similar symptoms?

Dietary Exposure to Infectious Agents

Undercooked poultry is a potential cause of *Salmonella* or *C. jejuni* diarrhea. Undercooked beef and unpasteurized milk are food sources that contain *E. coli* 0157:H7. Raw shellfish is a potential source of Norwalk virus. Food can be contaminated through bacteria that remain on incompletely cleaned food preparation surfaces.

Other Ill Persons

Food poisoning should be considered if diarrhea develops in two or more persons after ingestion of the same food. Such multiple occurrences suggest ingestion of infected food or toxic substances (e.g., lead, mercury).

Is there any family predisposition that can point to a cause?

Key Questions

- Have you or anyone in your family been diagnosed with cystic fibrosis?

- Does anyone in your family have a history of chronic diarrhea, ulcerative colitis, or inflammatory bowel disease?

Family History of Cystic Fibrosis

Cystic fibrosis is the most common genetic disease in Caucasians. It has an autosomal recessive mode of inheritance. The condition leads to fat malabsorption and produces fatty, foul-smelling diarrhea.

Family History of Diarrheal Illnesses

Inflammatory bowel disease is genetically linked.

DIAGNOSTIC REASONING: FOCUSED PHYSICAL EXAMINATION
Inspect General Appearance

Observe the patient's general appearance. Diarrhea should be considered a symptom in all instances, and principal attention should be directed to determination and correction of the cause.

Assess Hydration Status

Assessment of hydration status is the most important aspect of physical examination in the child. Dehydration in otherwise healthy adults is uncommon unless the diarrhea is very severe (Table 11-1). Hydration is also an important consideration in older adults and the chronically ill and in those persons who cannot replace fluid losses with oral intake. In the presence of hypernatremia, the state of dehydration can be found to be greater than suggested by physical examination because extracellular fluid volume tends to be preserved at the expense of intracellular volume.

Indicators of Hydration Status
Mucous Membranes

The earliest clinical sign of dehydration is dryness of mucous membranes. Hyperventilation with mouth-breathing can dry the mucous membranes of the mouth in the absence of dehydration. Recent vomiting makes the mucous membranes appear moist. The patient can also have halitosis.

Tissue Turgor

Turgor reflects the amount of fluid in the interstitial spaces and is best assessed on the thigh, chest, and abdomen. Abdominal testing alone can be misleading because distention can mask the loss of turgor. Obese

Table 11-1 Determining Hydration Status

SIGNS/SYMPTOMS	MILD DEHYDRATION	MODERATE DEHYDRATION	SEVERE DEHYDRATION
Estimated fluid deficit (% of body weight)*	<5	>6-9	>10
Estimated fluid deficit (mL/kg)	30-50	60-90	>100
Thirst	Increased	Marked increase	Very marked increase
Blood pressure	Normal	Postural drop only	Low or absent (peripherally)
Pulse (peripheral)	Normal	Rapid	Rapid, thready
Heart rate	Mildly elevated	Elevated	Greatly elevated
Mucous membranes	Thick saliva	Dry	Very dry
Eyes	Normal	Sunken	Deeply sunken
Tears when crying	Present	Absent	Absent
Skin turgor	Normal	Tenting	None
Fontanel	Normal	Sunken	Very sunken
Urine output	Mildly decreased	Decreased	Markedly decreased or absent
Affect/sensorium	Normal	Restlessness/irritability	Lethargy/coma

*Percent body weight loss = [(normal weight − present weight)/normal weight] × 100.

children often do not appear to have loss of skin turgor because of the elasticity of their skin.

Fontanel

The fontanel, if still open, is best assessed with the child in an upright position. The normal fontanel can feel tense in the infant who is supine. In the crying child, physiological bulging occurs only during expiration; this bulging disappears when the child relaxes or inspires. The fontanel will be sunken in a dehydrated state.

Peripheral Perfusion

Blanching of the nail bed (using the sternum in the infant) with pressure and quick refill of capillary blood in less than 2 seconds is normal. In dehydration, it takes longer for the blood to reappear in the tissue.

Urine Output/Specific Gravity

In a mildly dehydrated child, the output decreases with a slight increase in specific gravity. In a moderately dehydrated child, the urinary output is decreased and the specific gravity is increased. In a severely dehydrated child, the urinary output is decreased to oliguria and the specific gravity is markedly increased, up to 1.030.

Take Temperature

An elevated temperature increases insensible water loss and can lead to more rapid dehydration. The presence of a fever in a patient with acute diarrhea indicates viral or bacterial infection. Fever in a patient with chronic diarrhea points to inflammatory causes.

The generally accepted normal basal body temperature is 37° C (98.6° F) determined orally or 0.6° C (1° F) higher determined rectally. Fever is generally accepted as any oral temperature above 37.8° C (100° F).

Weigh Patient and Note Persistent or Involuntary Weight Loss

Lactose intolerance, cystic fibrosis, intestinal malabsorption, infectious diarrhea, and inflammatory bowel disease can cause weight loss. Persons with these conditions have adequate or even increased food intake, but they cannot absorb sufficient nutrients to sustain normal nutrition. In children, this can cause failure to thrive and interruption of growth. In adults, colonic neoplasm can cause partial obstruction and diarrhea, and weight loss can be evident.

Observe Abdominal Contour

Abdominal distention can be associated with an ileus as in enteritis or with gaseous dilation resulting from malabsorption. A scaphoid abdomen can be seen in children with severe dehydration.

Auscultate the Abdomen

The major objective is to detect the presence of bowel sounds anywhere in the abdomen. Listen in all four quadrants. The absence of bowel sounds is established only after 5 minutes of continuous listening. Bowel sounds that are high pitched are heard with peristaltic rushes found in enteritis and secretory diarrhea. Bowel sounds are diminished or absent with necrotizing enterocolitis.

Palpate the Abdomen for Tenderness

Peritonitis can cause diarrhea as a result of inflammation and local enteric irritation. Signs of peritoneal irritation include a rigid abdomen, rebound tenderness (Blumberg sign), and positive signs on the following tests: iliopsoas muscle test, obturator muscle test, and heel jar test (Markle sign) (see Chapter 2). Tenderness is uncommon in self-limiting diarrhea. Localized right lower quadrant tenderness in a "sick" patient with acute diarrhea can indicate appendicitis, Crohn disease, right-sided diverticulitis, or carcinoma. Localized left lower quadrant tenderness suggests diverticulitis, fecal impaction, colon cancer, and various causes of proctocolitis. Localized pain in chronic diarrhea can also occur with IBS.

Perform a Digital Rectal Examination

Look for fissures and lacerations and feel for impacted stool. Impacted stool can be felt as a puttylike mass that fills the rectum and extends upward. Also obtain a stool sample for occult blood testing and for laboratory studies. Observe stool on finger for color and the presence of blood.

Palpate Lymph Nodes

Evidence of systemic disease should be assessed. Chronic diarrhea in patients who have lymphadenopathy is associated with lymphoma and AIDS.

LABORATORY AND DIAGNOSTIC STUDIES

Laboratory or diagnostic studies are not necessary if the patient appears to have a viral or toxigenic bacterial infection because the disease is usually mild and self-limiting. Reserve stool cultures and examine for ova and parasites in patients who appear relatively ill, with signs of invasive diarrhea or persistent diarrhea, or who have a history of suspected parasite infection.

Fecal Leukocytes

Fecal leukocyte detection is an easy and inexpensive test that is 75% specific for bacterial diarrhea. Leukocytes are found in inflammatory diarrheal disease and are present in bacterial infections that invade the intestinal wall (*E. coli, Shigella,* and *Salmonella*). Leukocytes are also present in diarrhea from ulcerative colitis and Crohn disease as well as antibiotic-related diarrhea. They are not seen in viral gastroenteritis, parasitic diarrhea, *Salmonella* carrier states, or enterotoxigenic bacterial diarrheas. Obtain a small fleck of mucus or stool. Do not allow the specimen to dry. Place the specimen on a slide, add two drops of Löffler alkaline methylene blue stain, and wait 2 minutes. Microscopic white and red blood cells indicate the presence of *Shigella*, enterohemorrhagic *E. coli*, enteropathogenic *E. coli*, *Campylobacter*, *C. difficile*, or other inflammatory or invasive diarrhea.

Fecal Occult Blood Testing

Fecal occult blood testing (FOBT) is used to test for occult blood in the stool. A stool sample is placed on a filter paper, and an activating solution is applied. A positive test is indicated by the appearance of a color (usually blue or green). A positive result indicates the presence of occult blood. Red blood cells often appear in diarrhea caused by enteropathic bacteria or protozoa. A 3-day series of stool samples is used to screen for colon cancer and is recommended annually in adults ages 50 and older.

Fecal Immunochemical Test

Also called immunochemical FOBT (iFOBT), fecal immunochemical test (FIT) uses antibodies to human globin to detect a specific portion of a human blood protein. FIT does not react with non–human hemoglobin or peroxidase, so food restrictions before the test are not necessary. Immunochemical FOBTs are also more specific for lower GI tract bleeding as they target the globin portion of hemoglobin, which does not survive passage through the upper GI tract. This test is done essentially the same way as conventional FOBT, but is more specific and reduces the number of false positive results. Vitamins or foods do not affect the fecal immunochemical test, and some forms require only one or two stool specimens.

Fecal Fat

A 72-hour fecal fat analysis is done by instructing the patient to have a daily dietary intake of 100 g of fat for 3 days before and during a 72-hour period of stool collection. In children, a fat retention coefficient is determined. An abnormal result is greater than 6 g/day in the stool on an 80- to 100-g diet of fat and indicates a malabsorption syndrome.

D-Xylose Absorption Test

The D-xylose absorption test is used to determine whether diarrhea is caused by malabsorption or maldigestion. Blood is taken before the patient ingests the D-xylose. The patient is then asked to drink a fluid containing 25 g of D-xylose. Repeat venipuncture to obtain blood is performed in exactly 2 hours for adults and 1 hour for children. Urine is collected approximately 5 hours after ingestion of the fluid. Blood and urine levels are subsequently evaluated. An abnormal result is found if less than 4.5 g of the D-xylose is excreted in a 5-hour urine collection and blood levels are less than 25 to 40 mg/dL in adults (30 mg/dL in children). The abnormal result indicates the diarrhea is caused by malabsorption.

Stool pH

The pH of the stool specimen is determined by using litmus strips. A pH value of 5.5 indicates lactose or other carbohydrate malabsorption. Normal stool pH is neutral or weakly alkaline.

Wet Mount

Wet mounts are useful to assess for trophozoites, cysts, ova, and certain helminth larvae. Obtain a sample of feces on a wooden applicator stick, mix with a drop of saline, and add iodine contrast to view and examine under a microscope. *V. cholerae* can be identified by using dark-field microscopy. The characteristic darting motility of vibrios can be recognized in fresh wet preparations.

C. difficile Toxin Assay

This assay detects *C. difficile* toxin in the stool, which is diagnostic of clostridial enterocolitis. The clostridial bacterium releases a toxin that causes necrosis of the colonic epithelium.

Stool Culture

Stool culture is used to detect common bacteria such as *Enterococcus, E. coli, Proteus, Pseudomonas, Staphylococcus aureus, Candida albicans, Bacteroides,* and *Clostridia.* Special enriching techniques or media are necessary to look for some agents. Pathogenic bacteria are *Salmonella, Shigella,* *Campylobacter, Yersinia,* pathogenic *E. coli, Staphylococcus,* and *C. difficile.*

Stool for Ova and Parasites

Stool can be tested for the presence of ova and parasites (O & P). Fresh stool is required to preserve the trophozoites of some parasites. Common parasites are *Ascaris* (hookworm) and *Strongyloides* (tapeworm).

Giardia Antigen Test

Giardia antigen test is a solid phase immunoassay used for the detection of *Giardia* specific antigen 65. Only one stool specimen is required and the test result is available within 1 day.

Indirect Hemagglutinin Assay

The indirect hemagglutinin assay (IHA) detects antibodies to *E. histolytica.* A positive titer is greater than 1:128.

Complete Blood Count with Differential

A CBC with differential should be obtained in severely ill or dehydrated patients to screen for infection. Infection is indicated with increased leukocytes. Microcytic hypochromic anemia (mean corpuscular hemoglobin concentration [MCHC], <30 g/dL; mean corpuscular volume [MCV], >85 fl) can indicate the presence of chronic disease. Most bloody diarrhea produces an elevated platelet count as an acute-phase reactant in an inflammatory process. In hemolytic uremic syndrome (HUS), the platelet count can be normal or low.

Peripheral Blood Smear

A peripheral blood smear is an examination of the cellular contents of the blood under a microscope using a variety of stains. Hemoglobin can be roughly estimated by the depth of staining present. This quantitative analysis assists in characterizing a number of conditions, including hemolytic anemia associated with HUS. In HUS, the peripheral smear shows characteristic schistocytes.

Blood Urea Nitrogen and Creatinine

The blood urea nitrogen (BUN) and creatinine tests are indicated in severely ill or dehydrated patients to ascertain adequate kidney functioning. Dehydration is a cause of prerenal failure. HUS will cause impaired renal function.

Endoscopic Studies

Further endoscopic diagnostic studies such as flexible sigmoidoscopy or colonoscopy should be considered when the cause of diarrhea is not determined or when the diarrhea lasts for longer than 1 month.

DIFFERENTIAL DIAGNOSIS
Acute Diarrhea
Viral Gastroenteritis

Viral gastroenteritis presents with explosive onset of diarrhea, vomiting, low-grade fever, anorexia, and myalgia. Symptoms last for 1 week or less. Norwalk virus is a major causative agent and is usually seen in school-age children and adults. Rotavirus is the most common cause of diarrhea in children ages 6 to 24 months and is usually seen in the winter.

Shigella

Shigella presents with acute diarrhea that contains mucus and blood. The patient has up to 7 days of watery diarrhea; then toxins are produced that result in ulceration, mucosal irritability, and frequent bowel movements. Stools are yellow or green and contain undigested food, mucus, and blood. Leukocytes and red blood cells are seen in the stools. It is the second most common cause of diarrhea in children ages 6 to 10 years old and is common in day care settings. Upper respiratory tract infection symptoms can also be present.

Food Poisoning with *Staphylococcus* or *Bacillus aureus*

Staphylococcus or *Bacillus aureus* food poisoning causes explosive diarrhea 2 to 6 hours after eating. High attack rates are seen among persons eating contaminated food (improperly stored meats or custard-filled pastries). Cramping and vomiting in addition to diarrhea are present. There usually is no fever. The diarrhea lasts 18 to 24 hours, and the person recovers quickly. However, the condition could be life threatening in the elderly and in persons with other serious illness.

Food Poisoning with *Clostridium perfringens*

C. perfringens causes severe diarrhea 8 to 20 hours after eating. The patient reports crampy abdominal pain and diarrhea. The stool is watery and nonbloody. Nausea, vomiting, and fever can be present but are less common. The diarrhea usually lasts for less than 3 days.

Salmonella

Salmonella causes severe diarrhea and fever. It is seen 20 times more often in patients with AIDS, sickle cell disease, or reticuloendothelial dysfunction. The incubation period is 3 to 40 days with insidious or abrupt onset. The patient has fever, anorexia, and weight loss. GI symptoms occur first, followed by fever, abdominal cramps, and vomiting. Stools are green, loose, and slimy and have the odor of spoiled eggs. Rarely is blood present.

Campylobacter

Campylobacter infection causes fever, headache, and myalgia for 12 to 24 hours; then diarrhea develops. Roughly two thirds of patients have watery diarrhea and one third have bloody dysentery. The incubation period is 2 to 5 days. The patient has abdominal cramping, pain, and fever, and the diarrhea contains mucus and blood. The condition can mimic appendicitis because of mesenteric lymphadenitis. Toxic megacolon and colonic hemorrhages can occur, especially if antimotility agents have been used.

Vibrio cholerae

V. cholerae causes severe watery diarrhea without a preceding illness. It usually occurs in epidemics. The onset is acute, usually 8 to 18 hours after the ingestion of contaminated seafood, water, or food prepared in contaminated water. Diarrhea resolves in 3 to 5 days. The essential element in cholera is the speed at which fluid is lost. This quick loss of fluid and dehydration can lead to death within hours. Red and white blood cells are not seen on stool examination.

Enterotoxic E. coli

E. coli causes moderate amounts of nonbloody diarrhea. This develops acutely 8 to 18 hours after the ingestion of contaminated food/water and typically lasts for 24 to 48 hours. The patient experiences cramping and abdominal pain with the diarrhea. The organism (gram-negative rod) is transmitted via the fecal-oral route. It is spread through contaminated water or incompletely cooked food that was cleaned in contaminated water, or through incompletely cooked beef, especially ground hamburger meat. Enterotoxic *E. coli* is the leading cause of traveler's diarrhea. The diagnosis can be confirmed with fecal leukocytes or stool culture.

Entamoeba histolytica

A patient with diarrhea caused by this parasite presents with large amounts of bloody diarrhea and abdominal cramping and vomiting that develop acutely 12 to 24 hours after the ingestion of contaminated food or water. The diagnosis is confirmed through an IHA. Antibodies to *E. histolytica* are formed; a positive titer is greater than 1:128.

Antibiotic-Induced Diarrhea

This condition produces a mild, watery diarrhea and is caused by taking antibiotics, especially ampicillin, tetracycline, lincomycin, clindamycin, and chloramphenicol. The patient often reports crampy abdominal pain. Diagnosis is made through history and clinical findings.

Pseudomembranous Colitis

Pseudomembranous colitis is most often caused by *C. difficile*. This diarrhea is induced by antibiotics, most commonly ampicillin, clindamycin, or cephalosporins. An acute inflammatory bowel disorder occurs with symptoms that range from transient mild diarrhea to active colitis with bloody diarrhea, abdominal pain, fever, and leukocytosis. Symptoms usually begin during a course of antibiotic therapy but can begin 1 to 10 days after treatment is completed. The diagnosis is established with sigmoidoscopy or colonoscopy. The diagnosis is confirmed with *C. difficile* toxin assay or stool culture.

Necrotizing Enterocolitis

Necrotizing enterocolitis is an inflammatory bowel condition that occurs in newborns. The patient is usually a premature or low–birth-weight infant who presents with feeding intolerance, vomiting, abdominal distention, lethargy, and loose, bloody stools containing mucus. It is the most common cause of death in the second week of life for low–birth-weight infants. Radiography shows pneumatosis intestinalis, indicating air within the subserosal bowel wall, which is the radiological hallmark used to confirm the diagnosis.

Hemorrhagic Disease of the Newborn

Hemorrhagic disease of the newborn is due to a deficiency in coagulation factors dependent on vitamin K. Most newborns do not have adequate levels of vitamin K, but bleeding problems develop in only a few. GI bleeding occurs 2 to 3 days postnatally. Laboratory studies typically show markedly elevated prothrombin time (PT) and partial thromboplastin time (PTT) and depressed levels of vitamin K–dependent factors. The routine use of prophylactic vitamin K prevents most cases.

Hemolytic Uremic Syndrome

HUS is seen in children and is usually preceded by a GI illness. The leading bacterial cause of HUS in the United States is now *E. coli* 0157:H7. The patient presents with a history of bloody diarrhea, fever, and irritability. Initially, laboratory blood values are essentially normal except that the platelet count is normal or low. The stool culture is negative. A peripheral blood smear reveals schistocytes, confirming the diagnosis. Fragmented red blood cells are often seen on the peripheral smear before complications of renal involvement occur. The child can have a sudden onset of acute renal failure. Renal function test results will be altered.

Chronic Diarrhea
Irritable Bowel Syndrome

IBS is characterized by alternating periods of constipation and diarrhea. Patients often have mucus in their stools. It is commonly seen in young and middle-age women with a history of intermittent diarrhea. Patients often present with reports of constipation rather than diarrhea. The patient reports abdominal pain in the left lower quadrant, although it can occur anywhere. The pain seldom occurs at night, does not awaken the patient, and is commonly present in the morning. The patient can have rectal urgency and abdominal distention. There is no weight loss, the patient is afebrile, and the colon can be tender on palpation. IBS is a diagnosis of exclusion, and sigmoidoscopy or proctoscopy is used to rule out other disorders.

Ulcerative Colitis

Ulcerative colitis is an inflammatory bowel disease that causes proctitis with rectal bleeding, tenesmus, and the passage of mucopus. Abdominal cramping is common, but abdominal pain and tenderness are not common. The greater the extent of colon involvement, the more likely it is that the patient has diarrhea.

Crohn Disease

Crohn disease is an inflammatory bowel disease that presents with abdominal cramping, tenderness, rectal bleeding, and diarrhea. The disease can produce chronic, bloody diarrhea and cause failure to thrive in children. The patient can have a fever. Weight loss is common because of malabsorption or a reduced intake of food used to minimize postprandial symptoms. Diagnosis is made through colonoscopy and biopsy.

Carbohydrate Malabsorption and Lactose Intolerance

Malabsorption and/or lactose intolerance causes the patient to experience diarrhea, bloating, and increased flatus. The ingestion of specific disaccharides, such as lactose or sorbitol, exacerbates the episodes of diarrhea. A trial of elimination of offending foods often confirms the clinical diagnosis.

Fat Malabsorption

Fat malabsorption is seen with patients who have cystic fibrosis or vitamin A, D, or K deficiency. Patients with cystic fibrosis have foul, pale, bulky diarrhea that is greasy, oily, and consistent with steatorrhea. The diarrhea usually precedes lung involvement. Laboratory testing for fat malabsorption includes a 72-hour fecal fat analysis.

Toddler's Diarrhea

Toddler's diarrhea is described as the occurrence of abnormal amounts of formless stools with mucus in children ages 1 to 3 years. Symptoms rarely persist beyond age 4 to 5 years. The diarrhea is chronic and nonspecific, with three or four stools per day, some containing mucus. Physical examination and growth are within normal limits for the child's age. This is a diagnosis of exclusion, and other causes of chronic diarrhea must first be ruled out.

Celiac Sprue/Protein Hypersensitivity

This diarrhea causes increasing stool frequency, looseness, paleness, and bulkiness 3 to 6 months after dietary intake of wheat, rye, and other grains. Patients have a hypersensitivity reaction to the protein in wheat, rye, barley, and oats. Children appear lethargic, irritable, and anorexic.

Giardia

Giardia is the leading parasitic cause of chronic diarrhea in children in the United States and can be contracted through travel both in and outside of the country. Patients experience watery, foul-smelling diarrhea, abdominal pain, distention, and gas.

Cryptosporidium and Isospora belli

These parasites produce recurrent episodes of nonbloody diarrhea with varying amounts of water. The volume can be massive. The organisms are transmitted via the fecal-oral route and are spread through the ingestion of contaminated water or direct orofecal contact.

Postgastrectomy Dumping Syndrome

This syndrome occurs after GI surgery. The condition can occur whenever the pyloric mechanism is disrupted by pyloroplasty, gastroduodenostomy, or gastrojejunostomy. The diarrhea occurs after meals because of increased transit of food through the colon. Patients can experience associated symptoms, including diaphoresis and tachycardia.

Diabetic Enteropathy

Diabetic enteropathy occurs in patients with diabetes. Patients can experience nocturnal diarrhea, postprandial vomiting, and fatty stools from malabsorption. The condition is a diagnosis of exclusion in persons with diabetes.

HIV Enteropathy

HIV enteropathy has an insidious onset and is recurrent. Patients have large amounts of nonbloody diarrhea and mild to moderate nausea and vomiting. It is caused by direct infection of mucosa and neuronal cells in the GI system. Patients will demonstrate other HIV-related symptoms and lymphadenopathy.

Medication-Induced Diarrhea

Diarrhea can occur as a result of taking prescription or over-the-counter drugs; the most common ones are antacids that contain magnesium, antibiotics, methyldopa, digitalis, ß-blockers, systemic anti-inflammatory agents, colchicine, quinidine, phenothiazine, high-dose salicylates, and laxatives.

DIFFERENTIAL DIAGNOSIS OF *Common Causes of Acute Diarrhea*

CONDITION	HISTORY	PHYSICAL FINDINGS	DIAGNOSTIC STUDIES
Viral gastroenteritis (e.g., Norwalk or rotavirus viral agents)	Abrupt onset 6-12 hr after exposure; nonbloody, watery diarrhea; lasts <1 wk; nausea/vomiting, fever, abdominal pain, tenesmus	In children can see severe dehydration; hyperactive bowel sounds, diffuse pain on abdominal palpation	None
Shigella (gram-negative rod; fecal-oral transmission; common in day care setting; common in gay bowel syndrome)	Acute onset 12-24 hr after exposure; lasts 3-7 days; large amounts of bloody diarrhea with abdominal cramping and vomiting	Lower abdominal tenderness, hyperactive bowel sounds, no peritoneal irritation	Fecal leukocytes, positive stool culture
S. aureus food poisoning (gram-positive cocci; from improperly stored meats or custard-filled pies)	Acute onset 2-6 hr after ingestion; lasts 18-24 hr; large amounts of watery, nonbloody diarrhea; cramping and vomiting	Hyperactive bowel sounds	Fecal leukocytes, negative stool culture
Clostridium perfringens food poisoning (gram-positive rod; from contaminated food)	Acute onset 8-20 hr after ingestion; lasts 12-24 hr; large amounts of watery, nonbloody diarrhea; abdominal pain and cramping	Hyperactive bowel sounds, diffuse pain on abdominal palpation	Fecal leukocytes, negative anaerobic culture of stool
Salmonella food poisoning (gram-negative bacilli; ingestion of contaminated food, poultry, eggs)	Acute onset 12-24 hr after ingestion; lasts 2-5 days; moderate to large amounts of nonbloody diarrhea; abdominal cramping and vomiting	Fever of 38.3-38.9° C (101-102° F) common; hyperactive bowel sounds, diffuse abdominal pain	Fecal leukocytes, positive stool culture, WBC count normal
Campylobacter jejuni (gram-negative rod; fecal-oral transmission; household pet)	Acute onset 3-5 days after exposure; lasts 3-7 days; moderate amounts of bloody diarrhea	Fever, lower quadrant abdominal pain	Fecal leukocytes, positive stool culture
Vibrio cholerae (gram-negative rod; fecal-oral transmission; ingestion of contaminated water, seafood, or food)	Acute onset 8-24 hr after ingestion of contaminated food; lasts 3-5 days; large amounts of nonbloody, watery, painless diarrhea; can be mild or fulminate	Cyanotic, scaphoid abdomen, poor skin turgor, thready peripheral pulses, voice faint	Fecal leukocytes, negative stool culture
Enterotoxic *E. coli* (gram-negative rod; fecal-oral transmission; ingestion of contaminated water or food)	Acute onset 8-18 hr after ingestion of contaminated food/water; lasts 24-48 hr; moderate amounts of nonbloody diarrhea; pain, cramping, abdominal pain; adults in United States generally do not develop illness from enterotoxic *E. coli*	No fever; dehydration is major complication	Fecal leukocytes, positive stool culture
Entamoeba histolytica parasite (cysts in food and water, from feces)	Acute onset 12-24 hr after ingestion of contaminated food or water; large amounts of bloody diarrhea; abdominal cramping and vomiting	Right lower quadrant abdominal pain; in small number of cases hepatic abscess forms	IHA: antibodies to *E. histolytica;* positive titer is >1:128
Antibiotic-induced diarrhea (begins after taking antibiotics)	Mild, watery diarrhea; crampy abdominal pain	Diffuse abdominal pain on palpation, fever absent	Usually not needed
Pseudomembranous colitis (Antibiotic-induced *Clostridium difficile*)	Induced by antibiotics, most commonly ampicillin, clindamycin, or cephalosporins; symptoms range from transient mild diarrhea to active colitis with bloody diarrhea, abdominal pain, fever	Lower quadrant tenderness, fever	CBC: leukocytes; sigmoidoscopy/colonoscopy; *C. difficile* toxin assay or stool culture; *C. difficile* toxin

DIFFERENTIAL DIAGNOSIS OF *Common Causes of Acute Diarrhea—cont'd*

CONDITION	HISTORY	PHYSICAL FINDINGS	DIAGNOSTIC STUDIES
Hemolytic uremic syndrome (HUS) (primary cause of HUS in United States is *E. coli* O157:H7)	Children <4 yr with history of gastroenteritis; history of bloody diarrhea, fever, and irritability	Fever, irritability; can have oliguria or anuria	CBC, platelet count, renal function tests, peripheral blood smear; negative stool culture
Necrotizing enterocolitis	Premature or low–birth-weight infant who presents with feeding intolerance	Vomiting, abdominal distention, lethargy, loose, bloody, mucousy stools	Refer
Hemorrhagic disease of the newborn	GI bleeding 2-3 days postnatal; history of lack of vitamin K injection; history of mother on anticonvulsants prenatally	Bruising, ecchymoses, mild to moderate bleeding	Laboratory studies typically show markedly elevated PT and PTT with depressed levels of vitamin K–dependent factors

CBC, complete blood count; *IHA,* indirect hemagglutinin assay; *PT,* prothrombin time; *PTT,* partial thromboplastin time; *WBC,* white blood cells.

DIFFERENTIAL DIAGNOSIS OF *Common Causes of Chronic Diarrhea*

CONDITION	HISTORY	PHYSICAL FINDINGS	DIAGNOSTIC STUDIES
Irritable bowel syndrome (IBS)	Intermittent diarrhea alternating with constipation; mucus with stool; seldom occurs at night or awakens patient; commonly present in morning; can have rectal urgency; episodes usually triggered by stress or ingestion of food; affects women 3 times as often as men	Tender colon on palpation; can have abdominal distention; no weight loss; afebrile	Diagnosis of exclusion; sigmoidoscopy, proctoscopy
Ulcerative colitis (distal colon is most severely affected and rectum is involved)	History of severe diarrhea with gross blood in stools, no growth retardation; few reports of pain; age of onset second and third decades with small peak during adolescence; positive family history	Overt rectal bleeding; initially no fever, weight loss, or pain on palpation of abdomen; moderate colitis: weight loss, fever, abdominal tenderness	CBC shows leukocytosis or anemia, ESR elevated; stool cultures to rule out other causes of diarrhea; colonoscopy
Crohn disease (associated with uveitis, erythema nodosum)	History of chronic bloody diarrhea with abdominal cramping, tenderness, and rectal bleeding; in children a history of growth retardation, weight loss, moderate diarrhea, abdominal pain, and anorexia	Weight loss; rare gross rectal bleeding; fistulas common	Colonoscopy with biopsies
Carbohydrate malabsorption	Bloating, flatus, diarrhea exacerbated by ingestion of certain disaccharides (e.g., lactose, milk, milk products); can follow viral gastroenteritis	Diffuse abdominal pain	Trial elimination of offending foods
Fat malabsorption	Greasy, fatty, malodorous stools; associated with deficiencies of vitamins K, A, and D; cystic fibrosis	Rectal prolapse, poor weight gain, abdominal distention	73-hr fecal fats, sweat test
Toddler's diarrhea	3-4 stools/day; some contain mucus; rare past 4-5 yr of age	Physical examination and growth normal	Clinical diagnosis

Continued

DIFFERENTIAL DIAGNOSIS OF *Common Causes of Chronic Diarrhea—cont'd*

CONDITION	HISTORY	PHYSICAL FINDINGS	DIAGNOSTIC STUDIES
Celiac sprue/protein hypersensitivity (reaction to protein in wheat, rye, barley, and oats)	Increased stool frequency, looseness, paleness, and bulkiness of stool within 3-6 mo of dietary onset; children are lethargic, irritable, and anorectic; peak frequency 9-18 mo	Failure to thrive, abdominal distention, irritability, muscle wasting	Clinical findings, improvement on gluten-free diet, CBC, anemia, folate deficiency, radiography, biopsy
Giardia parasite (primary cause of chronic diarrhea in children)	Watery, foul diarrhea; common in day care, among travelers, and in male homosexuals	Low-grade fever, weight loss; chronic form: fatigue, growth retardation, steatorrhea	*Giardia* antigen test
Cryptosporidium species/*Isospora belli* protozoan parasites (fecal-oral transmission; ingestion of contaminated water or direct oral-anal contact)	Recurrent episodes; variable amounts watery, nonbloody diarrhea; amounts can be massive	Weight loss, severe right upper quadrant abdominal pain with biliary tract involvement	Stool for O & P
Postgastrectomy dumping syndrome	Following GI surgery, diarrhea occurs after meals because of increased transit of food through colon	Diaphoresis and tachycardia	Upper GI series
Diabetic enteropathy	Nocturnal diarrhea, postprandial vomiting, fatty stools from malabsorption	Findings associated with diabetes	Diagnosis of exclusion in diabetic persons
HIV enteropathy (direct infection of mucosa and neuronal cells in GI system)	Insidious onset, recurrent large amounts of nonbloody diarrhea, mild to moderate nausea/vomiting	Findings associated with HIV infection	Testing for HIV
Medication-induced diarrhea	Mild to moderately severe nonwatery, nonbloody diarrhea	No specific findings related to diarrhea	Usually none needed

CBC, complete blood count; *ESR,* erythrocyte sedimentation rate; *GI,* gastrointestinal; *HIV,* human immune deficiency virus; *O & P,* ova and parasites.

REFERENCES AND READINGS

American Academy of Pediatrics: The use and misuse of fruit juice in pediatrics, *Pediatrics* 107:1210, 2001.

Aranda-Michel J, Giannella RA: Acute diarrhea: a practical review, *Am J Med* 106:67, 1999.

Armon K, Stephenson T, MacFaul R, Eccleston P, Werneke U: An evidence and consensus based guideline for acute diarrhoea management, *Arch Dis Child* 85:132, 2001.

Carollo AA, Schiller LR: Chronic diarrhea: differential diagnosis and initial management, *Consultant* December:1604, 2005.

Casper C: Detecting and treating foodborne infections, *The Clinical Advisor* February:24, 2005.

Canavan A, Arant BS Jr: Diagnosis and management of dehydration in children, *Am Fam Physician* 80:692, 2009.

Corrigan JJ: Hemolytic uremic syndrome, *Pediatr Rev* 22:365, 2001.

Dennehy PH: Acute diarrheal disease in children: epidemiology, prevention, and treatment, *Infect Dis Clin North Am* 19:585, 2005.

Goodgame RW: Viral causes of diarrhea, *Gastroenterol Clin North Am* 30:779, 2001.

Keating J: Chronic diarrhea, *Pediatr Rev* 26:5, 2005.

Lawrence R, Schiller LR: Chronic diarrhea, *Gastroenterology* 127:287, 2004.

Montgomery L: What is the best way to evaluate acute diarrhea? *J Fam Pract* 51:575, 2002.

Practice parameter: The management of acute gastroenteritis in young children, *Pediatrics* 97:424, 1996.

Ramaswamy K: Infectious diarrhea in children, *Gastroenterol Clin North Am* 30:611, 2001.

Thielman NM, Guerrant RL: Acute infectious diarrhea, *N Engl J Med* 350:38, 2004.

Tobillo ET, Schwartz SM: Acute diarrhea, *Adv Nurse Pract* 6:38, 1998.

Turgeon DK: Laboratory approaches to infectious diarrhea, *Gastroenterol Clin North Am* 30:693, 2001.

Dizziness

izziness is a symptom of a variety of conditions, including vertigo, lightheadedness, and loss of balance. In children the symptom is frequently a new sensation, and is usually poorly defined. Family members often state that the child has trouble walking or is irritable or that the child's behavior is different. Older children, like adults, tend to categorize everything from lightheadedness and unsteadiness to spinning and falling as dizziness. This chapter is limited to the discussion of vertigo. Patients with vertigo have the sensation of either their body moving (subjective vertigo) or their environment moving around them (objective), usually described as a spinning or rotary motion.

The sensation of balance depends on interconnections among the visual, vestibular, and sensory systems. Vertigo can be thought of as a disruption of one of these three systems. Vertigo can be central, involving the brainstem or cerebellum; be peripheral, involving the inner ear or vestibular apparatus; or result from systemic causes.

Central vertigo is generally either neoplastic or vascular in origin, although any central nervous system disorder, such as multiple sclerosis, that disrupts the pathway between the vestibular apparatus and the brain can result in dizziness. Common vascular causes include recurrent intermittent vascular insufficiency, transient ischemic attack, or stroke. Migraine headache is a vascular-related central cause of vertigo.

Peripheral vertigo is typically produced by disruption of the inner ear or vestibular apparatus. Common causes include idiopathic etiologies, vestibular nerve inflammation, inner ear inflammation or infection, or tumor. Systemic origins include psychogenic, cardiovascular, and metabolic causes. Mixed or other causes include trauma and ototoxicity.

DIAGNOSTIC REASONING: FOCUSED HISTORY

What does the patient mean by dizziness?

Key Questions
- Can you describe how you feel when you are dizzy?
- Do you feel as though you or the room is spinning?
- Do you feel as though your balance is off?
- Do you feel like you are about to faint?

Sensation

Vertigo produces the sensation of either the patient spinning or the environment spinning around the patient. Some patients describe a sensation of their body moving forward or accelerating.

Patients can also report loss of equilibrium accompanying the vertigo. Neoplasms and progressive vestibule loss typically produce a change in vestibular function that is slow in onset and manifested as imbalance.

Loss of balance and lack of coordination in the absence of vertigo can be the result of degenerative, neoplastic, vascular, or metabolic disorders. With these symptoms, look for other nervous system abnormalities. Imbalance can also occur in adults as a result of impaired sensory input, either visual or kinetic, such as occurs with peripheral neuropathy.

Children who have a vague sense of unsteadiness can have peripheral neuropathy or a dysfunction of the vestibular or cerebellar system, whereas children who report a feeling of motion are more likely to have an abnormality of the vestibular system.

In contrast to dizziness and imbalance, lightheadedness is the feeling that one is about to faint (near syncope). Some patients describe it as a generalized weakness and the feeling that they are about to pass out if they do not lie down. True syncope, or a sudden transient loss of consciousness with concurrent loss of postural tone, always has a spontaneous recovery (see Chapter 30).

Orthostatic hypotension is a frequent cause of lightheadedness and is most common in elderly persons, occurring as a result of abnormal regulation of blood pressure. Neurological causes of orthostatic hypotension are less common and are usually accompanied by neurological findings.

In both children and adults, a report of lightheadedness can accompany anemia, hypoglycemia, or hyperventilation syndrome.

Does the vertigo result from a systemic cause?

Key Questions

- What other medical problems do you have?
- Would you describe yourself as anxious or nervous?
- Do the episodes occur with any specific activity or movement?

Other Medical Problems

Cardiovascular problems are a common cause of vertigo that is systemic in origin. The mechanism of vertigo can include vasomotor instability that decreases systemic vascular resistance, venous return, or both; severe reduction in cardiac output that obstructs blood flow within the heart or pulmonary circulation; or cardiac dysrhythmia that leads to transient decline in cardiac output. Patients with hypertension can experience vertigo while taking antihypertensive or potassium-depleting medications or as a result of postural hypotension.

Anxiety

Psychogenic dizziness is one of the most common causes of vertigo. Symptoms tend to be vague and can include other symptoms such as fatigue, fullness in the head, lightheadedness, and a sense of feeling apart from the environment. Patients can describe themselves as anxious or nervous. Patients can also have other psychiatric diagnoses. Stressors and tensions affecting children, such as divorce, custody battles, and day care, can cause vertiginous-like symptoms in the older child. Anxiety with hyperventilation can cause lightheadedness in a child, who then reports the symptom as dizziness.

Relationship to Activity or Movement

Dizziness when turning, especially when rolling over in bed, is usually due to vertigo. However, unsteadiness while walking is often considered to be disequilibrium, which can be caused by many factors. Dizziness on standing can be the result of decreased cerebral perfusion.

In children, attacks that occur with sudden changes of posture can be the result of hypotension, vascular disease, or positional vertigo.

Is the vertigo central (brainstem or cerebellar) or peripheral (vestibular) in origin?

Key Questions

- Do you have migraine headaches?
- Do you have other symptoms that bother you?
- Do you have nausea and vomiting?
- When do the episodes occur?

Headaches

Headache is a vascular-related cause of central vertigo. Approximately one third of patients with migraine headaches experience vertigo. The vertigo can appear as an aura, occurring during the headache, or can occur separately. Some of these persons have additional symptoms that are consistent with vertebrobasilar circulation abnormalities. Migraine both with and without headache is recognized as a source of dizziness in children.

Other Symptoms

Patients with central vertigo nearly always have neurological symptoms, such as double vision, facial numbness, and hemiparesis.

Cerebellar causes can produce other symptoms, such as loss of balance, that closely resemble those of a peripheral disorder; therefore neurological examination findings are important in differentiating the two. Pay particular attention to reports of motor dysfunction or lack of coordination.

Vertigo that is peripheral in origin does not produce additional neurological symptoms or signs. If the patient has nausea and vomiting, suspect a peripheral vestibular apparatus problem rather than a central cause. Nausea and vomiting are common with vestibular neuronitis and labyrinthitis and occur less often with brainstem lesions.

Timing

Vertigo that occurs on first arising in the morning is usually the result of a vestibular disorder. Vertigo that occurs while turning over in bed is characteristic of benign paroxysmal positional vertigo (BPPV) (peripheral).

What do characteristics of the episodes tell me?

Key Questions

- How long do the episodes of dizziness last?
- Is the onset sudden or gradual?
- Do you have any hearing loss?
- Do you have ringing in your ears?

Duration of Episodes

Episodes that last a few seconds are typically caused by BPPV and are usually elicited by a rapid head movement. Episodes lasting minutes to hours can be caused by Meniere disease or recurrent vestibulopathy.

Episodes that last days or weeks are commonly produced by vestibular neuronitis. Patients can feel better when they lie completely still. Stroke can also produce long-lasting episodes. The two can be differentiated based on medical history and physical examination findings.

Sudden onset of prolonged dizziness (lasting ≥60 minutes) suggests central causes, such as infection, brainstem infarction, inflammation, or vestibular hemorrhage. Trauma can also produce prolonged dizziness.

The child with chronic recurrent dizziness (episodes lasting <30 minutes) can have central causes, such as seizure problems or migraine headache. The cause can also be peripheral, such as BPPV. Chronic persistent episodes can indicate brainstem lesions, anemia, diabetes, thyrotoxicosis, or a psychosomatic disorder.

Onset

A gradual onset of dizziness is typical of an acoustic neuroma or other neoplastic process that is slow-growing. BPPV can also have a gradual onset.

Acute or sudden onset of vertigo is characteristic of labyrinthitis, Meniere disease, stroke, or vertebro-basilar causes.

Recurrent episodes are typical of BPPV, vertebro-basilar causes, and Meniere disease.

Hearing Loss and Tinnitus

A classic triad of symptoms—vertigo, hearing loss, and tinnitus—defines Meniere disease. Patients can also report a sensation of fullness in the ears. The hearing loss can be unilateral or bilateral. Patients with secondary or early tertiary syphilis can have symptoms identical to those of Meniere disease. Tinnitus, hearing loss, and pain in the ear point to lesions in the inner ear or cranial nerve VIII.

Patients with labyrinthitis and perilymphatic fistulas can also experience hearing loss but without tinnitus. An acoustic neuroma will produce unilateral hearing loss with tinnitus. Patients with recurrent vestibulopathy usually do not report hearing loss.

What else should I consider?

Key Questions

- What medications are you taking?
- Are you now or have you recently been ill?
- Have you had any recent injury to your head? Did you have dizziness before the head injury?
- Have you had any previous ear surgery?

Medications

Mediations that are salt-retaining or ototoxic can produce vertigo, lightheadedness, or unsteadiness. Salt-retaining drugs include steroids and phenylbutazone. Ototoxic medications include ethacrynic acid, streptomycin, gentamicin, aminoglycosides, aspirin, and furosemide.

Psychotropic drugs can also produce vertigo. Antihypertensive drugs can cause hypotension leading to lightheadedness. Sedatives, alcohol, and anticonvulsants can cause a sense of disequilibrium.

Current or Recent Illness

Vestibular neuronitis is associated with recent viral infection, often an upper respiratory tract infection. If a patient is currently ill, consider labyrinthitis because it is frequently associated with concomitant bacterial and viral infection. Current ear or sinus infection can produce dysfunction of the vestibular apparatus, resulting in vertigo. Recent abnormalities of middle ear ventilation and middle ear effusion are the most common cause of balance disturbance in childhood. In balance disturbance, transmission of pressure gradients through the labyrinthine windows to the inner ear fluids and the vestibular sensory receptors is altered.

History of Head Trauma

Trauma to the head or ear can cause disturbance of both peripheral and central balance mechanisms. Certain traumas can cause acute destruction of the inner ear and produce vertigo. Direct trauma can occur to the labyrinth from a temporal bone fracture. A blow to the head or a whiplash injury can also produce a concussive effect on the labyrinth. Children who have a history of head trauma can present with vertigo caused by labyrinthine damage.

Vertigo often occurs as a residual symptom and usually gradually improves over the course of a year. Trauma can also produce a fistula between the middle and inner ear, causing tympanic membrane (TM) damage and ossicle disruption.

Previous Otology History and Procedures

Patients with cholesteatoma usually have a history of chronic middle ear infection, otorrhea, and conductive hearing loss. Prior surgical procedures of the ear can produce peripheral vertigo through disruption of the vestibular apparatus or through formation of a perilymph fistula.

DIAGNOSTIC REASONING: FOCUSED PHYSICAL EXAMINATION
Take Vital Signs and Note Blood Pressure

Assess orthostatic blood pressure to rule out postural hypotension as the cause of vertigo. Assessment is made by measuring the blood pressure in both the supine and standing positions. A drop in arterial blood pressure of at least 30 systolic and 20 diastolic mm Hg when the patient changes from the supine to the standing position indicates orthostatic hypotension.

Note General Appearance

In a patient who is currently ill, suspect labyrinthitis. In a patient who is acutely nauseated and vomiting, suspect vestibular neuronitis.

Have Patient Hyperventilate and Perform Valsalva Maneuver

Perform this testing if you suspect psychogenic vertigo because the maneuver can reproduce the vertigo in these patients. Ask the patient to perform a Valsalva maneuver and to breathe in and out or blow vigorously for 1 to 3 minutes.

Perform Vision Examination

A recent change in visual acuity or new corrective lenses can cause transient episodes of imbalance.

Perform Ear Examination

Look for the presence of effusion or infection that signals serous otitis or otitis media. Look for the presence of a cholesteatoma. It will appear as a shiny white irregular mass; foul-smelling discharge can also be present. Note the integrity of the TM; trauma can sometimes cause its disruption. Perform pneumatic otoscopy (see Chapter 14), which will enable you to determine whether changes in pressure trigger an episode of vertigo. If the patient has a fistula, changes in pressure transmitted directly to the inner ear will cause a sudden episode of vertigo.

Perform Screening Hearing Tests

Perform Rinne (AC:BC) and Weber (lateralization) tests. Expect sensorineural loss with Meniere disease, labyrinthitis, perilymph fistula, and acoustic neuroma. In sensorineural loss, the sound lateralizes to the unaffected ear. With sensorineural hearing loss, bone and air conductions are both reduced in Rinne tests, but the ratio remains the same (AC:BC). Patients with a cholesteatoma, serous otitis, or otitis media can demonstrate a conductive hearing loss (see differential diagnosis table).

Perform Positional Nystagmus Testing/Provoking Maneuvers

A test for nystagmus assesses the function of the vestibular branch of the acoustic nerve (cranial nerve VIII). The presence and characteristics of nystagmus are important in determining central versus peripheral causes of vertigo. Nystagmus is defined by the axis on which it occurs (horizontal, vertical, rotary, or mixed) and by the direction in which it occurs. Nystagmus is composed of quick and slow components that can be observed. With the eye fixated, a slow drift away from the position of fixation is corrected by a quick movement back to the original position. The direction of the nystagmus is determined by the quick component because it is easier to see. The quick component depends on the interaction between the vestibular system and the cerebral cortex and represents the compensatory response to vestibular stimulation. The slow component moves in the direction of the movement of the endolymph, a clear fluid within the membranous labyrinth of the inner ear.

Fixed nystagmus, which always beats in the same direction, occurs with peripheral disorders of BPPV, Meniere disease, vestibular neuronitis, or labyrinthitis. Vestibular nystagmus typically consists of a horizontal-rotary, jerk motion of both the slow and fast components. The nystagmus associated with central causes can be horizontal, vertical, rotary, or inconsistent. Pronounced rotary, unidirectional upgaze or downgaze nystagmus always arises from central processes. Nystagmus that is equally rapid in both directions is characteristic of central causes. In vertigo of peripheral origin, nystagmus generally resolves on fixation within 24 to 48 hours, whereas nystagmus associated with central vertigo does not. See Table 12-1 for a comparison of characteristics.

Positional Maneuvers (Bárány or Dix-Hallpike Maneuvers)

To determine the origin of vertigo and accompanying nystagmus, seat the patient on the table with the patient's head turned to the left or right. Quickly lower the patient to a lying position with the head lower than the table edge so that the ear faces the floor. Repeat, with the head turned to the other side and then again with the head in the midline. The maneuver produces intense vertigo in patients with vestibular problems and can cause mild vertigo in patients with central causes. Watch for nystagmus during this maneuver. The patient's eyes should be kept open to observe the duration and direction of the nystagmus. The nystagmus associated with peripheral causes has a 3- to 10-second delay in onset, lessens with repetition, and is in a fixed direction. In contrast, the nystagmus associated with central causes begins immediately, does not fatigue with repetition, and can be in any and changing directions. With inner ear damage, the rapid phase of nystagmus is always in the same direction regardless of the direction of gaze (see Evidence-Based Practice box).

Provocation Maneuvers

In patients who experience vertigo associated with position changes or rapid movement of the head, provoke nystagmus and vertigo by having the patient assume the positions that cause the vertigo. Provocation assists in the diagnosis of BPPV. If you suspect a perilymph fistula, perform pneumatic otoscopy. The pressure applied to the middle ear can provoke nystagmus and vertigo.

Perform Neurological Examination

Look for brainstem or cerebellar dysfunction, which could cause abnormal neurological findings. Specifically test cranial nerves, looking for sensory and/or motor deficits. With the exception of hearing loss, cranial nerve function should be normal in patients with peripheral vertigo. Patients with brainstem dysfunction typically have diplopia as well as changes in sensory and motor function.

Table 12-1	**Comparison of Nystagmus in Central and Peripheral Vertigo**	
CHARACTERISTICS	**CENTRAL**	**PERIPHERAL**
Severity	Can be disproportionate to vertigo	Proportionate to vertigo
Axis	Horizontal, vertical, rotary; unidirectional upgaze or downgaze	Horizontal, rotary
Consistency of direction	Can be inconsistent	Consistent; always beats in same direction
Type	Irregular or rapid in both directions	Has both slow and quick components

◎ EVIDENCE-BASED PRACTICE *Dix-Hallpike Maneuver*

The Dix-Hallpike maneuver has a positive predictive value of 83% and a negative predictive value of 52% for the diagnosis of BPPV. After the initial test, the induced symptoms are typically less intense in peripheral vertigo; the intensity stays about the same in central vertigo. The combination of a positive Dix-Hallpike maneuver and a history of vertigo or vomiting suggests a peripheral vestibular disorder. Laboratory tests identify the etiology of vertigo in less than 1% of patients with vertigo.

Data from Labuguen RH: Initial evaluation of vertigo, *Am Fam Physician* 73:244, 2006.

Test cerebellar function. Testing gait differences while blindfolded can be helpful. Ataxia from bilateral vestibular loss is worsened by loss of visual input, whereas ataxia from cerebellar disease remains about the same. The sensitivity of gait testing is increased by watching tandem gait (heel to toe). When trying to walk a straight line, the patient with a cerebellar lesion will tend to fall toward the side of the lesion. However, gait disturbances can also be present with peripheral vertigo.

Test the patient's ability to perform rapid alternating movements (RAMs) either through pronation-supination or through touching thumb to fingers sequentially. Movements should be smooth and rhythmic, and the patient should be able to gradually increase speed. Stiff, slowed, or jerky movements indicate cerebellar dysfunction.

Perform the past-pointing test. Have the patient sit with arm extended forward and index finger pointed while you sit in the same position facing the patient. The tips of your fingers should touch. Then ask the patient to close the eyes, raise the arm above the head, and bring the arm and finger back to the same position. In patients with central lesions or unilateral vestibular abnormalities, the arm will deviate toward the side of the lesion.

Test sensory and motor function. Look for focal deficits that can occur with central vertigo. Many patients with vertigo also report generalized weakness; therefore it is important to distinguish between generalized weakness and focal motor impairment caused by brainstem disorder.

Perform Cardiovascular Evaluation

Note the heart rate and rhythm and attempt to detect dysrhythmias. Auscultate carotid and temporal arteries for bruits that can alert you to a cardiovascular cause for the vertigo.

Congenital heart disease can produce episodes of syncope that might be falsely interpreted as vertiginous episodes (see Chapter 30).

LABORATORY AND DIAGNOSTIC STUDIES
Audiometry

Audiometry is used to quantify hearing loss. The patient is tested at specific frequencies (pure tones) and specific intensities. Hearing loss is measured in decibels. Audiometry is used anytime the patient presents with both vertigo and hearing loss (i.e., Meniere disease, acoustic neuroma, labyrinthitis, perilymph fistula, or use of ototoxic medications) (see Chapter 14).

Electronystagmography

Electronystagmography (ENG) electronically detects nystagmus that cannot be detected visually. Vestibular function is evaluated using gaze testing, positional changes, and caloric stimulation. Eye movements are recorded electronically. Caloric stimulation is produced by ear irrigation with warm and then cool water.

ENG is most useful in diagnosing chronic peripheral disorders (i.e., Meniere disease and persistent BPPV) to determine the degree and progression of the vestibular deficit. It can also be useful in patients with psychogenic vertigo to provide reassurance that no organic disease is present.

Magnetic Resonance Imaging

Magnetic resonance imaging (MRI) of the brain is indicated when the history and physical examination point to acoustic neuroma or a central cause of the vertigo. Consider urgent MRI if vertigo is of sudden onset; is accompanied by severe headache, direction-changing nystagmus, or neurological signs; or if the patient has risk factors for stroke.

Computed Tomography

Computed tomography (CT) scanning of the brain is indicated whenever there is persistent vertigo and in all cases with additional signs of neurological disturbance. In patients with medical conditions such as renal failure, hypertension, or a hematological malignancy who have sudden onset of vertigo, CT scan is used to look for hemorrhage into the cerebellum, brainstem, or labyrinth.

Electroencephalography

An electroencephalogram (EEG) should be obtained for patients who have vertigo associated with alterations of consciousness.

Cardiac Monitoring

An electrocardiogram (ECG) or Holter monitoring can provide confirmatory information on cardiovascular causes of vertigo.

Hematology and Urinalysis

Complete blood count (CBC) can reveal anemia, which can cause presyncopal lightheadedness. Urine or serum glucose levels will detect diabetes mellitus, which can produce vertigo. Urine testing and blood urea nitrogen (BUN) level can reveal renal failure, which can also be associated with vertigo.

Serological Testing for Syphilis

Because secondary syphilis or early tertiary syphilis can produce the same symptoms that occur in Meniere disease, screening is advocated by some to rule out syphilis as a cause.

DIFFERENTIAL DIAGNOSIS

Central Causes

Brainstem Dysfunction and Cerebellar Dysfunction

Central vertigo produced by disorders of the brainstem and cerebellum is usually caused by neoplastic or vascular processes, including recurrent intermittent vascular insufficiency, transient ischemic attack, and stroke. Neoplasms are usually slow growing; therefore vestibular dysfunction is of gradual onset and usually manifests as a problem with equilibrium.

Vascular causes are more common and can produce acute-onset, long-lasting, or recurrent transient episodes of vertigo. Patients usually manifest other neurological deficits. With brainstem disorders, patients can have reports of diplopia, dysarthria, dysphagia, and paresthesia. They can demonstrate sensory and motor deficits. Cerebellar dysfunction usually results in gait disturbance and difficulties in fine-motor coordination, including rapid alternating movements (RAM) and finger-to-finger testing.

Multiple Sclerosis

Multiple sclerosis can produce a range of neurological symptoms. Vertigo occurs in up to 50% of patients with multiple sclerosis. Disease onset is usually in the third or fourth decade of life. MRI shows characteristic demyelinating plaques.

Migraine Headache

Approximately 30% of persons with migraine headaches have vertigo. It can be present before the headache begins, during the headache, or independent of the headache. Patients can have other symptoms consistent with vertebrobasilar vascular abnormalities such as visual changes, tinnitus, decreased hearing, ataxia, or paresthesia. Diagnosis is usually made on the basis of the history.

Peripheral Causes

Benign Paroxysmal Positional Vertigo

Episodes of BPPV are characterized by acute onset of vertigo associated with rapid head movement or position changes. Many women report dizziness with position change around the time of their menses. The episodes are brief, lasting a few seconds. Nystagmus can be elicited by positional testing. Testing positional changes can provoke the vertigo. There is no hearing loss. Diagnosis is made on the basis of the history and clinical findings. This is one of the most common causes of vertigo, especially in older adults.

Benign Paroxysmal Vertigo of Childhood

Benign paroxysmal vertigo (BPV) of childhood occurs most often in children 2-3 years old. The disorder tends to be recurrent with one to four attacks per month. The episodes occur suddenly, and the child cries out for help. Vomiting, pallor, sweating, and nystagmus are common during the episode. The neurological and audiological examinations are entirely normal. Some children can have a hypoactive or absent response to caloric testing (ear irrigation with warm and then cool water).

Meniere Disease

Meniere disease is characterized by a classic triad of symptoms—vertigo, hearing loss, and tinnitus. A sensation of ear fullness can also be present. The attacks are abrupt and recurrent and last for minutes to several hours. The interval between attacks can be weeks or months. Between episodes, the patient is asymptomatic. On physical examination, sensorineural hearing loss is present in the affected ear, or it can be bilateral.

Vestibular Neuronitis

Vestibular neuronitis is frequently preceded by an acute viral infection. These patients usually present with severe vertigo, nausea, and vomiting. The vertigo lasts for days to weeks. Remaining completely motionless can help the symptoms. Auditory function is not affected. Physical examination reveals nystagmus that intensifies in amplitude when the gaze is directed away from the affected ear. Visual fixation minimizes the nystagmus.

Labyrinthitis

Frequently associated with a concurrent viral or bacterial illness, labyrinthitis produces severe vertigo that lasts for several days. Labyrinthitis can be a complication of otitis media or meningitis. This condition is distinguished from vestibular neuronitis by the accompanying hearing loss that occurs as a result of destruction of the inner ear.

Acoustic Neuroma

Also called a vestibular schwannoma, acoustic neuroma is a benign tumor that originates most often in the vestibular portion of cranial nerve VIII (acoustic). It usually causes unilateral sensorineural hearing loss, tinnitus, and loss of equilibrium. The neuroma grows slowly; therefore loss of equilibrium is more often a symptom than is vertigo. Acoustic neuroma can also occur in cranial nerve V (trigeminal) with symptoms of paresthesia consistent with the nerve distribution. Large tumors of cranial nerve VI (abducens) can compress the brainstem.

Perilymph Fistula

Fistula formation can occur as a result of ear trauma, from a direct blow, secondary to otologic surgery, or indirectly from straining, coughing, or pressure changes. In this condition there is leakage of perilymph from either the round or the oval window into the middle ear. Sensorineural hearing loss is frequently present as well as vertigo. The fistula will often heal spontaneously but sometimes can require surgery.

Sinusitis and Otitis

Serous otitis, otitis media, and sinusitis can cause disruption of the vestibular apparatus, producing vertigo. History and physical examination findings will be consistent with the specific disorder (see Chapters 14 and 22).

Cholesteatoma

Collection of squamous debris often associated with chronic middle ear infection can form a cholesteatoma, which enlarges and destroys structures in its way. On physical examination, the cholesteatoma will appear as a shiny white irregular mass. Foul-smelling discharge can be evident, and there can be visible bone destruction. A conductive hearing loss can be present.

Systemic Causes
Psychogenic

Psychogenic causes of vertigo are common. Patients often describe themselves as anxious or nervous and can have psychiatric diagnoses (see Chapter 3). Their symptoms are vague and imprecise. Neurological examination is normal. No nystagmus is present or elicited. The vertigo can be reproduced with hyperventilation. MRI can be useful to provide reassurance.

Cardiovascular

Orthostatic hypotension and cardiac dysrhythmias can produce vertigo. The diagnosis of postural hypotension can be made by taking orthostatic blood pressure readings. The diagnosis of cardiac conditions can involve CBC, blood chemistry, ECG, cardiac stress testing, and echocardiography.

Neurosyphilis

Secondary or early tertiary syphilis can present with symptoms similar to those of Meniere disease. The patient demonstrates various clinical symptoms, including papilledema, aphasia, monoplegia or hemiplegia, cranial nerve (CN) palsies, pupillary abnormalities, or focal neurological deficits. The Argyll Robertson pupil, which occurs almost exclusively in neurosyphilis, is a small irregular pupil that reacts normally to accommodation but not to light. Serological testing will be positive for syphilis.

Other Causes
Ototoxic Drugs and Drugs Causing Salt Retention

Medications that are ototoxic, salt-retentive, or psychotropic can produce vertigo, lightheadedness, or unsteadiness. Drugs causing salt retention include steroids and phenylbutazone. Ototoxic medications include aspirin, ethacrynic acid, streptomycin, gentamicin, aminoglycosides, and furosemide. Psychotropic drugs can also produce vertigo. Ototoxic drugs can produce a sensorineural hearing loss. Audiometry should be performed with any noted hearing loss.

Trauma

Injury to the head or ear from labyrinthine concussion, temporal bone fracture, or perilymph fistula can produce disturbance of the vestibular apparatus and result in vertigo. Head trauma can also produce cerebral concussion involving the anterior tip of the temporal lobe. Trauma from otologic procedures can also cause vertigo.

DIFFERENTIAL DIAGNOSIS OF *Common Causes of Dizziness*

CONDITION	HISTORY	PHYSICAL FINDINGS	DIAGNOSTIC STUDIES
Central Causes			
Brainstem dysfunction/ cerebellar dysfunction	Elderly; acute-onset; recurrent vertigo; tinnitus; hearing OK	Symptoms of brainstem/ vertebrobasilar vascular abnormality: ataxia, double vision; lack of coordination; sensory/ motor deficits; vertical, lateral, rotary nystagmus; hearing normal; cerebellar: impaired RAM, finger-to-finger testing	MRI
Multiple sclerosis	Onset is often in third or fourth decade of life	Can have no other findings or can have other neurological symptoms	MRI
Migraine headache	Headache history; other migraine symptoms	Can have symptoms of vertebrobasilar vascular abnormalities, as above	None
Peripheral Causes			
Benign paroxysmal positional vertigo (BPPV)	Adults: associated with positional changes; recurrent episodes; lasts seconds to minutes; some relief if motionless	Lateral or rotary nystagmus; no tinnitus or hearing loss	Provoke nystagmus and vertigo by position that causes response; Dix-Hallpike maneuver; ENG
Benign paroxysmal vertigo of childhood	Children: usually 2-3 years of age, sudden onset with crying by child	Vomiting, pallor, sweating, and nystagmus common; no loss of consciousness; neurological and audiological examination can be normal	Can have hypoactive or absent response to caloric testing
Meniere disease	Sudden onset; lasts hours, recurrent; tinnitus and fullness in ears	Lateral or rotary nystagmus; fluctuating hearing loss: low tones; sensorineural	Positional maneuvers, audiometry, ENG
Vestibular neuronitis	Sudden onset; antecedent viral infection	Nausea and vomiting; nystagmus; no hearing loss, loss of equilibrium always to the same side	Positional maneuvers
Labyrinthitis	Sudden onset, lasts hours to days	Can currently be ill; lateral nystagmus; hearing loss; rarely tinnitus; nausea and vomiting can be present	Positional maneuvers, audiometry
Acoustic neuroma	Adults; gradual onset; mild vertigo; persistent tinnitus; facial numbness, weakness	Unilateral hearing loss, poor speech discrimination	MRI; audiometry
Perilymph fistula	History of trauma; hearing loss	Nystagmus and vertigo with pneumatic otoscopy; sensorineural hearing loss	Audiometry
Otitis/sinusitis	Pain in ear or face; history of ear or sinus infections; gradual onset of vertigo	Serous otitis, otitis media; tenderness over sinuses; purulent nasal discharge; no nystagmus	See Chapters 14 and 22
Cholesteatoma	History of chronic middle ear infections	Shiny white irregular mass on otoscopic examination; foul-smelling discharge can be present; bone destruction can be visible; conductive hearing loss can be present	Audiometry

Continued

DIFFERENTIAL DIAGNOSIS OF *Common Causes of Dizziness—cont'd*

CONDITION	HISTORY	PHYSICAL FINDINGS	DIAGNOSTIC STUDIES
Systemic Causes			
Psychogenic	Vague symptoms; recurrent; can describe self as anxious; can have other psychiatric diagnoses	Normal neurological and auditory examinations	Hyperventilation to reproduce the vertigo
Cardiovascular	CV history; antihypertensive medications	Orthostatic blood pressure; dysrhythmias; carotid or temporal bruits	Depends on client condition and symptoms
Neurosyphilis	Vertigo, tinnitus, fullness in ears	Various clinical symptoms; papilledema, aphasia, monoplegia or hemiplegia, central nervous palsies, pupillary abnormalities, Argyll Robertson pupil; focal neurological deficits	Serology for syphilis
Other Causes			
Ototoxic and salt-retaining drugs	Medication history: steroids, phenylbutazone, ethacrynic acid, aspirin, streptomycin, gentamicin, aminoglycosides, furosemide, psychotropic drugs	Sensorineural hearing loss	Audiometry
Trauma	History of trauma to head or ear	Depends on nature and location of injury; can exhibit peripheral or central symptoms	MRI/CT

CT, computed tomography; *ENG,* electronystagmography; *MRI,* magnetic resonance imaging; *RAM,* rapid alternating movements.

REFERENCES AND READINGS

Casselbrant M, Mandel E: Balance disorders in children, *Neurol Clin* 23:805, 2005.

Clark MM: How to sort out a complaint of dizziness, *Patient Care* 37:44, 2003.

Fetter M: Assessing vestibular function: which tests, when? *J Neurol* 247:335, 2000.

Goebel JA: The ten-minute examination of the dizzy patient, *Semin Neurol* 21:391, 2001.

Hanley K, O'Dowd T, Considine N: A systematic review of vertigo in primary care, *Br J Gen Pract* 51:666, 2001.

Kerber KA: Vertigo and dizziness in the emergency department, *Emerg Med Clin North Am* 27:39, 2009.

Koelliker P, Summers RL, Hawkins B: Benign paroxysmal positional vertigo: diagnosis and treatment in the emergency department—a review of the literature and discussion of canalith-repositioning maneuvers, *Ann Emerg Med* 37:392, 2001.

Labuguen R: Initial evaluation of vertigo, *Am Fam Physician* 73:245, 2006.

Maarsingh OR, Dros J, Schellevis FG, van Weert HC, van der Windt DA, ter Riet G: Causes of persistent dizziness in elderly patients in primary care, *Ann Fam Med* 8:196, 2010.

MacGregor D: Vertigo, *Pediatr Rev* 23:10, 2002.

Sloane PD, Coeytaux RR, Beck RS, Dallara J: Dizziness: state of the science, *Ann Intern Med* 134:823, 2001.

Wiener-Vacher S: Vestibular disorders in children, *Int J Audiol* 47:578, 2008.

Dyspnea

Dyspnea, or shortness of breath, is a subjective sensation of air hunger that results in labored breathing. True dyspnea results from three general causes: (1) an increased awareness of normal breathing, such as with hyperventilation; (2) an increase in the work of breathing, such as in airway obstruction or restricted volume; and (3) abnormalities in the ventilatory system, such as in neurological disorders, diseases of the muscles, and chest wall abnormalities. In disease states it is usually a result of pulmonary or cardiac pathology. When eliciting the history, it is helpful to determine if this is new-onset acute dyspnea, chronic progressive dyspnea, or chronic recurrent dyspnea. Carefully directed questioning will provide essential clues for identifying the differential diagnoses. In children younger than 3 years, who usually cannot express the sensation, caregivers can observe tachypnea, retractions, stridor, nasal flaring, or feeding difficulty.

DIAGNOSTIC REASONING: FOCUSED HISTORY

Is this an emergency?

Severe dyspnea is a medical emergency. If not treated immediately, respiratory failure and death can occur. Assess the adequacy of the airway first. Emergency measures should be instituted to establish ventilation. When the patient is stabilized, search for the underlying cause of the dyspnea.

Key Questions

- Did this occur suddenly, or has it been developing gradually? Over what period of time (hours, days, weeks) has it developed?
- What were you (or the child) doing just before having difficulty in breathing?
- Do you (or the child) have other symptoms, such as itching or swelling?

Onset

New-onset acute dyspnea in a patient in acute distress can signal a life-threatening problem. In the patient with no previous history of heart or lung disease, dyspnea can indicate several conditions that require immediate treatment, such as aspiration of a foreign body, anaphylaxis, pulmonary embolism (PE), and pneumonia. A common cause of acute-onset dyspnea is left ventricular dysfunction.

Acute upper or lower airway obstruction in children has the greatest potential to cause serious morbidity or mortality and therefore must initially be ruled out. The most serious problem is hypoxemia caused by the inability to transport oxygen past a blocked upper airway, such as with epiglottitis, croup, or a foreign body.

Acute dyspnea requires immediate assessment of the airway and ventilatory status with oxygen and cardiac monitoring. Often this must occur before a definitive diagnostic evaluation has been completed.

Acute epiglottitis in children is caused by *Haemophilus influenzae*. Inflammation of the epiglottis causes edema that obstructs the tracheal airway. The onset is sudden and the course of the disease is rapid. The patient's presenting symptoms usually include drooling, dysphonia, dysphagia, and respiratory distress with inspiratory stridor. The child looks anxious and sits up and forward with the jaw open to assist in air intake.

Status asthmaticus is a progressive bronchospasm from an increase in airflow resistance in children who are having an asthma event that does not respond to pharmacological intervention. Fever can be present, and pulse rate and respirations are increased. The use of accessory respiratory muscles is seen. Sometimes wheezing is not heard because of lack of air movement. The combination of hypoxia, hypercapnia, and acidosis can result in cardiovascular depression and cardiopulmonary arrest.

Foreign Body Aspiration

The adult patient with foreign body aspiration reports that dyspnea occurred while eating solid foods or drinking large amounts of alcohol. Children who put small objects in their mouth are at risk for aspiration of the object into the airway and subsequent airway obstruction. The patient or the care provider gives a history of sudden onset of choking, coughing, or wheezing, without preceding upper respiratory tract infection. Often the child has been playing on the floor or outside at the time of the onset of symptoms.

Anaphylaxis

Anaphylaxis can follow insect bites or the ingestion of medication or other potential allergens (e.g., shellfish, peanuts). Primary symptoms include flushing, generalized pruritus, fear, faintness, and sneezing. An allergic response can lead to shock, cardiac arrythmia, laryngeal edema, and death within minutes. The sooner the symptoms occur, the more severe the reaction.

Is the dyspnea caused by a secondary obstruction in the lower respiratory tract?

Key Questions

- Have you had cough or recent cold?
- Do you have a history of asthma?
- Is there a family history of asthma?

Cough

Secondary partial airway obstruction caused by small airway disease contributes to hypoxemia via intrapulmonary shunting. The pulmonary obstruction can be intraluminal (distal foreign objects, asthma); intramural (edema, bronchomalacia, bronchiolitis); or extramural (compression from tumor, lymph nodes). The narrowing increases both airway resistance and turbulence of airflow. The imbalance between pulmonary ventilation and perfusion affects oxygen exchange. This causes the patient to work harder to maintain adequate ventilation, resulting in dyspnea.

History of Asthma

Both adults and children can experience airway obstruction caused by reactive airways disease or asthma. Personal or family history of asthma increases the risk of dyspnea from acute bronchospasm.

Is the dyspnea caused by trauma to the chest?

Key Question

- Have you experienced any trauma to the chest?

Trauma

Limitation of motion of the thoracic cage because of pain and/or trauma can be associated with severe alveolar hypoventilation and subsequent dyspnea.

Pneumothorax occurs most frequently in young persons during strenuous activity. Spontaneous pneumothorax results in sudden loss of lung volume, hypoxia, hypercapnia, and significant shortness of breath (SOB). Blunt chest trauma can be caused by a fall or motor vehicle accident.

Is the dyspnea caused by a pulmonary embolus?

Key Questions

- Have you recently been confined to bed or been sitting for a long period of time?
- Have you had recent surgery?
- Have you recently sustained a fracture?
- Are you taking birth control pills or estrogen?
- Do you smoke?
- What medications are you taking?
- Are you feeling anxious or scared?

The person with PE is usually in acute distress and reports significant SOB, localized pleuritic chest pain, apprehension, bloody sputum production, diaphoresis, fever, and history of conditions causing risk for emboli. These risk factors include age of greater than 60 years, pulmonary hypertension, congestive heart failure, chronic lung disease, ischemic heart disease, stroke, and cancer. Predisposing factors that can contribute to thrombus formation include (1) venous stasis, (2) hypercoagulability, and (3) endothelial injury with inflammation to the vessel lining. Trauma, muscle spasm, or clot dissolution can cause the thrombus to dislodge, creating an embolus. Emboli circulate in the blood to the right side of the heart and enter the lungs via the pulmonary artery. If the clot is not dissolved within the lungs, it occludes the pulmonary artery and obstructs blood flow and perfusion of the lungs. Patients with suspected PE are referred for emergency pulmonary/vascular consultation.

Confinement, Surgery, and Fracture

Persons with a history of deep vein thrombosis or prolonged immobility are at greater risk for PE. Vascular lung disease is characterized by a decrease in the size of the pulmonary vascular bed. When emboli reach the pulmonary artery, the reduced blood flow through the lungs results in arterial hypoxemia and hypercapnia. These lead to symptoms of dyspnea. Dyspnea resulting from PE is usually accompanied by fever, chest pain, and restlessness.

Trauma to Leg

There is an increased risk of PE in adolescents who have sustained traumatic injury to their lower limbs.

Anxiety

People with PE feel a sense of impending doom. Significant oxygen deprivation can contribute to this symptom.

Oral Contraceptives/Estrogen

The estrogen in oral contraceptives causes increased coagulation of red blood cells, which increases the risk for PE. In addition, the risk of PE increases with the combination of smoking and oral contraceptives, especially in women older than age 35.

Medications

A complete medication history can provide clues to a possible hypercoagulability state. Patients who are taking anticoagulants and are underdosed can be at risk for PE. Patients taking medication for heart failure, such as digitalis or angiotensin-converting enzyme (ACE) inhibitors, are at risk because of chronic heart failure. Serum estrogen receptor modulators (tamoxifen, raloxifene) increase the risk for PE.

Is the dyspnea related to a preexisting disease?

Key Questions

- Do you have a history of heart problems, lung problems (asthma), or anemia?
- Do you have any numbness or tingling in your body? Where?
- Have you noticed any other symptoms?

Past History of Disease

History of coronary artery disease (CAD), heart failure, valvular heart disease, chronic obstructive pulmonary disease (COPD), or asthma should raise the level of suspicion for recurrence or complications of that disease. Myocardial infarction (MI) can cause sudden dyspnea in persons with or without prior history of CAD. Careful questioning regarding associated symptoms and risk factors can reveal characteristics of probable MI (see Chapter 7).

Progressively increasing SOB is frequently a symptom of worsening COPD. It is often associated with cough that is worse in the morning, clear to yellow color sputum, exercise intolerance, and fatigue. Chronic progressive dyspnea in the patient with a history of heart failure or cardiac valve disease is most frequently a symptom of heart failure. Associated symptoms include peripheral edema, ascites, cough possibly with frothy sputum production, chest pain, and fatigue. Orthopnea (difficulty breathing when lying flat) and paroxysmal nocturnal dyspnea (PND) (a sudden onset of SOB when lying flat) are most often associated with heart failure.

In children with heart disease, dyspnea occurs because of insufficient blood being pumped to the lungs as a result of congenital structural anomaly or pump failure or secondary to pulmonary hypertension. Simple respiratory tract infections can cause severe respiratory insufficiency in the child who has cardiopulmonary disease. Associated symptoms include retractions (including abdominal muscles), tachypnea, nasal flaring and grunting, peripheral edema, ascites, cough, and fatigue.

Chronic progressive dyspnea because of lung involvement can also be present in patients with a history of systemic illnesses, such as sarcoidosis, rheumatological disease (rheumatoid lungs), cystic fibrosis, or Goodpasture syndrome (a rare syndrome of progressive glomerulonephritis, hemoptysis, and hemosiderosis).

Periodic recurrent dyspnea is most often the result of bronchospasm and inflamed bronchi caused by asthma. Persons with asthma can be relatively symptom free between episodes and can often identify the cause of their SOB with little prompting. Symptoms are frequently associated with recent respiratory tract infection, exercise, or exposure to allergens. The patient or parent may report audible wheezes, decreased exercise tolerance, and frequent cough. Wheezing is extremely unusual in the neonatal period and implies intrathoracic airway obstruction due to intraluminal obstruction, fixed airway narrowing, variable narrowing, or external compression. All of these factors lead to turbulent expiratory flow and audible wheeze.

Hematological diseases can affect the oxygen-carrying capacity of the blood, resulting in tissue hypoxia and a decrease in arterial pH, which stimulates the central nervous system to cause the symptom of dyspnea. Severe anemia from any cause can result in this reaction. Also, whenever the oxygen-carrying capacity of the blood is decreased because of the inability of hemoglobin to bind oxygen, dyspnea can occur. Carbon monoxide poisoning, cyanide poisoning, and methemoglobinemia are examples.

The progressive dyspnea of anemia is usually associated with fatigue, palpitations, lightheadedness, or dizziness.

Hyperventilation

Hyperventilation syndrome, a nonemergent but frightening experience, is usually accompanied by paresthesias around the mouth and of the distal extremities. Anxiety-related dyspnea should not be diagnosed until one has ruled out more serious causes.

When dyspnea is caused by pulmonary or cardiac conditions, the SOB worsens with increasing activity and improves with rest. Dyspnea caused by anxiety does not improve, and can worsen, with rest.

What factors precipitate or aggravate the dyspnea?

Key Questions

- What activities are associated with shortness of breath?
- Do you take any medication?
- Do you have any known allergies (to trees, dust, pollen, animals)? Have you been exposed to these recently?
- Is there anything you can do to help yourself feel less short of breath, such as sit up, stay indoors, lie down, or use medication?

Precipitating Factors

Chronic dyspnea of pulmonary origin is most frequently precipitated and aggravated by exposure to smoke. This is true for both progressive and recurrent

dyspnea. Progressive dyspnea manifested in COPD is often exacerbated by exertion and is alleviated or improved with rest. As the disease progresses, less and less intense exercise, even talking, can result in increased SOB. In addition, respiratory tract infections are frequent causes of increased SOB for these patients. Exercise-induced asthma will cause dyspnea related to activity and is relieved with rest or use of bronchodilators.

Medication Use

The dyspnea related to asthma is relieved by use of bronchodilator agents and steroids.

Allergies

Exposure to cold and/or allergens, exercise, and viral respiratory tract infections frequently precipitate chronic recurrent dyspnea associated with asthma.

Recumbence, missed medications, high sodium intake, and exertion often precipitate chronic dyspnea associated with heart failure. This applies to both progressive and recurrent chronic dyspnea.

Alleviating Factors

Alleviating factors for dyspnea include sitting upright, taking diuretic medications, using bronchodilators, and resting for a prolonged period.

Is the dyspnea caused by a neuromuscular problem?

Key Questions

- Are your immunizations up to date?
- If a child: Has the child eaten any honey?
- Do you live on a farm?
- If a child: Is the child at risk for lead poisoning?
- Do you have a headache, muscle weakness, or visual changes?

Neuromuscular Effects

Abnormalities of neural or neuromuscular transmission to the respiratory muscles can result in paresis or paralysis, leading to alveolar hypoventilation. Direct involvement of the respiratory muscles affected by systemic musculoskeletal diseases can lead to reduction of vital capacity and total lung capacity and result in hypercapnic hypoventilation and dyspnea. Examples of neuromuscular health problems leading to dyspnea include infections, such as poliomyelitis or tetanus, or a central nervous system insult.

Immunizations

Lack of childhood or adult immunizations for poliomyelitis or tetanus can lead to paralysis or tetany of the respiratory musculature, resulting in dyspnea and subsequent respiratory distress.

Honey

Honey is a common source of contamination of *Clostridium botulinum*, which can cause respiratory distress in infants and small children. The incubation period is only a few hours. Nausea, vomiting, and diarrhea result, followed by cranial nerve involvement, diplopia, weak suck, facial weakness, and absent gag reflex. Generalized hypotonia and weakness then develop and can progress to respiratory failure.

Farm Residence

Organophosphate chemicals that are commonly used as insecticides can cause a myasthenia-like syndrome in children exposed to these toxins. Children residing on farms are most at risk.

Neuromuscular Affects

In children, some causes that affect the primary respiratory center are myasthenia gravis, myopathies, insecticide poisoning, and lead poisoning.

Secondary Causes

Diseases that affect the central nervous system and produce respiratory distress include meningoencephalitis, seizures, and central nervous system lesions.

> **Does the patient have any pertinent risk factors that will point me in the right direction?**

Key Questions

- Do you smoke? Have you ever smoked? Are you regularly exposed to cigarette smoke?
- What type of work do you do?
- Have you had a recent weight gain?
- Have you ever had eczema?

Risk Factors

Persons at risk for developing dyspnea are those with a history of pulmonary and/or heart disease, cigarette smokers and those persons subjected to passive exposure or second-hand smoke, persons exposed to noxious environmental pollutants, and persons with a predisposition to allergies or asthma.

Work

Occupational exposure to asbestos, silicon, paint and chemical fumes, and coal dust place the patient at risk for lung disease with resultant dyspnea.

Obesity

Physically deconditioned and obese persons report dyspnea on exertion more frequently than their non-obese counterparts. Obese persons can report dyspnea, especially during exercise. This is caused by an increase in the metabolic requirement for a given amount of work. In addition, the diaphragm moves against increased abdominal pressure, and the chest wall is heavier, resulting in more energy required to maintain ventilation.

Eczema History

Asthma occurs in 20% to 40% of children with a history of atopic dermatitis.

DIAGNOSTIC REASONING: FOCUSED PHYSICAL EXAMINATION
Note General Appearance and Observe Posture

Patients who appear in acute distress with manifestations of severe oxygen deprivation require emergent evaluation and treatment. Assess vital signs immediately. Tachypnea, eupnea, and hypopnea are critical clues to impending respiratory failure. Use of accessory muscles to breathe, posturing, and chest retraction all point to severe dyspnea. The severity of the dyspnea almost always correlates with the severity of the problem. In such situations consider pulmonary embolism, anaphylaxis, foreign body aspiration, pneumothorax, status asthmaticus, and severe heart failure. Persons presenting with COPD, anemia, mild asthma, and mild heart failure appear less acutely ill.

Determine if the patient has to lean forward or sit up to breathe comfortably. With severe respiratory distress or upper airway obstruction, an infant can adopt a posture of hyperextension of the trunk and neck. A child with epiglottitis prefers to sit up and lean forward.

A child who is in acute respiratory distress, sitting forward, and perhaps speaking with a muffled voice or drooling may have epiglottitis, and immediate assistance should be secured. Do not attempt to lay the child down or inspect the throat because this can occlude the airway.

Assess Level of Consciousness

Diminished level of consciousness, confusion, and restlessness are manifestations of hypoxia in a patient experiencing respiratory problems. Frequently the patient with a PE expresses a sense of impending doom.

An acutely ill child can have an alteration in level of consciousness, restlessness, mouth breathing, and flaring of the nostrils.

Observe Chest Movement

Place the patient in a sitting or side-lying position with the chest exposed. The chest cannot be adequately viewed through clothing. Many respiratory abnormalities are unilateral or localized. Compare findings on one side of the body with those on the other. Also compare front to back. Pneumothorax and PE can cause unequal expansion of the chest.

Inspect the Shape and Symmetry of the Chest

Cardinal features of restrictive pulmonary disease are deformities of the chest wall and reduction in lung volume and pulmonary compliance secondary to pathological changes in the lung parenchyma or pleura. Examples of deformities that cause decreased lung volume include kyphosis, scoliosis, and kyphoscoliosis. Decreased volume necessitates an increase in respiratory rate to maintain a normal volume. The work of breathing must be increased to overcome the reduced compliance.

Kyphoscoliosis is associated with marked structural abnormality of the thoracic cage, leading to abnormal positioning and functioning of the respiratory muscles. The lungs are compressed by the thoracic deformity, leading to a small lung volume. Breathing entails a high work and energy cost, and dyspnea can appear.

An increased anteroposterior (AP) diameter indicates air trapping. This is a frequent finding in persons with COPD. Other musculoskeletal chest abnormalities to note include pectus excavatum and pectus carinatum. These conditions can contribute to chest infection and respiratory failure because of decreased lung volume and ability to cough. Also, bronchomalacia, a softening of the bronchial tissue, is an abnormality associated with pectus excavatum. Pectus carinatum is associated with chronic lung disease

such as asthma or with cystic fibrosis, heart disease, and idiopathic scoliosis. Harrison sulci are exaggerated grooves running parallel to the subcostal margins, produced by prolonged diaphragmatic traction, and are associated with chronic airway disease or rickets.

In the presence of neuromuscular disease, chest movement in children should be examined in both the supine and sitting positions. Diaphragmatic weakness leads to paradoxical abdominal movements in the supine position, which can be missed if the child is examined only in the sitting position.

Respiratory distress triggered by placing the child in the supine position can be the only subtle abnormality in older children with mediastinal compression of the trachea.

Look for Retractions

In normal breathing, inspiration is the work necessary to overcome the elastic forces of the lung, the tissue viscosity of the lung and chest wall, and airway resistance. When there is a problem with any of these, the accessory muscles (sternocleidomastoid, anterior serratus, and external intercostal) are recruited to help. Contraction of these muscles causes forceful expansion of the thorax, resulting in increased negative pressure that draws in the soft tissues of the chest wall and results in retractions. Retractions begin in lower intercostal spaces and then move up to the higher spaces. In an infant, head-bobbing in time with respiration reflects use of the accessory muscles of respiration.

Observe the Rate, Rhythm, and Depth of Respiration for 1 Full Minute

In children, the respiratory rate should be counted while the child sleeps, if possible.

Tachypnea is an early sign of most pulmonary, parenchymal, cardiac, or systemic causes of respiratory distress. Hyperventilation can occur secondary to acidosis or central nervous system disease. Slow respirations can indicate central nervous system depression, hypoxemia, shock, or systemic infection.

Exhaling should take about twice as long as inhaling, but in patients with COPD, it can take up to four times longer. Rhythm should be even, with occasional sighs. Shallow respirations, which are rapid, indicate that restrictive forces must be overcome. Box 13-1 describes abnormal breathing patterns.

Box 13-1 **Abnormal Breathing Patterns**

Cheyne-Stokes respirations are manifested by rhythmic increase and decrease in depth, punctuated by regular episodes of apnea. This can be a sign of severe heart failure or neurological disease.

Tachypnea is rapid breathing with no change in depth and can be caused by hypoxia, pain, fever, or anxiety. Consider pulmonary embolism, foreign body aspiration, anaphylaxis, pneumothorax, heart failure, asthma, or pneumonia.

Asymmetrical chest movement with respirations can be observed in lobar pneumonia, pleural effusion, or any condition that affects just one side of the chest.

Use of accessory muscles indicates respiratory distress. Observe for bulging or retraction of the intercostals, sternocleidomastoid, and/or trapezius muscles. Nasal flaring is an objective manifestation of hypoxia.

Listen for Stridor

Stridor is caused by extrathoracic inspiratory dynamic narrowing of the airway in the oropharynx, glottis, subglottic region, or mid-trachea. Any condition that causes further decrease in the lumen of the airway will obstruct airflow and produce stridor. Inspiratory stridor usually indicates a supraglottic obstruction. If the obstruction varies or is extrathoracic (above the vocal cords), inspiration is affected more because the negative intraairway pressure during inspiration tends to collapse the extrathoracic airway. If the obstruction varies and affects the intrathoracic airways, expiration is prolonged because the positive intrathoracic pressure tends to collapse these airways during expiration. Expiratory or biphasic respiratory stridor generally indicates an obstruction at or below the larynx.

With severe narrowing of the air passage, stridor can be audible on both inspiration and expiration but is worse during inspiration. Biphasic or expiratory stridor alone usually indicates a more significant obstruction. Supraglottic stridor is usually quiet and wet and is associated with a muffled voice, dysphasia, and a preference to sit. Subglottic lesions produce a loud stridor, often causing a hoarse voice, barky cough, and possibly facial edema. Inspiratory stridor can be a sign of incomplete obstruction of the airway by a foreign body.

Infants younger than 6 months who present with stridor can have an underlying anatomical abnormality that can be symptomatic secondary to an acute illness. Common anomalies that predispose the infant to upper airway obstruction are anomalous vascular rings, laryngeal webs, laryngomalacia, or tracheomalacia. Stridor in older children can indicate foreign body aspiration, infection, inflammation, trauma, or tumor.

Listen for Audible Wheeze

Expiratory wheezing is a high-pitched musical sound caused by partial airway obstruction. It is commonly associated with disorders of the lower respiratory tract that cause inflammation, infection, or bronchoconstriction such as asthma and bronchitis.

Increased inspiratory effort suggests disease in the upper airways, whereas increased expiratory effort suggests disease in the smaller airways or lower respiratory tract.

Listen for Voice Changes

Voice changes can occur in association with upper airway obstruction. Paralysis of the vocal cords results in dysphonia. Subglottic stenosis results in decreased volume of the voice because a much smaller column of air is making the vocal cords vibrate. Involvement of the supraglottic area, proximal to the vocal cords, can result in a hyponasal or muffled voice such as in tonsillitis and epiglottitis). A normal voice with stridor can indicate a subglottic or tracheal lesion (see Chapter 19).

Take Pulse, Temperature, and Blood Pressure

Palpate the radial, femoral, popliteal, and pedal pulses for rate and quality.

Tachycardia increases cardiac output. It occurs either as a result of primary heart disease or as a secondary process in response to oxygen deprivation because of PE, pneumonia, fever, and/or heart failure. Tachycardia and drowsiness can indicate a metabolic acidosis. Bradycardia is usually seen late in respiratory disease.

Tachycardia can occur with an irregular pulse, signaling heart failure from atrial fibrillation and/or heart block. Diminished peripheral pulses indicate possible atherosclerotic vessel disease or decreased cardiac output.

Fever can indicate epiglottitis or any other upper and/or lower respiratory tract infection.

Orthostatic hypotension can be secondary to dehydration associated with pneumonia or status asthmaticus. Anaphylaxis is also manifested by severe hypotension.

Pulsus paradoxus, an inspiratory drop in systolic blood pressure of more than 10 mm Hg, is caused by greater inspiratory effort from increased airway resistance. Negative intrathoracic pressure is associated with increased afterload and low systolic blood pressure. In heart failure, decreased stroke volume reduces the systolic blood pressure. Compensatory vasoconstriction maintains a constant diastolic pressure and along with the decreased systolic pressure can produce a decreased pulse pressure.

Inspect the Oral Cavity

First observe the oropharyngeal cavity for any evidence of a foreign body obstructing the airway. Also, evidence of vomitus can indicate possible aspiration. Note the color of the tongue and mucous membranes for signs of central cyanosis.

Inspect the posterior pharynx for peritonsillar cellulitis, retropharyngeal abscess, or other intraoral pathology that might be causing obstruction. Lift the jaw forward. Obstruction of the airway associated with micrognathia, depressed airway reflexes, or an enlarged tongue will diminish with this maneuver because the tongue will be lifted off the posterior pharynx. If epiglottitis is suspected, do not examine the oral cavity.

Inspect the Nose

Assess the patency of the nares. Fifty percent of airway resistance comes from the nose. Check for nasal flaring. An infant who has nasal flaring is using a compensatory mechanism to decrease airway resistance. Noisy, difficult breathing in an infant, especially while feeding, can signal choanal atresia. A deviated septum compromises the patency of one side of the nose when there is mucosal swelling.

Palpate the Neck

Neck masses caused by intraoral, paratracheal, or intrathoracic malignant disease can cause respiratory distress. Inspect the position of the trachea. To assess the trachea for lateral displacement, position your index finger first on the right side of the suprasternal notch and then on the left. If the trachea has shifted to the side, you will feel the wall on one side but only soft tissue on the other. This is most likely to occur with pneumothorax. Observe the neck for jugular venous distention; this is a sign of heart failure.

Examine the Skin and Extremities

Note cyanosis. Bluish color seen in the lips and mucous membranes of the mouth (central cyanosis) is associated with low arterial saturation and can result from inadequate gas exchange in the lungs or from cardiac shunting. Cyanosis implies more than 5 g/100 mL of desaturated hemoglobin, but its absence does not imply that hypoxemia is not present. Dark-skinned patients' mucous membranes can appear gray with central cyanosis. Central cyanosis can also be seen in persons with COPD. Bluish color of extremities (peripheral cyanosis) can be observed in Caucasians and is associated with low venous saturation, resulting from vasoconstriction, vascular occlusion, or reduced cardiac output.

Pallor can be a manifestation of severe anemia.

Note clubbing, which is characterized by the loss of the angle between the skin and nail bed. This is a manifestation of chronic tissue hypoxia that occurs with lung cancer and other chronic lung diseases. It is uncommon in children other than those with cystic fibrosis or cyanotic congenital heart disease. Clubbing develops rapidly with infective endocarditis.

Test for peripheral edema. Edema of the lower extremities can be a sign of increased right-heart filling pressure caused by primary lung disease or left-ventricular failure. Make note of how high the edema extends up the extremity. In children, the location of peripheral edema is age dependent. In young infants, edema occurs as hepatomegaly and periorbital or flank edema. In older children, lower extremity edema can occur.

Note any angioedema. The presence of generalized or local giant urticaria is objective evidence of probable anaphylaxis.

Check skin perfusion by pressing on the skin of a finger or sole of a foot and saying "capillary refill" after removing the pressure. A normal finding is that the color returns to the skin in 2 seconds or before you can finish saying the words.

Feel the skin for diaphoresis. When respiratory muscles are working at their maximum level to overcome increased resistive and elastic forces, the child will sweat, especially on the forehead and above the lip.

Palpate the Chest

Using the palmar surface of the hands, palpate the entire chest for tenderness, depressions, bulges, and crepitus (presence of air in the subcutaneous tissues).

Crepitus can indicate a chest injury, pneumothorax, or emphysema.

Pneumothorax, atelectasis, pneumonia, and partial paralysis of the diaphragm will result in reduced expansion of one side of the chest wall, and chest wall motion will be decreased.

Assess for Vocal Fremitus

Fremitus is diminished in pneumothorax, asthma, emphysema, and other conditions that trap air in the lung. Vocal fremitus intensity can be increased in pneumonia, heart failure, and tumor, all conditions that increase the lung density.

Percuss the Chest

Sounds produced by percussion indicate the density of lung tissue (see Chapter 10). In children, transmission of a percussion note and assessment of the quality of transmitted sound are useful to reveal an area of consolidation or effusion that would be difficult to auscultate with an uncooperative child.

Auscultate Breath Sounds

Auscultation of bronchial or bronchovesicular breath sounds over the peripheral lungs can indicate consolidation, which occurs when lungs fill with exudate. Young children normally have bronchovesicular sounds because of the thinness of their chest wall.

If breath sounds are diminished over all lung fields, suspect shallow breathing, lack of air movement, neuromuscular diseases, obesity, or COPD. Breath sounds will be inaudible in areas of pneumothorax.

Abnormal lung sounds are superimposed on normal sounds and can be auscultated over any area of the lung field during inspiration or expiration. Documentation of abnormal lung sounds should include type of sound, location where it is heard, and the phase(s) of respiration in which it is noted. In small children it can be difficult to distinguish upper and lower airway sounds. Listening with the stethoscope over the nose or mouth and then returning to the lungs can help to identify the findings.

Crackles or rales are discontinuous popping sounds heard most often during inspiration. They are caused by the explosive equalization of gas pressure between two compartments of the lung when a closed section of the airway that separates them suddenly opens. They indicate the presence of fluid, mucus, or pus in the smaller airways. Fine crackles are soft and high pitched. Medium crackles are louder and lower pitched. Coarse crackles are moist and more explosive.

The frequency and timing of crackles are the important parts of assessment. In resolving pneumonia, crackling is heard on inspiration caused by a mix between the aerated and nonaerated alveoli and bronchioles. In airways that are swollen and narrowed, such as in asthma bronchiolitis, generalized medium or coarse crackles are heard throughout both phases of respiration. Early inspiratory crackles are heard in COPD. Mid to late inspiratory crackles are more likely a sign of interstitial lung disease or heart failure. Crackles can be heard over the site of a pulmonary embolus.

Wheezing is frequently described as a whistling sound and can be heard during inspiration, expiration, or both. The sound is high pitched and musical. Wheezing indicates that there is fluid in the large airways such as in severe heart failure or, more often, heralds bronchospasm, as seen in asthma. In addition, localized wheezing can accompany incomplete obstruction of the airway by a foreign body.

A wheeze of fixed pitch occurring with inspiration and expiration suggests a localized abnormality. Wheezes of varying pitch occurring predominantly throughout expiration reflect the narrowing of airways of different calibers.

Rhonchi are continuous, deep-pitched, coarse breath sounds usually heard during expiration. Rhonchi are frequently present when the patient has bronchitis or pneumonia.

Pleural friction rub is a grating or squeaking sound usually heard in the lateral lung fields during inspiration and expiration. It indicates that parietal and visceral pleural linings are inflamed and are rubbing together as can occur with pneumonia, pleural effusion, pleuritis, and tumors. It is often accompanied by limited chest expansion because of pain.

If abnormal lung sounds are detected, additional auscultation for bronchophony, egophony, and whispered pectoriloquy is indicated. Consolidation will produce positive findings for each of these tests. To test for bronchophony, instruct the patient to say "ninety-nine." The words are heard louder and clearer than usual. In egophony, instruct the patient to say "ee." This sound is transmitted as "ay" if consolidation is present. To test whispered pectoriloquy, instruct the patient to whisper a sentence. Whispered sounds are louder and clearer than normal.

Auscultate Heart Sounds

In COPD, lung hyperinflation can muffle heart sounds. Poor tissue oxygenation can result in tachycardia. In children, muffled heart sounds can indicate pericarditis.

In heart failure, S1 and S2 can equal rapid pulse rate or can indicate a pulse deficit. S3 (ventricular gallop) is an early sign of heart failure and is heard best at the apex of the heart. S4 (atrial gallop) typically indicates a stressed heart and heart failure in children. In adults it can be the result of hypertension, MI, or CAD causing heart failure. A summation gallop can also occur with heart failure; this is the result of S3, S4, and rapid rate.

Listen for the presence of any murmurs and note their location, grade of loudness, timing, or radiation. Incompetent heart valves can be the cause of heart failure.

LABORATORY AND DIAGNOSTIC STUDIES

Diagnostic tests are indicated in almost all initial evaluations of the patient presenting with SOB. Posteroanterior (PA) and lateral chest radiographs, hemoglobin level, and spirometry are useful preliminary tests.

Transcutaneous Pulse Oximetry

Oximetry measures the fraction of oxygen carried in hemoglobin and provides noninvasive information about the delivery of oxygen from the atmosphere to the pulmonary capillaries. The partial pressure of oxygen in arterial blood (PaO_2) in healthy adults ranges from 80 to 103 mm Hg, and more than 95% saturation of hemoglobin is considered normal. In children, a pulse oximetry reading of 95% to 98% is normal, 90% to 95% is mild hypoxia, 85% to 90% is moderate hypoxemia, and less than 85% is severe hypoxemia.

Chest Radiography

Chest radiographs are essential in the diagnosis of dyspnea and can show pneumothorax, pneumonia, malignant disease, pleural disease, foreign body, or pulmonary edema. They can also provide clues to other causes of dyspnea, such as cardiomegaly, deformities of the chest bones and musculature, and the position of the diaphragm. When a foreign body is suspected, both inspiratory and expiratory chest films can be helpful.

Electrocardiography

An electrocardiogram (ECG) can provide important information about myocardial ischemia, arrhythmias, pericarditis, or the presence of pulmonary disease. Cardiopulmonary exercise testing can be done if the severity of the dyspnea is disproportionate to objective tests, there are coexisting cardiac and pulmonary causes, or deconditioning, obesity, or psychological factors are suspected.

Echocardiography

An echocardiogram is performed when cardiac disease is suspected; this test can define the cause of dyspnea related to heart chamber size, valves, pericardial disease, and ventricular function.

Hemoglobin and Hematocrit

Significantly decreased hemoglobin and hematocrit levels suggest anemia as a possible cause of dyspnea. Erythrocytosis can indicate chronic hypoxia resulting from a number of causes, including COPD.

Spirometry

Spirometry is indicated if the dyspnea is related to obstructive or restrictive lung disease. Spirometry measures forced vital capacity (FVC), 1-second forced expiratory volume (FEV1), the FEV1/FVC ratio, and the peak expiratory flow rate (PEFR). In obstructive lung disease (i.e., asthma and COPD), the FEV1 and the FEV1/FVC ratio are less than predicted. In restrictive lung disease (i.e., pneumonia, pneumothorax, pleural effusion), the FVC is reduced and the ratio is normal or elevated.

Additional Testing

Additional diagnostic tests may be indicated after the initial data gathering and can include the following:

- Computed tomography (CT) provides more detailed assessment of mass lesions.
- Pulmonary angiography confirms PE.
- Complete blood count with differential is used to determine the presence of bacterial infection.
- Blood urea nitrogen and creatinine levels help assess renal function. Renal insufficiency frequently presents with dyspnea as a result of the combined effects of volume overload and anemia.
- Arterial blood gases (ABGs) should be determined in an acutely ill patient with dyspnea and tachypnea.

- If sputum is present, a sputum culture should be obtained to determine the presence of an infectious agent.

DIFFERENTIAL DIAGNOSIS

When a patient reports severe dyspnea and manifests significant oxygen deprivation, emergent assessment and referral are indicated. The following health problems can be the cause of the emergent situation.

Emergent Conditions Manifested by Dyspnea

Pulmonary Embolus

A patient reporting severe dyspnea, cough, fever, hemoptysis, chest pain, history of deep vein thrombosis, and/or history of recent immobilization should be evaluated for possible PE (see Chapter 7).

Foreign Body Aspiration

Foreign body aspiration occurs most frequently in children and the elderly. If the event was witnessed, history of aspiration is usually clear. If the person is found after the event, the history cannot be as revealing. Generally, the onset of cough is sudden and unexpected. If the foreign body is obstructing the airway, the patient is in acute respiratory distress and immediate intubation or bronchoscopy is indicated to remove the foreign body and open the airway. Partial obstruction of the airway can cause stridor, cyanosis, labored respirations, and/or wheezing. Lateral neck and chest radiographs can reveal the location and size of the obstructing object (see Chapter 10).

Anaphylaxis

Anaphylaxis is an emergent situation. History can include insect bite, drug ingestion, or recent meal containing exposure to known allergens. Early symptoms include pruritic rash, feeling of warmth, wheezing, fatigue, lightheadedness, and dyspnea. On examination, persons in anaphylaxis manifest angioedema, tachypnea, clammy skin, hypotension, wheezes, and tachycardia. Immediate treatment and support of ventilation can be necessary.

Pneumothorax

History of blunt chest trauma often seen after a motor vehicle accident or a fall can cause pneumothorax, hemothorax, or pulmonary contusion. Cystic fibrosis can cause a spontaneous pneumothorax from rupture of subpleural blebs located at the apex of the upper lobe or in the superior segment of the lower lobe. Spontaneous pneumothorax can also occur, with the highest incidence in tall, thin males between the ages of 15 and 30 years. There is sudden severe chest pain and dyspnea aggravated by normal respiratory movement. Absent or decreased breath sounds are found on the side of the pneumothorax. Chest radiography can be diagnostic.

Croup

Croup, or laryngotracheobronchitis, is a viral infection that is usually preceded by symptoms of an upper respiratory tract infection. The illness is usually gradual in onset and includes a hoarse, seal-bark cough and fever. The degree of respiratory distress is variable.

Acute Epiglottitis

Acute epiglottitis is a serious, life-threatening bacterial infection caused primarily by *H. influenzae*. It typically has a rapid onset with stridor, high fever, drooling, muffled voice, and sore throat. A child will appear anxious and can be sitting forward. Parents should be asked if a child has received an *H. influenzae* B, or HiB, immunization. This condition is rare in children who have been immunized.

Bacterial Tracheitis

Bacterial tracheitis is usually a secondary infection caused by *Staphylococcus aureus* or *H. influenzae* that inflames the trachea after a viral infection. It is a subglottic lesion and mimics croup; however, a high fever and toxic appearance are present. Frequently there is a copious amount of purulent sputum present.

Status Asthmaticus

Acute bronchoconstriction in a patient with asthma can develop as a result of a respiratory tract infection, exposure to allergens, inhalation of fumes or other airway irritants, or environmental factors. Airway obstruction is caused not only by bronchial smooth muscle constriction but also by mucosal edema and excessive mucus production. Predominant symptoms include breathlessness, wheezing, and coughing. Absence of wheezing in a child with asthma can indicate severe airway obstruction with poor air exchange.

Botulism

Botulism poisoning can occur after ingestion of the toxin in inadequately cooked or improperly canned food. Infant botulism is caused by ingestion of the spores of *C. botulinum* rather than the exotoxin. It occurs before the first year of life, and honey has been implicated in 20% of patients. Symptoms occur 1 to 2 days after ingestion of contaminated food. Weakness and respiratory dyspnea and failure often accompany visual problems. Infant botulism begins with constipation, and the infant becomes weaker and listless. Respiratory arrest can be sudden.

Nonemergent Conditions Manifested by Dyspnea

Chronic progressive dyspnea is most often caused by COPD, heart failure, and obesity. It is seen less often in severe anemia and carcinoma of the pulmonary system. These patients report gradual onset of SOB over days or weeks.

Chronic Obstructive Pulmonary Disease

COPD is associated with frequent cough that is worse in the morning, sputum production that is clear to yellow in color, decreasing exercise tolerance, and mild to moderate fatigue. History of smoking is present in most instances. Exposure to asbestos, coal dust, and other significant environmental pollutants can also be reported. Objective manifestations of COPD include rapid, shallow respirations, reddish complexion, increased AP diameter, use of accessory muscles to breathe, pursed-lip breathing, decreased tactile fremitus, decreased respiratory excursion bilaterally, hyperresonant lungs, distant breath sounds, prolonged expiration, occasional wheezes, and muffled heart sounds. Chest radiography, pulmonary function tests, and possible exercise tests are indicated to confirm the diagnosis of COPD.

Heart Failure

Persons reporting history of heart disease or heart valve disease, dyspnea, orthopnea, PND, peripheral edema, weight gain, cough with frothy sputum, fatigue, and palpitations must be further assessed for acute heart failure. Physical examination findings can include altered level of consciousness, anxiety, jugular venous distention, tachypnea, rales, rhonchi, tachycardia, displaced point of maximum impulse, S3, S4, and possible ascites. Symptoms in children also include sweating on the forehead or upper lip. An ECG and chest radiograph will show increased heart size, oximetry will reveal a decreased arterial PO2, and an echocardiogram will display a significantly reduced ejection fraction.

Anemia

Patients reporting dyspnea (especially on exertion), fatigue, lightheadedness, palpitations, and possible history of chronic disease should have blood tests to measure the oxygen-carrying capacity of their blood (hemoglobin and hematocrit levels). Hematological diseases affect the oxygen-carrying capacity of the blood, with resulting tissue hypoxia. A decrease in arterial pH stimulates the central nervous system and dyspnea is seen. Objective signs of anemia include tachycardia and pallor.

Poor Physical Conditioning

Poor physical conditioning can cause the patient to experience SOB with exertion. Associated symptoms can include cardiac palpitations and history of excessive weight and sedentary lifestyle. The physical examination is often normal except for tachycardia and possible obesity. Exercise stress tests can be done for an adult with cardiovascular risk factors or a history of cardiovascular disease.

Asthma

Asthma is the most frequent cause of recurrent dyspnea. Persons usually report a history of asthma and possibly allergies, and can be taking prescribed inhaled bronchodilators and/or inhaled steroids. Paroxysmal cough and audible wheeze often accompany dyspnea. They can report recent respiratory tract infection, exposure to known allergens, or strenuous exercise. Objective manifestation on physical examination includes restlessness, tachypnea, use of accessory muscles to breathe, intercostal retraction, decreased vocal fremitus, decreased breath sounds, and inspiratory and possible expiratory wheezes. Pulse oximetry and spirometry testing will provide confirming evidence of asthma. ABGs are indicated in the patient manifesting acute O_2 deprivation, and chest radiographs are indicated if a lower respiratory tract infection is suspected. If the patient does not have a history of asthma and the spirometry test result is normal, a methacholine challenge test can be diagnostic.

The lessening or absence of wheezes in a person with asthma can indicate mucus plugging and an impending episode of status asthmaticus.

Pneumonia

Pneumonia is usually associated with dyspnea, pleuritic chest pain, cough with greenish or rust-colored sputum, fever, and chills. In children, irritability, feeding problems, and lack of playfulness can also be seen. Objective manifestations of pneumonia include fever, tachycardia, tachypnea, inspiratory crackles, asynchronous breathing, vocal fremitus, dull percussion sound over area of consolidation, and bronchophony. Pneumonia can be confirmed by chest radiography and sputum cultures.

Hyperventilation Syndrome

Hyperventilation syndrome is a common cause of recurrent faintness without actual loss of consciousness. Dyspnea, lightheadedness, palpitations, and paresthesias (perioral and extremities) occur. Restlessness, anxiety, and a normal cardiovascular examination are present. Recumbency does not relieve the symptoms. Chest radiography is normal.

Laryngomalacia

Laryngomalacia is the most common cause of persistent stridor in infancy. Onset of the stridor is almost always within the first 4 weeks of life, commonly in the first week (with preterm neonates who were on ventilation at high risk). Occasionally parents become aware of the condition when a respiratory tract infection is present. Stridor is predominantly inspiratory, and the sound can change with change in position of the infant. The cry and cough are normal. Direct visualization of the larynx is performed for diagnosis.

Vascular Ring

Tracheal compression from vascular anomalies can cause stridor and dyspnea in infants. The main symptom is soft inspiratory stridor with expiratory wheeze. Frequently a brassy cough and difficulty swallowing may be present. Barium swallow followed by echocardiography is done to establish the diagnosis.

DIFFERENTIAL DIAGNOSIS OF *Emergent Conditions Manifested by Dyspnea*

CONDITION	HISTORY	PHYSICAL FINDINGS	DIAGNOSTIC STUDIES
Pulmonary embolus	Acute-onset dyspnea, cough, mild to severe chest pain, sense of impending doom; hemoptysis; history of DVT, recent surgery, oral contraceptive, smoker, hypercoagulability states	Restlessness, fever, tachycardia, tachypnea, diminished breath sounds, crackles, wheezing, pleural friction rub	ABGs, chest radiograph, ECG, ventilation/ perfusion scans, D-dimer, CTPA
Foreign body aspiration	Acute-onset dyspnea; history of drinking large amounts of alcohol; in children, history of putting small objects in mouth; possible cough	Apnea or tachypnea, restlessness, suprasternal retractions, intoxication, inspiratory stridor, localized wheeze	Lateral neck radiograph, chest radiograph, bronchoscopy
Anaphylaxis	Acute-onset dyspnea; history of insect sting, ingestion of drug, or allergen	Angioedema, tachypnea, clammy skin, hypotension, bilateral wheezes, tachycardia	None; emergency measures necessary
Pneumothorax	Acute-onset dyspnea; sharp, tearing chest pain; pain can radiate to ipsilateral shoulder	Tachycardia, diminished breath sounds, decreased tactile fremitus, hyperresonance of lung area affected; possible hypertension and tracheal shift	Chest radiograph, ABGs
Croup	History of upper respiratory tract infection	Hoarse, seal-bark cough, fever (variable)	None initially; if respiratory distress increases, pulse oximeter and referral

Continued

DIFFERENTIAL DIAGNOSIS OF *Emergent Conditions Manifested by Dyspnea—cont'd*

CONDITION	HISTORY	PHYSICAL FINDINGS	DIAGNOSTIC STUDIES
Acute epiglottitis	Positional sitting forward; sore throat, anxious, toxic child	High fever, drooling, stridor, muffled voice	Admit; life threatening
Bacterial tracheitis	Recent viral infection	Fever, stridor, purulent sputum	Radiography of airway, WBC increased, tracheal culture
Status asthmaticus	Recent URI, exposure to allergens, breathlessness	Wheezing, coughing, tachycardia, tachypnea	Peak flows, chest radiograph, ABGs
Botulism	Honey ingestion in infant, contaminated food ingestion	Hypoventilation, drooling, weak cry, ptosis, ophthalmoplegia, loss of head control	Pulmonary function testing, chest radiograph, fluoroscopy, stool culture

ABG, Arterial blood gas; *ECG,* electrocardiogram; *DVT,* deep vein thrombosis.

DIFFERENTIAL DIAGNOSIS OF *Nonemergent Conditions Manifested by Dyspnea*

CONDITION	HISTORY	PHYSICAL FINDINGS	DIAGNOSTIC STUDIES
Pneumonia	Dyspnea, cough, sputum production (green, rust, or red), pleuritic chest pain, chills; in infants and children: irritability and feeding problems	Fever, tachycardia, tachypnea, inspiratory crackles, asynchronous breathing, vocal fremitus, percussion dull or flat over area of consolidation, bronchophony, egophony	Chest radiograph, sputum cultures, ABGs, WBC
Hyperventilation syndrome	Dyspnea, lightheadedness, palpitations, paresthesias (perioral and extremities)	Restlessness, anxiety, normal CV examination	Chest radiograph
Laryngomalacia	Neonate, infant: history of stridor, history of URI	Inspiratory stridor; normal cough, cry	Refer for visualization of larynx
Vascular ring	Infant: dyspnea, brassy cough, difficulty swallowing	Inspiratory stridor with expiratory wheeze	Barium swallow, echocardiography
Heart failure	Chronic progressive dyspnea, cough, frothy sputum, fatigue, lightheadedness, syncope, weight gain, ankle swelling, palpitations, PND, orthopnea, history of heart disease; in children: chronic progressive dyspnea, sweating above lip and forehead, especially while eating	Altered level of consciousness, restlessness, jugular venous distention, tachypnea, use of accessory muscles to breathe, rales, rhonchi, wheezes, tachycardia, decreased peripheral pulses, cool extremities, displaced PMI, S3, S4, ascites, liver enlargement	ECG, chest radiograph, ABGs, echocardiogram
Anemia	Dyspnea on exertion, fatigue, palpitations, lightheadedness, history of chronic disease	Pallor, tachypnea, cool dry skin of extremities, possible orthostatic hypotension	CBC, iron studies
Poor physical conditioning	Dyspnea on exertion, weight gain, palpitation on exertion, sedentary lifestyle, cigarette smoker	Overweight, tachycardia	Cardiac stress test
Asthma	Dyspnea, paroxysmal cough, audible wheeze, history of asthma or allergies	Restlessness, tachypnea, use of accessory muscles to breathe, intercostal retractions, decreased vocal fremitus, decreased breath sounds, inspiratory and possibly expiratory wheezes	Spirometry, chest radiograph, ABGs

DIFFERENTIAL DIAGNOSIS OF *Nonemergent Conditions Manifested by Dyspnea—cont'd*

CONDITION	HISTORY	PHYSICAL FINDINGS	DIAGNOSTIC STUDIES
COPD	Chronic progressive dyspnea, dyspnea on exertion, persistent cough, minimal sputum, easy fatigue, history of smoking	Rapid shallow respirations, reddish complexion, increased AP diameter of thorax, use of accessory muscles to breathe, pursed-lip breathing, decreased tactile fremitus, decreased respiratory excursion bilaterally, lungs hyperresonant, distant breath sounds, prolonged expiration, occasional wheezes, possible tachycardia, muffled heart sounds	Chest radiograph, pulmonary function tests, exercise tests, ABGs

ABGs, Arterial blood gases; *AP,* anteroposterior; *COPD,* chronic obstructive pulmonary disease; *CV,* cerebrovascular; *ECG,* electrocardiogram; *PMI,* point of maximal impulse; *PND,* paroxysmal nocturnal dyspnea; *URI,* upper respiratory tract infection; *WBC,* white blood cell count.

REFERENCES AND READINGS

Bettmann MA, Lyders EM, Yucel EK, Khan A, Haramati LB, Ho VB et al: Expert Panel on Cardiac Imaging. Acute chest pain—suspected pulmonary embolism [online publication]. Reston (VA): American College of Radiology (ACR); 2006.

Evans SE, Scanlon PD: Current practice in pulmonary function testing, *Mayo Clinic Proceedings* 78:758, 2003.

Fedullo PF, Tapson VF: The evaluation of suspected pulmonary embolism, *N Engl J Med* 349:1247, 2003.

Karnani NG, Reisfield GM, Wilson GR: Evaluation of chronic dyspnea, *Am Fam Physician* 71:8, 2005.

Leung AKC, Kellner JD, Johnson DW: Viral croup: a current perspective, *J Pediatr Health Care* 18:297, 2004.

Meek PM: Measurement of dyspnea in chronic obstructive pulmonary disease: what is the tool telling you? *Chron Respir Dis* 1:1, 2004.

Owens S: Exercise intolerance, *Pediatr Rev* 21:6, 2000.

Schwartzstein RM: Evaluation of the patient with chronic dyspnea: clinical application of pathophysiologic principles, *Prim Care Case Rev* 3:201, 2000.

Weinberger M, Abu-Hasan M: Perceptions and pathophysiology of dyspnea and exercise intolerance, *Pediatr Clin N Am* 56:33, 2009.

Werner HA: Status asthmaticus in children: a review, *Chest* 119:1913, 2001.

Zoorob R, Campbell J: Acute dyspnea in the office, *Am Fam Physician* 68:1803, 2003.

Earache

Otalgia, or ear pain, is generally caused by an inflammatory process. In children, inflammation most commonly occurs in the middle ear. Adults more often have an earache from external ear conditions or from referred pain from other head and neck structures. Acute otitis media (AOM) refers to any inflammation of the middle ear and encompasses a variety of clinical conditions. Otitis media with effusion is a collection of fluid in the middle ear. This condition is also known as serous otitis media, secretory otitis, or nonsuppurative otitis. External or middle ear disorders can often be distinguished after a brief history and physical examination. If the physical findings are normal, referred pain is a likely cause. About 50% of referred pain is caused by dental problems, although other causes may include temporomandibular joint (TMJ) disorder, parotitis, pharyngitis, or cervical, mouth, or facial disorders. The most serious, although least common, cause of referred pain is nasopharyngeal cancer, a condition more common in Asians. Figure 14-1 illustrates the structures of the ear.

DIAGNOSTIC REASONING: FOCUSED HISTORY

Is this an acute infection?

Key Questions

- How old are you?
- Have you had a fever?
- Have you had an upper respiratory infection?
- Have you had ear infections before?
- Is there a family history of ear infections?

Age

The occurrence of AOM declines significantly after age 6. Increased age raises the likelihood of secondary otalgia caused by disorders of the head, face, and neck; by sinus or periodontal disease; and by malignancy.

Fever

Fever is present in 60% of all children with AOM. In infants younger than 2 months, fever with AOM is uncommon. A high fever accompanying otitis is more likely to indicate a systemic illness, such as pneumonia or meningitis.

Upper Respiratory Infection

A URI occurs when the mucous membranes of the nasopharynx and/or sinuses become infected and organisms are forced up the lumen of the eustachian tube. Inflammation of the mucosa or enlarged adenoids obstruct the eustachian opening so that the air in the middle ear is absorbed and replaced by mucus. This mucus creates a mechanical obstruction and can serve as a medium for bacterial growth.

Previous Infections

Infants younger than 3 months who have their first AOM run a high risk of recurrence. Seventy-one percent of children younger than age 3 years have had at least one episode, and one third have had an average of three episodes. Chronic otitis media can result in anatomical changes to the tympanic membrane (TM) and middle ear ossicles, which may predispose the patient to additional ear infections.

Family History

Having a sibling or parent with chronic otitis media makes it twice as likely for the illness to develop in the child. The presence of chronic otitis media may also be related to child-care practices, such as bottle propping, or environmental exposures, such as second-hand cigarette smoke.

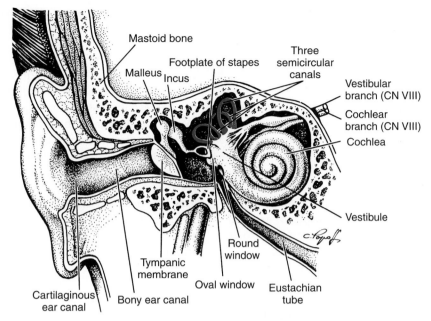

FIGURE 14-1 External auditory canal, middle ear, inner ear. (From Barkauskas VH, Baumann L, Darling-Fisher C: *Health and physical assessment,* ed 3, St Louis, 2002, Mosby.)

What environmental conditions might suggest increased risk?

Key Questions

- Does anyone around you smoke? Do you smoke?
- If a child: Does the child attend day care?
- If a child: Does the infant take a bottle lying down?
- Have you been swimming recently?
- Have you recently been in an airplane or been scuba diving?

Smoke Exposure

Second-hand cigarette smoke exposure has been associated with a two- to threefold increased risk of otitis media. Cigarette smoking leads to functional eustachian tube obstruction and decreases the protective ciliary action in the tube.

Attending Day Care

Attending a day care with other children is associated with an increased incidence rate of otitis media because of exposure to organisms.

Bottle Propping

In very young children, lying supine while drinking from a bottle has been associated with AOM. It is postulated that swallowing while lying down allows nasopharyngeal fluid to enter the middle ear, with subsequent infection.

Swimming

Repeated or prolonged immersion in water results in loss of protective cerumen and chronic irritation with maceration from excessive moisture in the canal. This leads to an increased occurrence of otitis externa, also called swimmer's ear.

Airplane Travelers, Divers

Barotrauma is a cause of acute serous otitis related to pressure changes from flying or scuba diving. This is often aggravated by recent upper respiratory tract infection or nasal congestion. Failure of the eustachian tube to open and equilibrate during descent results in a collection of serosanguineous fluid in the middle ear. This may be felt as ear pressure that can lead to pain, tinnitus, and temporary deafness. Swallowing, chewing, or blowing out the nose with the mouth and nose occluded can relieve symptoms.

Could this be related to a systemic disease?

Key Questions

■ Do you have diabetes?
■ Have you ever had dermatitis, eczema, or psoriasis?
■ If a child: Does the child have a nonrepaired cleft palate?

Diabetes Mellitus

Diabetes mellitus predisposes adults to malignant otitis externa, which is cellulitis involving the ear and surrounding tissue. Persons with diabetes are also at increased risk for otitis media and mastoiditis.

History of Seborrheic Dermatitis or Psoriasis

Chronic inflammatory dermatitis from overproduction of sebum can occur in the external canal and cause otitis externa.

Cleft Palate

Nonrepaired anomalies anatomically predispose a child to otitis media because of functional obstruction of the eustachian tubes.

What does the presence of pain tell me?

Key Questions

■ Where specifically is the pain felt?
■ Is it in one ear or both?
■ How severe is the pain?
■ Does it interfere with sleeping, eating, or other activities?
■ How long have you had this pain?
■ Is the pain constant or intermittent? If intermittent, how long does it last?
■ Does the pain travel (radiate) to other areas?

Location of the Pain

Pain of otitis externa is described as tenderness around the outer ear or opening to the ear canal that worsens with manipulation of the pinna. Mastoiditis is often associated with severe pain or tenderness over the mastoid bone. If the pain is bilateral, suspect otitis externa. Referred pain or pain of AOM is usually unilateral. Infants cannot assist in location of the ear pain; instead, they exhibit behavioral changes that may indicate pain, such

as irritability, lethargy, poor appetite, vomiting, and diarrhea. Young children may pull or tug at their ears.

Quality of the Pain

The pain of AOM is often described as a deep pain or a blockage of the ear. Serous otitis is often painless or may be described as a bubbling, popping, or stuffy sensation in the ear. Otitis externa involves a tenderness of the outer ear or ear canal that can be accompanied by itching. A cerumen impaction creates a milder pain or vague discomfort of stuffed ears.

Quantity and Severity of the Pain

The pain of AOM is severe enough to interfere with sleep and may be suddenly relieved if the eardrum perforates. Chronic ear pain that is unresponsive to treatment may indicate a tumor.

Onset, Timing, and Duration of the Pain

TMJ pain is often described as severe pain lasting a few minutes and recurring three or four times per day, sometimes associated with headache. It is worse in the morning because nighttime teeth grinding is associated with this condition. The pain is intermittent but can be acute, and is related to trauma or overextension of the mouth. Chronic pain may be related to dental malocclusion or rheumatoid arthritis.

Crying when sucking is often an infant's only indication of pain with compression and increased pressure in the ears. Nocturnal onset of otalgia from a developing infection is caused by increased vascular pressure in the reclined position, causing the TM to bulge and to stimulate pain sensation.

What does the presence of discharge or itching tell me?

Key Questions

■ Do you have any itching in the ear?
■ Do you have any discharge from the ear?

Itching or Drainage

Itching or drainage from the ear usually indicates an infection or inflammation of the external canal. Itching can also be a precursor to herpes zoster of the trigeminal nerve (CN V). Drainage may also be present after the TM ruptures from increased middle ear pressure, or it may be from exudate secondary to mastoiditis. Cholesteatoma is an epidermal inclusion cyst of the middle ear or mastoid. A perforation of the TM and associated foul-smelling discharge may occur.

What does a history of trauma or injury tell me?

Key Questions

- Have you had any recent trauma to the ear?
- Have you had any head trauma?
- How do you clean your ears? Do you use cotton-tipped swabs?
- Do you have a history of excessive earwax?
- If a child: Does the child have a history of putting objects in the ears?
- Have you had any recent insect bites around the ear?
- Have you been exposed to any loud noise?

Ear Trauma

Perforation of the eardrum can be caused by blunt or penetrating trauma. Blunt trauma might include a slap to the ear or barotrauma. Penetrating trauma to the canal or TM may be self-induced with cotton-tipped swabs or other sharp objects used to remove cerumen or to scratch the canal.

Head Trauma

Direct injury to the inner ear by fracture of the petrous temporal bone located at the base of the skull also destroys the inner ear.

Cerumen Impaction

Cerumen is a naturally wet, sticky, honey-colored wax that serves as a lubricant to protect the external ear canal. In some individuals it occurs in a dark, scaly form and accumulates in the ear canal. This accumulation may cause hearing loss, tinnitus, pressure sensation, vertigo, and infection. Self-cleaning practices can produce trauma to the canal, and cerumen-softening solutions can cause chemical irritation to the canal tissue.

Foreign Bodies

Foreign bodies, such as feathers, beads, and insects (especially cockroaches), can produce ear pain and inflammation. Children often self-insert objects.

Insect Bites

Insect bites can lead to acute pain and tenderness of the external canal and may develop into a secondary infection.

Loud Noise

Exposure to high-pitched and loud noise for a prolonged period of time destroys the cochlear hair cells. Exposure to noisy work environments, to the operation of heavy machinery, and to loud music increases the risk of injury and eventual hearing loss.

Is hearing loss a clue?

Key Questions

- Do you have any difficulty in hearing?
- Do you have any dizziness?
- Do you have any ringing in the ear?
- If a child: Do you think the child can hear normally?
- If a child: Does the child turn his or her head to listen?

Difficulty in Hearing

Reports of hearing loss or "difficulty hearing" can indicate blockage of the ear canal by cerumen or a foreign body, inflammation of the middle or inner ear, or a neoplasm. The most frequent cause is conductive hearing loss caused by blockage of the external canal, usually by cerumen. Chronic otitis media is usually a condition of adults who have a chronic infection that may destroy the ossicles and spread to the mastoid, labyrinth, and intracranial structures, causing hearing loss. Chronic ear pain is often associated with hearing loss and ear discharge secondary to a perforated nonhealing TM.

Hearing Loss in Children

Chronic otitis media with effusion causes a conductive hearing loss in children. This loss may be caused by negative middle ear pressure, the presence of an effusion in the middle ear, or structural damage to the TM or ossicles.

Dizziness, Ringing in Ear

Hearing loss associated with dizziness, vertigo, or tinnitus may indicate a serious inner ear condition. Abnormal middle ear ventilation and middle ear effusion are the most common causes of balance disturbance in children. These symptoms are caused by reestablishment of aeration in the middle ear cavity as the effusion clears.

DIAGNOSTIC REASONING: FOCUSED PHYSICAL EXAMINATION

A correct diagnosis of ear pain requires a good view of the TM and external ear canal. Cerumen obstruction should be removed through lavage or by separating an impaction with an ear curette so that irrigation fluid can penetrate behind the impaction. The curette must be manipulated cautiously because trauma to or inflammation of the sensitive perichondrium, which lies immediately below a thin layer of epithelium in the ear canal, elicits excruciating pain and easy bleeding.

Lavage should not be performed if the medical history suggests perforation of the TM. Without visualization of the TM, however, otitis media cannot be ruled out. Lavage solution helps to soften the cerumen and can be purchased commercially in kits or a solution can be made of hydrogen peroxide and water (1:1).

Note Behaviors in Children

Otitis media is the most common childhood disorder. Young infants may exhibit nonspecific signs of irritability, poor feeding, congestion, and fever. Older infants and young toddlers are irritable, pull on the painful ear, or bang their head on the affected side. Older children will report an earache.

Inspect External Ears

General inspection should begin with the pinna and condition of the skin around the ear, face, and scalp. Hemorrhage over the mastoid bone (Battle sign) may occur with a basal skull fracture. Eczematous seborrhea or psoriasis manifests as redness and scaling of the skin that can extend into the external ear canal. Pain in the opening of the ear canal and inflamed skin may suggest a bacterial infection. Fungal and yeast infections appear as white or dark patches. Furuncles or lesions secondary to trauma or irritation appear as localized areas of tenderness or swelling. A hot, swollen, and erythematous ear and surrounding skin indicate cellulitis. Redness and painful swelling over the mastoid process is a sign of infection in the mastoid air cells.

Palpate External Ears

Palpate the pinna and tragus for tenderness. In mastoiditis, the pinna is displaced forward and swelling may be present behind the ear. Palpation of the mastoid process elicits severe tenderness. Otitis externa is associated with pain on manipulation of the pinna. With referred pain, the structures will appear normal, although palpation over the TMJ may elicit tenderness, and movement of the jaw may create a clicking sound.

Palpate the preauricular and postauricular areas on the right and left simultaneously to elicit pain. Palpate anterior and posterior cervical lymph nodes and over the mastoid process. Preauricular nodes may be enlarged in AOM and otitis externa. Postauricular swelling may indicate extension of infection into the mastoid cavity.

Inspect Ear Canals

With the otoscope, observe for the patency of the canal, the condition of the skin of the ear canal, and the presence of cerumen. With cerumen impaction, no structures can be visualized. A foreign body is easily visualized. Vesicles on the external ear canal and auricle may indicate herpes zoster (Ramsay Hunt syndrome).

Visualize any discharge, noting color, consistency, and odor. Discharge is usually indicative of an active infection. However, cranial trauma with cerebrospinal fluid leakage must be kept in mind. Cheesy, green-blue, or gray discharge can be seen with otitis externa.

Inspect Tympanic Membranes

Visualize the TM, noting light reflex and anatomical structures. A normal TM is translucent and pearly gray in color. Mild diffuse redness can occur from crying or coughing. Mild vascularity is sometimes seen in the normal eardrum, especially on the handle of the malleus. Localized redness is a sign of inflammation. Scarring and effusion can cause whitening and opacification of the TM.

The contour of the normal TM is somewhat concave. Fullness or bulging indicates either increased air pressure or, more commonly, increased hydrostatic pressure within the middle ear. Fullness of the eardrum is seen first around the periphery of the TM. As pressure increases, central fullness becomes visible. Concavity or retraction of the eardrum is associated with negative middle ear pressure or postinflammatory adhesions. As the eardrum retracts, the handle of the malleus short process becomes more visible.

Myringitis is a red, inflamed eardrum without effusion. Bullous myringitis describes an extremely painful condition of small blisters on the TM caused by bacterial otitis media. Figure 14-2 illustrates the usual landmarks of a normal right TM. Chronic otitis media can lead to cholesteatoma, or a cyst-like mass behind the eardrum, caused by the proliferation of squamous epithelium. The mass can grow to cause necrosis of the ossicles. Examination will reveal a

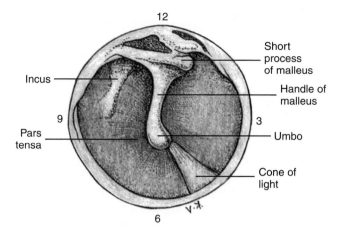

12

Incus

9

Pars
tensa

6

Short
process
of malleus

Handle of
malleus

3

Umbo

Cone of
light

FIGURE 14-2 Usual landmarks of the right tympanic membrane with a "clock" superimposed. (Modified from Potter PA, Perry AG: *Basic nursing: essentials for practice,* ed 6, St Louis, 2006, Mosby.)

collection of white granulation tissue with perforation of the TM.

Perform Pneumatic Otoscopy (Insufflation)

The normal eardrum is suspended from its margins and responds to slight pressure changes. Insufflation tests the mobility of the TM. It can be an insensitive test for otitis media if poor technique fails to create a seal. Properly performed, however, it is more reliable than visualization alone.

To perform insufflation, a large speculum is needed to create a seal. A normal finding elicits a slight motion of the TM when air is insufflated. This movement is compared with the opposite ear. A TM that has been retracted as a result of negative middle ear pressure or adhesions does not move with inflation, but rebound mobility is seen when the bulb is released. Any accumulation of liquid in the middle ear (e.g., effusion) or scarring of the TM inhibits movement when air is insufflated.

Test Hearing Acuity

Hearing acuity is tested using the whisper test and the tuning fork for the Rinne and Weber tests. The sensory function of the acoustic nerve (CN VIII) should be tested to determine whether air or bone conduction loss is present with ear pain.

The Weber test is performed with a 512-hertz (Hz) or higher frequency tuning fork. To perform the test, firmly place the vibrating tuning fork on a midline point of the skull. If there is unilateral conductive hearing loss, sound will lateralize to the ear with loss because the better ear is being distracted by ambient noise. Alternately, if the patient has unilateral sensorineural loss, the sound will lateralize to the better ear because the neural pathway is interrupted on the affected side. Equal perception of vibration can indicate normal hearing or bilateral hearing loss. The Rinne test compares air conduction with bone conduction; the ratio should be 2:1. A 20- to 30-decibel (dB) conductive loss would result in better sound transmission through bone than through air. Conductive hearing loss results when sound transmission is impaired through the external or middle ear. Sensorineural hearing loss results from a defect in the inner ear.

Examine Related Body Systems

Examine other regional body systems of the head and neck, including inspection of the conjunctivae, examination of the mucosa and patency of the nose, percussion and palpation of the frontal and maxillary sinuses for tenderness, and inspection of the posterior pharynx for lymphedema, color, and presence of exudate. Inspection of the condition of the oral mucosa—teeth and gums—will provide information about possible causes of referred pain. A focused physical examination for head and neck symptoms should include palpation of cervicofacial lymph nodes, especially the preauricular and postauricular nodes.

Perform an Intraotic Manipulation

If referred pain is suspected, conduct a more extensive neurological examination and assess for TMJ disorder. TMJ pain can be replicated by instructing the patient to open the mouth wide. Face the patient, insert a single fingertip in each ear, and pull the patient toward you as the patient is instructed to open and close the mouth. Pain will be elicited in 90% of patients with TMJ disorder.

Evaluate Cranial Nerves V, VII, and IX

Observe jaw and facial muscle movement for symmetry and strength by palpating over the masseter muscles and asking the patient to bite and clench the teeth (CN V). Assess intactness of sensation to pain and light touch using a sharp/dull stimulus over the three branches of CN V. Both CN VII (anterior two thirds) and CN IX (posterior one third) innervate taste sensation to the tongue as well as sensation to the external ear. Test taste sensation by having the patient protrude the tongue and apply sweet and salty substances separately to each half of the tongue to test CN VII and bitter and sour substances to test CN IX.

LABORATORY AND DIAGNOSTIC STUDIES

Tympanometry

Tympanometry involves inserting a probe into the external ear canal while continually changing pressure against the eardrum to assess the mobility of the TM. The tympanogram provides an indirect measure of pressure in the middle ear. Under normal middle ear pressure, the TM absorbs the sound energy waves and produces a bell-shaped pattern that peaks when sound pressure is introduced. With positive or negative middle ear pressure, the tympanogram results in a flat pattern or an early peak pressure. Figure 14-3 illustrates examples of various tympanogram results.

Audiometry

Audiometry assesses both the frequency and the intensity of sound that can be perceived. An air conduction audiometer transmits via earphones a pure tone that has

FIGURE 14-3 Middle ear evaluation with pneumatic otoscopy and impedance tympanograms. (From Daeschner CW Jr: *Pediatrics: an approach to independent learning*, New York, 1983, John Wiley & Sons.)

variable frequency and intensity settings to test each ear separately. The goal of audiometry is to test the lowest decibel intensity that can be heard for each frequency tested. An individual trained in the proper technique will produce reliable, reproducible, and valid test results. A threshold of up to 20 dB is considered normal. At a higher level, hearing loss is graded as mild, moderate, moderately severe, severe, or profound.

Mastoid Process Radiography

Radiographs of the mastoid bone show clouding of the air cells when otitis media is present. Chronic mastoiditis may reveal decalcification of the bony wall between the mastoid air cells.

Computed Tomography Scanning

A computed tomography (CT) scan of the temporal bone is helpful in diagnosing cholesteatoma and congenital syndromes.

DIFFERENTIAL DIAGNOSIS
External Otitis

External otitis is more common in adults than in children and often presents as bilateral pain that worsens with manipulation of the pinna. The patient reports a stuffed ear, and occasionally conductive hearing loss occurs. Discharge and itching that occur 1 to 2 days after swimming may be associated with otitis externa. The affected canal may be swollen shut. Palpation will often disclose enlarged preauricular or postauricular nodes.

Acute Otitis Media

AOM most often occurs in children younger than 6 years and is associated with an upper respiratory tract infection. It is an acute infection associated with ear pain and a bulging, red eardrum. The pain of otitis media is severe enough to interfere with sleep and may be suddenly relieved if the eardrum perforates. Swelling of the preauricular node is sometimes seen in children with AOM.

Otitis Media with Effusion

Otitis media with effusion commonly occurs in children and is by definition painless. It is caused by a mechanical process or eustachian tube blockage that leads to inadequate ventilation of the middle ear. On exam, a collection of fluid that resembles mucus, air bubbles, or a fluid level is seen. Associated conductive hearing loss is usually present. The TM may be injected and immobile, either bulging or retracted, as noted by the shape of the cone of

light reflex and pneumatic otoscopy. Associated recent upper respiratory tract infection is a common finding in adults.

Cholesteatoma

Cholesteatoma is an epidermal inclusion cyst formation in the middle ear and mastoid cavity. It is often the sequel of chronic otitis media. The formation occurs with chronic negative middle ear pressure, causing the migration of skin cells from the external ear canal through a perforation in the TM. Once established in the middle ear, the cells desquamate and form the cholesteatoma. This condition is life threatening if left untreated because it will continue to erode away medially to impinge on intracranial structures. A cholesteatoma can also occur congenitally. A cholesteatoma appears as a cyst or collection of granulation tissue on the TM, commonly located in the pars flaccida area in the superior anterior quadrant of the TM.

Mastoiditis

Mastoiditis is an infection of the soft tissue surrounding the air spaces in the mastoid bone and is connected to the middle ear space. Mastoiditis usually occurs with bacterial otitis media and is associated with fever. More advanced mastoiditis is manifested by swelling, erythema, and tenderness over the mastoid bone. Swelling can displace the position of the auricle. The swelling can extend to the facial nerve, causing paralysis, or to the labyrinth or cerebrospinal fluid, causing meningitis or brain abscess. Advanced mastoiditis requires immediate referral and surgical management.

Foreign Bodies

Foreign bodies are easily visualized on examination of the ear canal and can produce foul-smelling ear drainage secondary to infection or abscess.

Cerumen Impaction

Impaction of cerumen is likely if the patient reports a stuffed-up ear or decreased hearing acuity. An impaction may also produce pain if cerumen is pressed against the TM. Examination will reveal cerumen that occludes the external canal.

Barotrauma

Barotrauma produces an acute serous otitis that is caused by pressure changes (e.g., in divers or airplane travelers) and is often aggravated by a recent upper respiratory tract infection or nasal congestion. Serosanguineous fluid collects in the middle ear; during descent this may be felt as ear pressure, pain, tinnitus, or temporary deafness. Swallowing, chewing, or blowing out the nose with the mouth and nose occluded can relieve symptoms.

Trauma

Blunt or penetrating trauma can perforate the TM. A hole in the TM is visible on examination, or the examiner may notice an absence of normal landmarks. A perforated eardrum does not significantly impair hearing or result in vertigo and usually heals within 4 to 6 weeks without sequelae. Assess the extent of other damage to the ear when perforation is identified.

Cervical Lymphadenitis

Anterior cervical lymphadenitis is a common cause of referred ear pain in children. This may be seen with strep throat, as well as in cases of mononucleosis with extensive cervical node swelling in adolescents or young adults.

Referred Pain from Cervical Nerves

CN II and CN III innervate the skin and muscles of the neck and include the great auricular nerve, which supplies the external canals and posterior auricular area. Pain is perceived in these areas. The ear examination will be normal.

Referred Pain from Cranial Nerves

CNs associated with referred ear pain include V, VII, IX, and X. The trigeminal nerve (CN V) supplies the anterior portion of the auricle and tragus, the anterior and superior auditory canal, and the anterior TM. The facial (CN VII), the vagus (CN X), and the glossopharyngeal (CN IX) nerves innervate the posterior portion of the TM and the external auditory canal. Inflammation of CN X is associated with lesions of the larynx, esophagus, trachea, and thyroid. With referred pain, the structures of the ear will appear normal.

Temporomandibular Joint Disorder

TMJ disorder is a common secondary cause of ear pain. Diagnosis of the disorder is likely if palpation over the TMJ elicits tenderness and movement of the joint creates a clicking sound. Results of examination of the ear are normal. Pain also increases with intraotic manipulation. TMJ pain is often worse in the morning. The pain can be acute (related to trauma or overextension of the mouth) or chronic (related to dental malocclusion or rheumatoid arthritis).

DIFFERENTIAL DIAGNOSIS OF *Common Causes of Ear Pain*

CONDITION	HISTORY	PHYSICAL FINDINGS	DIAGNOSTIC STUDIES
External otitis	More common in adults, especially those with diabetes, ear pickers, or swimmers; bilateral itching; pain	Discharge; inflamed, swollen external canal; pain with movement of pinna; TM normal or not visible	None
Acute otitis media	More common in children <6 years; those with smoke exposure, recent URI; severe or deep pain; unilateral; sensation of fullness	Red, bulging TM; fever; decreased light reflex; opaque TM; decreased TM mobility	None initially
Otitis media with effusion	More common in children but occurs in adults with recent URI; unilateral pain; sensation of crackling or decreased hearing	Fluid line or air observed behind TM; conductive hearing loss; decreased TM mobility	Tympanogram
Cholesteatoma	Hearing loss; recent perforated TM	Pearly white lesion on or behind TM	Immediate referral
Mastoiditis	History of recent otitis media; chronic otitis pain behind ear	Swelling over mastoid process; fever, palpable tenderness, and erythema over mastoid process	Radiograph of mastoid sinuses reveals cloudiness; referral

DIFFERENTIAL DIAGNOSIS OF *Common Causes of Ear Pain—cont'd*

CONDITION	HISTORY	PHYSICAL FINDINGS	DIAGNOSTIC STUDIES
Foreign body or cerumen impaction	Both children and adults have pain or vague sensation of discomfort; decreased hearing	Visualize foreign body or cerumen; may detect foul odor; conductive hearing loss	None
Barotrauma	History of flying, diving; severe pain; hearing loss; sensation of fullness; history of recent nasal congestion	Retraction or bulging of TM; perforation of TM; fluid in canal	Tympanogram
Trauma	History of blunt trauma, penetrating trauma	Perforation of TM	Radiographs/CT scan as directed by injury
Cervical lymphadenitis	History of cervical node swelling; pain in ear common in children	Enlarged, tender, cervical lymph nodes; may see early onset of AOM in children	Throat culture if indicated; in adolescents Monospot if indicated
Cervical nerves II and III (referred pain)	Pain in skin and muscles of neck and in ear canal	Dermatome evaluation for cervical nerve involvement	None
Cranial nerves (referred pain)	History, depending on CN involved	Test function of CNs V, VII, IX, and X; ear examination normal	Radiography/CT scan, directed by CN involvement
TMJ disorder	More common in adults; 50% related to dental problems; discomfort to severe pain; unilateral; pain worse in morning	Malocclusion; bruxism; normal external and middle ear structures and function; jaw click; abnormal CN function; ear examination normal	None

AOM, acute otitis media; *CN*, cranial nerve; *CT*, computed tomography; *TM*, tympanic membrane; *URI*, upper respiratory tract infection.

REFERENCES AND READINGS

American Academy of Pediatrics and American Academy of Family Physicians: Diagnosis and management of acute otitis media, *Pediatrics* 113:1451, 2004.

Ishiyama A: Why does air travel cause earache? *West J Med* 171:106, 1999.

Li J, Brunk J: Otalgia, *Emedicine*. Available at http://emedicine.medscape.com/article/845173-overview. Accessed October 6, 2010.

Majumdar S, Wu K, Bateman ND, Ray J: Diagnosis and management of otalgia in children, *Arch Dis Child Educ Pract Ed: 94:*33, 2009.

O'Neill P: Acute otitis media, *BMJ* 319:833, 1999.

Pelton SI: Otitis media: re-evaluation of diagnosis and treatment in the era of antimicrobial resistance, pneumococcal conjugate vaccine, and evolving morbidity, *Pediatr Clin North Am* 52:711, 2005.

Pichichero ME: Acute otitis media, part I: improving diagnostic accuracy, *Am Fam Physician* 61:2051, 2000.

Fatigue

Fatigue, also called asthenia, is a constitutional symptom that can be the result of normal physiological consequences of exertion or a symptom of illness. It is a sensation of profound tiredness that is not relieved by rest or sleep without an objective finding of muscle weakness. Fatigue can result from any disruption of energy production. Anemia, decreased oxygenation of blood, or reduced blood flow limits the amount of oxygen available to cells. Other factors that contribute to fatigue interfere with restorative mechanisms provided by sleep and rest, nutritional state, and mechanisms to remove or regulate wastes of metabolism. When fatigue is associated with cardiovascular or respiratory symptoms, clues are present that may point to the cause. However, most patients who have the symptom of fatigue have a normal physical examination and psychological factors are often a contributing cause.

Fatigue is classified as physiological, psychological, and acute or chronic. Physiological fatigue is the result of normal activities that lead to overwork or exhaustion. Psychological fatigue is often related to a stressful event. Organic causes can produce acute or chronic fatigue. Acute fatigue lasts less than 6 months and is often a prodrome to other illnesses, most often infections, such as endocarditis, hepatitis, or other acute bacterial or viral illnesses. However, fatigue can also indicate a disease state, most often related to hyperthyroidism, hypothyroidism, heart failure, anemia, chronic obstructive pulmonary disease (COPD), sleep apnea, autoimmune disorder, or cancer.

Chronic fatigue lasts longer than 6 months, and its onset is usually slow and progressive. Chronic fatigue may be an indication of depression, chronic infection, or systemic disease, or it may be secondary to alcohol or medication use. Chronic fatigue syndrome is a distinct clinical entity characterized by fatigue that is persistent or relapses, is not alleviated with rest, and affects the patient's ability to function.

Fatigue is uncommon in very young children; the younger the child, the more likely the cause is organic. Most cases of fatigue in school-age children are related to acute infection. Fatigue is common in adolescents because of lifestyle factors, as well as in older adults.

DIAGNOSTIC REASONING: FOCUSED HISTORY

Is this really fatigue?

Key Question
- Can you tell me what you mean by fatigue?

Fatigue Versus Weakness

It is important to discriminate between weakness and fatigue. Often, patients describe muscle weakness when speaking about fatigue such as, "I am tired all the time and I feel weak." In children with weakness, parents will say the child is floppy or "doesn't run in gym like the other children." An individual tends to tire easily with metabolic or neuromuscular diseases, such as hypothyroidism or myasthenia gravis.

Young children tend not to have vocabulary that describes fatigue; often it is the parent who brings the child to the clinic. Parents may state that the child is "lying around" or "I can't get the child to do anything" or "she just doesn't have any energy." Adolescents will say they are "always" tired.

Is the fatigue physiological?

Key Questions
- Can you tell me about your lifestyle habits (e.g., exercise and diet)?
- Can you tell me about your sleep pattern?
- Do you require naps?
- Do you feel rested when you wake up in the morning?
- When was your last menstrual period?

Lifestyle Habits

A history of the patient's daily living and working habits may reveal a physiological cause for exhaustion. Erratic eating patterns, dieting, and missed meals may result in undernutrition or overnutrition. High levels of caffeine can affect the amount of energy a person has and can affect the sleep cycle, causing fatigue. Academic stress, athletic participation, and employment further contribute to fatigue in adolescents.

Sleep Pattern

Lack of adequate amounts of sleep is often the cause of fatigue (see Chapter 28). Adults need at least 6 to 8 hours of sleep for adequate rest; adolescents, 8 to 9 hours; and children, 10 hours. Patients with sleep apnea, which is more common in men older than 45 years, may report waking up and not being refreshed. Heart failure causes postural nocturnal dyspnea, leading to difficulty breathing at night and disturbed sleep. Early morning wakening is a symptom of depression, as is excessive sleeping during the day.

Last Normal Menstrual Period

Fatigue is a common symptom in women. Fatigue is an early sign of pregnancy, a symptom post childbirth, and a symptom associated with menopause. Perimenopausal women may have fatigue as a result of disrupted sleep because of night sweats or hot flashes.

Do I need to consider an organic cause?

Key Questions

- Do you practice safe sex (if sexually active)?
- Have you ever had hepatitis?
- What medications do you take?
- Do you drink alcohol or use street drugs?

Exposure to Body Fluids

Fatigue may be the initial and most prominent symptom of hepatitis, human immunodeficiency virus (HIV) infection, or acquired immunodeficiency syndrome (AIDS). Hepatitis B can be a sexually transmitted infection through semen or contracted from exposure to contaminated blood. Sexual practices that traumatize mucous membranes, such as anal intercourse, increase the risk of transmission of organisms. The person with HIV/AIDS experiences cognitive impairment that includes difficulty processing complex information.

These impairments are correlated with the severity of fatigue.

Medications

Almost any drug can have fatigue as a side effect. The most common drugs that cause fatigue are antihypertensive drugs, cardiovascular medications, psychotropic medications, and opiates. Side effects also occur with drugs such as sedatives and antihistamines. Many drugs that cause fatigue are over-the-counter preparations.

Alcohol and Drug Use

Alcohol abuse and use of illicit drugs may be overlooked as a cause of chronic fatigue in adolescents and school-age children. This fatigue is due directly to the substance, usually alcohol or marijuana, and to secondary factors such as associated poor lifestyle habits related to sleep, rest, and nutrition. Family and friends may express the greatest concerns about fatigue that affects the patient's ability to function. The CAGE questionnaire is a useful screening tool to assess for alcohol abuse (see Box 3-3).

What other clues can help me rule out an organic cause?

Key Questions

- Have you noticed a change in appetite?
- Do you have any joint tenderness or pain?
- Have you noticed increased urination?
- What other symptoms have you experienced?

Appetite

An increased appetite may indicate hypoglycemia. A decreased appetite may indicate an infectious process.

Weight Loss

Weight loss may indicate malignancy, infection, or poor nutrition related to depression or lack of information about a healthy and balanced diet.

Increased Urination

Diabetes mellitus, especially type 2, often presents with fatigue along with polydipsia, polyphagia, and polyuria.

Joint Tenderness

In children with juvenile rheumatoid arthritis (JRA), severe fatigue that seems to be more than expected with the degree of joint involvement is seen. In young and middle-aged patients, chronic fatigue syndrome can involve multiple tender points on the body that are over joints.

Associated Symptoms

Psychological fatigue is often associated with non-specific and multiple symptoms, such as muscle aching, abdominal pain, and general lethargy. Organic causes of fatigue are associated with a few specific symptoms that worsen over time, such as dry skin and nails with hypothyroidism or shortness of breath with exertion or when lying flat with congestive heart failure.

Could this have an environmental cause?

Key Questions

- Where do you work?
- Have you been exposed to any toxins?
- Have you been camping?

Occupational Exposure

Heavy metals and pesticides may cause fatigue and other neurological symptoms. Soldiers returning from combat zones, such as the Gulf War, have been found to have unrelenting fatigue from an unknown cause.

Camping

Lyme disease is carried by the deer tick and may present with a history of weeks of malaise and chronic fatigue before any skin manifestations appear.

What else do I need to know about the fatigue?

Key Questions

- Can you describe the onset and pattern of your fatigue?
- When did you first notice this?
- How severe is the fatigue?
- What makes the fatigue better or worse?
- Have you had a fever?
- Have you had any bleeding?

Onset and Pattern

The onset of psychological fatigue is often related to a stressful event and may have a sudden onset. Fatigue associated with metabolic causes may have a slow and progressive onset. Significant fatigue is considered to last more than 2 weeks and is experienced by about 25% of adults. Fatigue may be an early sign of pregnancy.

Severity

Clinically significant fatigue may vary throughout the day but never completely disappears. Children with Lyme disease and JRA experience severe fatigue that is in excess of the degree of disease involvement. The patient may need to limit social functioning and recreational activities as a result of fatigue, which may then exacerbate mood disturbances, which in turn contributes to fatigue.

Aggravating/Alleviating Factors

Psychological fatigue is usually worse in the morning and physical activity may relieve the fatigue. Organic fatigue is not associated with intensity or duration of activity and is not relieved with rest or sleep.

Fever

Fever generally accompanies infectious diseases, which are common causes of fatigue (see Chapter 16). Prolonged fever may indicate chronic infection, inflammatory disease, or malignancy.

Bleeding

Heavy menstrual flow may lead to anemia (see Chapter 33). Other sources of bleeding, such as gastrointestinal ulcers, polyps, or cancer of the bowel, may result in occult blood loss and fatigue.

If I suspect a psychological cause, what else do I need to know?

Key Questions

- Can you describe your stress level and how you cope with stress in your life?
- Have you recently had a stressful event in your life?
- Do you or does anyone in your family have a problem with anxiety or depression?
- How are you doing in school?

Stress

Stressful life events increase the risk of depression in some adolescents and adults. In the presence of organic disease, stress may be secondary to pain or discomfort that may disrupt sleep and rest patterns. Deconditioning secondary to muscle atrophy with inactivity or bed rest can lead to fatigue (see Chapter 3).

Anxiety and Depression

Children who have family members with depression are at a greater risk for depression. Generally, the first episode of major depression occurs between the ages of 20 and 30 and more often affects women. Major depressive disorder may have a genetic component. Diagnostic criteria will point to depression or anxiety as a cause.

School Performance

Decreased academic performance and decreased productivity may be an early sign of low self-esteem and early depression. Children also may overachieve academically to compensate for their lower self-esteem and hide their depression.

DIAGNOSTIC REASONING: FOCUSED PHYSICAL EXAMINATION

A general physical examination, including psychological screening for depression and anxiety, is needed to make a differential diagnosis of fatigue. The majority of patients will have a normal physical examination, but clues can be found for the presence of systemic disease.

Note General Appearance

Observe the patient entering the examination room to note any abnormality of gait that may indicate neurological involvement or generalized weakness. Observe the patient's demeanor and appearance for signs of neglect or a facial expression that might indicate depression or generalized anxiety. In the presence of organic disease, the patient will appear ill; with psychological stress, the patient may appear depressed or anxious. Children may appear sad or irritable.

Take Vital Signs

The presence of fever suggests inflammation or infection. Blood pressure reading, pulse rate, and respiratory rate reflect the function of the cardiorespiratory system. An elevated pulse rate may be associated with anxiety, anemia, or hyperthyroidism. Evaluate the patient for orthostatic hypotension. Weigh and measure the patient to obtain the body mass index (BMI); a BMI outside the normal range can indicate poor nutritional status as well as cardiovascular risk.

Inspect Skin, Hair, and Nails

Observe for signs of thyroid dysfunction. Hypothyroidism is associated with coarse, dry hair and skin and thickening of nails. Hyperthyroidism is characterized by fine, limp hair and warm skin. Look for skin lesions or rashes that may indicate infection or inflammation. A faint maculopapular rash is sometimes associated with mononucleosis. Lyme disease is associated with a macular lesion with a clear center. Atrophic skin of the lower extremities is an indication of arterial insufficiency and underlying arteriovascular disease. Patients with anxiety disorders may bite their nails or self-inflict excoriation lesions, usually over the face and extremities.

Examine the Nose, Eyes, Mouth, and Throat

Inspect for any signs of infection or inflammation secondary to an allergic response. Petechiae on the palate may be seen with mononucleosis. Palpate for cervicofacial nodes. Lymphadenopathy is seen with HIV, malignancy, and mononucleosis. Inspect mucous membranes for lesions and moisture. Dry, cracked, and ulcerated mucosa can indicate a nutritional deficiency or dehydration.

Conduct a Cardiovascular Examination

Palpate the anterior thorax for the location of the point of maximal impulse (PMI) and for lifts or heaves. Listen for carotid and thyroid bruits. Auscultate the heart, listening carefully for rate, rhythm, and murmurs, especially a late systolic murmur heard loudest over the mitral area, which may indicate mitral prolapse. An audible S_3 or S_4 in an adult may indicate heart failure.

Examine the Lungs

First, observe the patient for ease of breathing and respiratory rate. Note the anteroposterior (AP)/lateral diameter of the thorax. An increased AP diameter indicates chronic obstructive pulmonary disease (COPD). Test for egophony, and palpate and percuss the anterior and posterior thorax to listen for resonance (normal) or consolidation. Tactile fremitus will increase over areas of consolidated lung. Listen for rales and wheezes. Bilateral basilar rales indicate congestive heart failure.

Barely audible breath sounds are associated with COPD.

Examine the Abdomen

Begin the examination by observing the abdomen (see Chapter 2). Observe the intactness and condition of the skin. A rigid abdomen suggests peritoneal irritation. Generalized symmetrical distention may occur with obesity, enlarged organs, fluid, or gas. Dehydration or malnutrition may present as a concave contour of the abdomen.

Listen for bowel sounds. Anxiety, gastrointestinal irritation, and hunger can increase the frequency and loudness of bowel sounds. Depression can decrease bowel sounds.

Perform general light palpation to assess the skin and abdominal musculature. Note the patient's response to the examination. Perform deep palpation over the liver, spleen, and right kidney. Fist palpation over the posterior thorax tests for kidney tenderness associated with pyelonephritis.

Perform a Musculoskeletal Examination

Observe and palpate joints for inflammation and swelling. Bilateral tenderness over the major trigger points is diagnostic of fibromyalgia. Test stamina by asking the patient to perform certain musculoskeletal movements or to walk a certain distance to evaluate changes in fatigue level. For example, ask the patient to walk a distance for 3 minutes as far and as fast as they can comfortably and then assess fatigue level.

Conduct a Neurological Examination

Assess both cognitive and physical function to evaluate attention span, judgment, memory, and affect. Abnormalities may suggest a psychiatric disorder or brain pathology. Dementia is also seen in persons with HIV/AIDS. Test cranial nerves. A change in deep tendon reflexes (DTRs) may indicate thyroid dysfunction. Cerebellar and motor testing will rule out weakness or any associated neurological pathology.

LABORATORY AND DIAGNOSTIC STUDIES
Complete Blood Count with Indices and Differential

A complete blood count (CBC) with indices will provide information about the degree and cause of anemia. Hematocrit and hemoglobin levels reflect the degree of anemia and the indices point to a cause. Microcytic hypochromic anemia reflects chronic blood loss, whereas normocytic normochromic anemia suggests an acute blood loss.

A white blood cell (WBC) count of greater than 12,000/μl indicates inflammation or infection. Normally the circulating neutrophils are in a mature form, known as segs because the cell nuclei are segmented. Immature forms are known as bands. Infection will increase the total number of neutrophils with an increase in the number of immature cells or bands.

Ferritin

Ferritin is a protein that stores iron in bone marrow, and ferritin levels most accurately reflect total body iron stores. Ferritin levels are low with iron deficiency anemia. In contrast, ferritin levels may be elevated or normal in anemia of chronic disease or in thalassemias, caused by a reduction in the life cycle of a red blood cell (RBC) and the bone marrow failing to compensate for the loss by increasing RBC production.

Total Iron-Binding Capacity

Iron is transported in plasma bound with transferrin, a serum protein synthesized in the liver. Total iron-binding capacity (TIBC) of serum is an indirect measure of transferrin. This capacity may be increased in iron deficiency anemia because although the capacity to bind with iron is high, hemoglobin is decreased and both mean corpuscular volume (MCV) and mean corpuscular hemoglobin concentration (MCHC) are decreased (e.g., microcytic, hypochromic anemia). TIBC is normal or low in chronic disease, often because of the shorter life cycle of an RBC and the body's inability to compensate.

Urinalysis

Dipstick urinalysis can rule out or point to infection or systemic disease as a cause of the incontinence. Note hematuria, pyuria, bacteriuria, or the presence of leukocyte esterase or nitrites as indicators of urinary tract infection. Glycosuria or proteinuria suggests diabetes mellitus or renal disease. The presence of bacteria, RBC casts, and WBCs on microscopic examination indicates urinary tract infection (see Chapter 32).

Erythrocyte Sedimentation Rate

The erythrocyte sedimentation rate (ESR) measures the rate at which RBCs settle in a tube of anticoagulated blood. An increase in plasma globulins or fibrinogen causes the cells to stick together and fall faster than normal. An increased ESR is a general indication of an inflammatory process and does not identify the source. The ESR is often elevated as a result of acute or chronic infection or inflammatory conditions such as rheumatoid arthritis or temporal arteritis.

Fasting Blood Glucose

A fasting blood glucose level ≥ 126 mg/dL will identify a patient who is at risk for diabetes.

Hepatic Function

Obtain aspartate aminotransferase (AST) and alanine aminotransferase (ALT) values to assess for general inflammation of the liver, associated with hepatitis.

Thyroid-Stimulating Hormone

A serum thyroid-stimulating hormone (TSH) level identifies hypothyroidism.

HIV Infection

An enzyme-linked immunosorbent assay (ELISA) will rule out HIV infection as a cause.

Tuberculin Skin Testing

A Mantoux test is used to test for tuberculosis antibodies. See Chapter 10 for a more thorough description of skin testing for tuberculosis.

Monospot

The Monospot is a rapid slide test that detects heterophil antibody agglutination. It is not specific for Epstein-Barr virus (EBV). It is most sensitive 1 to 2 weeks after symptoms appear and remains positive for up to 1 year. If chronic fatigue syndrome is being considered as a differential diagnosis, specific EBV antibody tests should be considered.

Chest Radiograph

A chest radiograph can reveal the presence of pneumonia, a lesion in the lungs, heart size, or the presence of fluid in the lungs as a result of congestive heart failure.

DIFFERENTIAL DIAGNOSIS
Physiological Causes
Poor Sleep and Rest

In general, total sleep time is greatest during infancy, decreases in childhood, may increase again during parts of adolescence, remains relatively stable during the adult years, and declines during the late years of adulthood (see Chapter 28).

Total sleep time for the newborn is 14 to 18 hours a day. As the child matures, the sleep cycle increases in length and the total sleep time decreases. Sleep patterns of 8 to 10 hours develop during childhood. Many adolescents need increased amounts of sleep.

Most healthy adults spend 7 to 9 hours sleeping each day. Older adults sleep less, and may experience more frequent awakenings during the night; some need to compensate for this with rest periods during the day.

Poor Nutritional Status

Assessment of nutritional risk is determined by data from the history and physical examination, food recall data, BMI (BMI <18.5 = underweight; BMI 18.5 to 24.9 = healthy weight; BMI 25 to <30 = overweight; BMI >30 = obesity), and waist circumference.

According to Dietary Guidelines for Americans 2010, adults are advised to do the following:

- Eat a variety of fruits and vegetables. Choose five or more servings a day.
- Eat a variety of grain products, including whole grain. Choose six or more servings a day.
- Include fat-free and low-fat milk products, fish, legumes, skinless poultry, and lean meats.
- Restrict total fat intake to 20% to 35% of calories, with the majority of fats consisting of polyunsaturated and monounsaturated fatty acids.
- Balance the number of calories you eat with the number of calories you burn.
- Engage in regular physical activity of moderate intensity for at least 30 minutes on most days.
- Limit your intake of high-calorie, low-nutrition foods.
- Limit your intake of foods high in saturated and trans-fatty acids.
- Eat less than 2300 mg (1 teaspoon of salt) of sodium per day.
- Drink no more than one alcohol drink a day if a woman and no more than two drinks a day if a man.
- Clean hands when handling food; cook foods to safe temperatures; chill foods promptly; and defrost foods properly.

Psychological Causes
Depression

About 30% of primary care patients will have depressive symptoms. The adult patient will most often present with a loss of interest in usual activities, feelings of worthlessness and guilt, and thoughts of suicide for more than 2 weeks' duration. The practitioner must assess the risk of suicide and intervene or refer to a mental health specialist (see differential diagnosis box in Chapter 3).

Other symptoms include sleep and appetite disturbances, malaise, and decreased libido. Patients with bipolar disease may reveal a history of a manic episode associated with increased activity, increased libido, and feelings of grandiosity. The physical examination is usually normal.

Children will appear sad, angry, or irritable. They may have somatic complaints or low self-esteem and have problems with school performance. Adolescents may exhibit euphoria, hypersomnia, and lack of interest in activities.

Anxiety

Diagnostic and statistical manual of mental disorders, ed 4, text revision (DSM-IV-TR) diagnostic criteria for anxiety will guide the diagnosis of anxiety disorder or panic attack. Patients will report a sense of doom and fear of losing control, dyspnea and chest discomfort, fatigue, restlessness, and sleep disturbance. Physical findings will include tachycardia, palpitations, and diaphoresis (see differential diagnosis table in Chapter 3).

Organic Causes of Acute Fatigue
Infection

The prodrome stage of many viral infections may produce fatigue before other symptoms, such as sore throat, nasal congestion, and myalgia. Acute hepatitis A and B can cause fatigue before symptoms of jaundice or abdominal discomfort appear. Endocarditis, an infection of the heart valves, can cause fatigue.

Drugs

Alcoholism is one of the most common causes of acute fatigue related to organic causes. Chronic alcohol abuse is associated with undernutrition, a contributing factor to fatigue.

Anemia

The fatigue associated with anemia is secondary to the body's compensation to increase oxygen in blood that is oxygen-deprived because of abnormal size or quantity of RBCs. The body compensates by increasing the heart rate but may not be able to make up for this deficit, which leads to increased breathlessness with activity.

A diet history may show inadequate dietary intake of iron or heavy menstrual bleeding. Early symptoms are fatigue, weakness, and shortness of breath. A CBC will identify the cause of anemia. Serum iron, serum ferritin, and transferrin levels may also support the diagnosis of anemia.

Hypothyroidism (Myxedema)

Patients report cold intolerance, constipation, weight gain, hoarseness, depression, and fatigue. Physical examination reveals bradycardia, dry skin, generalized edema, and delayed recovery of deep tendon reflexes. An elevated TSH level is present in primary hypothyroidism.

Hyperthyroidism (Graves Disease)

This disorder is associated with increased sweating, heat intolerance, weight loss, irritability, disturbed sleep, and menstrual irregularity. The physical examination may disclose tachycardia, atrial fibrillation, tremor, warm moist skin, and lid lag. Graves disease is associated with exophthalmos. Radioiodine uptake scan will differentiate Graves disease, toxic nodule, and thyroiditis.

Organic Causes of Chronic Fatigue
Sleep Apnea

This disorder most often affects middle-age and older men. Risk factors include obesity and hypertension. Patients describe excessive daytime fatigue, morning headaches, and erectile dysfunction. Bed partners of patients report restless sleep, loud snoring, and periods of apnea for at least 30 seconds during the night.

Medication

Antihypertensive medications and cardiac medications, such as ß-blockers, often are associated with fatigue. Fatigue is a side effect of some pain medications, antihistamines, and many other medications.

Heart Failure

Heart failure is associated with dyspnea, orthopnea, paroxysmal nocturnal dyspnea, peripheral edema, weight gain, cough with frothy sputum, palpitations, and fatigue (see Chapter 10). Persons with a history of heart disease or valvular disease are at greater risk. Physical examination may reveal an altered level of consciousness, anxiety, jugular venous distention, tachypnea, rales and rhonchi, and a displaced

PMI. An S_3 and S_4 can be heard on cardiac auscultation. Chest radiographs will disclose basilar consolidation and increased heart size. An echocardiogram shows a reduced ejection fraction.

Cancer

Lymphoma and leukemia may first be detected by unexplained fatigue that increases with activity and worsens over time. A CBC with differential will show blood dyscrasias. Gastrointestinal cancer may produce occult blood loss that leads to anemia and fatigue.

Mononucleosis

Mononucleosis is often a disease of young adults that is caused by Epstein-Barr virus in 90% of cases. History discloses a gradual onset of low-grade fever, mild sore throat, posterior cervical lymphadenopathy, and fatigue and malaise. Splenomegaly occurs in 50% of cases, and palatine petechiae are a less common sign. Diagnosis can be confirmed with a positive Monospot test and a CBC that shows greater than 50% lymphocytosis. Ten percent of patients may also have concurrent ß-hemolytic streptococcal pharyngitis.

Hepatitis

Generally associated with hepatitis B or C, patients will report a history of malaise, fatigue, flulike symptoms, arthralgia, and an aversion to smoking. A health history will reveal risky sexual behavior, exposure to body secretions through blood transfusion or injectable drug use, or exposure to contaminated food or water. Physical findings may include jaundice, fever, and an enlarged and tender liver. Hepatitis serology for hepatitis A, B, and C will determine the causative agent.

Fibromyalgia

This condition occurs most often in women 20 to 50 years old. It is associated with chronic pain and stiffness of the trunk and extremities, especially the neck, shoulders, low back, and hips. Patients will report fatigue, headaches, sleep disturbance, and irritable bowel symptoms. To diagnose fibromyalgia, 11 of 18 bilateral tender points must be confirmed by physical examination.

Chronic Fatigue Syndrome

There is no single pathological mechanism to explain this condition that appears as an infectious or autoimmune disorder that has neurological, affective, and cognitive symptoms. Chronic fatigue syndrome is severe fatigue lasting longer than 6 months in association with (1) impaired memory or concentration, (2) sore throat, (3) tender cervical or axillary lymph nodes, (4) muscle pain, (5) multiple joint pain, (6) new-onset headaches, (7) nonrestorative sleep, and (8) postexertional malaise.

DIFFERENTIAL DIAGNOSIS OF *Common Causes of Fatigue*

CONDITION	HISTORY	PHYSICAL FINDINGS	DIAGNOSTIC STUDIES
Physiological Causes			
Poor sleep and rest	Adolescent and younger adult; history of overwork, psychological stress, disturbed sleep	Normal examination	None
Poor nutritional status	Depression, decreased appetite, lack of balanced nutrient intake, excessive alcohol intake	BMI reflecting underweight or overweight	Hematocrit increased or decreased, low serum ferritin
Psychological Causes			
Depression: children	Feeling sad, angry, irritable Decrease in academic performance Somatic complaints	None	DSM-PC, DSM-IV
Depression: adults	Loss of interest in usual activities Feelings of worthlessness Sleep problems	Depressed affect; normal examination	Depression screening instrument
Anxiety	Numerous somatic complaints, breathlessness	Tachycardia, palpitations, diaphoresis	None

Continued

DIFFERENTIAL DIAGNOSIS OF *Common Causes of Fatigue—cont'd*

CONDITION	HISTORY	PHYSICAL FINDINGS	DIAGNOSTIC STUDIES
Organic Causes: Acute Fatigue			
Infection	Sudden onset; history of exposure; recent viral illness	Fever; lymphadenopathy, localized signs of erythema, edema	CBC, ESR, Monospot
Drugs and alcohol	History of smoking, alcohol use; antihistamines, analgesics, antihypertensive medications	Bilaterally enhanced or depressed DTRs; pupillary changes; reduced attention span, judgment	CAGE alcohol screening
Anemia	Breathlessness with exertion; menstruating female; recent surgery, delivery	Increased pulse rate; pale mucosa; smooth red tongue	CBC with indices, serum iron, ferritin, transferrin
Hypothyroidism (myxedema)	Poor appetite, fatigue, weight gain, cold intolerance	Decreased pulse rate; dry skin, coarse dry hair; thyroid possibly enlarged, hoarseness	T_4 low, T_3 low, TSH elevated
Hyperthyroidism (Graves disease)	Hyperactivity, heat intolerance, sleep problems	Lid lag, fine thinning hair, tachycardia	T_4 increased, T_3 increased, TSH depressed
Organic Causes: Chronic Fatigue			
Sleep apnea	Male, middle-age or older; partner reports periods of no breathing during sleep, fatigue	Hypertension, obesity, narrowed upper airway	Sleep studies
Medications	History of allergies treated with antihistamines; medications for hypertension, heart disease, chronic pain	Nasal congestion, cough, injected conjunctiva	Evaluate medication choices
Heart failure	Dyspnea, weight gain, fatigue, cough	Anxiety, jugular venous distention, displaced PMI, rales	ECG, chest radiograph, ABGs
Cancer	Fatigue, unexplained weight loss	Observe, palpate, and percuss all systems for lumps, lesions, or consolidation; physical examination may be normal	CBC to rule out anemia; leukocyte count
Mononucleosis (Epstein-Barr virus)	Young adult; slow onset of malaise, low-grade fever, mild sore throat	Palatine petechiae, posterior cervical lymphadenopathy, splenomegaly	Positive Monospot; CBC with differential; >50% leukocytes
Hepatitis	Jaundice, anorexia, fatigue; fever may be reported	Jaundice, weight loss, arthralgia, skin rash	Bilirubin increased; hepatitis panel
Fibromyalgia	Female 20 to 50 yr; history of depression, sleep disturbance, chronic fatigue, general muscle and joint aches	Palpation of trigger points will produce pain; normal physical examination	None
Chronic fatigue syndrome	Fatigue lasting longer than 6 mo; sudden onset of flulike symptoms that persist or recur	Physical examination may be normal; cervical and axillary lymphadenopathy	CBC, ESR

ABGs, arterial blood gases; *BMI,* body mass index; *CBC,* complete blood count; *DTR,* deep tendon reflex; *ECG,* echocardiogram; *PMI,* point of maximal impulse; T_3, triiodothyronine; T_4, thyroxine; *TSH,* thyroid-stimulating hormone.

REFERENCES AND READINGS

American Diabetes Association (ADA): Clinical practice recommendations, *Diabetes Care* 31:S1, 2008.

Cavanaugh R: Evaluating adolescents with fatigue: ever get tired of it? *Pediatr Rev* 23:337, 2002.

Centers for Disease Control and Prevention: Chronic fatigue syndrome, http://www.cdc.gov/cfs/general/symptoms/index.html. Accessed October 7, 2010.

Craig T, Kakumanu S: Chronic fatigue syndrome: evaluation and treatment, *Am Fam Physician* 65:1083, 2002.

Morrison RE: Fatigue in primary care, *Obstet Gynecol Clin North Am* 28:225, 2001.

Pinching A: Chronic fatigue syndrome: believing in ME, *Nurse Prescribing* 7:358, 2009.

Rodriguez T: The challenge of evaluating fatigue, *J Am Acad Nurs Pract* 12:329, 2000.

Rosenthal TC, Majeroni BA, Pretorius R, Malik K: Fatigue: an overview, *Am Fam Physician* 78:1173, 2008.

Sheperd C: The debate: myalgic encephalomyelitis and chronic fatigue syndrome, *Br J Nurs* 15:662, 2006.

Solomon L, Reeves WC: Factors influencing the diagnosis of chronic fatigue syndrome, *Arch Intern Med* 164:2241, 2004.

U.S. Department of Agriculture: The dietary guidelines for Americans 2010, Washington, DC, 2010. Available online at www.cnpp.usda.gov/dietaryguidelines.htm. Accessed January 17, 2011.

16

Fever

Fever is an elevation of temperature above the normal daily variation and is a symptom of an underlying process. The major common cause of fever is infection; however, noninfectious processes may present with fever. Fever of unknown origin (FUO) occurs in a small percentage of cases. These fevers are usually caused by an infection that has not yet been identified. A meticulous history and physical examination supported by laboratory investigation are necessary to find the origin of the fever.

There are three types of fevers, each caused by a specific pathophysiological process. The first involves the raising of the hypothalamic set point. The receptors in the area of the hypothalamus regulating body temperature are triggered to reset at a higher core body temperature. This results in an elevation of the helper T-cell production and an elevation in the effectiveness of interferon. Infection, collagen disease, vascular disease, and malignancy are commonly responsible for these fevers.

A second type of fever is a result of heat production exceeding heat loss. Here the set point is normal, and heat loss mechanisms are active. Fever occurs either because the body raises its metabolic heat production or because the environmental heat load exceeds normal heat loss mechanisms. Aspirin overdose, malignant hyperthermia, hyperthyroidism, or hypernatremia may cause this type of fever.

A third type of fever is caused by a defective heat loss mechanism that cannot cope with normal heat load. Heat stroke, poisoning with anticholinergic drugs, ectodermal dysplasia, and burns are causes of this kind of fever.

For the first type of fever, antipyretics are given to lower the hypothalamic set point. Antipyretics are ineffective for the second and third types of fever.

DIAGNOSTIC REASONING: FOCUSED HISTORY

Is this really a fever?

Key Questions

- How do you know you have a fever?
- Have you taken your temperature?
- How did you measure it?

Occurrence of Fever

Fever is a common presenting problem and a cardinal manifestation of disease. Patients often report a subjective fever (i.e., clinical symptoms, such as flushing, chills, shaking chills, headache, malaise, or muscle aches) that is assumed by the patient to be a fever although not validated with a thermometer. Nevertheless, the absence of fever in a single patient visit does not eliminate a febrile illness.

Measurement of Temperature

Many people use touch to determine whether a fever is present. Although not a precise indication, touch can signal a high fever. During the early stages of fever, perfusion to the skin is decreased and skin temperature falls. In later stages, when temperature within the muscles has risen significantly, increased body temperature is reflected by increased skin temperature. In children, hands and feet should not be used to gauge a fever because they may be vasoconstricted and feel cold. Accurate temperature should be measured using a thermometer. Because of the diurnal variation in normal body temperature and the effect of physiological factors and body rhythms, frequent recordings throughout the day are needed to monitor fever.

Should sepsis or meningitis be of concern?

Key Questions

- Have you had any recent head trauma?
- Do you have recurrent ear infections?
- Have you had contact with anyone who has been ill?
- Have you had a headache, lethargy, confusion, or a stiff neck?
- If an infant: How old is the baby?

Head Trauma, Otitis Media, and Contact

Recent head trauma, especially at the base of the skull, may provide an entrance for infectious organisms. Children with recurrent or chronic otitis media may have mastoiditis spreading to the meninges. Contact with anyone with meningococcal disease and/or *Haemophilus influenzae* places the individual at risk for contracting the disease.

Headache, Vomiting, Lethargy, or Stiff Neck

Meningitis is characterized by headache, fever, lethargy, confusion, vomiting, and stiff neck. However, the presentation is highly variable. Any patient with even minimal neurological signs and symptoms should be evaluated for meningitis.

Infant

Fever in children less than 2 months of age is uncommon but must be viewed as serious. Generally neonates and young infants are less able to mount a febrile response; when they do, it is a significant finding. Fever can be viral or bacterial in nature. Fevers in the neonate may also be an indication of an underlying anatomical defect. Urinary tract infection and bacteremia are often the first indications of a structural abnormality of the urinary tract. Also, infants with galactosemia may present in the first weeks to 1 month of life with gram-negative sepsis. Occasionally, infants present with sepsis associated with delivery (prolonged rupture of membranes); acquired from instrumentation used during delivery, such as scalp electrodes; or from a procedure performed in a neonatal intensive care unit.

All infants younger than 2 months with fever are considered to have sepsis or meningitis until proven otherwise.

What does the pattern of fever tell me?

Key Questions

- How long have you had the fever?
- What has been the highest temperature reading? When did this occur?

Duration of Fever

In adults, fevers from an acute process usually resolve in 1 to 2 weeks. Fevers that last 3 weeks or longer, that exceed temperatures of 38.4° C (101.1° F), and that remain undiagnosed after 1 week of intensive diagnostic study are classified as FUOs.

Fevers in children can be grouped into three categories: short-term fever, fever without localizing signs, and fever of unknown origin. Short-term fever is defined as a fever of short duration, readily diagnosed, that resolves within 1 week. Fever without localizing signs is a fever with no localizing sign and of brief duration (usually <10 days) that is not explained by findings on history or physical examination. FUO is a fever usually greater than 38.5° C (101.2° F) that lasts longer than 2 weeks on more than four occasions.

Height of Fever

Dehydration and febrile seizures are related to the height of the fever. Generally, body temperatures greater than 41.1° C (106° F) are seen in heat illness, central nervous system disease, or either of these in combination with infection. The higher the fever, the greater is the likelihood of bacteremia.

Is the fever caused by a localized infection?

Key Questions

- Do you have frequency, burning, or urgency with urination?
- Are you having unusual vaginal/penile discharge?
- Do you have face or sinus pain?
- Do you have nasal discharge? If so, what color is the discharge?
- Do you have a cough? Is it productive? What color is the sputum?
- Do you have ear pain?
- Is your throat sore?
- Do you have any sores (aphthous ulcers) in your mouth?

- Are you having any nausea/vomiting or diarrhea?
- Do any of your joints hurt?

Location of Symptoms

Localizing symptoms will point to the site of the infection. These diagnostic clues include headache or sinus pain, purulent nasal discharge, ear pain, toothache, sore throat, breast tenderness, chest pain, cough, dyspnea, abdominal pain, flank pain, dysuria, vaginal discharge, pelvic pain, rectal pain, testicle pain, calf pain, neck stiffness, joint stiffness, pain or heat, or focal neurological deficits (see appropriate chapters).

Genitourinary Tract

Upper urinary tract infection (UTI) in adults commonly produces systemic symptoms with flank pain and fever (see Chapters 17, 31, and 32). Fever with cystitis is uncommon in adults, but children with UTIs present with systemic rather than localized signs and symptoms. UTI is the most common infection in girls younger than 2 years who present with a high fever and in all infants younger than 90 days with fever. Pelvic inflammatory disease in women may cause fever as well as an increased amount of vaginal discharge and bleeding after intercourse. Men who have an acute UTI often present with chills, high fever, urinary frequency and urgency, perineal pain, and low back pain. They may also have penile discharge.

Ear, Nose, and Throat Symptoms

Viral infections of the upper respiratory tract are common and usually produce fever (see Chapters 14, 22, and 29). Otitis media is common in children. Fever may accompany both viral and bacterial pharyngitis. Pharyngitis is frequently manifested only by fever, with the infection localizing 1 or 2 days later. Acute sinusitis can produce a fever. Aphthous ulcers with pharyngitis and cervical lymphadenopathy are seen in children with periodic fevers.

Respiratory or Gastrointestinal Symptoms

Most febrile illnesses are caused by viral upper respiratory infection (URI), lower respiratory infection (LRI) (see Chapters 10 and 13), or gastrointestinal (GI) tract infection (see Chapter 2). Localized symptoms can help pinpoint the cause of the fever. Vomiting occasionally signals pneumonia.

Joint Pain

Joint pain may indicate connective tissue disorders in adults and in children more than 6 years of age (see Chapter 20). Osteomyelitis or septic arthritis may also produce fever.

Can I narrow the diagnostic possibilities or eliminate a cause?

Key Questions

- Have you noticed a rash?
- Do you ache all over?

Skin Rash

The prodromal period of a rash is an important historical clue to diagnosis (see Chapter 25). Fever and rash usually appear together 1-5 days after infection. Common eruption periods are as follows:

- Varicella, rubella, erythema infectiosum—1 day
- Scarlet fever—2 days
- Rocky Mountain spotted fever—3 days
- Measles—4 days
- Roseola infantum—5 days

Ache

Fevers localized to a site without general body manifestations are often bacterial in nature. Fevers accompanied by muscle aches (myalgias), malaise, and/or respiratory symptoms are often viral in nature.

Does the patient have an increased risk for complications?

Key Questions

- Do you have any chronic health problems?
- Have you had recent surgery?
- Have you been diagnosed with an infectious disease recently?
- Are you sexually active? If so, how many partners do you have?
- Are your immunizations up to date?
- Does anyone in the family have tuberculosis (TB) or hepatitis?

Chronic Disease

Chronic conditions and systemic disorders (such as diabetes mellitus, human immunodeficiency virus [HIV], malignancies, neutropenia, and sickle cell anemia) compromise host resistance and increase susceptibility to infection. Prosthetic devices, such as heart valves or joint prostheses, also increase susceptibility to infection.

Health Problems, Surgery, and Recent Infection

Current health problems, recurrent infection, or incomplete treatment of infection may be the cause of fever. Such risk factors as diabetes mellitus, neutropenia, and sickle cell anemia heighten the likelihood of bacterial infection. Patients with a past history of infection (such as URI or streptococcal pharyngitis) may be prone to relapse or recurrence. Recent surgical procedures can provide a locus for occult infection; however, a surgical procedure can also induce an inflammatory response, which causes a fever without infection.

Sexual Activity

High-risk sexual activity may raise the index of suspicion for HIV infection and additionally for pelvic inflammatory disease (PID) in women.

Immunizations

Children and adults who have not been properly immunized are at greater risk for infectious diseases.

Tuberculosis or Hepatitis Exposure

Exposure to populations with a high incidence of TB or viral hepatitis increases the risk of infection. Inquire further about constitutional symptoms, such as cough or night sweats (TB) or malaise and abdominal discomfort (hepatitis).

Does the parent report a behavior change in the child?

Key Questions

■ Is the child sleepier than normal?
■ Is the child more irritable?
■ How is the child's behavior?

In infants and children, behavior changes may be the only indication that the child is ill. Mildly ill infants may act alert, be active, smile, and feed well. Moderately ill infants may be fussy or irritable but continue to feed, be consolable, and may smile. Severely ill infants appear listless, cannot be consoled, and feed poorly or not at all.

Could the fever be caused by something acquired while traveling?

Key Questions

■ Have you been out of the country recently?
■ Have you spent time in the woods or been camping recently?

Travel

Patients can be exposed to an emerging infectious disease based on their travel activities. A history of travel out of the country presents the possibility of infection with amebiasis, malaria, schistosomiasis, typhoid fever, or hepatitis A and B. Dengue is the most common vector-borne disease worldwide and is a differential diagnosis for acute febrile illnesses in patients who live or have recently traveled to the tropics or subtropical areas of the United States. Epidemiological surveillance data continually provide updates on patterns of occurrence of infections such as severe acute respiratory syndrome (SARS), avian influenza or "bird flu," and West Nile virus (see Box 16-1).

Camping

Camping or exposure to wooded areas may indicate exposure to ticks, Q fever, tularemia, Rocky Mountain spotted fever, *Giardia*, or Lyme disease.

Could the fever be medication-related or caused by poisoning?

Key Questions

■ What medications have you taken recently?
■ Can you tell me what foods you have eaten in the past 3 days?
■ Could the child have eaten a poisonous plant?

Medications

Medications may hide an occult infection. Many drugs (e.g., penicillin, atropine, sulfonamides, streptomycin, and diphenylhydantoin) can induce fever in predisposed individuals. The fever starts about 7 days after the drug is taken for the first time or soon after the first dose in a patient previously sensitized. Any patient who is taking immunosuppressive agents is at a higher risk for infection. Some medications interfere with thirst recognition (e.g., sedatives, haloperidol) or sweating (e.g., anticholinergics, phenothiazines).

Emerging Infectious Diseases Associated with Fever

Avian Influenza ("Bird Flu")

A highly pathogenic strain of avian influenza A virus, H5N1, infects birds and mutates rapidly to acquire genes from viruses infecting other animal species. "Bird flu" is transmitted to humans usually through the slaughtering and processing of infected birds. Symptoms of infection can range from flulike symptoms (e.g., fever, cough, sore throat, muscle aches) to pneumonia and severe respiratory distress. Outbreaks that began in Asia in 2003 have spread to parts of Europe. Suspect infection in persons showing flulike symptoms, such as high fever and cough, who have confirmed contact with birds in an area where confirmed outbreaks have occurred. Clinical deterioration is rapid over 4 to 13 days. Laboratory findings include leukopenia, thrombocytopenia, and elevated levels of aminotransferases. Although avian influenza is a rare disease, more than half of reported cases have been fatal and there is great potential for this virus to evolve into a world pandemic.

SARS (Severe Acute Respiratory Syndrome)

SARS is a febrile severe lower respiratory tract illness that is caused by infection with SARS-associated coronavirus (SARS-CoV). From 2002 through 2003, the World Health Organization received reports of more than 8000 cases and nearly 800 deaths. No specific laboratory test distinguishes SARS-CoV from other febrile respiratory illness. Lymphopenia and elevated levels of hepatic transaminases, creatinine, and C-reactive protein have been seen in some patients. Diagnosis is based on clinical features (e.g., fever, difficulty breathing, pneumonia) and epidemiologic history of exposure either to a SARS patient or to a setting in which the SARS-CoV transmission is occurring.

West Nile Virus (WNV)

WNV is a potentially serious illness most often caused by the bite of an infected mosquito. It occurs most often in summer and fall in North America. Symptoms develop 3 to 14 days after being bitten. Approximately 80% of people who are infected with WNV will not show symptoms; however, up to 20% have symptoms called West Nile fever, characterized by fever, headache, fatigue, truncal rash, lymphadenopathy, and eye pain lasting from days to several weeks. People more than 50 years of age are more likely to develop serious symptoms. A positive IgM antibody test of serum or cerebral spinal fluid is needed to confirm the disease. The test is positive in most patients within 8 days of onset of symptoms.

NOTE: The most current information on these diseases can be found online at the Centers for Disease Control and Prevention, http://cdc.gov, and The World Health Organization, http://who.int.

Aspirin overdose can also cause fever. Earliest signs are vertigo and tinnitus, but fever can occur shortly thereafter and may be the only symptom that patients recognize.

Food Poisoning

Food poisoning fevers may occur up to 72 hours after ingestion of contaminated food.

Plants

Plants containing alkaloid atropine (deadly nightshade, jessamine, and thornapple) cause dilated pupils, flushed skin, and fever because they interfere with the normal heat loss mechanism.

Could exposure to animals explain the fever?

Key Questions

- Has a cat scratched you recently?
- Have you been around any animals?

Cat-Scratch Disease

Cat-scratch disease, or toxoplasmosis, is a bacterial infection transmitted by cats. The etiological agent is a gram-negative bacillus. Single-node or regional adenopathy is the dominant clinical feature. A low-grade fever is also present.

Animal Exposure

Also possible are brucellosis and leptospirosis from dogs; tularemia from rabbits; ornithosis, histoplasmosis, or psittacosis from birds; and lymphocytic choriomeningitis from hamsters or cats. Exposure to infected animals can produce infection and fever in humans. Occupational exposure to pathogens, such as brucellosis, should be investigated in patients who work with animals or animal products.

Could this be the result of a recent immunization?

Key Question

- What immunizations have you had recently?

Immunization Reactions

Adverse effects of immunization are rare but do occur. History of recent immunization followed by 4 hours of high temperature (39.5° C, 103° F) may indicate such an adverse reaction. Measles/mumps/rubella (MMR) immunization may cause elevation of temperature 10 to 14 days after the inoculation.

Could the fever be caused by heat exposure?

Key Questions

- Were you overdressed? If an infant: Is the infant overbundled?
- Do you have air conditioning or windows that open?
- How warm is (are) the room(s) in which you live/sleep?

Overdressing

Classic heatstroke occurs when the person is unable to dissipate the environmental heat burden. Mothers may inadvertently overdress children or cover them in blankets; the elderly may not be able to get out of bed when hot. Obese persons have extra adipose tissue that insulates the body, preventing loss of heat. Some cultures treat illnesses with bundling, which can cause high fevers.

Air Conditioning and Room Temperature

During heat waves, persons may become overheated in homes without air conditioning or with windows that will not open or are not opened because of safety concerns. The high ambient temperatures in those homes produce elevations in core body temperature that cannot be compensated for, leading to hyperthermia. The elderly and persons with impaired mobility are most at risk.

DIAGNOSTIC REASONING: FOCUSED PHYSICAL EXAMINATION

Most fevers have an obvious cause, so look initially for localizing symptoms or clusters of symptoms that point to the cause. Remember that in both children and adults, bacterial and viral URIs, LRIs, and GI tract infections are the most common causes of fevers. Look for and rule out the common causes before investigating more unlikely causes. Boxes 16-2 and 16-3 list the common causes of fever in children and adults.

Fever in a Child Less Than 2 Months Old

The younger the child, the greater is the cause for concern in the presence of fever. Neonates and young infants are less able to mount a febrile response and therefore are more vulnerable to meningitis and other hematogenous complications. The infrequency of high fever in this age-group relates to innate differences in the ability to mount a febrile response. The data suggest that fever in the first 2 to 3 months of life is rela-

---

| Box 16-2 | **Common Causes of Fever in Children** |

Acute Fever
- Upper respiratory tract disorders
  - Viral respiratory tract diseases
  - Otitis media
  - Sinusitis
- Lower respiratory tract disorders
  - Bronchiolitis
  - Pneumonia
- Gastrointestinal disorders
  - Bacterial gastroenteritis
  - Viral gastroenteritis
- Musculoskeletal infections
  - Septic arthritis
- Osteomyelitis
- Cellulitis
- Urinary tract infections
- Bacteremia
- Meningitis

Fever of Unknown Origin
- Infectious diseases (localized and systemic)
- Collagen/inflammatory diseases
- Neoplastic diseases
- Miscellaneous disorders
  - Drug fever
  - Factitious fever
  - Kawasaki disease
  - Inflammatory bowel disease
  - Immunodeficiency
  - Central nervous system dysfunction

---

tively uncommon but that when it does occur, it is usually significant and often ominous.

Observe the Patient

General appearance is a most important aspect of physical examination. Note how the patient looks—does he or she appear acutely ill, look dehydrated, seem lethargic, respond appropriately?

Responsiveness in children older than 2 months of age has been used by pediatricians to identify febrile children with serious illness. The Yale Observation Scale for severity of illness in children is commonly used to quantify observations (Table 16-1). The scale has six general areas related to the child's appearance and behavior. Two thirds of children with acute illness have scores of less than 10 and, of these, only 3% were found to have serious illness. Scores greater than 10 predicted serious illness, and a score of 16 was associated with serious illness 92% of the time.

Box 16-3	Common Causes of Fever in Adults

Acute Fever
- Upper respiratory tract infections
  - Tonsillitis
  - Sinusitis
  - Pneumonia
- Gastrointestinal disorders
  - Bacterial gastroenteritis
  - Viral gastroenteritis
  - Acute abdomen
- Urinary tract infection
- Pelvic inflammatory disease
- Prostatitis
- Drug reactions
- Alcohol withdrawal

Fever of Unknown Origin
- Infectious disease
- Neoplasm
- Collagen/vascular; other multisystem disease
- Drug fever
- Factitious fever

Take Vital Signs and Note Temperature

The incidence of bacteremia, as well as specific infections, increases with the magnitude of fever. A temperature greater than 40° C (104° F) seems to be the marker for occult bacteria. However, many patients with high fever do not have major diseases. In adults, take an oral temperature; in infants and children, a rectal temperature is more reliable.

Most infectious diseases produce temperatures between 37.2° C and 41° C (99° F and 106° F, respectively). However, some patients with infectious diseases remain afebrile; these include neonates, immunocompromised hosts, patients with chronic renal insufficiency, and the elderly. Extreme pyrexia (i.e., temperatures exceeding 41.5° C) rarely occurs with an infectious disease. Conditions in which extreme pyrexia is seen include drug fevers, central nervous system injury, malignant hyperthermia, stroke, and HIV.

Hypothermia is always an unfavorable prognostic sign in the presence of infectious disease. This condition is seen with overwhelming sepsis (most commonly in the elderly and neonates), uremia, cold exposure, and hypothyroidism.

Observe Skin and Mucous Membranes

A macular/papular rash may indicate a viral exanthema, infectious disease, or a drug sensitivity reaction (see Chapter 25). Vesicular rashes occur with viral infection. A petechial skin rash indicates meningococcemia or Rocky Mountain spotted fever. Petechial eruptions on the hard and soft palate may indicate mononucleosis. Splinter hemorrhages found in

Table 16-1	Yale Observation Scale Predictive Model: Six Observation Items and Their Scales		
OBSERVATION ITEM	**1 NORMAL**	**3 MODERATE IMPAIRMENT**	**5 SEVERE IMPAIRMENT**
Quality of cry	Strong with normal tone *or* content and not crying	Whimpering *or* sobbing	Weak *or* moaning *or* high-pitched
Reaction to parent stimulation	Cries briefly and then stops *or* content and not crying	Cries on and off	Continual cry *or* hardly responds
State variation	If awake, stays awake *or* if asleep and stimulated, wakes up quickly	Eyes close briefly, not awake *or* awakes with prolonged stimulation	Falls to sleep *or* will not rouse
Color	Pink	Pale extremities *or* acrocyanosis	Pale *or* cyanotic *or* mottled *or* ashen
Hydration	Skin normal, eyes normal, *and* mucous membranes moist	Skin and eyes normal *and* mouth slightly dry	Skin doughy or tented *and* dry mucous membranes *and/or* sunken eyes
Response (talk, smile) to social overtures	Smiles *or* alerts (<2 mo)	Brief smile *or* alerts (<2 mo)	No smile, face anxious, dull, expressionless *or* no alerting (<2 mo)

From McCarthy PL, Sharpe MR, Spiesel SZ, Dolan TF, Forsyth BW, DeWitt TG, et al: Observation scales to identify serious illness in febrile children, *Pediatrics* 70:806, 1982.

the nail beds and petechiae of the conjunctivae indicate endocarditis.

The presence of a petechial skin rash indicates a serious infection that requires immediate referral and hospitalization.

Examine the Head and Neck

Percuss the sinuses and transilluminate for evidence of sinusitis (see Chapter 22). Examine and palpate the teeth for abscesses. Palpate the salivary glands for tenderness. Examine the throat and tonsils for signs of infection, specifically enlarged or red tonsils, lymphadenopathy, or tonsillar or pharyngeal exudate. Examine the mouth for aphthous ulcers.

Inspect the ears and tympanic membrane (TM) for effusion, erythema, fluid, or purulent secretion. Inspect the optic fundi for changes associated with infectious endocarditis (i.e., Roth spots—small, pale retinal lesions with areas of hemorrhage with white centers, usually located near the optic disc).

In the infant, feel for a tense or bulging anterior fontanel. This is best noted if the patient is in the sitting position. The normal fontanel may feel questionably tense if the infant is supine. Tenseness may be noted in the crying child but only during expiration; this physiological bulging disappears when the patient relaxes or inspires.

Palpate the Lymph Nodes

Palpate all lymph nodes for enlargement and tenderness.
- Anterior cervical—Suspect viral or bacterial pharyngitis.
- Preauricular or postauricular—Suspect ear infection.
- Posterior cervical—Suspect mononucleosis.
- Supraclavicular—Suspect neoplasms.
- Axillary—Suspect breast inflammation, local infection, or neoplasm.
- Localized lymphadenopathy—Suspect local infectious process.
- Generalized lymphadenopathy—Suspect immunosuppression, such as being HIV positive, or neoplasm.

Examine the Lungs and Chest

Percuss and auscultate the lungs (see Chapters 10 and 13). Adventitious sounds, decreased breath sounds, or areas of consolidation may indicate LRI or pneumonia.

Examine the sputum for color, consistency, and presence of blood or odor.
- Yellow/green sputum—Suspect bacterial infection.
- Brown sputum—Check smoking history.
- Blood-streaked sputum—Suspect URI or bronchitis.
- Hemoptysis—Suspect tumor, trauma, or pulmonary embolism.

Palpate Breasts if Indicated

Inspect the breasts for signs of inflammation (see Chapter 5). Palpate for masses, tenderness, and discharge. Palpate axillary lymph nodes for presence of tenderness.

Examine Genitourinary System if Indicated

Palpate for suprapubic tenderness, which may indicate PID or UTI, and for costovertebral angle (CVA) tenderness, which suggests pyelonephritis (see Chapters 24, 32, and 34). Perform a pelvic examination in women without another obvious source of fever. Cervical motion tenderness, discharge, or adnexal tenderness and lower abdominal tenderness may indicate PID. In men, examine for penile discharge, suggesting a sexually transmitted disease, UTI, or prostatitis.

Perform a rectal examination to evaluate for tenderness and discharge, which may indicate rectal abscess or infection, as well as retrocecal appendicitis.

Perform a prostate examination in men without another obvious source of fever because prostatitis may be the cause. If you suspect prostatitis, do not perform a vigorous examination or massage the prostate as this can release bacteria and produce septicemia.

Examine Musculoskeletal System if Indicated

Examination may suggest inflammation or infection of bones or joints if there is swelling, increased warmth, or tenderness (see Chapters 20 and 21). Infants may present with poor feeding, irritability, fever, or vomiting. Examination should reveal decreased mobility of the affected bone or joint area, increased heat, tenderness, and swelling.

Examine the lower extremities for asymmetrical swelling, calf tenderness, or palpable vessels as an indicator of deep vein phlebitis.

Osteomyelitis may occur in young children, most commonly between 3 and 10 years of age. Septic arthritis can occur in children under the age of 3 and in young women who are sexually active.

Perform Neurological/Mental Status Examination

Evaluate for signs of meningeal irritation (see Chapters 12 and 18). Inflammation of the meninges from infection or blood evokes reflex spasm in the paravertebral muscles. In the cervical area, this manifests as neck stiffness. Normally the chin can be flexed passively to touch the chest. If neck stiffness is present, this maneuver is not possible. With the patient supine, attempts to flex the neck cause the knees and hips to rise from the bed (Brudzinski sign) to reduce the pull on the meninges. In the lumbar region, meningeal irritation also causes spasm and can be demonstrated by passive movement of the lower limbs. Attempts to extend the knee joint when the hip joint is flexed are resisted, and the other limb may flex at the hip (Kernig sign). Neck stiffness (nuchal rigidity) or resistance to neck flexion or rotation is a late sign and not a true sign of meningitis in infants less than 3 months old, the very old, or the severely obtunded patient. Vomiting, headache, and photophobia may also be present.

Note the presence of focal deficits, which suggests vascular occlusion or abscess formation. Assess for disturbances in mentation, irritability, lethargy, somnolence, or coma, which indicates increased intracranial pressure. Seizures occur in 20% to 30% of children with meningitis.

A seizure in a febrile infant less than 6 months old suggests meningitis rather than a simple febrile seizure. Benign febrile seizure is uncommon in very young infants.

LABORATORY AND DIAGNOSTIC STUDIES

Laboratory studies can be used selectively to confirm or negate the clinical diagnosis, especially if the history and physical examination findings provide strong indication of a particular infectious process. In patients with obvious viral URI, no studies are necessary. Patients with a sore throat may require a throat culture, Monospot, or rapid strep test, depending on the clinical findings. In patients with urinary symptoms, a urinalysis and culture may be sufficient unless clinical findings indicate an upper UTI, which would warrant further diagnostic testing such as radiography, ultrasonography, or intravenous pyelography.

Also see appropriate chapters for specific presenting problems and discussion of diagnostic tests.

Complete Blood Count

Leukocytosis with a left shift suggests a bacterial infection. Atypical lymphocytes are characteristic of systemic viral infection. Immature neutrophils suggest leukemia.

Anemia may be seen in inflammatory conditions, such as juvenile arthritis, malaria, and parvovirus B19 infections. Low platelet counts may be associated with Epstein-Barr virus infection, histoplasmosis, tuberculosis (TB), and spirochetal infections or may be drug induced. Thrombocytosis is common in Kawasaki disease (an acute febrile illness in children that resembles scarlet fever) and some viral infections.

Erythrocyte Sedimentation Rate

An elevated erythrocyte sedimentation rate (ESR) indicates an inflammatory condition. However, the test is nonspecific and does not indicate the source or cause of inflammation.

Antistreptolysin Titer

An increase in the antistreptolysin (ASO) titer is detectable by comparing two blood samples more than 2 weeks apart (see Chapter 29). An elevated titer indicates immunological response of the host after exposure to streptococcal antigen.

HIV Testing

There are two tests used to diagnose HIV infection. The enzyme-linked immunosorbent assay (ELISA) detects the presence of HIV-specific antibodies that the body produces in response to the virus. A positive test may be confirmed by a second test, the Western blot. Newer, more rapid tests are being developed.

Urinalysis

Use a dipstick urinalysis (U/A) to screen for upper or lower UTI, which would reveal the presence of nitrites and leukocyte esterase (see Chapter 32). Microscopic evaluation discloses the presence of cells (white and red blood cells) and blood casts.

Urine Culture and Sensitivity

Performed on a clean catch of urine, this test will confirm a diagnosis of UTI and isolate the organism(s) (see Chapter 32).

Stool for Leukocytes

The presence of white blood cells (WBCs) may suggest invasive bacterial gastroenteritis (see Chapter 11).

Stool Culture and Sensitivity

Use stool culture and sensitivity to detect the presence of *Salmonella* or *Shigella* (see Chapter 11).

Stool Sample for Ova and Parasites

Have the patient collect three stool samples over a 5-day period (see Chapter 11). The first morning stool is preferred and must be delivered to the laboratory in 30 minutes or less after defecation.

Sputum for Acid-Fast Bacilli

A sputum sample to test for acid-fast bacilli (AFB) is used to diagnose respiratory TB (see Chapter 10). A smear is prepared from a series of three first-morning specimens collected on three separate days to catch the sporadic discharge of the bacilli from the tubercle.

Sputum for Gram Staining

A smear is prepared from a sputum sample and stained with Gram stain. Gram-positive organisms stain purple; gram-negative organisms stain red.

- Gram-positive cocci or diplococci indicate pneumococcal, staphylococcal, or streptococcal infections.
- Gram-negative cocci indicate meningococcal or gonococcal infections.
- Enteric gram-negative bacilli indicate *Escherichia coli*, *Proteus*, *Bacteroides*, *Klebsiella*, typhoid, *Salmonella*, or *Shigella*.
- Other gram-negative bacilli indicate *Haemophilus*, pertussis, chancroid, brucellosis, tularemia, or plague.

Sputum for Culture and Sensitivity

Use a sputum culture to isolate a specific organism (see Chapter 10). Have the patient rinse the mouth well with water without swallowing before coughing to produce a specimen; this decreases the amount of saliva present. Do not use mouthwash because this can kill the bacteria. An early morning sample is best. The sample must contain mucoid or mucopurulent material.

Cultures of Discharge

Cultures can be prepared from any source with a discharge (e.g., vaginal, urethral, wound). Place the culture in the transport medium indicated. Culture is used to isolate causative organisms.

Collect a specimen of vaginal or penile discharge on a sterile swab and place in the medium provided. For penile discharge, use a sterile urethral swab to collect a specimen from the anterior urethra by gentle insertion and scraping of the mucosa. For wound culture, use a sterile swab or aspirate with a sterile needle and syringe from the moist area. Bacteria from the center of a wound may be nonviable; culture near the periphery.

Molecular Testing for Infectious Organisms

Molecular testing using a sample taken from the vagina provides rapid, sensitive, and specific results. A number of products are available. Follow manufacturer directions to collect and transport the sample. Polymerase chain reaction (PCR) is a very specific test for detecting the presence of *Borrelia* DNA in Lyme disease and dengue fever. A positive PCR suggests presence of the specific organism.

DNA probes and nucleic acid amplification tests (NAATs) are available to test for *Chlamydia trachomatis* and *Neisseria gonorrhoeae*. Single or dual organism tests are available.

Blood Cultures

Two culture specimens are obtained at two different venipuncture sites. If one culture produces bacteria and the other does not, the positive culture is likely from a contaminant and not the infecting agent. Culture specimens drawn through an intravenous catheter are frequently contaminated. All cultures should be drawn before initiation of antibiotics if possible. Most organisms require approximately 24 hours for growth in the laboratory, and a preliminary report can be given at that time. Often 48 to 72 hours are required for growth and identification of organisms. Blood cultures may be positive in bacteremia.

Lumbar Puncture

A lumbar puncture is indicated if you suspect meningitis (see Chapter 18). Laboratory data on cerebrospinal fluid (CSF) always include leukocytes, protein, glucose,

Gram stain, cell count, and culture and sensitivity. In meningitis, expect cloudy CSF fluid with many polymorphonuclear cells containing bacteria. Glucose level in CSF is decreased compared with blood glucose level, protein is increased, and the culture will be positive.

Radiographic Imaging

Chest radiographs may detect infiltrates, effusions, masses, or nodes. Kidney, ureter, and bladder (KUB) and upright abdominal films can reveal air-fluid levels in the bowel. Computed tomography (CT) scan may be used to detect abscess or tumor. Radiographs are useful for detecting bone and joint involvement in osteomyelitis. Radionuclide scanning is also beneficial in detecting osteomyelitis.

DIFFERENTIAL DIAGNOSIS
Upper Respiratory Infection

Viral infections can occur in any age-group and are more prevalent during winter months (see Chapter 10). The temperature is usually less than 38.7° C (101.5° F). Systemic symptoms are common. Known contact with others who have had similar symptoms or illness is typical but not necessary. The patient usually has a cough; any sputum is nonpurulent. Pharyngitis may be present with erythema of the oral pharynx.

Gastroenteritis

Nausea, vomiting, and diarrhea are the hallmarks of a GI infection (see Chapter 11). Fever is usually mild. Abdominal cramping may be present.

Urinary Tract Infection

UTIs are more common in females (see Chapter 32). Localized urinary tract symptoms are common in adults; systemic symptoms are more common in children. CVA tenderness indicates upper UTI. The temperature associated with an upper UTI is likely to be a high fever, and the patient feels systemically ill. Urinalysis can support a clinical diagnosis of UTI. Urine for culture and sensitivity usually confirms the diagnosis.

Pelvic Inflammatory Disease

Suspect PID in women with a fever for which there is no other explanation (see Chapter 34). There may be vague reports of lower abdominal pain; suprapubic tenderness may be present on abdominal examination. Pelvic examination reveals cervical motion tenderness, discharge, and/or adnexal tenderness.

Prostatitis

In men without another obvious source of fever, suspect prostatitis (see Chapter 24). The prostate will be exquisitely tender to gentle palpation. Other system examinations will be normal.

Pharyngitis

The patient reports a sore throat. In children, fever may precede throat complaints by 1 or 2 days. The pharynx is red, and the tonsils may be enlarged or have exudate. For differential diagnosis of bacterial and viral pharyngitis, see Chapter 29. Mononucleosis occurs most often in young adults and may present with palatine petechiae, tonsillar exudate, and posterior cervical lymphadenopathy.

Sinusitis

Sinuses that are tender to percussion or do not transilluminate may indicate sinusitis, especially in the presence of purulent nasal discharge. Patients often report a frontal headache, which worsens as the patient leans forward (see Chapter 22). Patients sometimes experience a sore throat and cough from postnasal discharge, which may be apparent in the posterior pharynx.

Ear Infections

Otitis media is more common in children (see Chapter 14). The tympanic membrane will appear red and may bulge. The light reflex will be absent or diminished. Tympanic membrane mobility will be limited. The child may tug at the ear and act restless or irritable. The young child or infant may feed poorly. The temperature may be a high- or low-grade fever. Respiratory symptoms occur if the patient has a concomitant respiratory tract infection. Ear infections are commonly associated with other upper respiratory tract symptoms.

Meningitis

The signs and symptoms of meningitis are related to nonspecific findings associated with bacteremia or a systemic infection or to specific manifestation of meningeal irritation with central nervous system inflammation (see Chapter 18). Inspect the skin for petechiae, cyanosis, and state of hydration and peripheral perfusion. Nuchal rigidity, back pain, Kernig sign, Brudzinski sign, nausea, vomiting, and bulging fontanel (in infants) may be seen. Papilledema is rarely seen. If it is present, look for other processes, such as brain abscess or subdural empyema. Ataxia may be a presenting sign. Lumbar puncture confirms the diagnosis.

Osteomyelitis

Bone infection is usually caused by bacteria and may arise from a clinically evident infection or from general bacteremia (see Chapter 20). Patients report pain in the affected bone or joint and may exhibit soft tissue tenderness and swelling. Children demonstrate localized tenderness near the epiphysis. Diagnosis requires isolation of the responsible organism via blood cultures, pus from tissue abscesses, synovial fluid aspirate, or material from needle aspiration or bone biopsy. Radionuclide scanning, CT, or magnetic resonance imaging (MRI) may be helpful in determining the extent of infection and destruction.

Kawasaki Disease

Kawasaki disease is an acute mucocutaneous lymph node syndrome that is classified as a vasculitic syndrome (of which fever is only one sign) affecting infants and young children under age 9 (see Chapter 25). It is more common in males and often occurs in fall and spring. The etiology is unknown. Fevers are of a high-spiking remittent pattern in the range of 38° C to 40° C (100.4° F to 104° F, respectively, with some to 107° F) and persist despite the use of empiric antibiotics and antipyretics. Seizures may be present, and other neurological causes must be ruled out. The febrile phase lasts from 5 to 25 days with a mean of 10 days. Because of the rash associated with the fever, Kawasaki disease resembles scarlet fever.

To make the initial diagnosis of Kawasaki disease, fever lasting at least 5 days with at least four of the following signs, in the absence of a known diagnosis or infection, must be present:

- Bilateral conjunctival hyperemia
- Mouth lesions—dry fissured lips and injected pharynx or strawberry tongue
- Change in peripheral extremities, edema, erythema, desquamation of skin at 10 to 14 days
- Nonvesicular erythematous rash
- Cervical lymphadenopathy

Factitious Fever

Suspect factitious fever when there is a discrepancy between oral or rectal temperature and urine temperature. The pulse rate will be inconsistent with elevated temperature. The patient has no weight loss. Repeated monitored temperature-taking does not support previous readings.

Roseola Infantum

Roseola infantum is the most common exanthema of children younger than 3 years of age. Symptoms include an irritable child who has high fever, with rapid defervescence when the rash appears on day 3 or 4. The rash is maculopapular and lasts 1 to 2 days.

Fevers Without Localizing Signs

Often examination fails to disclose any specific signs or symptoms other than the fever itself. Most children who have a fever without localizing signs have neither an unusual nor a serious disease. In many cases, the fever will clear within a few days without a specific diagnosis. However, the longer the child has a fever without localizing signs, the less likely the fever is the result of infectious disease. Viral illness or malignancy must be considered.

Always investigate in the history and physical examination any abnormal growth suggesting any possibility of preexisting chronic disease. Morning stiffness suggests rheumatoid arthritis, weight loss or abdominal pain suggests inflammatory bowel disease, and frequent respiratory tract infection suggests cystic fibrosis or immunodeficiency.

Enterovirus

All enteroviruses may cause a mild, nonspecific, febrile illness that lasts 2 to 5 days. Most are seasonal, occurring in late summer and early fall. Herpangina, nonexudative pharyngitis with or without lymphadenopathy, generally occurs.

Occult Bacteremia

Occult bacteremia is diagnosed in children older than 3 months who have positive blood cultures but do not have the usual clinical manifestation of sepsis or septic shock. Occult means hidden from view; the child looks well. The majority of children who look well and are playful are at low risk for bacteremia despite fever. Those who look ill or toxic are at significant risk. The primary concern is the small but important percentage of those children who develop secondary complications from invasive bacterial disease (i.e., meningitis, bacterial sepsis, septic arthritis, or pneumonia). Peak ages for bacteremia are between 6 and 24 months, with

Streptococcus pneumoniae being the organism most commonly responsible.

Periodic Fever in Children

This condition is characterized by an abrupt fever that occurs in children 2 to 5 years of age on a regularly recurring basis, generally every 6 weeks. The fever lasts an average of 4 days. Besides the fever, the child has malaise, sore throat, cervical adenopathy, and aphthous stomatitis. The white blood cell count may be elevated (13,000/mm^3), as is the sedimentation rate. There are no associated diseases or other physical examination and laboratory findings. The child has normal growth and development.

DIFFERENTIAL DIAGNOSIS OF *Common Causes of Fever*

CONDITION	HISTORY	PHYSICAL FINDINGS	DIAGNOSTIC STUDIES
URI	Any age-group; systemic symptoms; often known contact with ill others	Fever <38.7° C (101.5° F); cough; nonpurulent sputum; erythema of pharynx; viral exanthema	None
Gastroenteritis	Nausea, vomiting, diarrhea; abdominal cramping	Mild fever; abdomen may be diffusely tender	None
UTI	Females more than males; burning urgency; frequency in adults; systemic symptoms/ bedwetting in children	CVA tenderness with upper UTI; fever with upper UTI	U/A; urine C & S; CBC if suspect upper UTI
PID	May have pelvic or lower abdominal pain	May have suprapubic tenderness; cervical discharge; CMT, adnexal tenderness	CBC; molecular testing
Pharyngitis	Sore throat; may or may not have other upper respiratory tract symptoms	Erythematous pharynx; may have pharyngeal or tonsillar exudates or ulcers; may have palatine petechiae in mononucleosis; lymphadenopathy	CBC; culture; rapid strep test if suspect strep; Monospot if suspect mononucleosis
Prostatitis	Perineal discomfort, frequent urination, chills and malaise	Prostate tender to palpation; fever	Segmental urine specimen; C & S of urine; C & S of prostate discharge
Sinusitis	Facial or sinus pressure or pain; headache	Purulent nasal discharge; sinuses tender to percussion; headache or pressure worsens on bending forward	Radiographs or CT scan of limited value
Ear infections	Earache, pain; may have upper respiratory tract symptoms; child tugs at ear	High- or low-grade fever; TM red, may bulge, landmarks absent; TM mobility impaired; child irritable/ restless	Pneumatic otoscopy
Meningitis	Nonspecific symptoms; nausea, vomiting, irritability	Petechiae, nuchal rigidity, positive Kernig's and Brudzinski's signs, petechiae; bulging fontanel in infant	Lumbar puncture
Osteomyelitis	Pain in affected bone or joint	Swelling or tenderness over affected area of joint	Culture; CBC; radionuclide scan, CT, MRI
Kawasaki disease	Under 5 yr of age; males more than females; fall and spring	High fever, spikes; persists despite antibiotic therapy; may have seizures; fever for 5 days with at least 4 of the following: bilateral conjunctival hyperemia, mouth lesions, edema, erythema, desquamation of skin, nonvesicular erythematous rash, cervical lymphadenopathy	WBC increased, shift to left; slight anemia; thrombocytosis; positive C-reactive protein; ESR increased; serum IgM, IgE increased

DIFFERENTIAL DIAGNOSIS OF *Common Causes of Fever—cont'd*

CONDITION	HISTORY	PHYSICAL FINDINGS	DIAGNOSTIC STUDIES
Factitious fever	Vague or no symptoms	Normal physical examination; no weight loss; pulse rate normal (not consistent with temperature elevation)	Discrepancy between oral/rectal temperature and urine temperature; repeated monitored temperature-taking does not support previous readings
Roseola infantum	Irritable child with fever for 4-5 days	Normal physical examination; when fever breaks, rash appears	None
Fevers without localizing signs	No other specific symptoms	Physical examination usually normal initially; repeat examination in 24 hr and as needed	U/A; urine C & S; chest x-ray; WBC; rule out systemic disease, malignancy
Enterovirus	Mild, nonspecific febrile illness lasting 2-5 days; summer and early fall peaks	Nonexudative pharyngitis with or without lymphadenopathy frequently observed	None
Occult bacteremia	Fever in children older than 3 mo	No localizing signs; child appears well	Blood culture; WBC
Periodic fever in children	Abrupt fever on periodic basis (about every 6 wk); lasts about 4 days; child aged 2-5 yr; malaise	Cervical adenopathy, aphthous stomatitis	WBC and ESR elevated

CBC, complete blood count; *CVA,* costovertebral angle; *C & S,* culture and sensitivity; *CT,* computed tomography; *ESR,* erythrocyte sedimentation rate; *MRI,* magnetic resonance imaging; *PID,* pelvic inflammatory disease; *TM,* tympanic membrane; *U/A,* urinalysis; *URI,* upper respiratory infection; *UTI,* urinary tract infection; *WBC,* white blood cell.

REFERENCES AND READINGS

Baraff LJ: Management of fever without source in infants and children, *Ann Emerg Med* 36:602, 2000.

Bentley DW, Bradley S, High K, Schoenbaum S, Taler G, Yoshikawa TT: Practice guideline for evaluation of fever and infection in long-term care facilities, *J Am Geriatr Soc* 49:210, 2001.

Centers for Disease Control and Prevention: Locally acquired dengue—Key West Florida, 2009-2010, *MMWR* 59:577, 2010.

Claudius I, Baraff L: Pediatric emergencies associated with fever, *Emerg Med Clin North Am* 28:67, 2010.

High KP, Bradley SF, Gravenstein DR, Quagliarello VJ, Richards C, Yoshikawa TT: Clinical practice guideline for the evaluation of fever and infection in older adult residents of long-term care facilities: 2008 update by the Infectious Diseases Society of America, *J Am Geriatr Soc* 57:375, 2009.

Long S: Distinguishing among prolonged, recurrent, and periodic fever syndromes: approach of a pediatric infectious diseases subspecialist, *Pediatr Clin North Am* 52:811, 2005.

McPhee SJ, Papdakis MA: *Current medical diagnosis and treatment,* ed 49, New York, McGraw Hill, 2010.

Norman DC: Fever in the elderly, *Clin Infect Dis* 31:148, 2000.

Genitourinary Problems in Males

Urinary tract problems in males represent a range of conditions from infections, inflammation, and urine outlet obstruction to congenital malformation, trauma, or neoplasm. Any part of the renal/urological/reproductive tract can be involved, and symptoms may often be localized to a single site. Symptoms may also be vague, reflect the involved area, or be referred from the actual site of involvement.

Dysuria in males is most commonly caused by urethritis, prostatitis, cystitis, or mechanical irritation of the urethra. Inflammation, although infrequent in young males, increases with age until elderly men are affected as frequently as elderly women.

Cystitis in men results from ascending infection of the urethra or prostate, or occurs secondary to urethral instrumentation. The most common cause of recurrent cystitis in men is chronic bacterial prostatitis. *Escherichia coli* is the usual gram-negative pathogen. *Chlamydia trachomatis* is the major cause of prostatitis and nongonococcal urethritis in men under age 40 and is sexually transmitted. Recurrent urinary tract infections (UTIs) may involve resistant gram-negative *Klebsiella*, *Enterobacter*, *Pseudomonas*, or *Proteus mirabilis*, or gram-positive *Enterococcus* and *Staphylococcus aureus*. Infection may involve the kidneys and cause pyelonephritis. Secondary infection can occur as the result of urinary stones.

The male patient with urinary problems may also present with symptoms involving urinary flow. Urine flow may be altered by compression of the urethra as it passes through an enlarged prostate, obstructing the flow of urine and producing hesitancy, slowing of the urinary stream, dribbling, and nocturia. Benign prostatic hyperplasia (BPH) is common in men older than 50 and progresses with age until 80% of men over 80 are affected. Patients with BPH are more prone to UTIs and incontinence. Urinary stones can occur anywhere in the urinary tract and are common causes of obstructive symptoms, bleeding, and pain.

Trauma to the urinary tract may be caused by penetrating, straddle, blunt, or crushing injuries or by surgery or instrumentation. Hematuria, oliguria, and pain are the most common symptoms.

Neoplasms occur more often in males than in females. Kidney, prostate, and bladder neoplasms are more common in elderly men. Kidney and bladder neoplasms often produce painless hematuria. Prostate cancer may produce symptoms of outlet obstruction.

Kidney problems can range from asymptomatic blood chemical changes to life-threatening abnormal renal function that could manifest in fluid-electrolyte and acid-base imbalances. Patients with renal insufficiency may present with nonspecific complaints such as fatigue, anorexia, or weakness. A discussion of renal insufficiency and renal failure is beyond the scope of this chapter.

DIAGNOSTIC REASONING: FOCUSED HISTORY

Are systemic or acute symptoms present?

Key Questions

- Have you had fever, chills, nausea, or vomiting?
- Are you positive for HIV infection or receiving chemotherapy?
- Are you having acute pain?
- Have you been able to pass any urine?

Fever and Chills

The presence of fever and/or chills suggests a systemic inflammatory response and indicates that the patient may be acutely ill and should be aggressively treated. Specifically, suspect pyelonephritis or lithiasis of the upper urinary tract or prostatitis, orchitis, or epididymitis of the lower urinary tract.

Immunocompromised Patients

Immunocompromised patients are susceptible to overwhelming infections by both common and atypical organisms, and aggressive investigation is warranted.

Acute Pain

Acute pain in the abdomen or flank is characteristic of bladder, ureter, and kidney involvement. Acute pain in the scrotum or testicles may indicate infection or pathology of the scrotal contents or it may be referred pain from other sites in the urinary tract. Pain in the scrotum or testicles is characteristic of inflammation of the testicles, epididymitis, or torsion of a testicle (see Chapter 24).

Anuria

A sudden decrease in urinary output may result from compromised renal blood supply (prerenal); damaged interstitia, glomeruli, or tubules (intrarenal); or obstructed urine flow (postrenal). Patients with prerenal failure usually have a history of volume depletion or a reduction in arterial blood volume, such as in low cardiac output states. Patients with intrarenal failure may present with history of renal damage from nephrotoxic agents. Postrenal failure is the least likely cause of anuria, but it should be ruled out first, because when failure results from obstructive causes, mechanical intervention may reestablish kidney function before permanent nephron damage occurs. Patients at greatest risk for acute renal failure are the elderly, diabetic patients, and those with a history of renal, heart, or liver disease.

Anuria may represent obstruction or renal failure.

Is there hematuria?

Key Questions

- Have you noticed blood in your urine?
- Is there blood every time you urinate or just occasionally?
- Does the blood start with the beginning of urination, continue throughout urination, or occur only at the end of urination? Is there blood without urinating?
- Do you have pain with the blood?

Hematuria

Blood can enter the urinary tract at any site. The most common source of isolated hematuria is extrarenal. A lesion of the bladder or lower urinary tract is demonstrated in more than 60% of patients. The most common causes of gross hematuria from the kidney are nephropathy and polycystic kidney disease. No cause for hematuria can be found in 10% to 15% of patients.

Timing

Initial hematuria becomes clear during voiding and is indicative of anterior urethral lesions, such as urethritis, stricture, or meatal stenosis. Terminal hematuria begins with clear urine and then becomes bloody and is suggestive of prostatic lesions or lesions in the prostatic urethra. Total hematuria is usually characteristic of lesions in the kidneys and ureters. Bladder lesions may produce bleeding independent of micturition. Recent trauma to the kidneys can also produce hematuria. Gross hematuria is often transient but may continue microscopically.

Pain

Hematuria with pain usually indicates the passage of a stone or sloughed renal papilla, often with concurrent infection. Painless gross hematuria is consistent with upper or lower tract tumor, systemic coagulopathy, or excessive anticoagulant effect. Less common causes include acute necrosis or sloughing of a papilla. In elderly men, painless hematuria may be a late presenting sign of renal cancer.

Can the symptoms be localized within the urinary tract?

Key Questions

- Do you have trouble starting to urinate (e.g., slow/weakened urinary stream, dribbling of urine)?
- Do you have low back, flank, or abdominal pain?
- Do you have aching in the perineal area?
- Do you have suprapubic discomfort?
- Have you had urinary incontinence?
- Do you have frequency, urgency, dysuria, or penile discharge?
- Do you urinate at night?
- Do you have an excessive volume of urine?

Hesitancy, Slow Urinary Stream, and Dribbling of Urine

In men older than 50, the presence of hesitancy, slow urinary stream, and dribbling of urine with a gradual onset over time indicates obstructive problems from benign prostatic hypertrophy. Have the patient complete the American Urological Association (AUA) Symptom Index (Table 17-1). Using the index, classify symptoms as mild (0 to 7), moderate (8 to 19), or severe (20 to 35).

Table 17-1 The American Urological Association Symptom Index

Patients rate their answers to each question on a scale of 0 to 5.

QUESTIONS	AUA SYMPTOM SCORE (CIRCLE ONE NUMBER ON EACH LINE)†					
	NOT AT ALL	LESS THAN 1 TIME IN 5	LESS THAN HALF THE TIME	ABOUT HALF THE TIME	MORE THAN HALF THE TIME	ALMOST ALWAYS
Over the past month, how often have you had a sensation of not emptying your bladder completely after you finished voiding?	0	1	2	3	4	5
Over the past month, how often have you had to urinate again less than 2 hours after you finished urinating?	0	1	2	3	4	5
Over the past month, how often have you found you stopped and started again several times when you urinated?	0	1	2	3	4	5
Over the past month, how often have you found it difficult to postpone urination?	0	1	2	3	4	5
Over the past month, how often have you had a weak urinary stream?	0	1	2	3	4	5
Over the past month, how often have you had to push or strain to begin urination?	0	1	2	3	4	5
Over the past month, how many times did you typically get up to urinate from the time you went to bed at night until the time you got up in the morning?	0	1	2	3	4	5

From Barry MJ, Fowler FJ Jr, O'Leary MP, Bruskewitz RC, Holtgrewe HL, Mebust WK, et al: The American Urological Association Symptom Index for benign prostatic hyperplasia. The Measurement Committee of the American Urological Association, *J Urol* 148:1549, 1992.

†AUA Symptom Score = sum of above circled numbers. Symptoms are classified as mild (0-7), moderate (8-19), or severe (20-35).

Low Back, Flank, or Abdominal Pain

Patient reports of low back, flank, or abdominal pain are often indicative of ureteral and kidney involvement. Renal tract pain may present with a constant dull ache in the costovertebral angle (CVA) area. Dislodged kidney stones will produce an acute ureteral pain that is colicky and cyclic in nature. Gross blood in the urine and infection may accompany the ureteral pain. The pain can radiate to the abdomen, testes, and penis. However, renal disorders do not frequently cause pain. True renal pain can originate from the calyces or renal pelvis. Pain can result from stretching of the kidney capsule, interstitial edema, or inflammation of the capsule.

Aching in the Perineal Area

Prostate pain is often interpreted by the patient as a vague ache in the perineal area. The usual cause of perineal aching is infection; another cause may be prostatic stones with infection.

Suprapubic Discomfort and Urinary Incontinence

Discomfort in the suprapubic area is indicative of bladder involvement, whereas urinary incontinence is characteristic of bladder neck irritability caused by inflammation. Bladder pain is most often caused by infection; however, it can also be produced by obstruction and bladder distention as the result of tumor or stones.

Penile Discharge with Frequency, Urgency, and Dysuria

Penile discharge with frequency, urgency, and dysuria is characteristic of anterior urethral irritation in males and of exposure to a sexually transmitted infection (STI) (see Chapter 24).

Nocturia

Primary bladder disease from infection, stones, or tumors can produce nocturia. Prostate enlargement characteristically produces nocturia. Most adults do not need to void during the night, but some may get up once during the night depending on the amount and timing of fluid ingestion.

Patients who report daytime frequency without nocturia are usually free of organic disease.

Polyuria

Polyuria is defined as a volume greater than 3 L of urine/day and depends on fluid intake and the patient's state of hydration. Polyuria may be an early indication of renal disease progression because of the kidneys' inability to concentrate urine. Taking a history of fluid intake is important to identify possible causes of polyuria. Pseudopolyuria results from increased fluid ingestion and may present with certain personality disorders. With the current emphasis on water ingestion, however, a large fluid intake can also produce pseudopolyuria. Alcohol ingestion inhibits antidiuretic hormone; glycosuria promotes excess solute excretion. Diabetes insipidus may also be implicated. Nocturia can occur with the mobilization of fluid during sleep, secondary to congestive heart failure.

Are there any specific risk factors to point me in the right direction?

Key Questions

- Have you had this or similar problems before?
- Do you have a family history of renal or kidney problems, prostatitis, or prostate cancer?
- How old are you? (What is the patient's age?)
- Have you been confined to bed (especially if elderly)?
- Are you sexually active? How many partners do you have?
- Do you ride an upright bicycle?

History of Similar Problems

Patients with previous urinary problems are at risk for chronic relapsing conditions, such as unresolved infections, resistant strains of organisms, or reinfection. Recurrent infections, pyelonephritis, or complications warrant urological referral for workup and evaluation.

Family History of Urinary Problems

A family history of renal or kidney problems or prostatitis places the patient at increased risk for urinary problems. Familial disorders that may be implicated in kidney disease include diabetes mellitus, hypertension, collagen vascular disease, nephrolithiasis, and polycystic kidney disease.

Age

The occurrence of UTIs in males increases with age. Slow development of prostatic obstruction is common in men older than 50 and is usually painless. Patients have difficulty starting the urine stream; the urine stream has decreased force; and urine often continues to dribble after voiding. Chlamydia is the major cause of prostatitis, epididymitis, and nongonococcal urethritis in males under 40 years of age. Adolescents who are sexually active are at particular risk for STIs.

Confinement to Bed

Elderly patients confined to bed are at an increased risk of infection. Likely mechanisms include urinary stasis and reflux.

Sexual Activity

Sexually active males, especially those who engage in unprotected sex, are at risk for STIs, which can produce urethritis. The risk increases with multiple partners.

Bicycle Riding

On an upright bicycle, the design of the seat puts pressure on the ischial tuberosities and perineum of the rider. The hip and pedaling motion of the rider contribute to neural symptoms by stretching the pudendal nerve, especially if the seat is not correctly fitted to the rider. Perineal and penile numbness, without pain, are symptoms frequently reported by long-distance cyclists.

What else could this be?

Key Questions

- Have you had recent instrumentation in the urethra or urinary tract?
- Have you had recent treatment for an STI?
- Have you been recently diagnosed with, but not treated for, an STI?
- What drugs have you taken (prescription, over the counter, or illicit)?
- What is your occupation?
- What are your hobbies (toxic exposure)?

Recent Instrumentation

Recent instrumentation in the urinary tract places the patient at risk for infections. Patients with indwelling catheters are also at risk for infection.

Recent Sexually Transmitted Infection

STIs can produce urethritis and urinary tract symptoms. Recent treatment for an STI may indicate treatment failure, a coinfection that was not covered by the prescribed drug, or a reinfection.

Drug Review or History

The most prevalent nephrotoxic drugs include aminoglycosides, nonsteroidal anti-inflammatory drugs, iodinated radiocontrast media, and angiotensin-converting enzyme inhibitors. Less prevalent are antibiotics (such as amphotericin B), chemotherapeutic agents, cocaine, H_2-receptor antagonists, phenytoin, sulfonamide diuretics, and volatile hydrocarbons.

Toxic Exposures

Occupational hazards that may cause kidney problems include exposure to volatile hydrocarbons, benzene, aniline, xylene, heavy metals, and ionizing radiation.

DIAGNOSTIC REASONING: FOCUSED PHYSICAL EXAMINATION
Note General Appearance

A patient who appears ill or who is in pain is likely to have an upper urinary tract problem, such as pyelonephritis, urolithiasis, or acute prostatitis. Patients with lower urinary tract problems usually do not present with signs of systemic involvement, are free of fever, and generally appear well.

Obtain Vital Signs

Hypertension is seen in patients with nephritis.

Inspect Skin and Mucous Membranes

A pale skin color may suggest anemia caused by poor nutrition or chronic renal failure. Yellow-colored to brown-colored skin without scleral icterus may indicate severe chronic uremia. Other skin changes seen with renal problems may range from rash to purpura.

Hypertension and edema are two findings that usually indicate renal problems; however, a physical examination may not provide much data because few physical signs found on examination indicate the presence of kidney disease.

Palpate and Percuss for Flank Pain at the Costovertebral Angle

Pain that is reproducible is indicative of renal capsule distention and characterizes acute pyelonephritis or acute ureteral obstruction. Perinephric abscess may cause flank swelling and redness.

Palpate and Percuss the Abdomen

Abdominal distention suggests ascites or fluid collection in the bowel. Pain in the lower quadrant indicates lower ureter involvement. Perform deep palpation to identify kidneys or other abdominal masses. Normal kidneys are usually not easily palpated. A distended bladder rises above the symphysis pubis and is characteristic of residual urine from incomplete bladder emptying. Palpation of an enlarged bladder may cause pain. Chronic bladder distention is usually painless and cannot always be determined by manual palpation alone.

If the patient is hypertensive, auscultate at the subcostal anterior abdomen for bruit, which could indicate a renovascular cause of hypertension.

Inspect and Palpate the External Genitalia

Inspect the skin and hair for inflammation, lesions, parasites, and dermatitis. Note hair pattern distribution and level of development of structures for age-group. Palpate the shaft of the penis for strictures. Observe for phimosis if uncircumcised and retract the foreskin. Note inflammation or presence of smegma. Inspect glans, corona, and frenulum areas for lesions. Note personal hygiene; phimosis in uncircumcised males; and presence of urine, discharge, and fecal stains on undergarments. Check position of urethral meatus. Strip or milk the penis from the base toward the glans or head of the penis. Note the color, consistency, and amount of any discharge.

Check scrotum skin surfaces and testicles for tenderness and masses; also check epididymis, spermatic cords, and inguinal canals. The left scrotal sac usually hangs lower than the right. Elevation of an affected testicle may relieve discomfort and is characteristic of epididymitis. A painful scrotal mass is usually associated with inflammation or testicular torsion.

Perform scrotal transillumination in a darkened room. Do not use a halogen light source because it may burn the patient. A solid mass prevents the passage of light and requires further examination. A hydrocele is a nontender firm mass that results from fluid accumulation. It will transilluminate but may make testicular palpation impossible. A spermatocele (a cystic swelling on the epididymis) is not as large as a hydrocele but does not transilluminate. Dilated veins in the scrotal sac, or varicocele, is the most common scrotal mass, usually occurring on the left side. A varicocele is often more prominent when the patient is standing and regresses with the patient in the prone position. It is classically described as a "bag of worms."

Observe Voiding

Observing the patient urinating may be useful to check for hesitancy in initiating the urine stream, force of stream, and dribbling at end of micturition. Observe the abdominal force used during urination. Patients will use abdominal muscles to increase the intraabdominal pressure to force urine from the bladder while holding their breath.

Perform Digital Rectal Prostate Examination

Digital rectal examination of the prostate is performed to identify irregularities of the prostate that are suggestive of cancer and to note any tenderness or inflammation. The size and consistency should be noted. The median sulcus and lateral margins should be palpated. Induration or firmness is characteristic of early prostate disease; a hard stony gland suggests advanced prostatic carcinoma. The gland may feel soft because of inflammation or infection. If hypertrophied, the prostate gland will extend into the rectal canal, and the median sulcus may be obliterated. Do not massage the prostate if acute prostatitis is suspected because of the possibility of spreading the infection. Document the amount of prostate extension into the rectum using an acceptable clinical scale, such as the following:

- Grade I: protrudes less than 1 cm into the rectum
- Grade II: protrudes 1 to 2 cm into the rectum
- Grade III: protrudes 2 to 3 cm into the rectum
- Grade IV: protrudes more than 3 cm into the rectum

LABORATORY AND DIAGNOSTIC STUDIES

The history and the findings of the physical examination determine the extent of diagnostic investigation. The symptoms reported by the patient are taken into account when ordering diagnostic tests to corroborate or verify the diagnosis. General screening tests can be used to provide additional data for patients with urinary tract problems.

Specific tests for kidney function include urinalysis, screening blood chemistry tests (such as urea nitrogen and serum creatinine), and hematological studies. Abnormal blood tests include elevated creatinine and blood urea nitrogen levels, hyperkalemia, and hypocalcemia.

Urine collected for urinalysis should be freshly voided and usually midstream. If not examined immediately, the specimen should be refrigerated because cells begin to disintegrate after 1 to 2 hours.

Urine Dipstick

Reagent strips can be used to screen urine in the clinical setting. See Chapter 32 for a complete discussion of each component. A positive leukocyte esterase or nitrite test result is indicative of urethritis. Urine that tests positive for leukocyte esterase should be cultured for bacteria. Proteinuria may indicate kidney involvement. Suspect proximal renal tubular damage if urine glucose is elevated while serum glucose levels are normal. Blood in the urine could be caused by acute or chronic prostatitis, urethritis, hemorrhagic cystitis, renal stones, or tumors of the kidney, renal pelvis, ureter, bladder, prostate, and urethra. Hematuria with proteinuria usually suggests a renal origin. Isolated hematuria is usually produced by sites outside the kidneys.

Urinalysis with Microscopic Examination

See Chapter 32 for a complete discussion of each component. Turbidity with a foul odor indicates infection. Color changes of the urine may result from various sources: hemoglobin from systemic red blood cell (RBC) lysis; myoglobin from damaged muscle cells or rhabdomyolysis; vegetable pigments from food, such as red beets; pigments from drugs, such as rifampin and phenazopyridine; and porphyrins from porphyria. RBCs indicate acute inflammatory or vascular disorders of the glomerulus. Casts indicate hemorrhage or conditions of the nephron. Red cell casts are characteristic of glomerular origin. The presence of abnormal cells, protein, hemoglobin, myoglobin, or other debris with a cast helps identify the type of renal disease. Significant proteinuria results from glomerulopathies, whereas tubular disorders cause little proteinuria. Therefore the sediment findings are helpful to correlate with the degree of proteinuria. Urinalysis is indicated for all males presenting with lower urinary tract symptoms.

Segmented Urine Collection (Meares-Stamey 4-Glass Test) for Gram Stain, Culture and Sensitivity, and Leukocyte Count

Segmented urine collection is used to identify the site along the urinary tract where the colonization of organisms is occurring. The standard method for specimen collection and labeling is the following:

- Voided bladder specimen 1 (VB 1): 5 to 10 mL of first-voided urine collected
- Voided bladder specimen 2 (VB 2): sterile midstream urine collected
- Expressed prostatic secretion (EPS): prostatic massage performed and prostatic secretion collected from meatal opening
- Voided bladder specimen 3 (VB 3): complete emptying of bladder; urine specimen collected

Another option is the premassage and postmassage urine test (PPMT) (see Evidence-Based Practice box: 4 Glasses or 2?). The following two urine samples are collected:

- A midstream urine specimen before prostatic massage
- A first-voided urine specimen immediately after prostatic massage

---

◎ EVIDENCE-BASED PRACTICE   *4 Glasses or 2?*

The Meares-Stamey 4-glass test is the standard method of assessing inflammation and the presence of bacteria in the lower urinary tract in men presenting with chronic prostatitis. However, evidence suggests that the simpler 2-glass premassage and postmassage urine test (PPMT) may be sufficient to detect inflammation and bacteria.

In a study of 353 men, the 2-glass PPMT was compared to the Meares-Stamey 4-glass test in detecting inflammation and bacteria in men with chronic prostatitis syndrome. The PPMT had strong concordance with the 4-glass test and predicted a correct diagnosis in more than 96% of subjects.

Data from Nickel J, Shoskes D, Wang Y, Alexander R, Fowler J, Zeitlin S, et al: How does the pre-massage and post-massage 2-glass test compare to the Meares-Stamey 4-glass test in men with chronic prostatitis/chronic pelvic pain syndrome? *J Urol* 17:119, 2006.

Label each of the specimens and perform culture and sensitivity or Gram staining. Positive bacterial culture in VB 1 (premassage) suggests urethritis. Positive bacterial culture in VB 2 (premassage) suggests cystitis. Positive bacterial culture in EPS or VB 3 (postmassage) in the absence of positive bacterial culture in premassage specimens or a bacterial culture at least 10 times higher in postmassage samples than in premassage samples suggests bacterial prostatitis.

On microscopic analysis, increased numbers of leukocytes in the EPS and VB are indicative of inflammation. The presence of white blood cells (WBCs) helps diagnose prostatitis and chronic pelvic pain syndrome (see Box 17-1).

Urine Flow Studies (Uroflowmetry)

Urine flow studies can be used as a screening tool to determine diminished force of urination and obstruction. Flow rate is defined as the volume of fluid expelled from the urethra per unit of time and is expressed in milliliters per second. The patient must have a full bladder because urine flow rate depends on voided volume. The patient urinates into an insert in the toilet, which measures the flow rate of the urine. The normal flow pattern exhibits a rapid increase to maximal flow rate, within one third of the ultimate voiding time. After achieving maximal rate, flow decreases more slowly; average flow rate should be approximately 50% of the maximal urine flow rate.

Gram Stain

Gram stain of urethral exudate or spun urine should be performed to determine inflammation (WBCs) and the presence of either gram-negative or gram-positive bacteria. Gram-negative bacteria stain pink-red; gram-positive bacteria stain dark blue to purple. The nuclei of polymorphonuclear neutrophils (PMNs) (leukocytes) stain pink-red. A Gram stain with more than 4 PMNs/high-power field (HPF) is indicative of urethritis (defined by the presence of 5 to 10 PMNs/HPF). Practically, however, any number of WBCs is suggestive of urethritis. A symptomatic patient with risk factors but no positive laboratory results should be retested using the first voided urine of the day.

If the stain is positive for PMNs, then the smear is examined for gram-negative intracellular diplococci (GNICDCs). If GNICDCs are found, the smear is considered positive for gonococcal urethritis. A smear that is equivocal or atypical indicates a mixed gonococcal and nongonococcal urethritis. If there are no GNICDCs, nongonococcal urethritis is indicated. The Gram stain has 95% specificity in gonococcal urethritis, with nearly 100% sensitivity in urethritis.

Culture and Sensitivity

Culture and sensitivity should be performed on specimens to identify the causative organism and its sensitivity to antibiotics. This is especially important in populations at increased risk for resistant organisms.

DNA Testing for Infectious Organisms

DNA testing using a sample taken from the urethra or first-voided urine provides rapid, sensitive, and specific results. Follow manufacturer's directions to collect and transport the sample.

Nucleic acid amplification tests (NAATs) are available to test for *Chlamydia trachomatis* and *Neisseria gonorrhoeae*. Single or dual organism tests are available.

Creatinine and Blood Urea Nitrogen

Serum creatinine and blood urea nitrogen levels are used to indicate kidney function.

Box 17-1	**NIH Classification of Prostatitis**
I	Acute bacterial prostatitis (acute symptoms)
II	Chronic bacterial prostatitis (symptoms present for 3 months)
III	Chronic prostatitis/chronic pelvic pain syndrome (CPPS) (no bacterial cause)
IIIA	Inflammatory CPPS (WBCs found in semen, expressed prostatic secretions, or final voided specimen)
IIIB	Noninflammatory CPPS (no WBCs in semen, expressed prostatic secretions, or final voided specimen)
IV	Asymptomatic inflammatory prostatitis (no subjective symptoms; incidental detection of WBCs in expressed prostatic secretions or prostate tissue)

Modified from National Institute of Diabetes and Digestive and Kidney Diseases: Chronic prostatitis workshop, Bethesda, MD, December 7-8, 1995, National Institutes of Health. Available online at http://kidney.niddk.nih.gov/kudiseases/pubs/chronicprostatitis/index.htm. Accessed August 9, 2010.

Prostate-Specific Antigen

Tumor markers, such as prostate-specific antigen (PSA), may be used to detect or monitor prostate cancer. PSA results should be correlated with the digital rectal examination (DRE). For normal-risk males, levels of 1 to 4 ng/mL are considered within reference range, whereas 4 to 10 ng/mL are elevated levels that fall into a gray zone and may require other tests, such as transrectal ultrasound (TRUS) and prostate biopsy. PSA levels of 10 ng/mL or above are abnormal and indicate malignant activity of the prostate. The threshold level for African American males who are at risk may be lower than for other groups. The higher the PSA level, the more likely the presence of prostate cancer; however, men with prostate cancer can have a negative or borderline PSA level. In men taking finasteride, normal PSA is <2 ng/mL because finasteride halves the PSA level. A negative PSA and a negative DRE make the presence of cancer unlikely.

Currently the use of PSA testing to screen men is under debate. Some authorities recommend screening males older than 40 and those at risk (i.e., patients with a family history or African American males). Others do not recommend routine screening based on lack of empirical evidence of the benefit. In either case, the patient should be told of the potential benefits, known harms, and treatment options available, and should be assisted in making an individual decision about testing (see Evidence-Based Practice box: Prostate Cancer Screening).

Radiography

If microscopic hematuria is present and the patient is under 50 years of age, obtain a flat plate of the abdomen to identify structures of the kidney, ureters, and bladder (KUB). Urinary calculi are usually visible on radiographs (see Chapter 38).

Ultrasound

Ultrasonography is noninvasive and provides information on the kidneys, ureters, bladder, vascular structures, prostate, and testicles. Renal ultrasound is a good first test to determine kidney size and contour, and the presence of calculi. A urinary bladder sonogram is used to identify tumors of the bladder, thickening of the bladder wall, posterior masses behind the bladder, and obstruction of the lower urinary tract evidenced by residual urine. A scrotal sonogram is used to evaluate chronic scrotal swelling; it can be used to identify abscess, infected testes, tumor, hydrocele, spermatocele, adherent scrotal hernia, and chronic epididymitis. However, because it does not assess perfusion, it is less helpful in the initial examination of an acute condition of the scrotum, where a Doppler blood flow is more appropriate. Transrectal prostate ultrasound can be used to evaluate the prostate for tumors or nodules as well as to determine the volume of the prostate. It is also useful in diagnosing prostatitis, BPH, and cancer of the prostate.

◎ **EVIDENCE-BASED PRACTICE**   *Prostate Cancer Screening*

The decision to engage in prostate cancer screening is complex. There is no consensus and little evidence to direct when, who, and how to test, and specific guidelines vary. Authorities do agree that men should have a discussion with their health care providers, and the decision should be made after getting information about the uncertainties, risks, and potential benefits of prostate cancer screening. Men should not be screened unless they have received this information. Most authorities agree that prostate cancer screening should include both DRE and PSA testing.

Results from a large scale randomized clinical trial on prostate-cancer mortality showed no difference in mortality rates from prostate cancer between the screening group and the usual care group (Andiole, et al., 2009). Mortality from prostate cancer was low in both groups. Screening provided no reduction in death rates at 7 years and no indication of a benefit appeared with 67% of the subjects having completed 10 years of follow-up.

However, a European study (Schröder et al., 2009) reports contrary evidence. The study is a combination of seven European trials with different screening protocols and different ages of entry. The study demonstrated that the relative risk of death from prostate cancer was reduced by 20% in men aged 55 to 69 years who underwent serial PSA screening. The absolute risk difference was 0.71 death per 1000 men. This means that 1410 men would need to be screened and 48 additional cases of prostate cancer would need to be treated to prevent one death from prostate cancer.

Data from: Andiole G, Crawford E, Grubb R 3rd, Buys S, Chia D, Church T, et al: Mortality results from a randomized prostate-cancer screening trial, *N Engl J Med* 360:1310, 2009.
Schröder F, Hugosson J, Roobol M, Tammela T, Ciatto S, Nelen V, et al: Screening and prostate-cancer mortality in a randomized European study, *N Engl J Med 360*:1320, 2009.

Computed Tomography

Noncontrast helical (spiral) CT is the gold standard for evaluating kidney stones. It has 95% sensitivity and 98% specificity.

Doppler Flow Studies

Doppler blood flow studies are used to measure blood flow to the scrotal structures. Color Doppler provides a color image, depicting the direction of the flow and the velocity in shades of blue and red. It is useful in the differential diagnosis of testicular torsion and epididymitis. A Doppler of testicular torsion demonstrates reduced or absent blood flow, while epididymitis will show blood flow.

Biopsy

Biopsy of the prostate is necessary for definitive diagnosis of cancer. Guided biopsy is performed using transrectal ultrasound.

DIFFERENTIAL DIAGNOSIS
Cystitis/Urethritis

Males can have inflammation limited to the penile segment of the urethra. The history would include meatal burning and discharge. Classic symptoms are frequency, urgency, and dysuria. Nocturia with suprapubic or low back pain is common.

Screening can be done in most settings with urine dip strips. A positive leukocyte esterase and nitrate test indicates infection. Urine culture and sensitivity confirms diagnosis and identifies the causative organism(s). Urinalysis with microscopic examination can determine if 20 or more organisms/HPF are present, which is indicative of UTI. Less than 20 organisms/HPF merits further study, such as culture and sensitivity. Colonization has taken place if 103 or more organisms/mL are present in the culture.

Pyelonephritis

The patient with pyelonephritis has fever and chills, appears toxic, and reports back pain. Nausea and vomiting may be present. Some patients also report lower urinary tract symptoms, including frequency and dysuria. The patient feels and looks ill. On physical examination, CVA tenderness is usually present. The abdomen may also be tender. On microscopic examination, WBCs are usually present. White cell casts suggest pyelonephritis. Bacterial casts, although rare, are pathognomonic of pyelonephritis. Urine culture and sensitivity confirm the diagnosis and identify the pathogen, which is usually *E. coli, Klebsiella, Proteus mirabilis,* or *Enterobacter.*

Urolithiasis

Urinary stones can occur anywhere in the urinary tract and may produce symptoms of pain, hematuria, and secondary infection. Many calculi are "silent" and may cause only hematuria, either microscopic or gross. Renal calculi may occur when a stone obstructs the urinary tract. Typical symptoms of renal colic include severe flank pain that radiates along the pathway of the ureter to the scrotum or inner thigh. Chills, fever, and urinary frequency are common. The patient may have nausea, vomiting, and abdominal distention. There may be a history of hematuria. Painful hematuria is characteristic of a stone, and the pain is described as colicky. Evaluate if the hematuria occurs at the time of urine initiation, at termination of micturition, or throughout micturition. This may be helpful in localizing the stone.

The clinical diagnosis is supported by urinalysis and imaging findings. The urine may be normal; gross or microscopic hematuria is common. Pyuria (WBCs) with or without bacteria may be present. Crystalline structures may be present. Noncontrast helical (spiral) CT is the gold standard for evaluating kidney stones.

Acute Bacterial Prostatitis

The patient with acute prostatitis is obviously ill and presents with chills, high fever, urinary frequency and urgency, perineal pain, and low back pain. The patient may exhibit varying degrees of obstructive symptoms, dysuria or burning, nocturia, hematuria, arthralgia, and myalgia. On examination, the prostate gland is tender, swollen, indurated, and warm. Do not massage the gland because bacteremia can result from the expression of microorganisms. Urine or prostate secretion culture can confirm the diagnosis. The most common causative organism is *E. coli*. Other common organisms include species of *Klebsiella, Enterobacter,* and *Proteus*. (See Box 17-1 for the classification of prostatitis.)

Chronic Bacterial Prostatitis

Chronic prostatitis is a common cause of recurrent cystitis in men. The patient may present with recurrent urinary tract infections caused by the same pathogen.

Chronic bacterial prostatitis is caused by the same pathogens seen in acute prostatitis. Patients may be asymptomatic. Common symptoms, if evident, include low back pain and perineal discomfort, urinary frequency, and painful urination. Traditionally, symptoms are present for at least 3 months for a diagnosis of chronic prostatitis. Infection can involve the scrotal contents, producing epididymitis. Palpation of the prostate may reveal no specific findings. It may be moderately tender and irregularly indurated or boggy. Copious secretion may be present. Diagnosis is made on the basis of clinical symptoms and by culture of prostatic secretion or positive bacteria culture from postmassage urine. WBCs will be present in EPSs and VB 3.

Chronic Prostatitis/Chronic Pelvic Pain Syndrome

The diagnostic criterion for chronic prostatitis/chronic pelvic pain syndrome (CPPS) is pelvic pain that has been present for at least 3 of the preceding 6 months, with no bacterial cause. The pain may be accompanied by additional symptoms, such as dysuria, urgency, frequency, and backache. Patients may or may not have had obstructive voiding symptoms. Inflammatory CPPS is characterized by the absence of bacteria and the presence of WBCs in the semen, EPS, or VB 3. This category was previously called nonbacterial prostatitis. Noninflammatory CPPS is characterized by the absence of both bacteria and WBCs in the semen, EPS, or VB 3. This condition was formerly called prostadynia. The prostate may feel normal on clinical examination.

Asymptomatic Inflammatory Prostatitis

This condition is diagnosed in patients during the evaluation of another genitourinary (GU) problem, such as benign prostatic hypertrophy. These patients do not experience genitourinary pain. WBCs are found in the expressed prostatic secretions.

Epididymitis/Orchitis

The patient with epididymitis/orchitis is usually a sexually active young male, and pain is the likely presenting symptom. The patient may be febrile. The history usually indicates a slow onset of discomfort over hours or days compared with testicular torsion, which has a rapid onset of symptoms. Elevation of the affected testicle may reduce the discomfort. Swelling of the scrotum and testicle may be present. Palpable swelling of the epididymis is usually present. Doppler flow studies with color can locate hot spots and identify intact blood flow. Urethral discharge or an intraurethral swab specimen should be Gram stained for a diagnosis of urethritis. A nucleic acid amplification test (either on the intraurethral swab or with the first-void urine) should be used to test for *N. gonorrhoeae* and *C. trachomatis.*

Testicular Torsion

The patient with testicular torsion is usually a pubescent male with previous episodes of testicular pain. The history indicates a rapid onset of acute pain. Nausea and vomiting may have occurred or be present. Doppler blood flow studies may support the diagnosis by identifying lack of blood flow to the affected testicle. This is an emergent condition, and intervention must take place within the first 4 to 6 hours to salvage the testicle from infarction.

Benign Prostatic Hyperplasia

Prostatic hypertrophy is common in men over age 50. Presenting symptoms include hesitancy, slow urine stream, and dribbling. Digital rectal examination reveals an enlarged prostate with a reduced or obliterated median sulcus. Induration or firmness is characteristic of early prostate disease, and a hard stony gland suggests advanced prostatic carcinoma. The gland may feel soft because of inflammation or infection. The American Urological Association Symptom Index (see Table 17-1) is useful in determining treatment options based on severity of symptoms, ranging from mild to severe. Digital rectal examinations combined with PSA tests are done annually by many clinicians for men older than 50 and for men at risk, including African American males starting at age 40, to differentiate between BPH and prostate cancer.

Prostate Cancer

Patients with prostate cancer often present with the same obstructive symptoms as BPH but may also be asymptomatic. Males presenting with reports of lower abdominal pain probably represent extension of the cancer with metastasis. On examination, the prostate is stony hard and protrudes into the colon. PSA levels may be elevated, and TRUS indicates enlargement or nodules. An abnormal digital rectal examination or an elevated PSA necessitate further evaluation to determine or rule out prostate cancer (see Evidence Based Practice box: Prostate Cancer Screening).

Bladder or Kidney Tumor

Silent hematuria in elderly patients is often a late-presenting indication of cancer. It is more common in men than women. Patients often have a history of smoking or alcohol abuse.

Perineal Compression Syndrome

Compression of the pudendal nerve in long-distance cyclists can result in genital numbness without pain. An ill-fitting bicycle seat may contribute to the problem.

DIFFERENTIAL DIAGNOSIS OF *Common Causes of Genitourinary Problems in Males*

CONDITION	HISTORY	PHYSICAL FINDINGS	DIAGNOSTIC STUDIES
Cystitis/urethritis	Frequency, urgency, dysuria; nocturia with low back pain	Discharge may be present; may have suprapubic tenderness	Urine dipstick: positive leukocyte esterase; hematuria; urinalysis with microscopic examination; segmented urine collection; Gram stain; C & S; urine DNA test (NAATs)
Pyelonephritis	Fever, chills, back pain, nausea and vomiting, toxic appearance; some patients also have frequency and dysuria	Feels and looks ill; temperature >101° F; CVA tenderness; abdomen may be tender	Microscopic examination: WBCs may have white cell casts or bacterial casts; urine C & S; blood cultures
Urolithiasis	Pain, hematuria; may have symptoms of secondary infection; renal colic: pain that radiates to inner thigh; nausea, vomiting	May have CVA tenderness; looks ill during periods of acute pain; may have abdominal distention	Urinalysis: gross or microscopic hematuria; WBCs with or without bacteria; crystalline structures may be present; radiograph or ultrasound
Acute bacterial prostatitis	Chills, high fever, urinary frequency; urgency; perineal pain and low back pain; varying degrees of obstructive symptoms, dysuria or burning, nocturia, hematuria, arthralgia, and myalgia	Temperature >101° F; prostate gland tender, swollen, indurated, warm; do not massage as can cause bacteremia	Urinalysis; urine culture; prostate secretion culture
Chronic bacterial prostatitis	Common cause of recurrent cystitis in men; same pathogen as in prostate secretion; may be asymptomatic; commonly have low back pain and perineal pain, urinary frequency, and painful urination	Infection can involve scrotal contents, producing epididymitis; palpation of prostate reveals no specific findings; may be moderately tender and irregularly indurated or boggy; may have copious secretion	Culture prostatic secretion; culture postmassage urine; WBCs present in EPS and VB 3
Chronic prostatitis/ chronic pelvic pain syndrome (CPPS); can be inflammatory or noninflammatory	Pelvic pain present for at least 3 of preceding 6 months, with no bacterial cause; may be accompanied by additional symptoms such as dysuria, urgency, frequency, and backache; may or may not have had obstructive voiding symptoms	Normal prostate examination	Inflammatory: absence of bacteria and presence of WBCs in semen, EPS, or VB 3 Noninflammatory: absence of both bacteria and WBCs in semen, EPS, or VB 3
Asymptomatic inflammatory prostatitis	Symptoms of another genitourinary problem; no pain	Specific for another genitourinary disorder	WBCs found in expressed prostatic secretions

Continued

DIFFERENTIAL DIAGNOSIS OF *Common Causes of Genitourinary Problems in Males—cont'd*

CONDITION	HISTORY	PHYSICAL FINDINGS	DIAGNOSTIC STUDIES
Epididymitis/ orchitis	Abrupt onset over several hours; febrile; pain in scrotum and/or testicles	Tender, swollen epididymitis and/or testicles; elevation of affected testicle may lessen discomfort; may have fever	Doppler blood flow studies with color
Testicular torsion	Sudden onset of testicular pain that radiates to groin; may also have lower abdominal pain	Exquisitely tender testicle; testicle may ride high because of shortened spermatic cord; cremasteric reflex absent	Scrotal ultrasonography; this is a surgical emergency
Benign prostatic hyperplasia (BPH)	Hesitancy, slow urine stream, dribbling, nocturia	Prostate protrusion into rectum; median sulcus reduced; prostate boggy	TRUS; PSA
Prostate cancer	Hesitancy, slow urine stream, dribbling, nocturia; low back pain	Prostate protrusion into rectum; prostate hard	TRUS; PSA; biopsy
Bladder or kidney tumor	More common in men than women; patients often have history of smoking or alcohol abuse	Usually no signs other than silent hematuria	U/A: hematuria
Perineal compression syndrome	Genital numbness without pain; increase in training, miles, change in bicycle equipment	Usually no visible signs	Rule out cauda equina syndrome or other neuropathy; refrain from biking for three weeks, refit bike saddle

C & S, culture & sensitivity; *CVA,* costovertebral angle; *EPS,* expressed prostatic secretion; *NAAT,* nucleic acid amplification test; *PSA,* prostate-specific antigen; *TRUS,* transrectal ultrasound; *U/A,* urinalysis; *VB 3,* voided bladder specimen 3; *WBC,* white blood cell.

REFERENCES AND READINGS

Aldmen W, Joffe A: The adolescent male genital examination: what's normal and what's not, *Pediatr Rev* 20:125, 1999.

Asplund C, Barkdull T, Weiss B: Genitourinary problems in bicyclists, *Curr Sports Med Rep* 6:333, 2007.

American Urological Association: Guideline on the management of benign prostatic hyperplasia (BPH). Available online at http://www.auanet.org/content/guidelines-and-quality-care/clinical-guidelines.cfm. Accessed May 27, 2010.

American Urological Association: Prostate-specific antigen best practice statement: 2009 update, AUA. Available online at http://www.auanet.org/content/guidelines-and-quality-care/clinical-guidelines.cfm. Accessed May 27, 2010.

Bremnor JD, Sadovsky R: Evaluation of dysuria in adults, *Am Fam Physician* 65:1589, 2002.

Diaz-Parker C, Bratslavsky G: Male genitourinary disease: urethritis, epididymitis, and prostatitis, *Clin Rev* 15:40, 2005.

Edwards JL: Diagnosis and management of benign prostatic hyperplasia, *Am Fam Physician* 77:1403, 2008.

Epperly TD, Moore KE: Health issues in men, part I: common genitourinary disorders, *Am Fam Physician* 61:3657, 2000.

Fracchia MS, Pareek G, Armenakas N: Scrotal pathology in children: benign or serious? *Consultant* July:1114, 2004.

Grabe M, Bishop MC, Bjerklund-Johansen TE, Botto H, Çek M, Lobel B et al: Prostatitis and chronic pelvic pain syndrome. In: Guidelines on urological infections, European Association of Urology - Medical Specialty Society: 2008 Mar (revised 2009 Mar). Available online at http://www.guideline.gov/. Accessed May 27, 2010.

Grossfeld GD, Wolf JS, Litwin MS, Hricak H, Shuler CL, Agerter DC et al.: Asymptomatic microscopic hematuria in adults: Summary of the AUA Best Practice Policy Recommendations, *Am Fam Physician* 63:1145, 2001.

Lan G: Scrotal swelling in children, *Pediatr Rev* 21:311, 2000.

Mulle BA: Prostatitis: What NPs need to know about diagnosis and treatment, *Am J Nurse Pract* 9:33, 2005.

Nickel J, Shoskes D, Wang Y, Alexander R, Fowler J, Zeitlin S et al: How does the pre-massage and post-massage 2-glass test compare to the Meares-Stamey 4-glass test in men with chronic prostatitis/chronic pelvic pain syndrome? *J Urol* 176:119, 2006.

Stevemer JJ, Easley SK: Treatment of prostatitis, *Am Fam Physician* 61:3015, 2000.

Headache

Headache is a subjective feeling of pain caused by a variety of intracranial and extracranial factors. It is one of the most common complaints in adults and children, with most headaches being self-treated with an over-the-counter (OTC) analgesic. Most headaches are acute and self-limited and are not life threatening. One in ten people will have a migraine, and less than 1% of headaches are due to serious intracranial disease. The goals for the practitioner in evaluating a headache are to (1) identify life-threatening causes of headache, (2) diagnose treatable disease associated with some headaches, and (3) provide symptom relief. To accomplish these goals, the practitioner needs to conduct a careful history and physical examination, even though physical findings will be normal for the majority of patients with a headache.

Pain from headache arises from stimulation of pain-sensitive structures of the head and brain caused by traction, inflammation, vascular dilation, muscle contraction, or dysregulation of ascending brainstem serotonergic systems (Figure 18-1). Headaches can be categorized as primary or secondary. Primary headaches are characterized by the absence of structural pathology or systemic disease; they account for more than 90% of all headaches. Secondary headaches are attributed to an underlying disorder. Primary headaches are of five major types: migraine, tension-type headache (TTH), cluster headache, other trigeminal autonomic cephalalgias, and other primary headaches. Generally, pain arising from disordered function, damage, or inflammation of structures located anterior to and above the tentorium is felt in the front of the head, whereas pain felt in the back of the head arises from structures located below the tentorium. Extracranial structures that are sensitive to pain include the skin, scalp, blood vessels, facial muscles, eyes, ears, teeth, nasal cavity, mucous membranes of the mouth and pharynx, and the temporomandibular joint (TMJ). The substance of the brain itself is not sensitive to pain, but sensitive structures include the blood vessels, sensory nerves, and ganglia.

Cranial structures project pain to the surface close to the source of pain. Pain from extracranial structures is usually felt in the immediate region affected (Figure 18-2). The head is innervated extensively from the first branch of the trigeminal nerve (cranial nerve V). It has significant anatomical connections to the upper cervical roots C1-C3, which supply the posterior fossa and neck structures.

Headache has been divided by symptomatology into types using the diagnostic criteria revised in 2004 by the Headache Classification Committee of the International Headache Society.

Of the types classified, only a few are common (Box 18-1). Headaches can also be categorized into acute (new onset), subacute, or chronic. Acute headaches warrant close attention. The headache associated with subarachnoid hemorrhage (SAH) has an intense sudden onset. Subacute headaches are localized headaches preceding neurological findings, often caused by a vascular disorder or a space-occupying lesion. Headaches of greatest concern to clinicians are those that are persistent, severe, sudden in onset, and different from the patient's usual headache. The major clue to assessment of chronic headache is a change in the usual pattern of occurrence. Clinicians can ask patients to keep a headache diary that includes notes on timing, frequency, and association with sleep, diet, emotional episodes, and other potentially contributing factors.

DIAGNOSTIC REASONING: FOCUSED HISTORY

What clues indicate this is a potentially serious, life-threatening headache?

First assess whether the patient is fully oriented before proceeding with further history. A mental status screening can be performed using the Mini-Mental State Examination (see Chapter 8). If the patient shows a mental status deficit, immediate emergency treatment is indicated.

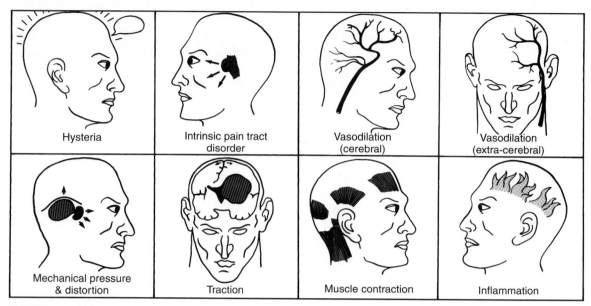

| Hysteria | Intrinsic pain tract disorder | Vasodilation (cerebral) | Vasodilation (extra-cerebral) |
| Mechanical pressure & distortion | Traction | Muscle contraction | Inflammation |

FIGURE 18-1 Mechanisms of cranial pain. (From Noble J et al: *Textbook of primary care medicine,* ed 3, St Louis, 2001, Mosby.)

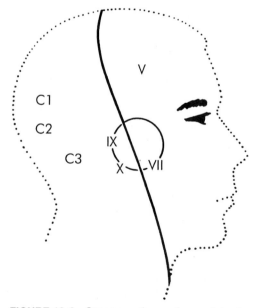

FIGURE 18-2 Sensory pathways for cranial pain.

Key Questions

■ How did the headache begin?
■ What is your age?
■ Have you had this type of headache before?

■ On a scale from 0 (no pain) to 10 (worst pain ever), how severe is the pain?
■ Do you have a history of recent trauma to the head?
■ Did you lose consciousness?
■ Do you notice other symptoms associated with the headache pain?
■ Do you have any chronic health problems?

Onset and Severity

Sudden onset of a severe headache without a history of chronic headache suggests an intracerebral hemorrhage (ICH) secondary to a ruptured aneurysm or vascular anomaly. Severity of headache is a very subjective measure and can sometimes be difficult to interpret. Headache of an ICH without a history of trauma is rare in children and adolescents, but the prevalence increases with age, especially in persons older than 50 years or those being treated with anticoagulation therapy.

Onset of sudden severe headache with neurological signs is an emergency; the patient needs immediate emergency treatment.

Subarachnoid hemorrhage (SAH) is often precipitated by physical activity and is described as the

Box 18-1	**First Level of the International Classification of Headache Disorders**

Primary Headaches
1. Migraine
2. Tension-type headache (TTH)
3. Cluster headache and other trigeminal autonomic encephalalgias
4. Other primary headaches

Secondary Headaches
5. Headache attributed to head/neck trauma
6. Headache attributed to cranial or cervical vascular disorder
7. Headache attributed to nonvascular intracranial disorder
8. Headache attributed to substance or its withdrawal
9. Headache attributed to infection
10. Headache attributed to disorder of homeostasis
11. Headache or facial pain attributed to disorder of cranium, neck, eyes, ears, nose, sinuses, teeth, mouth, or other facial or cranial structures
12. Headache attributed to psychiatric disorder

Cranial Neuralgias, Central and Primary Facial Pain, and Other Headaches
13. Cranial neuralgias and central causes of facial pain
14. Other headache, cranial neuralgia, central or primary facial pain

Data from the Headache Classification Committee of the International Headache Society: The International Classification of Headache Disorders, *Cephalalgia* 24:9, 2004.

"worst headache ever." Patients also report a stiff neck and may have a transient loss of consciousness, nausea and vomiting, photophobia, pupillary dilation, and seizure. Some patients who have a leaking aneurysm may report headache for several days but will subsequently have a worsening headache with neurological findings.

If SAH is suspected, the patient needs transport to an emergency center for a computed tomography (CT) scan and possible surgical intervention because early diagnosis and treatment improve prognosis.

History of Trauma

Trauma to the head may cause subdural or epidural bleeding. The patient may have a brief loss of consciousness followed by a period of lucidity that can last for minutes to days, with subsequent relapse and appearance of neurological signs. Epidural hematomas are often associated with skull fracture.

Minor head trauma may result in headache because of soft tissue or extracranial injury. Pain is often localized to the site of injury and is self-limiting. Anyone who has experienced head trauma should be carefully observed for at least 24 hours for signs of neurological damage.

Associated Symptoms

The entry of infectious organisms, chemical agents, and drugs into the subarachnoid space causes inflammation of meningeal structures and associated blood vessels, resulting in a headache. Headache associated with infection presents with fever and possibly meningismus (stiff neck), which can indicate meningitis or encephalitis. Unilateral upper or lower extremity weakness with loss of manual dexterity is seen in children with hemiplegic migraine.

An ICH presents as a sudden and severe "thunderclap" headache associated with confusion, vomiting, lethargy, and focal neurological signs; it is caused by a ruptured vascular anomaly or an aneurysm. Drowsiness or confusion can be produced by increased intracranial pressure secondary to meningitis or metabolic disorders.

Brain tumors in children, especially young children, are difficult to diagnose because of the child's inability to describe headache or diplopia until about 4 years of age. Signs are vague, and the developing skull in the infant may accommodate a pathological condition for some time. However, headache as the initial manifestation of brain tumor is followed quickly by neurological signs such as vomiting, recurrent morning headaches, reflex asymmetry, and papilledema.

Presence of Chronic Disease

Persons with AIDS are at increased risk for cryptococcal meningitis, encephalitis, and generalized sepsis. Persons being treated with anticoagulation therapy or the elderly are at increased risk for headache from a serious cause, such as an ICH or acute glaucoma. Headaches secondary to metabolic disorders can be the result of hyponatremia, uremia, hypoglycemia, and hypercapnia.

After determining the headache is not serious, how can I narrow down the causes?

Key Questions

- What does it feel like?
- Where does it hurt?
- What makes it worse?

- How long have you had this headache?
- Can you tell when a headache is developing?

Characteristics of the Pain

A moderately intense, constant throbbing headache is associated with dilation of the cervical arteries. Severe pain indicates an expanding lesion, such as a tumor or hematoma, edema, or enlargement of the ventricles secondary to hydrocephalus.

Migraine headache pain is caused by the production of various substances on dilated arteries that sensitize those arteries to pain. The pain is steady or throbbing and is usually limited to the same side. Migraine headaches are thought to result from an initial phase of inter-cranial or extracranial vasoconstriction, followed by a longer interval of vasodilation. Frequently the headache takes 3 to 4 hours to reach peak pain levels.

Cluster headaches (uncommon in children) are the result of an unknown vascular change that occurs within a period of 5 minutes. The pain of cluster headaches is described as explosive and severe.

Tension (muscle contraction) headaches usually occur at school or work and often disappear on weekends and vacations or during periods of relaxation.

Location

Pain secondary to trauma or inflammation is perceived as near the site of insult, such as the occipital area, nape of neck, bifrontal area, or generalized to the head. Noxious stimulation from any type of disease of the eye, ear, nose, or paranasal sinuses may spread to cause pain in the head.

Adults describe TTHs as a "hatband" distribution of pain, whereas children describe a generalized headache or discomfort. Most patients describe a cluster headache as sudden severe pain beginning over one eye and spreading rapidly to the same side of the face.

Orbital pain is seen with increased intraocular pressure. Periorbital pain may be present with sinusitis, migraine, or trigeminal neuralgia, or it may be a sign of ocular disease. TMJ pain is located in the frontotemporal or temporal regions and may be unilateral or bilateral. Nonpulsatile headache in the occipital and paracervical regions is often caused by contraction of muscles of the head and neck.

Aggravating Factors

Triggers are present in many patients with migraine and include sound, odor, and estrogen fluctuations associated with the menstrual cycle. The most common food triggers are red wine, chocolate, and ripe cheese—foods high in tyramine or tryptophan. Migraine is usually worse with activity, whereas patients with TTHs are able to continue their usual routine. Stress can trigger any type of primary headache and must be considered a comorbid condition.

Duration

Most TTHs last less than 24 hours, a similar duration as migraine headaches. Cluster headaches usually last less than 3 hours and tend to occur in cycles. A sub-acute headache persists for days and weeks.

Aura and Prodrome

In migraine with aura, visual symptoms predominate and range from nonspecific blurring to scintillating sco-tomata with zigzag patterns, diplopia, and stars or flashes. Aura often precedes the onset or is simultaneous with headache. Prodromal symptoms include fatigue, depressed or euphoric mood, increased or decreased appetite, constipation or diarrhea, and yawning.

What does the chronicity of pain suggest?

Key Questions

- How often do you get a headache?
- Can you describe any pattern to the headache?
- How long does the headache last?
- Have you had this kind of headache before?
- Do you drink alcohol? Do you take any medications?

Frequency

A patient with a persistent headache for more than 3 months may demonstrate physical findings such as papilledema, bilateral or unilateral cranial nerve VI (abducens) palsies, gait or balance disturbances, or spasticity of the lower extremities. As a rule, in the absence of such symptoms, a recurrent headache of more than 3 months' duration is rarely related to structural or systemic findings. If a headache has been present continuously for more than 4 weeks, without accompanying neurological signs or symptoms, it is most likely psychogenic in origin, especially if coupled with prolonged school or work absences, increased stress, and depression.

Pattern and Duration of Headache

Headaches that occur throughout the day suggest a tension type. Sinus headaches occur after arising and worsen as the day progresses, especially when the person bends forward, but are less painful in the evening. Headaches associated with severe hypertension are not common and occur only with a diastolic blood pressure reading of 130 mm Hg or greater. They are occipital, worse on arising, and lessen as the day progresses. Meningeal inflammation produces a pain that fluctuates throughout the day and night with no clear pattern. Migraine pain is episodic, occurring from several times a week to once a year. Cluster headache pain demonstrates a pattern of attacks that occur daily for several weeks with long periods of remission. The pain is short, often lasting less than 1 hour, but is intense.

Prior History of Headache

Headaches can be described as acute (new onset), subacute, or chronic. Acute-onset headaches must be evaluated for organic causes. Subacute and chronic headaches are usually caused by vascular inflammation or muscle tension. Chronic headaches are usually described as dull, bilateral, or bandlike. Chronic daily headaches may be mixed, produced by a combination of vascular and muscular causes.

Organic lesions may initially produce pain that is intermittent, but as the lesion progresses, the duration and frequency of the attack will increase.

Psychogenic headache pain is daily, constant, diffuse, and difficult to describe.

Age of Patient at First Onset

The age of onset of migraines can be as early as 5 years old. Usually migraine headaches begin at ages 10 to 30 years. New onset of migraine headaches in adults older than age 50 is unusual. Tension headaches have a usual first-onset age of 8 to 12 years. Cluster headaches have a usual first-onset age of 20 to 40 years.

Lifestyle Habits and Medications

Alcohol is an important trigger for migraine and cluster headaches although it may relieve a TTH. Smoking and second-hand smoke exposure can trigger headaches. Patients may be experiencing side effects of medications with headache.

What associated symptoms does the patient have?

Key Questions

- Do you have any nausea or vomiting?
- Do you notice any vision changes?
- Does light bother you?
- Are you dizzy?

Nausea and Vomiting

Nausea and abdominal pain are more common in children with migraines, whereas nausea and vomiting are more common in adults. Vomiting can be a sign of increased intracranial pressure. Headaches from tumors in the midline, cerebellar, and ventricular areas of the cranium obstruct the normal flow of the cerebrospinal fluid, producing hydrocephalus, headache, and early morning vomiting that usually occurs without nausea.

Vision Changes

Migraine headaches may have an aura that precedes them. A frequently reported visual aura is a scintillating scotoma or twinkling spots of brightly colored lights. In children, visual scintillation is the most common aura of migraine, often limited to one eye.

Cluster headaches are associated with ipsilateral conjunctival injection, lacrimation, and edema of the eyelid.

Photophobia

Photophobia is often present with migraine headaches but is not present with tension headaches. Patients with meningitis often report photophobia.

Dizziness

Approximately one third of patients with migraine headaches experience vertigo. The vertigo may appear as an aura, occur during the headache, or occur separately. A young child with vertigo may appear startled or have sudden ataxia.

What do the alleviating and aggravating factors suggest?

Key Questions

- Does anything make the headache better?
- Does anything make the headache worse?

Alleviating Factors

Patients with meningeal irritation obtain partial relief from being recumbent and lying quietly. Headaches that respond to mild analgesics are more likely to be tension headaches. Children obtain complete relief after a brief period of rest with a migraine headache, although rest does not affect a tension headache in children. Some adults experience migraine headache relief with sleep or rest, particularly in a dark, quiet environment.

Aggravating Factors

Increased headache with sneezing or coughing may indicate a benign headache or may be due to a lesion at the level of the foramen magnum long before clinical signs are present. Migraine headaches are made worse with exertion. Patients with cluster headaches have worse pain when lying down. Headaches that are much worse in the early morning and improve on arising may indicate tumor. Benign exertional headaches can occur during coitus. Trigeminal neuralgia pain can be triggered by stimulation of the affected nerve, produced by rubbing the face or chewing.

What does family history indicate?

Key Question

▪ Does anyone else in the family have headaches?

Family History

Tension-type headaches have no family history. Migraines have a positive family history.

Is there anything else that would help narrow the cause or causes?

Key Questions

▪ Have you been ill recently?
▪ Are you taking any medications or vitamins?
▪ Could you have been exposed to carbon monoxide?

Recent Health History

Any substance introduced iatrogenically into the ventricular and lumbar fluid spaces can lead to chemical meningitis. Radiographic contrast media, antibiotics, and steroids can cause headache. Lumbar puncture (LP) can cause a severe headache in 25% of patients. The headache is eased by lying down and aggravated by sitting or standing. Chronic infection, including otitis media, mastoiditis, sinusitis, dental or pulmonary infection, cardiovascular lesions with shunting, or endocarditis, predisposes to development of a brain abscess. Half of all brain abscesses occur in children with cyanotic congenital heart disease. Penetrating skull fractures can also be a portal of entry for bacteria and contribute to the occurrence of brain abscess. Melanomas may metastasize years after excision and may first be indicated by neurological changes.

History of Medications

Outdated tetracycline use can cause pseudotumor cerebri (increased intracranial pressure without any intracranial mass or hydrocephalus), as can excessive intake of vitamin A and substances found in some topical acne preparations. Oral contraceptives and overuse of over-the-counter analgesics can cause headache.

Withdrawal from certain substances, such as caffeine or nitrates, can also produce headache.

Exposures

Exposure to carbon monoxide (CO) may cause a severe, throbbing, generalized headache. Hemoglobin values less than 10 g/dL may cause headache as a result of hypoxia.

Assess occupational exposure to other toxins through an occupational history. Winter headaches may be caused by a faulty kerosene or gas heater.

DIAGNOSTIC REASONING: FOCUSED PHYSICAL EXAMINATION
Observe the Patient

Assess level of alertness and orientation to person, place, and time. Any patient who reports headache and exhibits an ataxic gait, uncoordinated movements, or reduced mental alertness should be immediately transported to an emergency center for neurological evaluation.

A patient who appears ill or toxic is a suspect for meningitis. The patient is usually lying down with the lights off (photophobia) and may report chills. Most toddlers cannot communicate the characteristics of a headache but instead become irritable and cranky and rub their eyes and head.

Muscle spasm may cause tilting of the head or lifting of the shoulder when there is a posterior fossa tumor, cervical spine disease, or whiplash injury. Ptosis of the eyelid may accompany a cluster headache or brain tumor. Blinking and squinting of the eyes indicate photophobia.

Take Vital Signs and Obtain Growth Parameters

Take temperature, blood pressure, and pulse measurements. Fever may be the only sign of infection. Bradycardia and narrowing of pulse pressure are signs of increased intracranial pressure. In children, if the plotted height and weight chart is significantly below average, consider a hypothalamic neoplasm. Plot head circumference to assess for normal skull growth. Macrocephaly may indicate hydrocephalus or brain tumor.

Palpate and Percuss the Skull

Palpate for symmetry of contour, tenderness, and lesions on the scalp, face, and neck. Palpate the temporal arteries for quality of pulse and tenderness. Focal tenderness and induration are seen in TTHs. Tenderness over nodular temporal arteries is a sign of temporal arteritis.

Brain abscesses cause pain by localized traction and produce tenderness on skull percussion over the area involved.

Auscultate the Cranium

Intracranial arteriovenous malformations may mimic migraine. Auscultate the orbit and skull to evaluate for cranial bruits.

Inspect the Ears, Eyes, Nose, Mouth, and TMJ

A thorough examination of the face, head, and neck structures is needed to detect organic disease. Examine the ears for signs of infection.

Ipsilateral lacrimation, ptosis, and pupillary constriction are seen with cluster headache. Test extraocular movement (EOM) in all fields of gaze. If a patient cannot look completely to the right or the left (lateral gaze), suspect a cranial nerve VI palsy, possibly the result of increased intracranial pressure. If EOMs are painful, consider optic neuritis.

Observe nasal mucosa for redness and swelling. Rhinorrhea and congestion are seen with sinus headaches. Observe teeth and oral mucosa because upper molar disease and poor dentition can cause headache. Tapping on the teeth or biting down on a tongue blade can elicit pain from sinusitis.

TMJ instability can cause headache pain. See Chapter 14 for a discussion of examination techniques.

Enlarged pupils seen during a headache indicate migraine; however, if they outlast a headache, then organic disease should be suspected.

Upper motor neuron facial weakness may be present in hemiplegic migraine.

Perform Ophthalmoscopy

On ophthalmoscopic examination, note contour of optic disc and clarity of margins. Note papilledema and inspect vasculature for hemorrhage or exudate, venous pulsations, and arterial spasm.

Papilledema is often caused by an expanding intracranial mass and increased intracranial pressure. Optic disc atrophy suggests a chronically increased intracranial pressure or a lesion in the optic chiasm.

Meningitis does not produce fundus changes. Retinal hemorrhage in children may indicate abuse.

Assess Cranial Nerve Function

A complete assessment of cranial nerve function may provide evidence for more serious causes of headaches secondary to inflammation, traction, or metabolic imbalance.

- Cranial nerve I—Assess for smell. The sense of smell may be lost when the olfactory nerve is damaged by head injury or by a tumor in the vicinity of the olfactory groove.
- Cranial nerve II—Check visual acuity. Rarely does poor vision contribute to a headache. Poor vision may contribute to eye pain, but children equate this with headache. Double vision may be the presenting ocular symptom of increased intracranial pressure caused by a unilateral cranial nerve VI palsy or a posterior fossa lesion.
- Cranial nerves III, IV, and VI—Check visual fields. Unilateral or homonymous hemianopsia, a loss of the same half of the visual field of both eyes, can occur with migraines or brain tumor headaches when the tumor is in the occipital lobes or adjacent to the visual pathways. A half-field defect is seen with parietal lobe tumor. Cranial nerve III palsy can cause an enlargement of the pupil from compression of the nerve by an expanding lesion. The dilated pupil is always on the side of the expanding lesion. Cranial nerve VI palsy (inability to move eyes in a lateral direction) may be found with acute hydrocephalus or cerebral edema. Nystagmus suggests a brainstem or cerebellar lesion and is usually ipsilateral. Lateral gaze nystagmus is also present with an elevated blood alcohol level. Vertical and rotatory nystagmus suggests central posterior fossa abnormality.
- Cranial nerve V—Test jaw strength, pain, and touch sensation to face. Trigeminal neuralgia pain can be triggered by stimulation of the affected nerve.
- Cranial nerve VII—Ask the patient to frown, raise eyebrows, show teeth, close eyes against resistance, and puff out cheeks. Test taste on the anterior two thirds of the tongue for sweet and salt discrimination. Salivary and lacrimal glands are innervated by cranial nerve VII.
- Cranial nerve VIII—Test hearing acuity. Unilateral deafness should be investigated to rule out acoustic neuroma.

- Cranial nerve IX, X—Observe swallowing; uvula rise.
- Cranial nerve XI—Test trapezius strength and sternocleidomastoid strength against resistance.
- Cranial nerve XII—Test tongue strength. An intracranial vascular event may cause a hemiplegia or hemiparesis that may be assessed by observing the protruded tongue drift laterally or by the inability to hold position against resistance.

Examine the Neck

Ask the patient to perform full range of motion (ROM) of the neck to observe for stiffness or difficulty with movement, which may indicate muscle tension or meningismus.

Test for Meningismus

Normally the chin can be flexed passively to touch the chest. If neck stiffness (nuchal rigidity) is present, this maneuver is not possible. With the patient supine, attempts to flex the neck cause involuntary hip flexion, and the hips rise (Brudzinski sign). Attempts to extend the knee joint when the hip joint is flexed may cause the other limb to flex at the hip (Kernig sign).

Assess Motor Strength and Coordination of Extremities

Asymmetrical increase in muscle tone on the affected side, contralateral to the hemisphere lesion, suggests a cerebral lesion.

Patients who exhibit forearm drift with arms extended and eyes closed may have a motor neuron or cerebellar disturbance with an expanding intracranial lesion.

Test Balance and Gait

Midline cerebellar abnormalities cause marked ataxia. The patient has difficulty standing on the ipsilateral leg and has a tendency to fall or stumble toward the side of the lesion. The gait is also wide-based and halting, and the patient turns with jerky movements. Minimal disturbance is observed when the patient hops on either foot or stands tandem (one foot behind the other).

Assess Deep Tendon Reflexes

Note asymmetry, absence, or hyperactive responses. Increase in or asymmetry of reflexes is seen with cerebral lesions. The plantar or Babinski response is often present with cerebral lesions.

Have Children Draw Pictures of Their Headaches

Having a child draw a headache is an inexpensive and accurate way to help diagnosis headaches. The child is given a plain piece of paper and asked to draw a picture of how his or her headache felt before any history of the headache is taken. These drawings help to diagnose migraine headaches. Drawings for migraines include visual images such as flashing. Photophobia is depicted by showing the lights out, a dark room, or a blanket over the head. The need to lie down is also associated with migraine headache. Images for nonmigraine headaches show pictures of pounding or tight headbands. Even very young children (age 4) are able to draw stick figures with significant detail.

LABORATORY AND DIAGNOSTIC STUDIES
Complete Blood Count

Complete blood count (CBC) is obtained to detect major blood dyscrasias. Hypoxia secondary to severe anemia can cause headache.

Blood Cultures

Blood cultures should be drawn in a patient who has a fever, headache, nuchal rigidity, and altered mental status.

Computed Tomography Scan

CT scan is the most common noninvasive initial diagnostic tool used to detect intracranial disease and should be done with new-onset severe headache or headache associated with abnormal neurological signs. A CT scan is done when brain abscess is suspected.

Lumbar Puncture

LP can directly measure cerebrospinal fluid pressure and be analyzed for normal values of components that are altered by disease, such as lymphocytes, glucose, protein, and presence of bacteria. An LP is performed when a central nervous system infection is suspected but is contraindicated if there is suspicion of increased intracranial pressure.

Erythrocyte Sedimentation Rate

Erythrocyte sedimentation rate (ESR) is a nonspecific test that is elevated in the presence of inflammation. An ESR should be performed when temporal arteritis is suspected.

Skull Radiograph

A radiograph of the skull is useful in posttraumatic headache. Specific views must be obtained to better observe intracranial structures, such as the pituitary gland or paranasal sinuses.

DIFFERENTIAL DIAGNOSIS
Primary Headaches

Tension-Type Headache (Muscle)

TTH is the most common type of headache in adults and occurs most often in women. The mechanism of tension headache is uncertain, but is thought to be related to sustained muscle contraction. Tension headache produces a bilateral pain, general or localized, often described as a frontotemporal bandlike distribution. The discomfort is described as a mild to moderate, nonthrobbing pain, tightness, or pressure with a gradual onset. It may last for hours or days, and recurrences may extend over weeks or months. It is associated with hunger, depression, or stress.

Migraine Without Aura (Common)

About 20% of adults experience migraines, and episodes are not uncommon in children as young as 5 years old. The headache is unilateral and throbbing, and most often accompanied by nausea, photophobia, and exacerbation from physical activity. The headache is usually frontal or periorbital. Onset is rapid and crescendo is within hours. Migraines may recur daily, weekly, or less often. Migraine headache is most commonly found in adults 25 to 34 years of age and are rare during pregnancy. Chronic migraine is present when attacks occur more than 15 days in a month.

Migraine with Aura (Classic)

Classic migraine headaches are preceded by neurological signs that indicate cortical and/or brainstem involvement. Headaches may be precipitated by bright lights, noise, or tension. Auras may include visual disturbances (e.g., scintillating scotoma—a pattern of twinkling colored lights), ascending paresthesias or numbness, weakness, and aphasia. The pain may be associated with photophobia, phonophobia (noise sensitivity), nausea, and vomiting. Aura usually precedes but may accompany a headache or occur without headache.

Mixed Headache

Mixed headaches are a combination of muscular contraction and vascular dysfunction. The headache is experienced as a throbbing, constant pain during waking hours with symptoms of tightness, pressure, and muscle contraction. Family history of migraine is not uncommon.

Cluster Headache

Cluster headaches are of vascular origin and are less common than migraines. The onset is abrupt, often during the night, and the severity increases steadily. The pain is unilateral, ocular, or periocular and described as burning, piercing, or neuralgic. Cluster headaches occur more often in men and last 15 minutes to 2 hours. The episodic recurrences are "clustered" in cycles of days or weeks, with remission lasting months to years. Associated symptoms include ipsilateral rhinorrhea, conjunctival injections, facial sweating, ptosis, and eyelid edema. Alcohol ingestion, stress, or vasodilation secondary to wind or heat exposure may precipitate the pain.

Benign Exertional Headache

These headaches occur suddenly and are related to coughing, sneezing, straining, running, or orgasm. Headache is the result of stretching the pain-sensitive structures in the posterior fossa. They are more common in men. The onset is sudden and "splitting," and pain may last from seconds up to 30 minutes. They should be distinguished from headache of SAH or arterial dissection.

Secondary Headaches
Infectious Origin

Sinusitis. Sinusitis is frequently associated with a sore throat irritated by postnasal discharge, facial or tooth pain, or a headache over the affected sinus that increases in intensity with coughing or bending forward. There frequently is a cough that worsens in a lying position, morning periorbital swelling, fever, malaise, and recent upper respiratory tract infection. The maxillary sinuses are the most often affected. Pain in the temporal and periorbital area suggests frontal sinusitis, whereas maxillary sinusitis produces pain below the eye, in the upper teeth, or both. Ethmoid sinusitis produces medial orbit pain.

Dental disorders. Patients with dental abscess, nerve root dysfunction, or infection may have headache and facial pain located near the site of the lesion.

Tenderness elicited by tapping on the maxillary teeth with a tongue blade may indicate dental root infection or maxillary sinusitis. Inspection of the mouth may reveal ulceration or infection of pain-sensitive structures in the oral mucosa and gingiva.

Pharyngitis. Bacterial infection may irritate pain-sensitive structures in the oropharynx, leading to headache.

Otitis media. Recurrent otitis media with sequelae of mastoiditis or chronic infection may result in headache. Signs of otitis will be seen on examination of the tympanic membrane.

Meningitis. Bacterial meningitis begins as bacteria colonize in the nasopharynx and enter the central nervous system through the dural venous sinuses or choroid plexus into the subarachnoid space. Common causal organisms in adults are *S. pneumoniae* and *meningitidis*. In children, common organisms are *S. pneumoniae* and *Haemophilus influenzae*; in neonates, group B *Streptococcus* and *Escherichia coli*. Bacterial meningitis is usually accompanied by severe systemic toxicity and mental status changes (encephalitis). In contrast, aseptic meningitis caused by enteroviruses or mumps virus produces a mild illness sometimes without fever. Photophobia and stiff neck are present in varying degrees. The person usually appears ill with a severe headache, fever, chills, myalgias, photophobia, and stiff neck. The Brudzinski and Kernig signs may be positive. A petechial skin rash may suggest meningeal disease. Patients may progress to coma and have seizures.

Neurogenic Origin

Trigeminal neuralgia. The pain associated with malfunction of the trigeminal nerve (cranial nerve V) is characterized by episodes of a series of bursts or jabs of sharp electrical, stabbing pain lasting seconds that occur repeatedly over minutes or hours with a minute or so of relief between episodes. The pain is limited to the distribution of the three branches of cranial nerve V. Headaches caused by trigeminal neuralgia are stimulated by sensory stimuli to the involved nerves, produced by rubbing or touching the face or swallowing. Trigeminal neuralgia usually occurs in women and persons more than 55 years old. In younger patients, episodes may suggest multiple sclerosis.

Optic neuritis. Optic neuritis refers to a variety of conditions that affect the optic nerve and reduce visual function. Disorders include demyelinating disease (such as multiple sclerosis), inflammation, viral illness, metabolic disorders, and toxin exposure. The patient has an acute onset of blurred vision with extraocular motion pain that precedes the visual changes by several days. Ophthalmoscopic examination reveals a slightly elevated (hyperemic) disc and a blurred disc margin. Treatment is focused on the underlying disease.

Cervical spine disorders. The three upper cervical nerves are sensory pathways for pain sensation felt in the posterior head and ipsilateral temporal and eye areas (see Figure 18-2). Disturbances in the neck may cause muscle spasms and pressure on other neck structures. Patients with neck-related headache have pain associated with motion of the neck. Downward pressure on the head makes the pain worse and may cause it to travel down the arms.

Temporal arteritis (giant cell arteritis). Temporal arteritis is a vasculitis of the ophthalmic and posterior ciliary branches of the internal carotid artery. It almost always afflicts persons more than 50 years old. It produces a sharp, localized pain over a tender, nodular temporal artery. Other symptoms include fever, malaise, anorexia, weight loss, and/or polymyalgia rheumatica. Ischemic jaw pain and face pain are rare but highly suggestive. Headaches precede the major danger of temporal arteritis—blindness—by weeks. Unilateral blindness may occur suddenly and is not reversible. Left untreated, blindness may occur in the other eye. An ESR >50 mm/hr is almost always present. Suspected temporal arteritis is an emergency, and the patient needs referral to an emergency center for immediate evaluation and treatment.

Metabolic Origin

Carbon monoxide poisoning. CO is a colorless, odorless gas with an affinity for binding with hemoglobin to produce carboxyhemoglobin (COHb), which impairs oxygen transport. Symptoms are nonspecific and are dose related. Low COHb levels may produce mild dyspnea and tightness across the head; however, as COHb concentration increases, the headache becomes more severe and is associated with dizziness, nausea, fatigue, and dimmed vision. As COHb levels rise, symptoms increase in severity and lead to loss of consciousness and seizures. Blood gases and COHb blood levels are diagnostic. History may suggest recent smoke inhalation or similar symptoms in multiple family members.

Severe hypoglycemia. Hypoglycemia is more likely to occur in persons with type 1 diabetes but can occur in anyone taking oral hypoglycemic agents, in younger persons who experience reactive hypoglycemia, or in persons who have ingested excessive amounts of alcohol. A dietary and medication history may lead to a specific causative factor. Headache is generalized and bilateral and is associated with dizziness and a sense of not feeling well. Some persons with diabetes may have nocturnal hypoglycemia and report nightmares and vivid dreams, night sweats, and a headache on awakening. Blood glucose levels can confirm the presence of hypoglycemia.

Drug withdrawal. Withdrawal from prolonged use of steroids may cause migrainous headaches. Nitrites may precipitate headache. Other drugs causing cranial dilation and an aftereffect of rebound vasoconstriction include hydralazine, alcohol, histamine, nicotinic acid, and caffeine.

Dietary ingestion. A mild to moderately severe generalized headache may occur after ingestion of tyramines (e.g., aged cheese, red wine), monosodium glutamate, and nitrites in smoked meats. A headache diary will help identify the pattern of headache related to specific foods.

Cerebrovascular Origin

Intracranial tumor. Intracranial tumors are more common in children than adults. Brain metastases from primary sites in the lung, breast, or kidney are more common in adults. Pain is constant and progressive, is felt in a discrete location, changes with head position, and awakens the person from sleep. Objective neurological signs are present in 98% of all children with brain tumors.

Hydrocephalus. Hydrocephalus is a collection of cerebrospinal fluid (CSF) in the ventricles of the brain and can be caused by tumors or cysts. If fontanels are still open, hydrocephalus will cause an enlargement of the head on measurement. Headache will be progressive and may be associated with neurological findings and mental status changes similar to those observed with dementia. Radiographic techniques are diagnostic, and LP may detect increased CSF pressure.

Subdural hematoma. Subdural hematoma produces a sudden, severe headache that is associated with a history of head trauma, exertional physical activity, or pharmacological anticoagulation. There is transient loss of consciousness, stiff neck, nausea, vomiting, photophobia, pupillary dilation, and pain over the eye. A thorough history of trauma is essential to obtain. Posttrauma headache can occur hours or a day after injury.

Pseudotumor cerebri. Teenagers being treated with topical acne preparations, menopausal women, and persons ingesting large amounts of vitamin A are at increased risk for pain from pseudotumor cerebri. Papilledema will be present in many cases, but, without it, the headache may be diagnosed as mixed type. A neurology referral is indicated to ensure that no local obstruction is present before an LP is done to assess for increased intracranial pressure. LP sometimes leads to herniation of the brainstem.

Brain abscess. Pain is of gradual onset, deep and aching in nature, often worse in morning, and aggravated by coughing or straining. Other signs of increased intracranial pressure may be present, such as papilledema and widening pulse pressure. There may be a recent history of head injury, infection, or assault to the central nervous system.

Intracerebral hemorrhage. ICH may result in a stroke or sudden coma and is associated with neurological findings defined by the site of bleeding. A person may present with a sudden-onset, severe headache, with or without a history of trauma. The severity of symptoms from bleeding intracranial aneurysms is correlated to the rate of hemorrhage and graded from I (asymptomatic to minimal headache with nuchal rigidity) to V (deep coma, decerebrate rigidity). Elderly persons with AIDS and persons prescribed anticoagulation therapy are at increased risk for ICH. CT scan is diagnostic.

DIFFERENTIAL DIAGNOSIS OF *Common Causes of Headache*

CONDITION	HISTORY	PHYSICAL FINDINGS	DIAGNOSTIC STUDIES
Primary Headaches Without Structural or Systemic Pathology			
Tension-type headache (muscle)	Common in adults; bilateral pain, general or localized in bandlike distribution; history of anxiety, stress, or depression	Normal physical examination; neck muscle tightness or fasciculations may be palpated	None
Migraine without aura (common)	More common in children; unilateral, throbbing pain; nausea	Photophobia and phonophobia	None
Migraine with aura (classic)	Pain precipitated by environmental stimuli; visual disturbances (scintillating scotoma) precede pain	Nausea and vomiting, photophobia and phonophobia	None
Mixed headache	Throbbing, constant pain during waking hours; muscle tightness; family history of migraine	Mix of findings related to tension and migraine headache pain	None
Cluster headache	Rare in children; abrupt, nighttime onset; unilateral periorbital pain that is severe	Ipsilateral rhinorrhea, nasal stuffiness, conjunctival injection, sweating, ptosis	None
Benign exertional headache	Sudden onset related to physical exertion, Valsalva, or coitus	Normal physical examination	May need to distinguish from subarachnoid hemorrhage with CT scan
Secondary Headaches with Structural or Systemic Pathology			
Infectious Origin			
Sinusitis	Frontal, upper molar, or periorbital pain; cough, rhinorrhea	Low to no fever; pain on palpation of frontal, maxillary sinuses; purulent nasal or postnasal discharge	Radiographs (Waters view)
Dental disorders	Localized pain in jaw and top of head	Malocclusion, caries, abscesses of teeth present, gum disease	Dental referral
Pharyngitis	Sore throat	Fever; infection of posterior pharynx	Throat culture
Otitis media	Ear pain, pain with swallowing	Fever; red, bulging tympanic membrane	None
Meningitis	Severe headache, chills, myalgias, stiff neck; toxic child or adult	Positive Kernig's and Brudzinski's signs; fever, photophobia, petechial rash may be present; mental status changes	Lumbar puncture
Neurogenic Origin			
Trigeminal neuralgia	Persons >55 yr; bursts of sharp pain over face innervated by affected nerve; triggered by stimulus to affected nerve	Normal physical examination; stimulation of triggers may provoke pain	None
Optic neuritis	Acute onset of pain with extraocular movement (EOM), followed by blurred vision	Diminished visual acuity, decreased papillary reflex, hyperemia of optic disc; pain with EOM	Ophthalmology referral
Cervical spine disorders	May have history of trauma; occipital pain, muscle stiffness	Normal physical examination or pain associated with neck motion	Cervical spine radiographs

DIFFERENTIAL DIAGNOSIS OF *Common Causes of Headache—cont'd*

CONDITION	HISTORY	PHYSICAL FINDINGS	DIAGNOSTIC STUDIES
Temporal arteritis	Age >50 yr; sharp, localized temporal pain; malaise, anorexia; history of polymyalgia rheumatica	Fever, weight loss; tender over a nodular temporal artery	Elevated ESR (>50); immediate referral for treatment
Metabolic Origin			
Carbon monoxide poisoning	History of exposure; throbbing headache, mild dyspnea	Nausea, vomiting, change in mental status, lethargy, loss of consciousness	Blood gases and carboxyhemoglobin level
Severe hypoglycemia	History of diabetes or medication, alcohol, and food ingestion; generalized headache, dizziness, sense of not feeling well	Normal physical examination or pallor, sweating, and weakness	Blood glucose level; may need self-monitoring of blood glucose to establish pattern
Drug withdrawal	Pattern of headache associated with stopping medication or substance use	Normal physical examination	Blood chemistry
Dietary ingestion	Mild to moderately severe headache after ingestion of foods or medication	Normal physical examination	Blood chemistry
Cerebrovascular Origin			
Intracranial tumor	Sudden-onset headache that is progressive, exacerbated by coughing or exercise; worse in morning; history of trauma increases risk	Papilledema, vomiting, asymmetrical reflexes, weakness, sensory deficit, or other neurological deficit	CT scan
Hydrocephalus	Progressive headache, vomiting, irritability	Rapid enlargement of head, bulging fontanels	CT scan and referral
Subdural hematoma	History of head trauma, bleeding disorders, child abuse; adult >35 yr; sudden onset of "worst headache ever," often over eye; transient loss of consciousness	Unequal pupils, photophobia, neurological changes, seizure	CT scan and neurosurgical referral
Pseudotumor cerebri	Teens, menopausal women; history of vitamin A or tetracycline ingestion; progressive headache	Papilledema may be present	CT scan, neurology referral to assess risk related to lumbar puncture
Brain abscess	History of chronic ear infection or cyanotic heart disease	Fever, seizures, focal neurological deficits	CT scan
Intracerebral hemorrhage	Risk factors: persons >50 yr, with AIDS, taking anticoagulation therapy	If conscious, abnormal neurological findings correlated with extent of lesion	Emergency transport for immediate evaluation or with hypertension (CT scan) and possible surgical treatment

AIDS, acquired immune deficiency syndrome; *CT*, computed tomography; *ESR*, erythrocyte sedimentation rate.

REFERENCES AND READINGS

American College of Emergency Physicians: Clinical policy: critical issues in the evaluation and management of patients presenting to the emergency department with acute headache, *Ann Emerg Med* 39:108, 2002.

Davenport R: Headache, *Pract Neurol* 8:33, 2008.

Dodick DW: Pearls: headache, *Semin Neurol* 30:74, 2010.

Kabbouche M, Cleves C: Evaluation and management of children and adolescents presenting in an acute setting, *Semin Pediatr Neurol* 17:105, 2010.

Kaniecki R: Headache assessment and management, *JAMA* 289:1430, 2003.

Lewis DW: Pediatric migraine, *Pediatr Rev* 28:43, 2007.

Lipton RB, Bigal ME, Steiner TJ, Silberstein SD, Olesen J: Classification of primary headaches, *Neurology* 63:427, 2004.

Manzoni GC, Torelli P: Headache screening and diagnosis, *Neurol Sci* 25: S255, 2004.

Purdy RA: Clinical evaluation of a patient presenting with headache, *Med Clin North Am* 85:847, 2001.

Smetana GW: The diagnostic value of historical features in primary headache syndromes, *Arch Intern Med* 160:2729, 2000.

Stafstrom CE, Rostasy K, Minster A: The usefulness of children's drawings in the diagnosis of headache, *Pediatrics* 109:460, 2002.

Hoarseness

Hoarseness is a disturbance of the normal voice pitch by an abnormal vibration of the vocal cords. It is a term used to describe an unnaturally rough, harsh, or deep voice. Voice is the sound produced when the vocal folds are approximated and expired airflow between the cords causes them to vibrate. The sound produced by the larynx is amplified by the pharynx, oral cavity, sinuses, and nasal cavity and is modified by movements of the tongue, uvula, and soft palate. Hoarseness may be an early sign of local disease or a manifestation of a systemic illness. Hoarseness is a cardinal symptom for laryngeal disease.

The larynx is a musculocartilaginous structure lined with a mucous membrane connected to the superior part of the trachea and to the pharynx inferior to the tongue and hyoid bone. It is the sphincter that guards the entrance into the trachea and functions secondarily as the organ of voice. Nine cartilages connected by ligaments and eight muscles form the larynx. The lower portion of the thyroarytenoid muscle forms the true vocal fold, or folds, which are highly elastic and account for the extraordinary versatility of the voice and the wide range of pitch, volume, and quality. The glottis is the triangular opening between the true vocal cords. The supraglottic area includes the ventricular folds (false vocal cords), aryepiglottic folds, and the epiglottis (Figure 19-1). The epiglottis is the lidlike cartilaginous structure that overhangs the entrance to the larynx and serves to prevent food from entering the larynx and trachea while swallowing.

Many benign conditions cause hoarseness, such as functional disorders from voice overuse. Functional causes are unrelated to organic disease and may have a psychosocial component, such as restraint in expressing anger, or crying, or a history of psychological trauma.

However, persistent hoarseness for more than 2 weeks in an adult and 1 week in a child may indicate secondary changes to the vocal cords. These changes may be caused by structural changes resulting from palsies, polyps, or cysts; laryngeal neoplasm; or congenital disorders of the larynx. Hoarseness may also be a symptom of systemic disease, such as hypothyroidism, or a symptom of inflammation caused by a variety of processes. Many forms of laryngitis that appear alike on physical examination have very different causes; critical clues to the specific etiology of laryngitis depend on a careful history.

DIAGNOSTIC REASONING: FOCUSED HISTORY

Is the hoarseness acute or chronic?

Key Questions

- How long has the symptom been present?
- Has this happened before? Is it recurrent?
- Is it getting better or worse?

Duration

Symptoms of less than 2 weeks' duration are considered to be acute; the most likely cause is a viral upper respiratory tract infection. Inflammations secondary to acute viral infection or voice overuse are the most common causes of acute laryngitis. Chronic symptoms suggest structural change in the larynx or hoarseness secondary to disorders, such as gastroesophageal reflux disease (GERD) or systemic disease. If the duration of hoarseness is longer than 2 weeks, referral to an ear, nose, and throat specialist is indicated to evaluate for neoplasm, most often squamous cell carcinoma, because chronic laryngitis is rarely of an infectious etiology.

Recurrence

Recurrent episodes of hoarseness may indicate allergies or sinusitis with postnasal drip.

Progression

Progressive hoarseness usually indicates a lesion, such as a laryngeal or hypopharyngeal cyst.

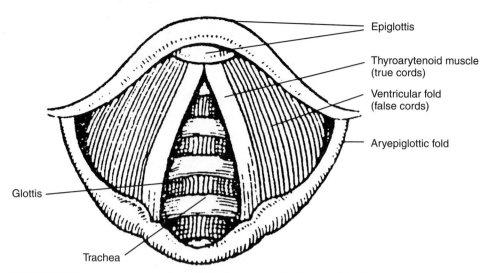

Epiglottis

Thyroarytenoid muscle
(true cords)

Ventricular fold
(false cords)

Aryepiglottic fold

Glottis

Trachea

FIGURE 19-1 Laryngoscopic view of the interior of the larynx. (Modified from Greene MCL, Mathieson L: *The voice and its disorders*, ed 5, London, 1989, Wiley. Copyright John Wiley & Sons Limited. Reproduced with permission.)

What does the onset of hoarseness tell me?

Key Questions

- How did the hoarseness develop?
- Is there any history of trauma to the throat?
- Have you had any recent surgery around the throat or neck?

Onset

Acute onset of hoarseness is usually the result of infection or trauma. The trauma can be from direct injury (foreign body, accidents) or overuse from screaming. The overuse can be gradual, resulting in progressive hoarseness and vocal cord changes. This hoarseness is worse in the afternoon or evening.

Hoarseness from birth may indicate a congenital problem, such as laryngeal web, cyst, palsy, or angioma. Newborns with aphonia or a hoarse cry that does not resolve may have a congenital anomaly, papilloma, or vocal cord paralysis.

Trauma

External trauma to the throat is a rare cause of hoarseness but can result in hematoma formation in the laryngeal soft tissues. There can also be mucosal lacerations, arytenoid cartilage dislocation, or fracture of the laryngeal cartilage. Internal trauma can occur with intubation associated with surgery, as occurs when an endotracheal tube catches on laryngeal structures and is pushed against resistance.

Surgical History

Tonsillectomy, thyroidectomy, or rhinoplasty can alter the quality of the voice secondary to structural change and scarring. Cardiac surgery has also been cited as a cause of injury when the vagus nerve (cranial nerve [CN] X) is damaged in its course around the aorta.

Does the presence of risk factors help narrow the diagnosis?

Key Questions

- Have you had a recent cold or upper respiratory tract infection?
- Do you have allergies or asthma?
- Do you smoke? How long have you been a smoker?
- How much alcohol do you drink?
- Can you describe your voice habits, such as singing, talking, and shouting?
- Are you frequently exposed to dust, fumes, or loud noise?
- Are your immunizations up to date?

Upper Respiratory Infection

Acute laryngitis, epiglottitis, and acute laryngotracheobronchitis (croup) are sequelae from a viral upper respiratory infection (URI) that can result in vocal cord inflammation. Postnasal discharge that is thick and purulent may pool around the larynx and cause chronic secondary edema. Nasal congestion that leads to mouth breathing produces laryngeal dryness, with resultant hoarseness on arising in the morning.

Children who have epiglottitis are not hoarse, but, as the epiglottis swells, the voice becomes muffled and drooling is observed.

Allergies and Asthma

Poorly controlled or undiagnosed asthma can result in a chronic cough with subsequent hoarseness. Allergies can cause chronic or recurrent irritation and swelling of both the upper and lower airways. Children who have a history of asthma and or allergies can develop vocal cord edema, inflammation, and hoarseness.

Smoking

Cigarette smoking is the most significant risk factor for laryngeal cancer. Smoking is also a risk factor for acute or chronic laryngitis because smoke irritates all mucous membranes and impairs ciliary function, causing pooling of secretions around the larynx.

Alcohol Consumption

Chronic consumption of hard liquor is a direct irritant to the throat and is associated with laryngeal cancer.

Voice Habits

Voice misuse occurs when the true vocal cords are forced to vibrate under undue stress and tension. Voice abuse is exuberant overuse and can lead to inflammation of the larynx and edema, hemorrhage, or vocal cord polyps. A gradual progression of hoarseness may go unnoticed by the patient. Often a precipitating incident (such as shouting, excessive speaking, or singing) produces acute laryngitis. Specific questions may need to be asked to make the patient aware of conditions that lead to voice abuse, such as the following:

- Have others noticed a change in the quality of your voice?
- Do you talk frequently to persons who are hard of hearing?

- Do you yell at children?
- Do you work in an environment that is noisy or contains dust or fumes?
- Have you attended a recent sporting event?

Exposures

Patients who are chronically exposed to work environments that contain dust, fumes, or a high noise level that leads to chronic voice abuse are at increased risk for laryngeal cancer.

Immunizations

Laryngeal diphtheria should be considered in patients who have failed to update their diphtheria immunizations. Updating the tetanus-diphtheria (Td) immunization is recommended every 10 years after the primary immunization series is completed. Laryngeal diphtheria usually develops as a downward progression of the tonsillar-pharyngeal membrane.

What other clues will help narrow the diagnostic possibilities?

Key Questions

- Does the hoarseness change during the day?
- Is it painful?
- What other symptoms are present?
- Do you have a neurological disorder?

Timing

Hoarseness that is altered by a position change suggests a mobile lesion, such as a pedunculated polyp. Patients with myasthenia gravis have a normal voice in the morning with progressive hoarseness throughout the day.

Pain

Pain may be associated with an inflammatory process, such as a viral URI or GERD. Pain occurs late in laryngeal cancer. Neurological and hormonal causes do not usually produce pain.

Associated Symptoms

The presence of cough, shortness of breath, weight loss, dysphagia, ear pain, or throat pain should raise concerns about neoplasm, systemic disease, or neurological causes. Hormonal disorders, such as hypothyroidism, will also produce signs and symptoms that vary in severity, according to the duration and degree of hormone deficiency. Early symptoms of hypothyroidism include cold intolerance, heavy menses, weight gain, dry skin, fatigue, and constipation. Later signs and symptoms include hoarseness, very dry skin, hair loss of lateral eyebrows, and neurological symptoms, such as delayed deep tendon reflex recovery, depression, and mental confusion.

Neurological Disease

Patients with Parkinson disease, myasthenia gravis, or amyotrophic lateral sclerosis have progressive dysarthria and dysphagia. As neurological disease progresses, patients will develop a chronic cough and throat clearing caused by microaspiration of pooled secretions.

Gastroesophageal Reflux Disease

Reflux of gastric contents causes inflammation of the posterior larynx, especially the arytenoid mucosa. The patient may also report a habit of frequent throat clearing and a sensation of a lump in the throat. Chronic cough or throat clearing further damages already irritated vocal folds. Generally patients have hoarseness in the morning and coughing at night. In children, GERD presents with dysphagia, vomiting, and failure to thrive.

DIAGNOSTIC REASONING: FOCUSED PHYSICAL EXAMINATION
Listen to the Quality of Voice

Acoustic evaluation criteria for voice include range (monotonic to extremely variable), loudness (soft to loud), pitch (low-pitched voice requires more effort to produce adequate volume; sudden changes in pitch), register (temporary loss of voice because of abductor spasm), and quality (roughness, breathiness, and hoarseness). Table 19-1 lists common criteria used in evaluating the voice.

Examine the Respiratory System

Assess the airway. Stridor, a high-pitched inspiratory sound caused by turbulent airway through a narrowed glottis secondary to inflammation or tumor, indicates an immediate referral to a specialist. If the patient is able to cough and laugh but cannot speak, this indicates a functional problem, because coughing and laughing require total adduction of the vocal cords. Auscultate the lungs for quality of breath sounds, asthmatic wheezing, and signs of consolidation.

Note any associated stridor in children. Inspiratory stridor may indicate an extrathoracic problem, such as supraglottic collapse or vocal fold paralysis. An intrathoracic lesion may cause an expiratory stridor.

Perform a General Inspection

Note hair distribution, especially signs of hair loss over lateral eyebrows and hair loss on scalp, to assess thyroid function. Look for the placement of the trachea and thyroid gland. Bulges or asymmetry of the neck suggest a tumor. A head and neck hemangioma or lymphangioma increases the possibility of a similar laryngeal lesion as the source of hoarseness.

Examine the Head and Neck

Examine the oral, pharyngeal, and nasal mucosa for signs of excessive dryness, inflammation, or infection. Excessive mucosal dryness, including the conjunctiva, may be secondary to medication use, such as decongestants and antidepressants, or may be a symptom of an autoimmune disorder, such as Sjögren syndrome.

Otoscopy may indicate otitis media with effusion, contributing to hearing loss, a factor to be considered in voice abuse. Inspect the nasal mucosa for color, edema, and purulent discharge, and examine

Table 19-1	Diagnostics Used in Evaluating Voice	
ACOUSTIC QUALITY	**MEASUREMENT**	**DISORDER**
Range	Monotonal to extremely variable	Monotonal: Parkinson disease, depression
Loudness	Soft to loud	Environmental, psychological, systemic disease
Pitch	Low to high; glottal, raspy to falsetto	Variable: puberty
		Low: male gender, overuse
Register	Presence of voice	Vocal fatigue, overuse
Quality	Breathy to resonant	Vocal cord mass, paresis, bowing, atrophy

the nasal septa for deviation that may cause obstruction. Hypertrophic tonsils and severe dental abnormalities (malocclusion, cleft palate) can contribute to hoarseness.

Any indication of airway obstruction associated with hoarseness is a potentially life-threatening situation. Do not perform a physical examination of the pharynx if you suspect acute epiglottitis. Examination may trigger laryngospasms and airway obstruction. Refer immediately for emergency treatment and airway support.

Examine the larynx indirectly using a laryngeal mirror. Patient cooperation is critical. Ask the patient to open the mouth wide and extend the neck while protruding the tongue. The mirror is advanced to contact and lift the uvula while the patient breathes through the mouth. Focus the light on the mirror after the mirror is angled to visualize the larynx. Ask the patient to say "e" or "a" to observe movement. Sometimes the epiglottis obscures visualization. Direct examination of the larynx with a laryngoscope requires the skill and experience of a specialist.

Observe the larynx for the presence of secretions and evidence of ulcers, polyps, masses, edema, or redness. Observe for vocal cord motion, especially adduction and abduction of vocal cords, and the presence of spasm or tremor.

Assess Cranial Nerve Function

Most of the CNs play a part in speech and voice production, and any disease process that affects neurological function, especially vocal cord paralysis, may affect the voice. Specifically examine CNs V, VII, VIII, IX, X, XI, and XII.

Assess Hearing (Cranial Nerve VIII)

Voice or whisper testing for hearing acuity is the first level of hearing screening. An audible whisper is approximately 20 decibels (dB), and normal speech is about 50 dB. Patients with neurosensory hearing loss may use abnormally loud speech.

Palpate Lymph Nodes

Palpate the cervicofacial lymph nodes. Tender nodes indicate inflammation; nontender nodes may indicate neoplasm. Enlarged nodes in the deep cervical chain in the absence of other symptoms may indicate laryngeal cancer.

Palpate Thyroid

Palpate the thyroid for size, tenderness, and crepitus by moving the thyroid cartilage across the cervical spine.

LABORATORY AND DIAGNOSTIC STUDIES
Flexible Fiberoptic Laryngoscopy

Laryngoscopy allows direct examination of the hypopharynx and larynx. A local anesthetic is applied to the oral or nasal mucosa, and the instrument is passed through the nose or oral cavity for excellent visualization of laryngeal structures. Laryngoscopy is also performed using a general anesthetic.

Radiography

Lateral view radiographs of soft tissues of the neck are used to evaluate structures for abnormalities.

Barium Esophagography

This contrast radiographic technique can be used to differentiate between mechanical lesions and motility disorders, providing important information about the latter in particular. For patients with esophageal dysphagia and a suspected motility disorder, barium esophagoscopy should be performed first.

DIFFERENTIAL DIAGNOSIS
Acute Laryngitis

Acute laryngitis is a self-limiting condition caused by a viral infection, environmental irritants, postnasal drainage secondary to poorly controlled allergic rhinitis, or voice overuse. The loudness and quality of voice are affected, and the patient may report a sore throat. Hoarseness often progresses throughout the course of the day. Indirect examination of the larynx reveals redness and edema of the vocal cords. Physical pathology may be absent in mild cases.

Acute Epiglottitis

Adults will report severe and rapidly progressing symptoms of sore throat, dyspnea, and hoarseness. In children, there is no cough or hoarseness, and drooling with a forward leaning posture is observed. This condition is most commonly associated with *Haemophilus influenzae* infection. Voice quality is frog-like. The patient will also have a high temperature and be anxious, fearful, and restless with respiratory distress.

Trauma

Any swelling in response to trauma, directly to the larynx or indirectly to the throat, will cause hoarseness. Swelling might be secondary to head and neck surgery, such as dental surgery, tonsillectomy, or thyroidectomy. Postintubation trauma may be acute if secondary to inflammation or chronic if neurological or structural damage is irreversible. Mucosal abrasion or ulcer may be caused by direct trauma to the larynx and is associated with painful phonation and a breathy voice.

Acute Laryngeal Edema

Laryngeal edema may be one symptom in a generalized allergic response that involves the lips, tongue, and other hypopharyngeal structures. Drug reactions and food allergies, especially to seafood and nuts, often precipitate this response. This condition is a medical emergency because of the high risk of airway obstruction.

Laryngotracheobronchitis (Croup)

Subglottic edema is caused by a viral infection, most often parainfluenza 1 virus, that can obstruct the airway. This condition is most common in children ages 3 months to 3 years of age and is more prevalent in the fall and winter. It is associated with a barking cough, dyspnea, wheezing, low-grade fever, and hoarseness. Inspiratory stridor occurs abruptly because of narrowing of the passage, causing negative pressures generated on inspiration. Physical examination can determine the degree of respiratory distress, such as color, stridor, nasal flaring, and level of consciousness.

Chronic Laryngitis

This condition is associated with a combination of chronic exposure to working conditions with high levels of dust, fumes, or noise; hard liquor consumption; cigarette smoking; and a history of frequent and persistent cough. Physical examination reveals edema or nodules of the vocal cords.

Polyps

Vocal cord polyps develop as a result of chronic inflammation from voice abuse, allergies, or GERD. The voice quality is breathy. With dependent polyps,

the patient may report that symptoms of hoarseness change with position.

Neoplasm

Laryngeal cancer usually occurs in patients who have a long history of cigarette smoking and alcohol consumption. Hoarseness is characterized by a raspy or harsh voice. Physical examination may reveal leukoplakia, or a white scaly appearance of the vocal cords. Patients do not usually report pain until carcinoma is advanced. Pain secondary to ulceration is late and is often perceived as ear pain, especially when swallowing.

Gastroesophageal Reflux Disease

Patients with GERD will report retrosternal burning (heartburn) that radiates upward. The regurgitation of gastric acid is exacerbated by consuming large meals, lying in a supine position, or bending over. Patients may describe a sour taste, experience salivary hypersecretion, have painful swallowing, or have a chronic cough or habit of throat clearing. Physical examination will be normal or epigastric tenderness may be elicited by abdominal examination. Inflammation or ulceration may be visible on the vocal cords.

Hypothyroidism

One symptom of hypothyroidism is a low, gravelly voice. The degree of hoarseness depends on the severity of thyroid deficiency. Usually the diagnosis of hypothyroidism is suspected when other symptoms are present, such as cold intolerance; rough, scaly skin texture; weight gain; and such signs as bradycardia and prolonged deep tendon reflex recovery. Risk factors for hypothyroidism include increased age, postpartum in women, and a family history of thyroid disease. The thyroid gland may be nonpalpable or enlarged. Examination of the larynx may reveal edema or polyps. An elevated serum thyroid-stimulating hormone (TSH) level will confirm the diagnosis.

Vocal Cord Paralysis

Paralysis is usually unilateral and produces a weak, breathy voice. Unilateral abductor paralysis on the left side is caused by pressure on the vagus or recurrent laryngeal nerve by a mass of malignant glands in the superior mediastinum or carcinoma of the thyroid or esophagus.

Psychogenic Hoarseness

Patients with psychogenic hoarseness will have a low, breathy voice caused by voluntarily abducting the vocal cords during phonation. Physical examination will be normal. Psychogenic hoarseness may follow a traumatic event.

Laryngeal Papillomas

These are the most common laryngeal lesions that occur during childhood. Most patients are between the ages of 2 and 7 and present with hoarseness. Occasionally papillomas, caused by the human papillomavirus, are seen in newborns.

DIFFERENTIAL DIAGNOSIS OF *Common Causes of Hoarseness*

CONDITION	HISTORY	PHYSICAL FINDINGS	DIAGNOSTIC STUDIES
Acute laryngitis	Voice overuse, exposure to environmental irritants, recent URI	Voice quality: aphonia, cervical lymphadenopathy; pharyngitis; edema and redness of vocal cords	None, if duration of hoarseness is <3 wk
Acute epiglottitis	Adults: rapid onset of sore throat, dyspnea, hoarseness; child: drooling, forward-leaning posture	Voice quality froglike; fever, signs of respiratory distress; drooling	Possible airway support; lateral and AP radiographic views of neck
Trauma	Hoarseness after intubation; direct throat trauma or foreign body	Subluxation of cricoarytenoid joint	Lateral and AP radiographic views of neck; laryngoscopy
Acute laryngeal edema	History of food or drug allergy	Edema of lips, tongue, and hypopharynx; observe for respiratory distress; voice quality breathy	Possible airway support
Laryngotracheobronchitis (croup)	Children 3 mo to 3 yr; recent URI	Barking cough, low-grade fever, wheezing, hoarseness; edema of vocal cords; observe for signs of respiratory distress	None initially, airway support may be necessary
Chronic laryngitis	Chronic history of smoking and alcohol use; exposure to environmental irritants; chronic cough; duration of hoarseness >3 wk	Edema of vocal cords; nodules may be present	Lateral and AP radiographic views of neck; laryngoscopy
Polyps	History of allergy; voice abuse, GERD, smoker; duration of symptoms >3 wk; progressive hoarseness, worse at end of day, but near normal in morning; hoarseness may change with position	Polyps visible on vocal cords	ENT referral for biopsy
Neoplasm	Smoking, airborne exposure, chronic alcohol use, history of chronic cough, hoarseness for >3 wk	Tracheal deviation; pain with advanced tumor; hoarseness may be only sign	ENT referral for biopsy

Continued

DIFFERENTIAL DIAGNOSIS OF *Common Causes of Hoarseness—cont'd*

CONDITION	HISTORY	PHYSICAL FINDINGS	DIAGNOSTIC STUDIES
GERD	History of upper GI burning; cough especially at night; chronic use of alcohol, NSAIDs, or aspirin; history of ulcer disease, smoker, age <45 yr; frequent throat clearing	May have epigastric tenderness on palpation; vocal cord inflammation or ulcers	Referral for endoscopy if symptoms not relieved with medication or dietary alterations
Hypothyroidism	Presence of systemic symptoms, such as cold intolerance, weight gain, fatigue; age >65 yr; postpartal women; family history of thyroid disease	Normal or enlarged thyroid gland, coarse hair, very dry skin, prolonged DTR recovery	TSH, free T_4 index
Vocal cord paralysis	Chronic cough; inspiratory or expiratory stridor with exertion	Breathy, weak, soft voice; abnormal movement (usually unilateral) of vocal cords; examination may suggest specific CN involvement	Refer for ENT evaluation
Psychogenic hoarseness	History of psychiatric illness or psychological trauma	Breathy, low voice; larynx will appear normal	As indicated to rule out other causes (i.e., lateral and AP radiographic views of neck); laryngoscopy
Laryngeal papillomas	Children 2-12 yr and may occur in infants; history of maternal human papillomavirus; may be recurrent, progressive	Faint cry, severe stridor, voice change, or complete aphonia	Refer for ENT evaluation

AP, anteroposterior; *CN,* cranial nerve; *DTR,* deep tendon reflex; *ENT,* ear, nose, and throat; *GERD,* gastroesophageal reflux disease; *GI,* gastrointestinal; *NSAIDs,* nonsteroidal anti-inflammatory drugs; T_4, thyroxine; *TSH,* thyroid-stimulating hormone; *URI,* upper respiratory tract infection.

REFERENCES AND READINGS

Banfield G, Tandon P, Solomons N: Hoarse voice: an early symptom of many conditions, *Practitioner* 244:267, 2000.

Dejonckere PH: Voice problems in children: pathogenesis and diagnosis, *Int J Pediatr Otorhinolaryngol* 49:S311, 1999.

Garrett CG, Ossoff RH: Hoarseness, *Med Clin North Am* 83:115, 1999.

Hartnick CJ, Cotton RT: Congenital laryngeal anomalies: laryngeal atresia, stenosis, webs, and clefts, *Otolaryngol Clin North Am* 33:1293, 2000.

McMurray JS: Disorders of phonation in children, *Ped Clin North Am* 50:2, 2003.

Schwartz SR, Cohen SM, Dailey SH, Rosenfeld RM, Deutsch ES, Gillespie MB et al: Clinical practice guideline: hoarseness (dysphonia), *Otolaryngol Head Neck Surg* 141:S1, 2009.

Sobol SE: Epiglottitis and croup, *Otolaryngol Clin North Am* 41:551, 2008.

Syed I, Daniels E, Blach NR: Hoarse voice in adults: an evidenced-based approach to 12 minute consultation, *Clin Otolarnygol* 34:54, 2009.

Van der Goten A: Evaluation of the patient with hoarseness, *Eur Radiol* 14:1406, 2004.

Wiatrak BJ: Congenital anomalies of the larynx and trachea, *Otolaryngol Clin North Am* 33:91, 2000.

Limb Pain

Reports of pain in a limb present a diagnostic challenge because of the many possible pathophysiological causes. Because of the broad range of differential diagnoses, it is best to use a framework of differentiating the pain as a symptom of musculoskeletal injury, musculoskeletal or joint disease, systemic disease, or a mixture of factors. Pain can be the result of a direct reaction in tissues, secondary reaction in adjacent tissues, or referral from a proximal or distal lesion or from organs such as the heart or kidney. In children, aches and pains in limbs are common; however, the presence, location, and intensity of the pain are often difficult to assess. Interpretation of pain is often made by the parents.

It is helpful to distinguish between limb pain that affects the bones, muscles, and tendons and injury/ inflammation of a joint that can affect surrounding musculature, nerves, and blood vessels. For example, lower extremity pain is often referred from the low back and emanates from irritated nerve roots or is secondary to myofascial syndromes of the low back, pelvic, and hip musculature.

DIAGNOSTIC REASONING: FOCUSED HISTORY

Is the pain related to an urgent problem that needs immediate treatment to avoid disability or death?

Key Questions

- Have you had a recent injury?
- Can you describe exactly how the injury occurred?
- Do you have any other symptoms, such as fatigue, fever, or swollen joints?
- What is the severity of the pain? Does it occur with exercise or rest?

Injury

Injuries to the musculoskeletal system can range from simple muscular strain to a significant fracture associated with nerve or vascular injury. Therefore, when a patient presents with a history of trauma, the priority is to assess the vascular integrity of the limb. Neurological integrity is next. Symptoms of coldness, severe pain, or paresthesia are signals that physical examination should begin immediately to assess the extent of injury and the need for emergency treatment. Acute pain and swelling that follow trauma usually indicate injury to a previously normal structure.

If the injury does not warrant urgent attention, obtain further history. Ask questions that specify the mechanism of injury, such as a direct blow or impact, landing position after a fall, twisting, jumping, running, overstretching, or overuse. When discussing the precipitating event, ask the patient to describe any noise such as snapping, popping, or breaking that may have occurred with the injury.

Constitutional Symptoms

The presence of generalized symptoms, such as fever, weight loss, general malaise, or hot swollen joints, suggests the presence of a systemic disorder such as infection or rheumatic disease. In addition, infection in a child causes systemic illness and the child appears ill.

Fever related to joint problems can be the result of hematogenous seeding by an organism, direct invasion as a result of trauma or puncture, or migration from an adjacent area of infection. In rheumatic fever, a ß-hemolytic streptococcal infection precedes the initial joint pain by 1 to 3 weeks. Often the hip joint may be the first of many joints affected before polyarticular migratory involvement occurs. The fever is sustained, not intermittent. Fever spikes are seen with chronic forms of arthritis in children.

Other systemic infections associated with polyarthritis include bacterial endocarditis, Lyme disease, syphilis, and such viruses as hepatitis B, rubella, cytomegalovirus, human immunodeficiency virus (HIV), Epstein-Barr virus, and varicella zoster.

Severity of Pain

Unrelenting diffuse pain, often occurring at night, is an indication of bone involvement, either through bone cancer or an infection such as osteomyelitis or septic hip. Claudication and neurogenic pain increase with activity and decrease with rest, more immediately for vascular causes and more slowly for neurogenic causes.

Lack of spontaneous movement of a limb in a child indicates pain and is often called *pseudoparalysis*.

What does the location of the pain tell me?

Key Questions

- Where does it hurt?
- Is the pain local or generalized?

Location

Location of pain provides a clue for identifying the site where the pain originates. Local pain receptors signal the site of irritation, and an increase in sensitivity (hyperesthesia) results. Referred pain generally involves the muscle chains, nerve pathways, and vessels. Unilateral, circumscribed limb or quadrant pain involves autonomic nerve fibers. Bilateral pain is more likely to originate from systemic involvement. Diffuse pain with inconsistent distribution may be the result of psychosomatic conditions such as depression and anxiety. Diffuse pain over trigger points is indicative of fibromyalgia. Collagen diseases and connective tissue diseases can affect one or more joints. The more vaguely defined the boundaries of the pain, the deeper or more central is the location of the somatic irritation. The obturator nerve has sensory branches that innervate the hip and skin on the medial aspect of the thigh, causing pain that comes from the hip to feel as though the pain is in the knee.

Could this be caused by a sprain or strain?

Key Questions

- Describe how the injury occurred.
- Did you hear a noise with the injury, such as a ripping or cracking sound?
- Were you able to use the limb after the injury?

Strain

A strain involves injury to muscles and tendons, whereas sprains involve injury to ligamentous structures. Both types of injuries can produce a ripping or tearing sound and range in severity from minor damage to a complete tear. Injuries are generally classified as mild, moderate, or severe. A moderate to severe strain/sprain may involve some loss of joint or ligament stability. Strains may be acute or chronic. Injury commonly occurs when lateral stress is applied while the joint is plantar flexed. This position is the least stable position of the ankle, and the overstretched ligaments are more susceptible to eversion or inversion forces.

Sprain

Sprains cause minimal to moderate pain increasing 1 to 2 days after the trauma when the inflammatory process begins. A complete disruption that severs the sensory nerve fibers within the structure will cause little pain, whereas a partial injury irritates sensory fibers and may produce intense pain.

In children, ligaments and joint capsules are two to five times stronger than the epiphysis; therefore, growth plate injuries are more common than sprains.

Fracture

A fracture produces diffuse swelling around the injured bone soon after injury. Deformity will be present if the fracture is displaced. A patient may report hearing a crack and being disabled by the increased severity of pain with weight bearing or movement of the limb. With stress fracture, there may be mild swelling and tenderness and pain with weight bearing.

If there is no history of trauma or a precipitating event, what else is causing the pain?

Key Questions

- Can you describe your usual daily activities at home, at work, and with hobbies?
- How does the pain affect your activities?
- Do you have other illnesses?

Overuse

Repetitive microtrauma results from cumulative injury or overuse. This type of trauma most often affects the fingers, wrists, and upper extremities. Persons who work on keyboards for long periods may complain of paresthesia of the fingers and pain and soreness of the wrists and fingers. Weekend hobbies or participation in sports may result in overuse of certain muscle groups associated with those activities.

Activities

A person may adapt to chronic musculoskeletal problems by using an assistive device such as a cane or by limiting activities. Rheumatic disorders produce symmetrical discomfort and pain with inactivity. Noninflammatory conditions are often associated with asymmetrical pain after extended use. Children will often avoid walking on a limb that causes pain. Infants will have lack of movement of the limb as well as irritability and fussiness when the limb is moved passively.

Other Illnesses

The presence of coronary artery disease increases the risk of arterial insufficiency and associated claudication pain. Peripheral neuropathy associated with diabetes can produce a burning pain or "pins and needles" sensation, especially in the lower extremities.

In joint pain with injury, what do I need to know about the specific joints involved?

Upper Extremity: Shoulder, Wrist, Elbow

Key Questions

- Is the pain in your dominant limb?
- Did you fall on an outstretched hand or arm?
- Did you overuse a joint?

Pain in the dominant hand may indicate repetitive microtrauma or overuse. Breaking a fall with an outstretched arm is a common mechanism of injury for a fracture or dislocation of the hand or wrist.

Lower Extremity: Knee, Ankle

Key Questions

- How is the pain affected by weight bearing or activity?
- Did you feel a sense of "giving way"?
- Did you hear a pop, tear, or other sound?
- In what position was your leg when you hurt your knee?

Continuing with an activity means the injury did not totally disrupt any ligamentous structures. An inability to straighten or bend the knee suggests a mechanical

blockage, such as a patellar dislocation or meniscus tear. In chondromalacia, the patient can bend the knee, but the movement is usually painful.

A loud pop is virtually diagnostic of an anterior cruciate ligament (ACL) tear. A ripping sound suggests a meniscus injury. A cracking sound may signify a bony injury or dislocation of the patella.

A quick change in direction or a sudden stop may put more force on the ligaments than they can dissipate, resulting in acute rupture. A sudden twisting injury is likely to represent a meniscus tear and a serious ligament disruption. Running or jumping activities are commonly associated with knee and ankle injuries.

In children, 10% to 20% of knee symptoms are the result of a problem in the hip joint.

Could this be musculoskeletal or joint disease?

Key Question

- Can you describe the pain?

In general, sharp, piercing, stabbing, cutting, pinching, gnawing pain is most common with lesions of the nerves and skin. Dull, tearing, boring, burning, and cramping are common terms used to describe pain arising from deeper structures such as muscles, joints, and internal organs. Pulsating, pounding, throbbing, and hammering are common descriptions of vascular pain. Gradually increasing sensations of pressure, tension, heaviness, and calf pain indicate venous obstruction. Severe pain that develops over 1 to 4 days is typical of osteomyelitis or septic arthritis in children, which is an emergency condition.

Muscle pain is caused by receptors located in bursa, muscle fibers, ligaments, and tendon attachments. It is a diffuse, dull, gnawing, boring, or tearing pain that increases with use and decreases with rest.

Intraarticular pain arises from receptors of the synovial membrane, joint capsule, or the fibrochondral layers of the articular surfaces. Joint pain is either inflammatory or degenerative. Inflammatory joint pain radiates diffusely to surrounding tissues. It is intense, sharp, burning, boring, or pulsating (effusion) pain. It persists during rest and is evident especially at night, worsening in the morning with stiffness that lasts more than 45 minutes, and then improves throughout the day.

Degenerative joint pain radiates to the soft tissue structures around the joint (i.e., muscles, ligaments, tendons). It is dull, boring, and gnawing when associated with muscle pain, or it can be a sharp, acute pain that increases with overuse.

Bone lesions cause a dull ache; periosteal pain is sharp and not well localized, and increases in intensity with dependency of the extremity.

Neuralgic pain occurs in the distribution of a peripheral nerve or nerve root. The pain is stabbing or cutting and can also present as pricking or lacerating.

What does the history of swelling tell me?

Key Questions
- Is there any swelling?
- When did the swelling begin?

Swelling

Swelling around a joint is always abnormal. Children do not always recognize swelling; they often report that they cannot squat down or flex their knee fully because it feels "full or tight."

Generally, swelling that develops immediately or within 2 hours after an injury is the result of a fracture or hemarthrosis and indicates a severe injury. Swelling 6 to 24 hours after an injury is usually of synovial origin, such as a meniscal tear, subluxation, dislocation, or ligamentous damage. Swelling after 24 hours suggests an inflammatory response.

Is this an acute or a chronic problem?

Key Questions
- When did the pain first occur?
- When did you first notice a problem?

Pain experienced hours after an injury or physical activity is usually caused by acute extensor injury or overuse. Severe ligament sprain is manifested as an immediately disabling pain at the moment of the injury.

Determining if the complaint is acute or chronic helps to differentiate the cause. Chronic joint problems compound each other, whereas intermittent or episodic pain is characteristic of diseases of the musculoskeletal system. In children, limping or not using the extremity may be a signal that the child is experiencing pain. Parents will often note the loss of motion in an extremity or an awkward gait; they often report that the child is unable to perform routine activities.

Patients may report noticing pain, weakness, or difficulty in activities of daily living, such as using a hair dryer, opening jars, holding a pen, or handling eating utensils.

How is activity affected?

Key Questions
- What are your usual activities?
- What activity makes the pain worse?
- What movements make the pain worse?

A large percentage of musculoskeletal injuries are caused by repetitive motion that leads to microtrauma and eventually cumulative damage. Repetitive microtrauma in the lower extremities from inappropriate rate and intensity of training, shoe wear, or playing surfaces can cause stress fractures of the weight-bearing bones of the lower limbs. Pain is worse over the site of the fracture.

In children, pain in the groin or referred to the knee and anterior thigh, occurring intermittently after activity and gradually becoming constant, may indicate Legg-Calvé-Perthes disease (LCPD).

Intraarticular lesions usually worsen with joint motion and sports activities. Intraosseous tumors are less sensitive to joint motion.

In children with a septic hip, pain increases with movement.

What does joint stiffness or locking tell me?

Key Questions
- Have you had any joint stiffness?
- Does activity make the stiffness worse or better?
- Do you have locking of the knee?

Joint Stiffness or Locking

Stiffness is felt after being in one position for a long time. This complaint gets confused with locking of the knee, which is an abrupt occurrence where the patient complains that something "gets in the way" and is unable to fully extend the knee. Manipulation of the leg often results in an equally abrupt unlocking. This is usually a sign of a chronic unstable meniscus tear.

Stiffness is a common feature of any inflammatory arthropathy. It is important to know whether it is localized or generalized. The length of time the stiffness lasts in the morning is a useful index of active synovitis in disease states such as rheumatoid arthritis (RA) or systemic lupus erythematosus (SLE). With most inflammatory arthropathies, stiffness and pain are alleviated by activity, whereas mechanical problems are aggravated by activity. Musculoskeletal tumors commonly present with mild joint stiffness because of muscle involvement but rarely demonstrate instability.

What does the history of a limp tell me?

Key Questions

- Is there pain with the limp?
- Did the limp develop suddenly?
- Is the limp constant or intermittent?
- What is the effect of running or climbing stairs?

Limp

Limping is a pathological alteration of a smooth, regular gait pattern and is never normal. Gait can be divided into two phases: stance and swing. The stance phase starts with the foot in contact with the ground and ends with the toe being lifted off the ground; the limb supports all the body weight. The swing phase begins with the toe elevated from the ground and ends with the heel strike. During the swing phase, the foot is not touching the ground; the pelvis rotates forward and tilts slightly while the trunk maintains a neutral position. Limp after strenuous running may indicate a stress fracture.

Quadriceps weakness causes difficulty in climbing stairs. During ambulation, this weakness causes the knee to be unstable on heel strike, and assistance is needed to push the knee manually into an extended position.

Neuromuscular diseases can result in progressive and painless muscle weakness or spasticity that affects ambulation in a variety of ways.

Symptoms of pain and limping in children may be incorrectly attributed to trauma instead of a more serious problem such as neoplastic tumors or bone infections.

Could this be caused by systemic disease?

Key Questions

- Have you been treated with antibiotics recently?
- Have you had any recent immunizations?
- Does the pain awaken you at night?
- Is the pain worse at night?

Medications

Certain antibiotics can cause serum sickness in children, producing joint pain and fever.

Transient arthralgia may occur 6 to 8 weeks after receiving MMR (measles, mumps, rubella) immunization. Recurrent or permanent arthritis may follow rubella vaccination, especially in adult females.

In adults, fluoroquinolone antibiotics can produce tendinitis or tendon rupture.

Night Pain

Intense pain may occur at rest and during the night. At first the pain may occur only when the patient changes position while sleeping; however, as the pain increases, it will disrupt sleep. Report by an adolescent of night pain is a red flag for the intraosseous pain of a bone tumor. Pain in the lower limbs in children 6 to 12 who are in a rapid linear growth period may awaken a child at night. The cause of these "growing pains" is unknown, but they are thought to result from muscle structures that have to catch up with bone growth. The pains are usually bilateral with no objective findings.

Could the pain be caused by Lyme disease?

Key Questions

- Have you been camping or spending time in wooded areas?
- Have you noticed any skin rash?

Lyme Disease

Lyme disease is an infection caused by the tick-borne spirochete *Borrelia burgdorferi*. Early symptoms include diffuse arthralgias, myalgias, fever, chills, and a characteristic targetlike rash. Although the arthralgia may involve multiple joints, usually the knee is the affected joint. Joint manifestations occur 1 week to 2 years following the initial illness. Patients may or may not recall the antecedent tick bite or exposure.

What does the medical history tell me?

Key Questions

- Have you had anything like this before?
- Do you have a chronic disease?
- Could you have been exposed to any sexually transmitted infection?
- Have you been treated with cortisone?
- Have you had a recent upper respiratory tract infection?

Chronic diseases, such as sickle cell anemia, inflammatory bowel disease, Crohn disease, hypothyroidism and hyperthyroidism, and collagen vascular diseases, are frequently associated with skin rashes, psoriasis, and limb and joint pain.

Gonorrhea disseminates to the musculoskeletal system in 1% to 3% of individuals with the disease. Of these, more than 80% develop arthritis.

Patients with chronic illness that requires long-term administration of corticosteroids are at risk for cortisone-induced necrosis of the hip. Sickle cell anemia can cause hip pain during a sickle cell crisis. Viral infections may cause diffuse myalgia.

Is this a mixed condition?

Consider the possibility that a patient may have a condition that is a mix of factors, such as a systemic disorder that has resulted in an acute injury. Clues to mixed etiology might include an injury that seems out of proportion to the extent of the precipitating activity or the presence of a chronic condition or other symptoms that might point to an undetected chronic condition. It is important to evaluate the limb pain in the context of the whole person.

DIAGNOSTIC REASONING: FOCUSED PHYSICAL EXAMINATION

Evaluation of musculoskeletal injuries should include examination of joint stability, deformity, and function. Examination should be done as soon after an injury as possible for an accurate diagnosis. Always observe for symmetry, and then functionally assess limbs and joints bilaterally, beginning with the unaffected side. Order the examination so that the most painful tests will be done last. See Figures 20-1 through 20-4 for anatomical landmarks of the shoulder, elbow, knee, and ankle.

Observe Patient Walking, Removing Coat/Jacket, Getting Into a Seated Position

Subtle clues of child abuse must be considered when the patient history is not consistent with the type or extent of injury. Abuse should always be considered in an infant within the first year when symptoms and history suggest a fracture, multiple injuries, rotational injuries, or multiple bruises in different states of healing. Radiographs may show previous fractures.

Persons who have septic joints appear ill, and movement of the joint will increase the pain. Inspect the patient with minimal clothing obstructing your

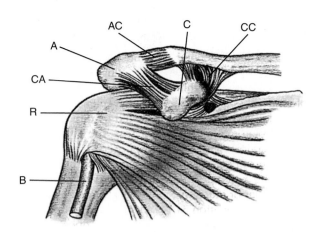

FIGURE 20-1 Bones and ligaments of the shoulder. *R,* Rotator cuff; *B,* long head of the biceps; *AC,* acromioclavicular joint capsule; *CC,* coracoclavicular ligaments; *A,* acromion; *C,* coracoid process; *CA,* coracoacromial ligaments. (From Mercier LR: *Practical orthopedics,* ed 6, St Louis, 2008, Mosby.)

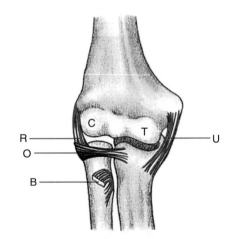

FIGURE 20-2 Bony and ligamentous anatomy of the elbow. *R,* Radial collateral ligament; *O,* orbicular ligament; *B,* biceps insertion; *U,* ulnar collateral ligament; *C,* capitellum; *T,* trochlea. (From Mercier LR: *Practical orthopedics,* ed 6, St Louis, 2008, Mosby.)

view of movements. A child with a septic hip lies with the thigh in a position of flexion, abduction, and external rotation and cries when a lower limb is moved.

In adults, an internally rotated abducted leg is the posture assumed with a posterior hip dislocation. An externally rotated hip and shortened lower extremity are signs of hip fracture.

General stiffness or limitation of motion of a single joint forces the surrounding joints to accommodate by

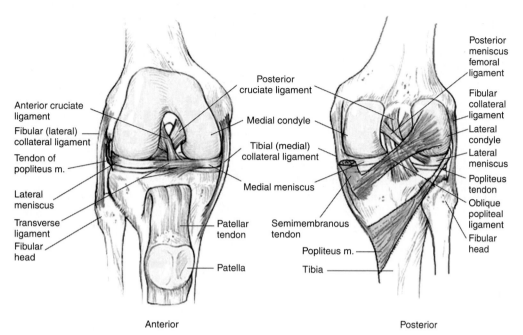

FIGURE 20-3 Basic anatomy of the right knee joint. (From Mathers LH et al: *Clinical anatomy principles*, St Louis, 1996, Mosby.)

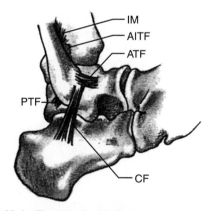

FIGURE 20-4 The lateral ankle ligaments—anterior and posterior talofibular (*ATF* and *PTF,* respectively) and calcaneofibular (*CF*). Also shown are the anterior inferior tibiofibular (*AITF*) ligament and the beginning of the interosseous membrane (*IM*). (From Mercier LR: *Practical orthopedics*, ed 6, St Louis, 2008, Mosby.)

moving with greater excursion or range of movement than usual. This makes the gait appear irregular or jerky.

Look for Limp

Pain, weakness, and deformity cause limping. Limping will be accentuated if the patient is asked to walk on the heels or tiptoes.

Common abnormal gaits related to limping are Trendelenburg gait, antalgic gait, and circumduction gait. Trendelenburg gait is a ducklike gait that reflects unilateral weakness of the gluteus medius muscle. The pelvis drops on the unaffected side during weight bearing on the affected side. In antalgic gait, there is an acute one-sided limp because the patient takes quick soft steps to shorten the period of weight bearing on the involved extremity. Stance time on the affected limb is decreased while stride length of the opposite side is shortened, allowing a quicker return of weight bearing to the unaffected limb. This is a reflex response to weight bearing on a painful limb.

Circumduction gait is seen with pathology of the foot or ankle and reduces discomfort by limiting movement of the ankle. The gait is characterized by a circular outward swing of the leg and external rotation of the foot that requires less ankle movement. External rotation of the entire extremity is seen with slipped capital femoral epiphysis.

Have the patient stand on one foot, and then the other. When standing on one leg, the gluteus medius on that side maintains the opposite side of the pelvis level, balancing the trunk over the weight-bearing hip. If the hip abductors are weak or painful, the opposite side of the pelvis dips down during the stance phase. With each step, the trunk shifts toward the side of a painful or weak extremity to decrease the force transmitted through the extremity to the hip.

Assessment of gait is best done either before or after examination, when patients are less aware that they are being observed.

Ankle plantar flexion and dorsiflexion are necessary for normal gait. If plantar flexion is restricted, there is no push-off and the forefoot and heel come off the floor at the same time. The result is a higher knee lift and the forefoot may slap against the floor. This condition is seen with weakness from peroneal nerve injury or with painful dorsiflexors associated with shin splints.

Observe the patient walking with and without shoes. If a child walks without difficulty with shoes off, the shoes are probably the problem. Inadequate shoe width is a common source of foot pain in children.

Have Patient Locate the Pain

Have the patient point to the area of pain. Location of pain and actual area of pathology may not be consistent. Hip pain often is referred to the knee area because the anterior branch of the obturator nerve passes close to the hip joint and, if irritated, provides a painful sensation to the medial side of the knee. True hip joint pain arises in the trochanteric bursa and is perceived in the groin area.

Shoulder pain from rotator cuff tendinitis is felt over the lateral aspect of the deltoid.

Swelling of the elbow may compress the ulnar nerve, producing a tingling sensation in the fourth and fifth fingers.

Pain in the groin, lateral hip, or knee in a child may indicate LCPD.

Pain in the groin, buttocks, or lateral hip in a child may indicate slipped femoral capital epiphysis.

Vague, nebulous discomfort in the front of the thighs, in the calves, and behind the knees located outside of the joints in a child may indicate growing pains.

Note Any Deformities

Fractures generally produce unilateral deformities or swelling in the extremities. Inflammatory and degenerative joint diseases produce observable joint swelling and deformity that usually occurs bilaterally.

Osteoarthritis typically involves the distal interphalangeal (DIP) and proximal interphalangeal (PIP) joints, spine, hips, knees, and first metatarsophalangeal (MTP) joints. Joints are enlarged with Heberden (DIP joints) and Bouchard (PIP joints) nodes. (See Figure 20-5.)

Joints affected by RA include PIPs, metacarpophalangeal (MCP), wrists, knees, elbows, cervical spine, and MTPs. Joints are swollen with a fusiform-shaped swelling of the PIP joints. Subluxation, ankylosis, and ulnar deviation may be observed as a result of joint destruction from chronic inflammation.

Assess Vital Signs

Elevated temperatures are seen with neoplastic, systemic, and infectious processes such as osteomyelitis, septic arthritis and septic hip in children, and rheumatic disease. Neonates may not exhibit a fever with a septic hip but may refuse to feed and will exhibit other symptoms of septicemia, such as lethargy and subnormal temperature. Palpate for quality and presence of pulses in any injured limb and compare to the opposite side. Assess peripheral pulses for presence, rate, regularity, strength, and equality.

Inspect the Skin and Nails

Inspect the skin for redness and inflammation. Chronic venous obstruction in the lower extremities causes a brownish coloring of the skin. Trophic skin changes from arterial insufficiency cause thin, shiny skin with an absence of hair and brittle nails.

Lyme disease usually presents with a rash before joint involvement; however, rash may occur concurrently. The rash, often characteristically found on the trunk, is an erythematous papule that develops into an

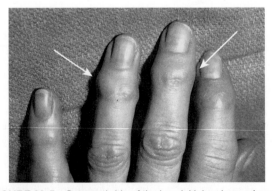

FIGURE 20-5 Osteoarthritis of the hand. Heberden nodes are shown at the DIP joints. (From Concannon MJ: *Common hand problems in primary care*, Philadelphia, 1999, Hanley & Belfus.)

annular lesion with a clear center. Concentric rings may develop, giving it a bull's-eye appearance (erythema migrans).

Look for a puncture or an abscess that could be the source of infection and seeding if a septic joint or osteomyelitis is suspected. Swelling and redness in a joint or in the midshaft of the tibia may be caused by osteomyelitis.

Look for an ingrown toenail that may alter gait. When the nails are trimmed by rounding off the edges, the hypertrophied and inflamed soft tissue fold can overlap the nail, and ingrowth at the distal margin will occur. Ingrown toenail pain is enhanced when tight-fitting shoes compress the soft tissues around the nail.

Look for ecchymosis and bruising. These indicate trauma as a source for pain as well as raise a suspicion of abuse. Ecchymosis indicates underlying bleeding and disruption of soft tissue or bone. Ecchymosis changes color over a period of days. Initially the color is dark red or violet, and in 1 to 3 days the bruise is blue-brown; in 1 week, it is yellow-green; and after 1 week, it is light brown. Ecchymosis resolves within 2 to 4 weeks.

Ecchymosis in the popliteal fossa after dislocation of the knee may be a sign of arterial disruption. Hemarthrosis, or bleeding into a joint, usually occurs within 1 to 2 hours after an injury and can occur secondary to hemophilia or other bleeding disorders, or it can be associated with visible ecchymoses caused by blood leaking into soft tissues.

Swelling and redness of a joint indicate underlying infection or inflammation. Edema will present as an asymmetrical area of swelling. Effusion, or fluid in the joint capsule, always distends the joint in a smooth, symmetrical manner.

Observe the muscles around the painful limb area. Decreased muscle tone or atrophy from disuse begins immediately after injury; however, it will not be clinically apparent for approximately 1 week.

Asymmetrical gluteal folds may indicate a congenital dislocated hip (Figure 20-6).

Measure Limb Circumference and Length

Use a tape measure to locate points at which to measure and compare limb circumference. Differences may be the result of muscle atrophy or edema. To measure leg length, have the patient lie supine with legs in comparable positions and measure the distance from the anterior iliac spines to the medial malleoli of the ankles. If a discrepancy is found, ask the patient to lie supine with knees flexed 90 degrees and feet flat on the table. If one knee is higher, the tibia of that extremity is longer. If one knee projects further anteriorly, the femur of that extremity is longer.

Palpate Extremities and Joints

Always palpate those areas that are suspected to be painless first and then compare with the affected limb.

Determine if there is edema (e.g., presence of interstitial fluid). Induration is interstitial swelling that has progressed and is now firm. An effusion is a collection of fluid in the joint capsule, which can be the result of rupture of a vascular structure or a synovial secretory response to an inflammatory process. The consistency of the fluid is noteworthy. Pus has a thick consistency and is less fluctuant than synovial fluid. Hematoma has a more gel-like consistency. Swelling in an ankle sprain is diffuse and nonfluctuant. Knee ligament sprain is much more fluctuant. To assess for fluid in the knee joint, press above the knee and watch the concave

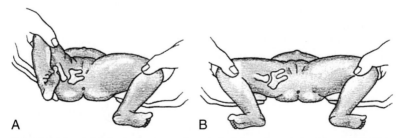

A   B

FIGURE 20-6 Ortolani sign for congenital dislocation of the hip. A "click" is palpable or audible as the hip is reduced by abduction. If the test is negative, the examination should always be repeated in 2 to 4 months. (From Mercier LR: *Practical orthopedics*, ed 6, St Louis, 2008, Mosby.)

or shallow areas of the joint become distended and bulge on either side of the kneecap. Note that swelling can extend above and below the point of pathology.

In severe knee trauma, rupture of the capsule allows fluid to escape into surrounding tissues, and less distention may be more apparent than with lesser injuries.

Palpate for fluid bulge if the knee is painful. Milk the fluid up into the suprapatellar pouch and then bring the hand down the lateral aspect of the knee looking for a medial fluid bulge. Palpate deeply to detect muscle fibrillation, fasciculation, or tumors.

Feel for heat in the affected joint, which can indicate an inflammatory or infectious process. Evaluate the joint for crepitus, both palpable and auditory. Tendinitis can produce a grating sensation on palpation of the ligament or a grating sound with movement.

Perform Passive/Active Range of Motion of All Limbs

Range of motion (ROM) may be limited because of pain, weakness, or deformity.

If pathology is in the joint, pain will be the same with active and passive motion. If the disease is outside the joint or extraarticular, passive motion may be painless while active motion produces pain. During passive tests, move the joint until an end point or end range is felt to help determine the affected structure and the severity of the injury.

There are six end points to note when assessing joint movement: (1) bone-to-bone sensation, felt with an osteophyte or abnormal bone development; (2) spasm, which can indicate severe ligamentous injury; (3) capsular feel or a firm arrested movement, with some give to it, which can indicate chronic joint effusion, arthritis, or capsular scarring; (4) spring block, or joint rebound at the end of range of movement, caused by an articular derangement or an intraarticular body; (5) tissue approximation, a normal end feel caused by tissue limiting further movement, such as the biceps muscle limiting elbow flexion; and (6) empty end feel, present when there is no tissue resistance, but the patient stops the movement because of pain. This last condition indicates bursitis, extraarticular abscess, or tumor.

Test for Muscle Strength

Test for flexor and extensor strength against resistance of both the proximal and distal muscle groups. Proximal muscle weakness is seen in myopathic disorders. Distal muscle weakness is seen secondary to a neuropathic process. Generally, if the opposite side is normal, strength should be compared to it. A scale of 0 to 5 is used to rate muscle strength (Table 20-1).

In the presence of significant pain, muscle strength may be unreliable. If the contraction is strong and painful, the pathology is caused by mild musculotendinous damage. If the contraction is weak and painful, the pathology is the result of severe musculotendinous damage. If the contraction is weak and painless, the pathology results from a neurological lesion (paresis).

Perform a Neurological Examination

A complete assessment of sensory and motor function and deep tendon reflexes should be done on the affected and contralateral limbs. If systemic illness is suspected, perform a complete neurological examination. A referral is indicated if initial treatment does not adequately control pain, if function loss is progressing, or if the patient is immunocompromised.

LABORATORY AND DIAGNOSTIC STUDIES
Complete Blood Count

A complete blood count (CBC) is obtained to evaluate for anemia associated with chronic disease, infection, or neoplasm. An altered white blood cell (WBC) count may indicate infection or leukemia.

Erythrocyte Sedimentation Rate

An erythrocyte sedimentation rate (ESR) is elevated when inflammation is present. It is a nonspecific test.

Table 20-1	Muscle Strength Test	
GRADE	**MUSCLE STRENGTH**	**TERM**
0	No palpable contraction	Zero
1	Muscle contracts but part does not move	Trace
2	Muscle moves part but not against gravity	Poor
3	Muscle moves part through range against gravity	Fair
4	Muscle moves part even with resistance	Good
5	Normal strength against resistance present	Excellent

Joint Aspiration

Joint aspiration is performed to assess synovial fluid for elevated WBC count, Gram stain, culture and sensitivity, crystal analysis, presence of glucose, and consistency or "string test." This procedure is performed using local anesthesia under sterile technique. Synovial fluid will flow easily when the joint capsule is penetrated.

Radiography

Obtain at least two radiographic views, anteroposterior and lateral, because injuries are not always apparent on a single view. Any evidence of fracture or dislocation will require orthopedic attention. Sometimes radiographic comparisons with the opposite limb may be useful. Traumatic knee injuries should include four radiographic views: anteroposterior, lateral, tunnel (intracondylar notch), and a 30-degree sunrise (patella). Other diagnostic imaging techniques such as magnetic resonance imaging (MRI), computed tomography (CT), or bone scanning are usually ordered by a specialist. MRI is usually used in spine, joint, and soft tissue imaging. CT scans are usually performed for bone visualization.

Antinuclear Antibodies

Antinuclear antibody (ANA) tests are positive with high titers in RA and SLE; however, other conditions, such as aging, medications, and other connective tissue disease, can produce positive antibody titers.

Rheumatoid Factor

Rheumatoid factor (RF) is the single most useful test to confirm a diagnosis of RA and is positive in 80% of patients with this disease.

C4 Complement

C4 complement determines serum hemolytic complement activity, a protein that binds antigen-antibody complexes for the purpose of lysis. Complement is increased in active inflammatory disease and in autoimmune disorders such as juvenile RA.

C-Reactive Protein

C-reactive protein (CRP) indicates the presence of abnormal plasma protein or a nonspecific response to inflammation caused by both infectious and noninfectious processes. CRP is elevated in RA and infection.

Lyme Titer Enzyme-Linked Immunosorbent Assay Serology

Enzyme-linked immunosorbent assay (ELISA) detects antibodies against *B. burgdorferi*, which causes Lyme disease. However, the ELISA may not detect antibodies for several weeks after the onset of infection.

DIFFERENTIAL DIAGNOSIS
Musculoskeletal Inflammation
Tenosynovitis (Tendinitis)

Soft tissue disorders of tendinitis, bursitis, and fibrositis tend to co-occur. Tenosynovitis is a term that refers to inflammation of the tendon and tendon sheath. In an acute inflammation, usually caused by trauma related to recreational or occupational activities, effusion may accumulate and result in swelling; with chronic inflammation, ROM will be limited by fibrosis of the tendon sheath.

The patient's chief complaint will be pain that is worse with movement and swelling around the affected area. Occupational and recreational history will provide vital clues to a traumatic or overuse cause of pain. Persons with arthritis may have tendinitis secondary to joint disease. Crepitus may be felt on palpation of the tendon.

Bursitis

Bursitis is inflammation of a sac lined with synovial fluid, most often secondary to traumatic tenosynovitis of the shoulder, hip, knee, and elbow. Numerous bursae lie over bony prominences and reduce friction from motion of fascial planes. Bursitis is caused by overuse and trauma and may be associated with RA. If isometric contraction of a group of muscles causes pain, the muscles or tendons, or both, may be involved. Bursitis causes an aching pain that radiates to points of tendon insertion or further along the limb. Muscle weakness may also be present. Palpation reveals local tenderness and swelling without full range of joint motion.

Fibrositis (Myofascitis, Fibromyositis)

Fibromyositis is a response to underlying conditions, such as polymyalgia rheumatica, RA, ankylosing spondylitis, hypothyroidism, neuritis, and viral infection, that generate major muscle tension around a large, weight-bearing proximal joint. Fatty and fibrous nodules may be palpable, and painful trigger sites can be located throughout the shoulder and pelvic girdles or lower extremities. Patients complain of stress and anxiety, sleep disturbance, painful trigger points, and joint stiffness.

Osteomyelitis

The presentation of osteomyelitis, a pyogenic infection of bone, depends on the age of the patient as well as the bone involved. This condition should be suspected in any patient who complains of pain in long or flat bones and walks with an antalgic limp. Fever, chills, and vomiting are usually present in acute osteomyelitis but may not occur in the neonate or young infant. Chronic osteomyelitis is characterized by relapse of pain, erythema, swelling, or evidence of purulent discharge. The hallmark is a constant local pain that progressively worsens. The slightest motion of the limb aggravates the pain. The child keeps the limb motionless. Laboratory findings show increased WBCs, ESR, and CRP. Radiographs may show bone destruction or deep soft tissue swelling at the site of infection.

Joint Inflammation
Osteoarthritis

Osteoarthritis (OA) is a degenerative disease of joint cartilage that results in osteophyte (spur) development and synovial inflammation. It is the most common form of arthritis and is present to some extent in all elderly persons. Patients will complain of joint stiffness, pain, and limited movement, most often of the spine (cervical and lumbar), large proximal joints (e.g., knee, hip), and PIP joints. Symptoms may be asymmetrical. Heberden nodes develop on the DIP joints. Patients at increased risk have a history of performing repetitive weight-lifting tasks, have sustained some form of joint trauma, are obese, or have been diagnosed with diabetes mellitus. Acute arthritis is associated with an increased ESR, and radiographs will show spurs, joint deformity, and erosive changes.

Rheumatoid Arthritis

RA is a systemic polyarthritis with a wide spectrum of clinical presentation. Symptoms of RA include morning stiffness of symmetrical small joints in the hands and feet, swelling, and progressive fatigue. Other symptoms include fever, weight loss, anorexia, and diaphoresis. Rheumatoid nodules are soft and spongy and appear on the elbows, forearms, and hands. Pericarditis, pleuritis, and vasculitis are associated conditions. Laboratory data may disclose a normochromic, normocytic anemia, an elevated ESR, and a positive rheumatoid factor in 75% to 90% of patients. Radiographs may show bony erosion at the joint margins and joint deformities. Box 20-1 lists criteria for the diagnosis of RA.

Juvenile Rheumatoid Arthritis

Juvenile rheumatoid arthritis (JRA), the most common connective tissue disease in children, presents with fatigue, low-grade fever, weight loss, and failure to grow. Night pain and morning stiffness that improve with activity are common symptoms. Younger children may present with irritability, refusal to walk, or guarding of a joint. The disease may be systemic, affect fewer than four joints (pauciarticular), or affect more than four joints (polyarticular). Laboratory findings show anemia, leukocytosis, and thrombocytosis. Rheumatoid factor and ANA may be negative. ESR is elevated.

Septic Arthritis

Septic arthritis is sudden pain and inflammation of a single joint, sometimes associated with systemic signs such as fever, malaise, and diaphoresis. The hip is a common site of blood-borne joint infection in neonates, infants, and young children. The presentation depends on the age of the child. A neonate may be afebrile but irritable, refusing to feed and failing to gain weight. In the older child, the onset of pain and fever is acute, and the child refuses to bear weight. ROM of the hip is markedly restricted and very painful.

In adults, migratory joint pain and tenosynovitis may follow 2 to 4 weeks after a mucosal site infection with *Neisseria gonorrhoeae*. Knee, wrist, ankle, and

---

Box 20-1	**Diagnostic Criteria for Rheumatoid Arthritis (Four Criteria Must Be Present)**

- Morning stiffness at least 1 hour before improvement for more than 6 weeks
- Arthritis of three or more joints for more than 6 weeks
- Arthritis of hand joints for more than 6 weeks
- Symmetrical arthritis of same joint
- Rheumatoid nodules
- Positive serum rheumatoid factor
- Radiographic changes showing erosions or bony decalcification

Modified from Arnett FC, Edworthy SM, Bloch DA, McShane DJ, Fries JF, Cooper NS et al: The American Rheumatism Association 1987 revised criteria for the classification of rheumatoid arthritis, *Arthritis Rheum* 31:315, 1988.

hand joints are most commonly affected. Joint aspiration shows increased WBCs, and culture of fluid or pus may reveal bacterial, tubercular, fungal, syphilitic, and viral organisms. The ESR and CRP are also elevated. With hip involvement, ultrasound shows marked distention of the hip joint, with varying degrees of femoral hip displacement. Septic arthritis is an emergency situation, and treatment must be initiated immediately.

Gout

Gout is a joint inflammation caused by deposits of urate crystals and is associated with an inborn error of uric acid secretion or with metabolic disorders (e.g., hemolytic anemia, renal insufficiency, sarcoidosis). Males older than 30 years and persons with a family history of gout are most often affected. The patient reports a recurrent, sudden onset of pain early in the morning that subsides over several days, especially of the first MTP joint. The joint is warm, tender, and red; tophi—chalky subcutaneous deposits of sodium urate—may be present on extensor surfaces. Gout can be differentiated from pseudogout by the presence of calcium pyrophosphate crystals, involvement of large joints, and secondary osteoarthritis. Laboratory findings during an acute attack show elevated serum uric acid levels, ESR, and WBC levels. The joint may be aspirated for fluid to observe uric acid crystals and cultured to exclude septic arthritis.

Musculoskeletal Pain Related to Trauma or Overuse
Shoulder

Dislocation (glenohumeral joint instability). A patient with shoulder dislocation presents with anterior and/or posterior joint pain, periarticular muscle spasm, anxiety, and limited movement. An anterior dislocation causes inability to internally rotate and abduct the humerus. Posterior dislocation causes limitation of external rotation, arm abduction, and hand supination with the shoulder flexed forward. Radiographs of the shoulder (anteroposterior, lateral, and axillary views) will exclude fracture of surrounding bones.

Acromioclavicular joint injury. Acromioclavicular joint injuries usually result from sports injuries or motor vehicle accidents. Injury occurs when the acromion, scapula, and upper extremity are driven inferiorly, and the supporting ligamentous structures are sprained or torn. The severity of injury is classified into three grades: partial tear (dislocation) of the acromioclavicular ligament (I); partial tear of the acromioclavicular

and coracoclavicular ligaments (II); and complete rupture of the acromioclavicular and coracoclavicular ligaments and joint separation (III). History will reveal the nature of the injury. The patient will have pain and limited shoulder movement and may present with obvious deformity if there is a severe injury.

Bicipital tendinitis. Bicipital tendinitis is an overuse syndrome of the biceps brachii muscle that ends in two tendons—one attached to the radial tuberosity (arm adduction) and one to the forearm fascia (arm abduction and internal rotation). The syndrome may be associated with other shoulder disorders, such as impingement syndrome. Children may have anomalies of the intertubercular groove, and younger individuals report repeated trauma from swimming, volleyball, baseball, or golf. Pain is localized to the intertubercular groove, is aggravated by the offending movement, and subsides with rest. A Yergason test can indicate bicipital tendinitis. A positive test is characterized by pain in the intertubercular groove with resistance to supination of the forearm while the elbow is flexed 90 degrees. A Fisk radiographic view enables the examiner to determine the size of the intertubercular groove.

Rotator cuff tear. Rotator cuff tears are acute injuries in children and young adults but occur as chronic injuries in older adults. In acute tears, the shoulder pain is severe, and the patient is unable to raise the arm sideways because of pain. In a complete tear, attempts to raise the arm laterally will produce a shoulder shrug. In a partial tear, the patient can raise the arm but cannot maintain the position with any resistance. Inflammation secondary to injury can cause rotator cuff tendinitis that produces shoulder pain, weakness, and a grating sound with movement.

Chronic rotator cuff tears are most common in persons older than 50 years, the result of cumulative and repeated impingement processes. The onset of pain is insidious and is made worse with the arm in an overhead position. Patients experience shoulder pain with sleep and tenderness over the acromioclavicular joint. Examination may reveal minimal restriction in movement, crepitus, and weakness in external rotation of the shoulder. Radiographs will show any bony abnormality such as an acromial spur.

Elbow

Olecranon bursitis. Olecranon bursitis is commonly seen in patients who engage in contact sports, repetitive motion, rubbing or pressure to the elbow, or overuse. Pain is localized over the bursae, and swelling may be the result of hemorrhage in a traumatic injury. Range of joint motion is usually normal. The joint may be warm and red. When these signs are present, carefully examine the skin over the elbow to ensure intactness, because a penetrating injury may cause a septic bursitis. Radiography will exclude underlying bone infection and show the plane of soft tissue swelling.

Lateral humeral epicondylitis (tennis elbow). Epicondylitis is an aseptic inflammation of the bone-tendon junction, resulting from repetitive concentric contractions that transmit force via the muscles to the origin on the lateral epicondyle. Persons most at risk for tennis elbow are the nonathletes who have occupations that require repeated contractions of extensor and supinator muscles. Athletes at risk are tennis players, bowlers, and hockey players. Patients present with gradual onset of pain and tenderness over the lateral epicondyle that progresses in intensity. Palpation over the lateral epicondyle produces point tenderness, although elbow movement is not limited. Resisted forearm supination with the elbow flexed at 90 degrees will intensify symptoms.

Subluxation of the radial head (nursemaid's elbow). Subluxation of the radial head is caused by a rapid upward pulling of the child's hand or wrist. The radial head is pulled out of the annular ligament. This ligament then becomes caught between the radial head and the joint, causing the elbow to be flexed and pronated. The child cries at the event and then refuses to move the arm and may complain of pain in the elbow. Radiographs are normal.

Wrist and Hand

Wrist fracture. Wrist fractures usually are the result of falling on an outstretched hand and may involve a number of types of fracture. Patients present with a painful, swollen distal forearm and wrist and may complain of numbness if the median nerve is involved. Gently palpate to locate the site of maximal pain, particularly the navicular ("snuffbox") area located between the extensor pollicis longus and the extensor pollicis brevis tendons when the mechanism of injury is hyperextension of the wrist. Pain localized here indicates a scaphoid (navicular) fracture. Assess pulses, pain sensation, and motor function (range and strength). Radiographic views (posteroanterior, lateral, and oblique) will reveal the bone involved. In a Colles fracture, the distal radius is displaced dorsally and shows up as a "silver fork" deformity on lateral view radiographs.

Finger fracture. The most common fractures of the fingers are those of the metacarpals and phalanges, commonly seen in sports injuries. Older persons usually sustain fractures as a result of falls. Correct diagnosis of a fractured finger is important in preventing long-term disability of use. Patients will present with a history of trauma or injury. Physical examination includes assessment of vascular and neurological function, tenderness and swelling, ROM of each joint, and signs of joint instability or deformity. Three radiographic views (posteroanterior, lateral, and oblique) are needed for a complete evaluation.

Ganglion. Ganglions are cysts that contain a gelatinous fluid formed by outpouching of a joint capsule or tendon sheath. They most often occur on the dorsum of the wrist. A ganglion can be distinguished from a tumor by its soft consistency and transillumination.

Hip and Leg

Slipped capital femoral epiphysis. In children undergoing a rapid growth spurt, the onset of knee pain, an antalgic limp, and leg weakness may indicate a slipped capital femoral epiphysis (SCFE). Pain may be of several weeks' or months' duration and is exaggerated by strenuous physical activity. Examine the child in a prone position and assess the symmetry of medial rotation of the hip. A reduction of medial rotation may indicate SCFE. A widening of the epiphyseal plate can be visualized in a lateral view radiograph.

Transient synovitis of the hip. A nonspecific inflammatory condition of the hip, transient synovitis is the most common cause of a painful hip in children younger than 10 years. History may reveal a recent upper respiratory tract infection or minor injury. The child complains of pain in the anteromedial aspect of the thigh and knee and walks with an antalgic limp; there is tenderness on palpation over the anterior aspect of the hip joint. Movement of the hip causes pain and is limited. There may be a low-grade fever. Ultrasound should be used for diagnosis, comparing it with the good hip. WBC count is usually normal, although the ESR may be elevated.

Legg-Calvé-Perthes disease. This disease occurs as osteochondritis of the femoral head epiphysis and is characterized by a period of avascular necrosis of the femoral head, followed by revascularization and bone healing. It occurs most commonly in boys between the ages of 3 and 11 years. The child has groin or medial thigh pain and a limp. The pain may be recurring, and the child may have been limping for several months. The loss of medial hip motion is an early sign. There is a high incidence of hernia, undescended testicles, and kidney abnormalities in children with this condition. Radiographs show the ossific nucleus of the femoral head combined with the widened articular cartilage space compared with the opposite hip.

Iliopsoas tendinitis. This tendinitis is caused by frequent repetitive flexions of the hip joint and is common in weight lifters, oarsmen, and football players. The patient complains of mildly intense groin pain on the anterior hip, which worsens with movement. An acute injury involves forced extension of a flexed leg, and in younger age-groups, radiographic evaluation is done if evulsion of the epiphysis is suspected. Test for iliopsoas tendinitis by having the seated patient place the heel of the affected leg on the knee of the other leg. This movement will create pain and a tense iliopsoas muscle.

Proximal fibula fracture. Most proximal fibula fractures are caused by direct trauma to the lateral leg. However, some fractures can be the result of forces transferred from a lateral malleolar injury of the ankle, especially when the force is a combination of compressive and rotational trauma. The peroneal nerve and anterior tibial artery pass near the fibular head, thus injury to either of these structures can be a complication of a proximal fibular fracture. If foot drop is present or a diminished dorsalis pedal pulse is noted, the patient needs immediate referral to an orthopedic surgeon (Figure 20-7).

Stress fracture. Stress fractures occur in adolescents whose bodies are not able to accommodate an increase in intensity of training. Patients will note pain with activity several weeks after beginning a sport. Injury progresses from trabecular microfractures in the bone to the osteoclastic action exceeding the rate of osteoblastic bone formation resulting in the bone breaking. Plain radiographs may not demonstrate injury, so MRI used to identify location of injury and CT is used for follow up.

Knee

Chondromalacia patellae. Chondromalacia of the patella is a change in the patellofemoral joint cartilage, which most often occurs in adolescent females. The condition can be caused by trauma, anatomical anomalies, and misalignment of the patella. Softening of joint

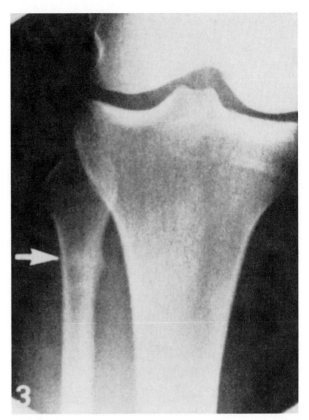

FIGURE 20-7 Typical appearance of a proximal fibular fracture. (From Crowther CL: *Primary orthopedic care*, ed 2, St Louis, 2004, Mosby.)

cartilage, tufts of patellar cartilage, fissures, or ulcers occur. Patients present with anterior knee pain that is worse while climbing stairs or biking. Radiographic studies of the knee, including tangential and sunrise views, show irregularities of the patellofemoral joint.

Patellar tendinitis (jumper's knee). This overuse syndrome is characterized by inflammation in the distal extensors of the knee joint. Patellar tendinitis is more common in athletes who habitually place excessive strain on their knees from jumping or running. Determine the quadriceps (Q) angle by measuring the angle between the center of the patella to the anterior superior iliac spine and from the center patella to the tibial tubercle. An angle greater than 10 degrees in males and 15 degrees in females suggests patellar tendinitis. Persons affected complain of dull, achy knee pain that may have associated clicking or popping. Associated malalignment from femoral anteversion or ankle varus may be present.

Medial collateral ligament sprain. Medial collateral ligament injuries are common and are the result of valgus stress to the knee. The patient limps soon after the injury and may or may not have pain. On physical examination, there is mild effusion and point tenderness over the medial collateral ligament. To test for stability of the medial collateral ligament, the knee is flexed about 30 degrees with the patient supine, and one hand is placed over the lateral knee with the other around the ankle. Apply medial pressure to the knee while pulling the ankle outward. An instability of the medial collateral ligament produces a sensation of opening the medial aspect of the joint. Applying lateral pressure in the same knee position tests for lateral ligament sprain. A radiograph is obtained to rule out fracture.

Medial meniscus tear. Medial meniscus injuries, more common than lateral meniscus injuries, occur after a twisting injury to the knee. The patient has pain, difficulty flexing the knee, and difficulty bearing weight. There often is a clicking or catching in the knee joint, and the joint may be swollen and tender. To examine for medial meniscus injury, perform the Mc-Murray test to assess for clicking, locking, or a springy end point of motion. With the patient supine, place one hand under the heel and flex the knee 90 degrees with slight abduction. Apply a lateral and medial force to the knee while extending and adducting it. A palpable or audible click indicates medial meniscus injury.

Anterior cruciate ligament tear. Ligaments may be stretched or torn if the knee is twisted or hyperextended. The ACL, located in the center of the knee, is one of the most common ligaments damaged in knee injuries. An ACL injury is often associated with an audible pop and a giving-way sensation in the knee, often with swelling from hemarthrosis. Physical examination reveals a positive Lachman test. With the patient supine and the knee flexed 20 to 30 degrees, anchor the patient's foot to the table; then pull the tibia forward. Anterior motion is a sensitive test for ACL laxity.

Osgood-Schlatter disease. This condition, most common in adolescent males, is a painful swelling of the anterior aspect of the tibial tubercle. It is caused by strenuous activity, especially of the quadriceps muscles. The patient will often limp, and the pain will be worse with activities such as stair climbing and kneeling. Examination will reveal a warm, swollen, tender tibial tubercle, and flexion and extension will increase pain intensity. Joint examination of the knee is normal.

Baker cyst (popliteal cyst). A popliteal cyst occurs when fluid from the knee joint enters the connecting bursa and becomes trapped. Patients complain of a fullness or swelling of the posterior knee and calf pain aggravated by walking and alleviated by rest. Examination of the knee focuses on assessment of a change in consistency of the mass on extension (hardening) and flexion (softening), called Foucher sign. Foucher sign is negative with a Baker cyst and positive with a tumor or popliteal aneurysm. The cyst can rupture and cause edema and tenderness of the lower extremity with a positive Homans sign. Ultrasound will detect the cyst or recently ruptured cyst.

Ankle and Foot

Ankle sprain (inversion or eversion). The most common mechanism of ankle injury is an inversion force that stresses the lateral ligamentous support of the joint. The lateral ligaments are of greater length than the medial ligaments and are more predisposed to injury. An audible pop or tear implies a rupture or tear of the ligament. Swelling of the ankle within minutes of injury indicates bleeding and soft tissue trauma. Patients with a ligamentous injury will generally be able to walk and bear weight on the injured foot, even though it may be uncomfortable. Examine the injured joint by palpating the course and attachment points of the ligaments and perform joint ROM to test for ligamentous integrity.

Shin splints (medial tibial stress syndrome). Shin splints are an inflammation of the origin of muscles on the shaft of the tibia caused by overuse, often by running athletes. Patients report achy pain and tenderness over the medial tibia that increases with exercise, especially running, and improves with rest. A radiograph of the tibia will exclude fracture.

Achilles tendinitis. The gastrocnemius and soleus muscles conjoin to form the Achilles tendon. Inflammation of this tendon creates pain and swelling where the tendon inserts into the calcaneus, and a patient will report a tightness of the tendon that makes walking or running difficult. Tendinitis may be caused by overuse, especially running, or by decreased vascularity to the tendon sheath. Examination reveals tenderness over the Achilles tendon with palpation and ankle ROM, especially with dorsiflexion, crepitus over the tendon with motion, and weakness of the calf muscles.

Plantar fasciitis. Plantar fasciitis, which affects women twice as often as men, is caused by chronic weight-bearing stress when laxity of foot structures allows the talus to slide forward and medially, the calcaneus to drop, and plantar ligaments and fascia to stretch. Persons who are obese or who engage in excessive standing are at greatest risk. Pain is worse on awakening and is relieved with non–weight-bearing activity. Tendons and joints become inflamed, and muscles spasm because of the misalignment of structures. Patients often complain of heel pain.

Muscle Pain (Myalgia)
Viral Infections
Viral infections can produce diffuse myalgias that are usually associated with fever, chills, upper respiratory tract symptoms, and malaise. A patient with influenza will have intense myalgia and high fever, and appear quite ill. Since viral illnesses are highly contagious, epidemics in both children and adults in a community may be a useful clue to diagnosis. A paraviral IgM titer is diagnostic of an acute parvovirus B19 infection.

Psychogenic
Pain that is diffuse, varies in pattern, and is unaffected by activity or rest may be psychogenic in origin. A careful history may reveal any secondary gain the patient may derive from the pain and suggest the presence of an anxiety or depression disorder. On examination, the patient may display facial expressions and descriptions of discomfort to palpation and movement that are inconsistent. This diagnosis involves excluding other causes.

Fibromyalgia
Fibromyalgia is a syndrome characterized by chronic fatigue, generalized musculoskeletal pain, and multiple trigger points of pain on physical examination. It affects primarily women between 20 and 50 years of age. Other symptoms associated with this syndrome include stage IV sleep disturbance, anxiety or depression, obsessive-compulsive behavior, and irritable bowel syndrome. Symptoms are exacerbated by stress. Physical examination shows focal tenderness without signs of synovitis.

Systemic Disorders
Acute Leukemia
Leukemia is the most common cancer in children, and bone and joint pain is the most common presenting complaint. The bone pain is diffuse and nonspecific, and may extend to adjacent joints. Laboratory findings may show the WBC count as elevated, depressed, or normal. Severe anemia is common as is a depressed platelet count. Radiographs of the limb at the distal end of the femur and the proximal end of the tibia show abnormal areas of radiolucency.

Sickle Cell Disease
Sickle cell disease is a genetic disorder characterized by production of hemoglobin S, an anemia secondary to short erythrocyte survival, and sickle-shaped erythrocytes. It affects mainly African American, Mediterranean, and Southeast Asian population groups. Sickle cell disease manifests itself after the first 6 months of life. The child presents with painful or vaso-occlusive crises characterized by symmetrical, painful swelling of the hands and feet. Older persons report pain in long bones and joints, abdominal pain, decreased appetite, fever, and malaise. The laboratory findings reveal a hemoglobin S genotype and anemia, but findings can vary depending on the hemoglobin genotype, age, gender, and presence of other organ involvement.

Systemic Lupus Erythematosus
SLE is a systemic inflammatory condition that occurs most often in women. It is characterized by arthritis that commonly involves the small joints of the hands, wrists, ankles, and knees, as well as malar rash, oral ulcers, glomerulonephritis, hematological disorders, and psychological symptoms. The pain is transient but severe. Laboratory findings show leukopenia with neutrophils predominating the peripheral count, and the ANA is positive.

Lyme Arthritis
The bite of the deer tick transmits the spirochete *B. burgdorferi*. Patients may not recall a tick bite but will have been in an endemic area. The presenting complaints in Lyme disease are diffuse joint pain and swelling, a targetlike skin rash (erythema migrans), fever, and chills. These symptoms may be present for weeks before the spirochete spreads via blood and lymph tissue to the myocardium and central nervous system. A chronic arthritis may appear months after the initial infection. The arthritis is asymmetrical and occurs in the large joints. The knee is a commonly affected joint. The patient has an antalgic limp with diffuse swelling and warmth of the knee joint anteriorly, as well as local

synovial thickening. Laboratory diagnosis reveals elevation of immunoglobulin M (IgM) titers and IgG antibodies against the spirochete. The ESR is elevated.

Neuroblastoma

Neuroblastoma is a malignant tumor that usually occurs in children under 5 years of age. It originates from cells in the sympathetic ganglia and adrenal medulla but can arise from any part of the sympathetic nervous system and metastasize to the bone. The presenting complaint may be varied, but bone pain, limp, pallor, and fatigue may be present. CT or MRI is used to identify the primary location of the tumor. In the urine, 3-methoxy-4-hydroxymandelic acid and homovanillic acid levels are elevated.

Osteogenic Sarcoma

Osteogenic sarcoma is a tumor that occurs in persons 10 to 25 years old, with the most common site being the distal femur or the proximal tibia. The patient initially complains of local intermittent pain that quickly progresses to a constant and severe pain, and an antalgic limp may develop. Palpation reveals tenderness over the area affected. Laboratory findings show an increase in serum alkaline phosphatase level; radiograph shows a "sunburst" image.

Nerve Entrapment Syndromes
Thoracic Outlet Syndrome

Thoracic outlet syndrome is the result of compression of nerve and vascular structures in the neck area. Arterial compression creates pallor and decreased pulses and weakness, with eventual skin and nail atrophy in the affected extremity. Nerve compression creates paresthesias, dysesthesias, and pain. History may disclose that the patient sleeps with the arm extended against the head, causing morning symptoms of pain and paresthesias. Reaching, working with the arm raised, and lifting exacerbate pain. Other risk factors include a rounded, sagging shoulder posture and shoulder muscle deformities. A common compression occurs with the cervical rib compressing the subclavian artery. A bruit may be heard over the supraclavicular fossa. Electromyographic studies help to delineate the specific nerve involvement; however, they may not identify the vascular involvement.

Carpal Tunnel Syndrome

Carpal tunnel syndrome involves entrapment of the median nerve in the dominant hand, resulting from repeated strain that causes thickening of the flexor tendon sheath. A dull, achy pain is felt across the wrist and forearm with paresthesia, weakness, or clumsiness of the hand; atrophy; dry skin; and skin color changes of the hand secondary to impaired nerve innervation. Symptoms are often worse at night. History reveals repetitive activity of the upper extremity. Carpal tunnel syndrome most often occurs in women and in persons older than 30 years. Examination discloses dry skin on the thumb, index finger, and middle finger (median nerve distribution). Thenar atrophy may be present. Tinel sign and Phalen test are positive (Table 20-2).

Peroneal Nerve Compression

Peroneal nerve compression can be caused by a cast, sports injury, or trauma. Pain is felt across the head of the fibula and can result in footdrop.

Tarsal Tunnel Syndrome

The posterior tibial nerve is involved, and pain is felt across the ankle and proximal foot. Tarsal tunnel syndrome is occasionally associated with motor weakness of the proximal toe flexors. Patients may not remember a specific onset but report pain and weakness of the foot muscles. Tapping the posterior tibial nerve posterior and inferior to the medial malleolus elicits pain. Ask the patient about shoe fit and use of any orthotic devices.

Neuritis

Vascular metabolism affected by systemic disorders such as diabetes mellitus can cause a nerve to become ischemic, producing toxins that can directly damage the nerve. Inflammation can be of the nerve axon, myelin sheath, or both. Soft tissue inflammation contributing to neuropathy can be caused by collagen disorders (e.g., SLE, scleroderma).

Diabetes mellitus is commonly associated with sensory peripheral neuropathy and results in pain and sensory loss that is more intense in the lower extremities.

Alcoholism is associated with distal, demyelinating neuropathy that may resolve with cessation of alcohol ingestion.

Table 20-2 Selected Tests Used to Assess for Musculoskeletal Disorders

TEST	DESCRIPTION	FINDINGS
Shoulder		
Yergason test	Have patient supinate forearm against resistance.	A positive test produces pain in bicipital groove and is suggestive of bicipital tendinitis.
Rotator cuff tear	Ask patient to externally rotate and abduct shoulder.	In a partial tear, patient can raise arm but cannot maintain position against resistance; in a complete tear, attempts to abduct arm will produce a shoulder shrug.
Elbow		
Tennis elbow	Have patient resist forearm supination with elbow flexed 90 degrees.	Pain with this movement indicates lateral humeral epicondylitis.
Wrist		
Finkelstein test	Have patient flex fingers over a clenched thumb; then passively deviate wrist ulnarly.	Movement produces pain in de Quervain disease (first dorsal compartment tenosynovitis).
Tinel sign	Tap over median nerve (palmar surface of wrist) to assess for compression neuropathy.	In a positive test, patient reports a tingling or prickling sensation distal to site tapped along first three digits, wrist pain, and weak grip.
Phalen test	Ask patient to maintain palmar flexion for 1 minute with dorsal surfaces of each hand pressed together.	Test is positive if maneuver produces numbness and paresthesia in fingers innervated by median nerve.
Leg/Hip		
Iliopsoas	Have seated patient place heel of affected leg on knee of other leg.	Pain with this movement indicates muscle iliopsoas tendinitis.
Knee		
Foucher sign	Look for change in consistency of a mass in popliteal fossa that hardens with extension and softens with flexion.	A positive sign indicates a popliteal tumor or aneurysm; a negative sign indicates a Baker cyst.
Bulge sign	Apply lateral pressure to area adjacent to patella.	Medial bulge will appear if fluid is in knee joint.
Drawer sign	With patient supine, flex knee 90 degrees and hip 45 degrees with foot on table; apply slow, steady anterior pull, and in same position gently push tibia back.	Tests for cruciate ligament stability; abnormal anterior or posterior movement of tibia on femur is a positive drawer sign and indicates ligamentous instability.
McMurray maneuver	With patient supine, maximally flex knee and hip; externally and internally rotate tibia with one hand on distal end of tibia; with other hand, palpate joint.	Pain and a palpable or audible click are positive findings and indicate a meniscus injury.
	Extend knee with slight lateral pressure with tibia internally rotated.	Positive finding in this position indicates a lateral meniscus injury.
	Extend knee with slight internal pressure on tibia externally rotated.	Positive finding in this position indicates a medial meniscus injury.
Collateral ligament test	Apply medial or lateral pressure when knee is flexed 30 degrees and when it is extended.	Medial or lateral collateral ligament sprain will show laxity in movement and no solid end points, depending on degree of sprain.
Lachman test (cruciate ligaments)	With knee flexed 30 degrees, pull tibia forward with one hand while other hand stabilizes femur.	Positive test is a mushy or soft end feel when tibia is moved forward, indicating damage to anterior cruciate ligament.

DIFFERENTIAL DIAGNOSIS OF *Common Causes of Limb Pain*

CONDITION	HISTORY	PHYSICAL FINDINGS	DIAGNOSTIC STUDIES
Musculoskeletal Inflammation			
Tenosynovitis (tendinitis)	Repetitive trauma activities; pain with movement	Swelling over tendon, crepitus	None
Bursitis	History of overuse; aching pain over affected bursae that radiates along limb	Local tenderness, swelling; limited joint motion; muscle weakness	None
Fibrositis	Pain in trigger sites throughout body, joint stiffness, disturbed sleep	Fatty, fibrous nodules in muscles; palpation of trigger points elicits pain	None
Osteomyelitis	Presentation depends on age, location of infection; history of infection, trauma, penetration, invasive procedure; refusal to bear weight (hip); constant pain	Fever, chills, vomiting; pain localized over affected area but progressively worsens; soft tissue injury or abscess	Increased WBCs, ESR, C-reactive protein; radiographs
Joint Inflammation			
Osteoarthritis	Older adults; asymmetrical joint pain and stiffness that improves throughout day; history of repetitive joint trauma; obesity	DIP, PIP joints enlarged; Heberden nodes; limited cervical spine ROM	ESR; radiograph may reveal osteophytes, loss of joint space
Rheumatoid arthritis	Morning stiffness of small joints; symmetrical involvement; anorexia, weight loss	Fever, rheumatoid nodules, ulnar deviation of wrists	Increased ESR, positive rheumatoid factor, anemia on CBC; radiograph shows bony erosion
Juvenile rheumatoid arthritis	Fatigue, weight loss, failure to thrive, refusal to walk, joint pain and stiffness	Fever, rash, guarding of joints, limited ROM; joint swelling, nodules	Elevated WBCs, ESR; positive rheumatoid factor and antinuclear antibody
Septic arthritis	History of systemic infection, malaise, diaphoresis, refusal to bear weight (hip), acute joint pain	Fever; red, swollen joint; limited range of motion	WBCs, culture of joint aspirate, ESR, C-reactive protein, ultrasound of joint
Gout	Acute pain of large joint, asymmetrical; males over 30 years, history of gout	Inflamed, swollen joint; tophi; sodium urate crystals	Increased serum uric acid level, ESR, WBCs
Musculoskeletal Pain Related to Trauma or Overuse			
Shoulder dislocation	History of trauma, pain	Limited rotation, arm abduction, and hand supination	Radiograph of shoulder with AP view and internal/external rotation
Acromioclavicular joint injury	History of trauma, pain	Limited shoulder movement; obvious deformity	Radiograph of shoulder with AP view and internal/external rotation
Bicipital tendinitis	History of overuse of biceps; pain worse with movement	Positive Yergason test; pain localized over intertubercular groove	Radiograph (Fisk view)
Rotator cuff tear	Acute: younger persons, history of trauma, severe pain; chronic: older, pain worse with overhead movement, sleep disturbance	Acute: inability to raise arm laterally, shrug shoulders; chronic: tenderness over AC joint, crepitus, weakness in external shoulder rotation	Radiograph may reveal humeral displacement or spurs; MRI

DIFFERENTIAL DIAGNOSIS OF *Common Causes of Limb Pain—cont'd*

CONDITION	HISTORY	PHYSICAL FINDINGS	DIAGNOSTIC STUDIES
Olecranon bursitis	Repetitive motion of or pressure to elbow; localized pain	Warmth, redness, and swelling over joint; full ROM	Radiograph to rule out fracture of olecranon process
Lateral humeral epicondylitis	History of repetitive contraction of extensor and supinator muscles; pain over lateral epicondyle that progresses	Tenderness over lateral epicondyle; palpation produces pain, motion does not; supination against resistance worsens pain	None
Subluxation of radial head	Occurs in children; pain in elbow or arm	Affected arm is flexed; child cries when attempts are made to move joint	Radiograph of elbow
Wrist fracture	History of fall on an outstretched hand; pain and swelling of forearm and wrist	Palpation of snuffbox increases pain; observe for joint deformity	Three-view radiographs to determine scaphoid or Colles fracture
Finger fracture	History of trauma or fall, joint tenderness	Joint swelling, instability	Three-view radiographs (PA, lateral, and oblique)
Ganglion	Noticeable lump on dorsal surface of wrist	Gelatinous filled nodule, soft, transilluminates	None
Slipped capital femoral epiphysis	Children: during rapid growth spurts; knee pain worse with activity	Limitation of medial hip rotation, limp	Radiograph of epiphyseal plate
Transient synovitis of hip	Children less than 10 yr; history of upper respiratory tract infection; limp, pain in anteromedial thigh and knee	Tenderness on palpation over anterior hip; hip movement increases pain and is limited; low-grade fever	Ultrasound, ESR
Legg-Calvé-Perthes disease (LCPD)	Boys 3-11 yr; groin or medial thigh pain, limp	Decreased hip ROM	AP and frog lateral radiographs of hip; LCPD may show increased density of femoral head
Iliopsoas tendinitis	History of repetitive flexion of hip; pain worse with movement	With patient sitting, place heel of affected leg on knee of other; test is positive if pain is elicited	None
Proximal fibular fracture	History of direct trauma to the fibula or ankle	Pain on weight bearing, edema and tenderness to palpation over fracture	Radiography, CT if soft tissue injury is suspected
Stress fracture	Younger ages, history of overuse of lower extremities	Pain with activity	Radiography, MRI
Chondromalacia patellae	Adolescent females; history of knee trauma or misalignment, knee pain worse with activity	Tenderness to palpation over knee	Four-view radiographs of knees to rule out arthritis
Patellar tendinitis	History of overuse, especially running or jumping; dull, achy knee pain; click	Q angle >10 degrees in males, 15 degrees in females; clicking or popping with knee movement	None
Medial collateral ligament sprain	History of valgus stress to knee; limp; pain	Effusion and point tenderness over knee; valgus and varus pressure to assess instability	AP and lateral radiographs may reveal a ligament avulsion of femoral origin

Continued

DIFFERENTIAL DIAGNOSIS OF *Common Causes of Limb Pain—cont'd*

CONDITION	HISTORY	PHYSICAL FINDINGS	DIAGNOSTIC STUDIES
Medial meniscus tear	History of twisting injury to the knee, pain, difficulty flexing, bearing weight, clicking or catching of knee with movement	Positive McMurray test, clicking or locking during joint movement	Four-knee view radiographs to rule out bony abnormality; MRI
Anterior cruciate ligament tear	History of twisting or extension knee injury; audible "pop"	Swelling; positive Lachman test	Radiograph to rule out fracture; MRI
Osgood-Schlatter disease	Adolescent males; knee pain and swelling aggravated by activity, limp	Tenderness, warmth, swelling over anterior tibial tubercle	Radiograph with knee rotated inward may show soft tissue swelling
Baker cyst	Fullness or swelling of posterior knee, aggravated by walking	Negative Foucher sign; normal joint examination; positive Homans sign in ruptured cyst	None
Ankle sprain	History of inversion stress with audible "pop," immediate swelling	Swelling, soft tissue trauma, able to perform active ROM with ligament sprain	Radiograph needed only with tenderness over the lateral malleolus to rule out fracture
Shin splints	Ache or pain over medial tibia that is worse with exercise, history of running	Tenderness over medial tibia	AP and lateral radiographs may show a stress fracture; a bone scan will be positive with increased uptake along the medial tibia
Achilles tendinitis	Pain and tightness over Achilles tendon, especially with walking or running	Tenderness over Achilles tendon; pain worse with dorsiflexion ankle; calf weakness	Lateral ankle radiograph reveals enlarged posterosuperior tuberosity of the calcaneus
Plantar fasciitis	History of chronic weight bearing; aching feet, muscle spasms, obesity	Misalignment of foot structures, especially talus, calcaneus, and plantar ligaments	None
Muscle Pain (Myalgia)			
Viral infections	History of upper respiratory tract infection; malaise, chills, cold symptoms, general muscle aches	Fever, ill-appearing adult or child	Viral serum titer
Psychogenic	Pain is diffuse; varies in pattern of activity, setting; history of depression or anxiety	Normal examination or patient response to examination maneuvers disproportionate to physical findings or subjective complaints	None
Fibromyalgia	Female 20-50 yr; history of depression, sleep disturbance, chronic fatigue, general muscle and joint aches	Palpation of trigger points will produce pain; normal physical examination	None

DIFFERENTIAL DIAGNOSIS OF *Common Causes of Limb Pain—cont'd*

CONDITION	HISTORY	PHYSICAL FINDINGS	DIAGNOSTIC STUDIES
Systemic Disorders			
Acute leukemia	Hip pain in children, refusal to walk	Fever, hepatosplenomegaly, bruising	CBC
Sickle cell disease	African American, family history; appears after 6 mo of age; acute pain with swelling of hands and feet, abdominal pain, decreased appetite, malaise	Normal examination	Hemoglobin S genotype
Systemic lupus erythematosus	Female; transient arthritis of small joints, malar rash	Normal examination may have joint tenderness on palpation	Kidney function tests, antinuclear antibody, CBC
Lyme arthritis	History of exposure to endemic areas of deer tick; chills, diffuse joint pain and swelling; often knee is affected	Asymmetrical swelling, warmth of joint; erythema migrans; may have myocardial involvement	Serum IgM and IgG antibodies, ESR
Neuroblastoma	Under 5 yr; pain in bones	Unexplained fever	Urine for vanillylmandelic or homovanillic acid; CT scan
Osteogenic sarcoma	Persons 10-25 yr; intermittent pain of lower femur, upper tibia; limp	Tenderness over affected area	Radiograph, serum alkaline phosphatase
Nerve Entrapment Syndromes			
Thoracic outlet syndrome	History of sleeping with arm against head; morning shoulder pain; pain worse with lifting; paresthesia, weakness, or clumsiness of hand; symptoms worse at night	Bruit over supraclavicular fossa; pallor, decreased pulses of upper extremity, weakness, skin and nail atrophy	None
Carpal tunnel syndrome	History of repetitive upper extremity motion; paresthesia, weakness, or clumsiness of hand; symptoms worse at night	Positive Phalen test and Tinel sign; weakness of hand; dry skin over distribution of median nerve	None
Peroneal compression	History of pressure to knee from a cast, sports injury, or trauma; pain over head of fibula; clumsy gait	Unilateral footdrop	None
Tarsal tunnel syndrome	Pain in ankle and proximal foot; weakness of toe flexors; ill-fitting shoes	Tapping posterior tibial nerve elicits pain	None
Neuritis	Pain and sensory loss, usually of lower extremities; history of alcohol ingestion, diabetes	Decreased sensory and pain sensation	Liver function tests, hemoglobin A_{1c} to rule out diabetes

AP, anteroposterior; *CBC*, complete blood cell count; *CT*, computed tomography; *DIP*, distal interphalangeal; *ESR*, erythrocyte sedimentation rate; *MRI*, magnetic resonance imaging; *PA*, posteroanterior; *PIP*, proximal interphalangeal; *ROM*, range of motion; *WBC*, white blood cell.

REFERENCES AND READINGS

Burbank KM, Stevenson JH, Czarnecki GR, Dorfman J: Chronic shoulder pain: part I. Evaluation and diagnosis, *Am Fam Physician* 77:453, 2008.

Edwards Jr PH, Wright ML, Hartman JF: A practical approach for the differential diagnosis of chronic leg pain in the athlete, *Am J Sports Med* 33:1241, 2005.

Fagan H: Approach to the patient with acute swollen/painful joint, *Clin Fam Pract* 7:305, 2005.

Garbez R, Puntillo K: Acute musculoskeletal pain in the emergency department: a review of the literature and implications for the advanced practice nurse, *AACN Clin Issues* 16:310, 2005.

Goolsby MJ: Evaluating acute musculoskeletal complaints, *J Acad Nurs Pract* 13:193, 2001.

Goroll AH, Mulley AG: *Primary care medicine*, ed 6, Philadelphia, 2009, Lippincott Williams & Wilkins.

Gutierrez K: Bone and joint infections in children, *Ped Clin North Am* 52:779, 2005.

Leung AK, Lemay JF: The limping child, *J Pediatr Health Care* 18:219, 2004.

Logan K: Stress fracture in adolescent athlete, *Ped. Ann* 36:738, 2007.

Lowe R, Hashkes P: Growing pains a noninflammatory pain syndrome in early childhood, *Nat Clin Pract Rheumatol* 4:542, 2008.

Roberts DM, Stallard TC: Emergency department evaluation and treatment of knee and leg injuries, *Emerg Med Clin North Am* 18:67, 2000.

Solomon DH, Simel DL, Bates DW, Katz JN, Schaffer JL: The rational clinical examination. Does this patient have a torn meniscus or ligament of the knee? Value of the physical examination, *JAMA* 286:1610, 2001.

Low Back Pain (Acute)

A report of acute low back pain (ALBP), although quite common, requires a thorough evaluation. The underlying pathophysiology of back pain is frequently multifactorial and includes both physiological and psychological components. The most common causes of ALBP relate to musculoligamentous injuries and age-related degenerative processes. About 90% of ALBP episodes in adults are related to mechanical causes that resolve within 4 weeks without serious sequelae. A smaller percentage of patients will continue to have chronic symptoms without organic pathology or will have underlying disease.

In children, the prevalence of back pain increases with age and with involvement in sports. Anthropometric variations in children place them at risk for excess strain on the spine, producing back pain. These variations include reduced hip mobility, decreased lumbar extension and increased lumbar flexion, poor abdominal muscle strength, tight hamstring muscles, and lumbar hyperlordosis.

ALBP is defined as activity intolerance producing lower back or back-related leg symptoms of less than 3 months' duration. The Agency for Healthcare Research and Quality (AHRQ) guidelines provide the following framework for causes of ALBP:

- Potentially serious conditions (e.g., spinal fracture, tumor or infection, or cauda equina syndrome)
- Sciatica, or leg pain and numbness of the lateral thigh, leg, and foot, suggesting nerve root compression (Figure 21-1)
- Nonspecific back problems such as musculoskeletal strain, diskogenic pain, or bony deformity secondary to inflammatory disease
- Nonspinal causes secondary to abdominal involvement (e.g., gallbladder, liver, renal, pelvic inflammatory disease; prostate tumor; ovarian cyst; uterine fibroids; aortic aneurysm; or thoracic disease)
- Psychological causes such as stress, work environment (e.g., disability, workers' compensation, secondary gains)

When evaluating ALBP, the goal of the clinician is to first identify signs and symptoms of potentially serious conditions through a careful history and physical examination. A holistic approach to the patient is needed to appreciate the extent to which pain affects the patient's daily routine or work-related activities. Because ALBP is a common occupation-related complaint and a cause of disability and lost productivity, the clinician must gain insight into the psychosocial and economic situation of the patient to help arrive at a correct diagnosis.

DIAGNOSTIC REASONING: FOCUSED HISTORY

Is this a potentially serious cause of ALBP?

Key Questions
- Do you have a fever?
- Have you experienced any trauma to the spine or back?
- Do you have any other health problems?
- Have you been treated for cancer?
- What is your age?
- Have you had loss of control of your bowels or bladder?
- Are you taking any medications?

Fever
The presence of a fever indicates an inflammatory condition such as spondyloarthropathy or systemic infection. Infection is a likely diagnosis when there are chills and fever, weight loss, a recent history of bacterial infection, intravenous drug use, or an immunosuppressed patient. Ewing sarcoma is a malignant tumor and can mimic spinal infection, occurring as back pain that can be accompanied by fever. Children with diskitis will have a fever and refuse to walk because of back pain.

Nerve root	L4	L5	S1
Pain	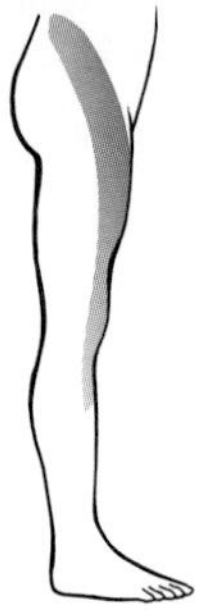	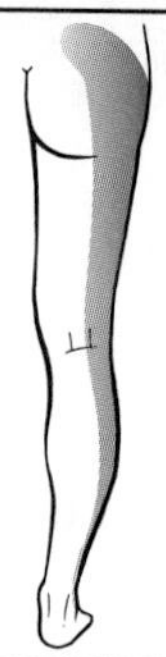	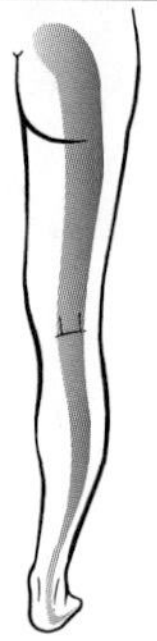
Numbness	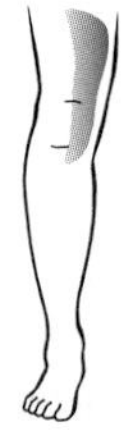	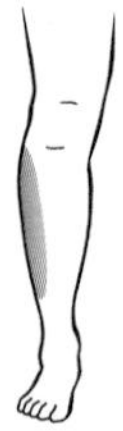	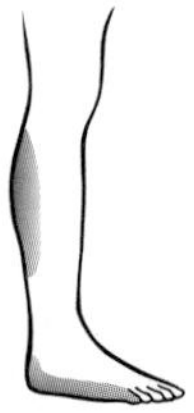
Motor weakness	Extension of quadriceps	Dorsiflexion of great toe and foot	Plantar flexion of great toe and foot
Screening exam	Squat and rise	Heel walking	Walking on toes
Reflexes	Knee jerk diminished	None reliable	Ankle jerk diminished

FIGURE 21-1   Testing for lumbar nerve root compromise. (From Bigos S et al: Acute low back problems in adults, clinical practice guidelines, Quick Reference Guide Number 14, Rockville, MD, 1994, Department of Health and Human Services, U.S. Public Health Service, Agency for Health Care Policy and Research, AHCPR Publication No. 95-0643.)

Trauma

Acute trauma to the spinal cord can result in fracture, dislocation, or misalignment of muscles, ligaments, and intervertebral disks. Trauma may be caused by blunt impact, repetitive injury, or sudden stress caused by lifting or pulling. Low back pain is the most common occupational injury reported. Injury to the back usually results in contusions and abrasions but can also cause spinal fracture if the force is major, such as that sustained in a motor vehicle accident or fall. In the elderly, an acute spinal fracture might result from strenuous lifting when osteoporosis is present. Injuries to the posterior structures of the spine account for most cases of low back pain in adolescents who are athletically active.

Injury to the spinal column should be suspected in anyone whose level of consciousness is impaired after an accident. Cervical spine fractures are sustained during flexion, extension, compression, rotation, or a combination of forces.

Age

In the absence of trauma, the sudden onset of severe low or middle back pain in persons older than 30 years might suggest a dissecting aortic aneurysm. The pain will not be alleviated by rest. Patients older than 50 years are at increased risk for compression fracture as well as cancer.

Systemic Disease

Metabolic disease, inflammatory disorders, and fibromyalgia can lead to back pain. Patients with a history of cancer may have increased risk of a spinal tumor. Neuroblastoma is common in young children, and although it occurs in the abdomen, metastases to the spine may produce back pain. Systemic disease may also be accompanied by unexplained weight loss. Persons younger than 20 years and older than 50 years are at increased risk for tumor, as are those with a history of cancer.

Bowel and Bladder Symptoms

Loss of urinary or stool continence indicates cauda equina or S1-S2 nerve root compromise secondary to a herniated disk, nerve root entrapment, spinal stenosis, infection, or tumor. Constant lumbar puncture with saddle anesthesia, urinary retention, and fecal incontinence are symptoms of cauda equina syndrome, which is considered a surgical emergency.

Children are embarrassed to talk about urinary or bowel habits and changes. Hidden spinal cord tumors might have a relationship to developmental delays in bladder and bowel control. Children under 4 years of age who have back pain should be evaluated for serious diseases, such as intraspinal tumors, dermoid cysts, and malignant astrocytomas.

Medications

Long-term use of corticosteroids can lead to compression fractures of the vertebrae. Use of intravenous drugs may suggest infection as a cause.

What does the location of pain tell me?

Key Question
■ Where does it hurt?

Location of Pain

In general, children are less specific than adults when describing location of pain. Traumatic lesions are more likely to occur in the cervical and lumbar portions of the spine, where there is more motion and less protection. Generalized pain or pain over a fairly wide anatomical area is frequently seen with overuse problems and inflammatory conditions.

Sciatica pain is a sharp, burning pain that radiates down the posterior and lateral leg to the foot or ankle. Back pain with neck stiffness can indicate cervical osteomyelitis. Rheumatoid arthritis produces pain in the upper back and neck. Localized pain is seen with spondylolysis and tumors. Flank pain in adults may indicate a kidney infection. Pain of gallbladder disease radiates to the subscapular areas. Compression fractures of vertebrae

associated with osteoporosis or malignancy may produce pain over the midthoracic area.

Children with traumatic low back derangement will have pain and muscle spasm in the lumbar area from the pressure and shock of an impact injury collision.

What does the pattern of pain tell me?

Key Questions
■ When did the pain start?
■ How long have you had this pain?
■ What does the pain feel like?
■ Does it interfere with sleep?
■ Have you had this pain before?

Onset

The onset of ALBP is sudden, and more than half of patients with this symptom do not associate it with a specific precipitating event or injury. The vast majority of cases of ALBP resolve with conservative treatment in 4 weeks, and radiographic or further diagnostic studies are not recommended until then.

Children are frequently poor historians and parents may have a difficult time remembering when the pain started. Association with events such as birthdays, holidays, and activities is helpful in establishing the onset of the pain. Pain that is mild and of short duration (1 to 2 weeks) is rarely serious.

Back pain lasting longer than 4 weeks needs to be reevaluated for further diagnostic studies.

Duration

Subacute back pain is of 6 to 12 weeks' duration. Chronic back pain is pain of more than 3 months' duration. In persons under 40 years of age, the cause may be postural or may indicate congenital spinal deformity, such as scoliosis or ankylosing spondylitis. In older persons, chronic back pain is more likely to indicate degenerative disease, such as spinal stenosis or disk herniation. In children, back pain present for more than 3 weeks is often due to organic and serious causes.

Pain Characteristics

In children, expression of pain depends on the child's ability to put feelings of pain into behavior; observing for these behaviors is important. Ask children to rate the pain using a 10-point pain scale with happy to sad faces (see Chapter 2). Ask adults to rate pain from 0 (no pain) to 10 (worst pain ever) and assess how much the pain interferes with daily activities. Intractable back pain, especially night pain with constitutional findings, is likely to indicate neoplastic disease. Painful scoliosis and stiffness are common presenting symptoms of a spinal tumor.

Night Pain

Nighttime back pain is a worrisome symptom that often signals a serious problem, such as tumor, infection, or inflammation. Generally, muscle pulls, overuse injuries, spondylolysis, spondylolisthesis, and Scheuermann disease (an exaggeration of the normal posterior convex curvature of the thoracic spine) produce less pain at night. Morning stiffness that improves as the day progresses suggests ankylosing spondylitis.

Nighttime back pain is unusual and indicates the need for a complete and thorough workup.

Recurring Pain

Back pain in young children who have had previous injuries or fractures may be a symptom of child abuse. In the older adult, it may be an indication of compression fractures of the spine. As with young children, it may also signal abuse by a caregiver.

What does the pain in relation to activity tell me?

Key Questions

- What makes the pain worse?
- What makes the pain better?

Aggravating Factors

Pain experienced in the lumbar area occurring after strenuous sporting activities is usually the result of trauma to the muscles and tendons, causing contusions and sprain. It occurs when the patient pushes the muscles and ligaments past the normal level of tolerance. Repeated injury can cause soft tissue scarring and shortening.

Stress and fatigue fractures of the pars interarticularis, the region between the superior and inferior articulating facets of the vertebra, occur when lumbar lordosis places more stress on the pars, such as in gymnastics and tennis.

Pain that is aggravated by activity is usually musculoskeletal in origin. Pain of ankylosing spondylitis is relieved with exercise. Spinal stenosis is associated with increased pain with standing, sneezing, or coughing.

Any child who has voluntarily given up a pleasurable activity because of back pain has a severe symptom.

Alleviating Factors

Back pain not associated with any activity and not relieved by rest may indicate tumor. Back pain relieved with aspirin or nonsteroidal anti-inflammatory drugs in children may indicate an inflammatory cause. Pain that is alleviated by rest and heat indicates a musculoskeletal cause. Pain of spinal stenosis is relieved on flexion of the spine.

Suspect spondylolisthesis, or forward slippage of one vertebra over another, if the onset of pain is during hyperextension, such as with a back handspring, butterfly stroke in swimming, or a tennis serve. The defect arises from a stress fracture or stress reaction of the isthmus of the pars interarticularis in the area of L5-S1. The pain localizes to the low back and occurs during a growth spurt and after engaging in sporting events. The pain improves with rest and is worse with standing.

What does radiation of pain tell me?

Key Questions

- Does the pain travel?
- Can you show me where the pain travels?

Radiation of Pain

Referred pain is of two types: (1) pain referred from the spine into areas lying within the lumbar and upper sacral dermatomes; and (2) pain referred from the pelvic and abdominal viscera to the spine. Pain from the upper lumbar spine usually radiates to the anterior aspects of the thighs and legs, and that of the lower lumbar spine radiates to the gluteal regions, posterior thighs, and calves.

Pain from visceral disease is usually felt within the abdomen or flanks. Gallbladder pain radiates around the trunk to the right scapula. Position does not affect the pain.

Persons with spondylolysis, a destruction of vertebral structure, or spondylolisthesis, an anterior displacement of a vertebra, report hamstring tightness and buttock discomfort as well as low back pain.

Pain that is sharp and burning and radiates down the lateral or posterior aspect of the leg to the lateral ankle or foot is called sciatica, and is a classic symptom of nerve root irritation most often caused by disk displacement.

Are there signs of neurological damage?

Key Questions

- Have you been stumbling?
- Have you noticed any change in your balance or coordination?
- Does the child frequently stumble or fall?
- Do you have numbness or tingling in your extremities?

Stumbling

Spinal cord tumors, such as astrocytoma or ependymoma, may present as a disturbance of movement, posture, or strength in the spine or extremities. Impairment of proprioception or sensation from an upper motor neuron lesion, exhibited by footdrop or ataxia, may produce stumbling.

Numbness and Tingling

Radiculopathy (nerve root pain) is sharp pain felt in a dermatomal pattern and is sometimes associated with numbness and tingling.

Is there a family history of back pain?

Key Question

- Does anyone in your family have scoliosis or a crooked spine?

Family History

Spondylolysis and scoliosis are often seen in families, with a 40% familial occurrence in Alaskan Eskimos.

Could this pain be caused by a systemic disease?

Key Question

- Have you been ill?

Illness

Pharyngitis or upper respiratory tract infections, such as pneumonia, can be the precursor to diskitis in children. The intervertebral disk in children receives its blood supply from the surface of the adjacent vertebral bodies, providing the mechanism necessary for infection. Uveitis and iritis may be associated with juvenile rheumatoid arthritis or juvenile ankylosing spondylitis.

A female patient with pelvic inflammatory disease may have mild to moderate dull, aching, lower abdominal, pelvic, or possibly back pain. With pyelonephritis, the patient may report fever, nausea and vomiting, headache, and back or flank pain.

DIAGNOSTIC REASONING: FOCUSED PHYSICAL EXAMINATION
Observe the Patient's General Appearance

Any person appearing ill with a fever, limp, or unwillingness to walk is highly suspect for having an infectious cause of back pain.

Observe for symmetry of posture and movement from a direct anterior, posterior, and lateral view of the patient. Note the amount of thoracic kyphosis (anteroposterior curve) and lumbar lordosis (anterior convexity) and the alignment of the head and neck above the center of gravity. Children with diskitis often protect their backs by sitting in a hyperextended position, using the arms as support, and may lie down and cry if they are made to sit.

Observe Gait

Shifting or leaning to one side (listing) and atypical scoliosis may indicate a tumor. Listing is caused by asymmetrical sustained muscle contraction. The spinal curvature serves to relieve the discomfort and reduce pressure on a nerve root.

Severely affected gait in spondylosis is caused by hamstring tightness and results in uneven stride length with a persistently fixed knee to prevent hip flexion, which would stretch the tight hamstring muscles and increase pain.

Assess Vital Signs

Fever may indicate systemic infection as well as diskitis. Unexplained weight loss may suggest neoplasm, infection, or depression.

Examine Skin

Dermal cysts and/or a hairy patch over the spine may indicate spinal anomaly or tumor.

A doughy, fatty mass in the midline of the back (sometimes covered with hair [Faun's beard]) is evidence of a lipoma, which may extend into the spinal cord and produce neurological symptoms.

Examine Eyes, Ears, Nose, and Mouth

Uveitis iritis is seen in juvenile rheumatoid arthritis and ankylosing spondylitis. Pharyngitis, otitis media, or infection of hematogenous origin may be the cause of diskitis in children.

Inspect the Back and Extremities

Observe for spinal alignment and symmetry of the tips of the scapula, iliac crests, and gluteal crease. If indicated, measure and compare leg lengths from the anterosuperior iliac crest to the medial malleolus. Measurements can be performed with the patient standing or supine. Legs should be of equal length or have less than 1-cm difference in length. Leg length differences are associated with sacroiliac, facet joint, and disk pathology.

From posterior and lateral viewpoints, observe the patient bending forward with feet together to detect scoliosis, kyphosis, or stiffness and guarding.

Percuss and Palpate Back and Spine

Painful scoliosis and stiffness are common in osteoid osteoma. Idiopathic scoliosis is usually painless without functional limitation. Point tenderness over the affected area is a finding associated with compression fracture of the vertebrae or an infection of the spine.

Palpate and percuss the back to determine if tenderness is in the paravertebral muscular or midline spinous processes, which may indicate diskitis in children or osteomyelitis. To rule out the sacroiliac joint as the site of origin of low back pain, conduct a FABER test. (Figure 21-2). Place the patient in the supine position. Flex the leg and put the foot of the tested leg on the opposite knee. The motion is that of **F**lexion, **Ab**duction, **E**xternal **R**otation at the hip. Slowly press down on the superior aspect of the tested knee joint lowering

the leg into further abduction. The test is positive if there is pain at the hip or sacral joint, or if the leg cannot lower to the point of being parallel to the opposite leg.

Use fist percussion over the costovertebral angles to discriminate flank pain caused by renal disease from spinal pathology. Apply fist percussion over the costovertebral angles and over the spine to localize tenderness.

Perform Range of Motion of the Spine

Ask the patient to flex, extend, rotate, and bend the spine laterally. Decreased mobility and back pain along the spine may indicate muscle spasm, neoplasm, or bony deformity. Pain with forward flexion usually indicates a mechanical cause. Back extension pain increases with spinal stenosis.

Look for compensating effects of hip motion on the spine. The absence of lumbar flexion may be totally masked by a normal range of hip flexion when the patient bends forward. Test lumbar flexion by placing a mark over the fourth lumbar vertebra and another over the sacrum. Lumbar flexion is demonstrated by an increased distance between these two marks when the patient bends forward.

Observe for limitation of motion on forward bending caused by hip flexion contracture. Lumbar lordosis does not flatten with forward bending and is an organic cause for back pain. In children, Scheuermann disease, an exaggeration of the normal posterior convex curvature of the thoracic spine, produces pain with forward flexion, and spondylolysis produces pain with hyperextension.

Perform Straight Leg Raising

The straight leg raising (SLR) test can assess sciatic (L5 and S1) nerve root tension. With the patient supine, place one hand above the knee, the other cupping

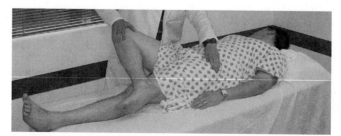

FIGURE 21-2 FABER maneuver. (Modified from Levin KH, Covington EC, Devereaux MW et al: Low back and neck pain, *Continuum: Lifelong Learning Neurol* 7:22, 2001.)

the heel, and slowly raise the limb. Instruct the patient to say when to stop because of pain. Observe for pelvic movement and the degree of leg elevation when the patient tells you to stop. Ask the patient to tell you the most distal point of pain sensation, such as the back, hip, thigh, or knee. While holding the leg at the limit of elevation, dorsiflexing the ankle and internally rotating will add tension to the neural structures and increase the pain if nerve root tension is present.

Pain below the knee at less than 70 degrees of elevation that is aggravated by dorsiflexing the ankle or hip rotation is a sign of L5 or S1 nerve root tension, suggestive of a herniated disk. This test can also be performed with the patient sitting. In a positive test, the patient will resist extension or will compensate with hyperextension of the spine.

Lift each leg in succession to detect contralateral pain in patients with nerve root compression.

An SLR test in children might be unremarkable with a tumor.

Check Hip Mobility

With the patient prone and supine, check active hip flexion, extension, internal and external rotation, and strength against resistance. Weakness of the gluteus maximus is associated with lumbar or referred pain from L5 nerve roots or gluteal nerve injury. In small children, check for congenital hip dysplasia with the child supine, abducting the hips (see Chapter 20). The knees should appear of equal height and should externally rotate equal degrees. The presence of a hip click, joint instability, uneven hip-to-knee length with hips and knees flexed, and uneven gluteal skinfolds suggests congenital hip dislocation.

Examine Feet

Perform active range of motion of the ankle, feet, and toes against resistance. Weakness, pain, or limitation of dorsiflexion movement indicates an L4 nerve root injury. Similar symptoms produced by plantar flexion indicate S1, S2 involvement. Deformities of the foot, such as talipes equinovarus (clubfoot) or hallux malleus (claw toes), may aggravate misalignment of back structures because of asymmetry.

Evaluate Muscle Strength

Evaluate strength against resistance of the lower extremity muscle groups. Test the patient's ability to stand on the toes and heels and to squat. A person with S1 nerve root involvement may have little motor weakness but may demonstrate difficulty in toe walking. Difficulty heel walking or squatting indicates involvement of L5 and L4 nerve roots. Leg extension at the knee against resistance tests L4 root function. In young children who are unable to cooperate for measurement of muscle strength, use measurements of like limb–girths as an estimate of the bilateral symmetry of muscle strength.

Measure Muscle Circumference

Differences in muscle circumference greater than 2 cm in two opposite limbs may signify atrophy secondary to neurological impairment.

Test Sensory Function

All neurological test results are evaluated by comparing the symmetry of responses or perceptions. Bilateral comparison is the simplest, most efficient way to determine the presence, location, and extent of any abnormality. A sensory examination is a general guide in determining the level of spinal cord involvement. Test for light touch and pain sensation in the sensory areas of L3-S1 dermatomes (see Figure 21-1). Dermatomes overlap and vary greatly in individuals; thus only gross changes can be detected by pinprick. Test 5 to 10 pinpricks in each dermatomal area if the patient reports numbness and tingling. Disk lesions rarely produce bilateral symptoms. It is sometimes difficult to distinguish numbness from cutaneous nerve versus dermatomal origin. Numbness from cutaneous nerve lesions does not occur in a dermatomal pattern. Numbness and tingling are uncommon symptoms in most children with back pain. When these symptoms are present, it suggests a serious problem.

Assess Deep Tendon Reflexes

Normal deep tendon reflexes (DTRs) are symmetrical. DTRs are increased when an upper motor neuron lesion is present and decreased with a lower motor neuron lesion. A positive Babinski sign indicates a disorder of upper motor neurons, affecting the motor area of the brain or corticospinal tracts, caused by spinal tumors or demyelinating disease. DTRs are decreased if a tumor is pressing on a peripheral nerve. Asymmetrical abdominal reflexes are seen in tumors of the spine.

An absent or a decreased ankle jerk reflex suggests an S1 nerve root lesion. An L3-4 disk herniation is the most common cause of a diminished knee-jerk reflex.

Palpate the Abdomen

Palpation of the abdomen is performed to detect possible visceral causes of back pain. In an elderly person, a ruptured aortic aneurysm can cause acute, severe, midthoracic back pain. If an aortic aneurysm is suspected, immediate surgical referral is critical.

Check Rectal Sphincter Tone

In cauda equina syndrome, the compression of S1-S2 nerve roots results in decreased sphincter tone and decreased sensation in the perianal area. This syndrome is a surgical emergency.

LABORATORY AND DIAGNOSTIC STUDIES

According to national practice guidelines, no diagnostic tests are warranted within the first 4 weeks for acute onset of low back pain without neurological signs.

Plain Radiographs

Radiographs are useful in localizing the area of discomfort and ruling out fracture, tumor, osteophytes (bone spurs), or vertebral infection.

Standing Anteroposterior and Lateral Views of the Spine

These views of the spine accentuate any deformity, such as scoliosis, and demonstrate vertebral integrity.

Oblique and Flexion Views of the Spine

These views increase the sensitivity for determining instability.

Spine Radiograph

A flat lumbosacral spinal radiograph is obtained when there is a history of trauma or in persons older than 50 years who have ALBP with signs of neurological deficit. Older persons may have a history of straining or lifting.

Bone Scan

Bone scan is a radioisotope technique indicating blood flow and bone formation or destruction and can reveal inflammatory and infiltrative processes and occult fractures. The distal wrist and lumbosacral spine can be scanned to assess bone mineral density and risk of osteoporosis.

Electromyography

Electromyography (EMG) is performed to assess the extent of nerve root compression and function of the peripheral nerves.

Diagnostic Imaging

Magnetic resonance imaging (MRI) is useful in evaluating soft tissue detail, such as disk herniations, tumors, and spinal cord pathology, especially in vertebral osteomyelitis. Computed tomography (CT) scans are usually used for bone visualization.

Urinalysis

Urinalysis is performed to assess kidney and metabolic function, including infectious processes, to rule out a visceral cause of back pain, such as the pain of pyelonephritis.

Erythrocyte Sedimentation Rate

The erythrocyte sedimentation rate (ESR) will be elevated in about 90% of patients with a serious musculoskeletal infection; however, there is no direct relationship between ESR and the severity of infection. The test is nonspecific.

Complete Blood Count

The complete blood count (CBC) will detect anemia as well as other conditions that might manifest as back pain, such as tumor or infection. The anemia of chronic disease is usually hypochromic or normochromic with low iron indices.

DIFFERENTIAL DIAGNOSIS
Potentially Serious Causes of Acute Low Back Pain
Spinal Fracture
The patient may relate a history of major trauma to the back from an impact or fall or, if elderly, a history of strenuous lifting or a minor fall. Pain is felt near the site of injury. Any suspicion of spinal fracture should be treated as an emergency. The patient is immobilized to prevent further damage and transported by emergency personnel for radiographs of the suspected area of fracture.

Tumor (Osteoblastoma, Spinal Metastasis, Osteoid Osteoma)

Primary tumors are a more common cause of back pain in children, whereas metastasis is a more common cause in adults. The lower thoracic and upper lumbar vertebrae are the most common sites of bony metastatic disease from marrow tumors. A health history and diagnostic tests may reveal other signs of general poor health, such as weight loss, fatigue, weakness, and anemia.

Infection (Osteomyelitis, Diskitis)

The spine is the most common site of osteomyelitis in adults, secondary to adjacent infection or following invasive instrumentation that results in bacterial seeding of the bone via the arterial blood. *Staphylococcus aureus* is the most frequently identified organism. Vertebral osteomyelitis causes stiffness and pain, usually localized over the site of infection. A tender spinous process, positive SLR test, and paravertebral muscle spasm may be seen in vertebral osteomyelitis or septic diskitis. Patients may have hip pain secondary to involvement of L2-S1.

Diskitis is usually a benign disorder in children that results in intervertebral disk inflammation. Children will be reluctant to walk, sit, or stand. Pain will be aggravated by motion and relieved by rest. History will reveal a recent bacterial infection, often secondary to pharyngitis or otitis media, intravenous drug use, diabetes mellitus, or immunosuppression. A small percentage of adults will report an acute onset of fever, weight loss, and general malaise; however, the majority will only have the symptom of back pain, present from 2 weeks to years.

Herniated Disk

Disk herniation causes nerve root irritation and produces low back pain that radiates down the buttock to below the knee. Pain is the prominent symptom, with numbness and weakness less common. Physical exam will reveal a positive straight leg raise test. If the pain persists longer than one month, an MRI or EMG is indicated.

Cauda Equina Syndrome

Compression of the S1 nerve root produces constant back pain with saddle distribution anesthesia (buttock and medial and posterior thighs), fecal incontinence, bladder dysfunction, motor weakness of the lower limbs, and radiculopathy. The patient may limp and guard lumbar spine movement, will not be able to heel walk or toe walk, and will have abnormal or asymmetrical knee and ankle deep tendon reflexes. SLR test will be positive. This syndrome is a surgical emergency.

Sciatic Problems
Sciatica

The most common cause of sciatica is herniated disk. History may disclose repetitive motion strain or strenuous lifting, twisting, and bending. Low back pain is associated with pain and burning that radiates along the lateral thigh, leg, and foot, sometimes associated with numbness along the dermatomal areas. SLR and sitting knee extension produce radicular pain below the knee at less than 60 degrees of limb elevation, and pain may be felt in the buttocks or posterior thigh. Bowel and bladder functions are normal.

Nonspecific Back Problems
Musculoskeletal Strain (Postural, Overuse)

Back structures such as muscles and ligaments can become inflamed from overuse or strain. History often reveals no precipitating event for the onset of pain. Patients may report that pain is alleviated by rest, especially in the supine position with hips and knees flexed, and by the application of heat or cold. Pain is aggravated by sitting, walking, standing, and with certain motions. On physical examination, palpation will localize the pain, and muscle spasms may be felt. Range of motion of the spine will increase the pain, especially forward flexion. Neurological examination shows no abnormalities.

Spondylolisthesis

Pain can be the result of disruption of the vertebral spinous process, where the disruption results in subluxation of the vertebral body onto adjacent structures. This usually occurs between L5 and S1. Pain is usually chronic. Examination of the spine may disclose a palpable, prominent spinous process. Forward flexion may be limited.

Ankylosing Spondylitis

Ankylosing spondylitis is a systemic inflammatory condition of the vertebral column and sacroiliac joints. Peak incidence is in persons 20 to 30 years old; males are most often affected. Patients report chronic low back pain, which is worse on morning rising and lessens as the day progresses. Examination shows an excessive thoracic kyphosis and rounding of the posterior thoracic spine with forward flexion of the head, neck, and lower back. About 30% of patients will have arthritis of other joints. Radiographs may reveal fusion of vertebrae, and ESR is elevated.

Spinal Stenosis

Spinal stenosis is a bony encroachment on the nerve roots of the lumbar spine and is the most common cause of low back pain in adults older than 50 years. Patients report low back pain associated with lumbosacral radiculopathy, pain with walking or standing, and pain relief with sitting. Neurogenic (pseudo) claudication pain of the lower extremities is made worse with prolonged standing, walking, bending, or hyperextending the back.

Scheuermann Disease

Adolescent males develop this disease as a result of anterior disk protrusion, causing wedging of the thoracic vertebrae and an exaggeration of the normal posterior convex curvature of the thoracic spine. The cause is unknown but may develop from excessive lifting or spinal flexion. The patient reports mild to moderate pain, worsening toward the end of the day or after physical activity but relieved by rest. Physical examination demonstrates an increase in thoracic kyphosis on lateral view, made sharper by forward bending.

Osteoporosis

Osteoporosis is loss of mineralized bone mass that can result in a compression fracture of the vertebral body, usually occurring in the thoracic area. Back pain is often chronic and poorly localized. Multiple compression fractures may produce dorsal kyphosis and cervical lordosis. Persons at greatest risk are postmenopausal Caucasian women, especially those slight in build who have a history of inactivity. It is also common in persons older than 70 years who have age-related reduction in vitamin D synthesis. Osteoporosis can also be secondary to endocrine imbalance (such as hyperthyroidism), organ disease, drugs (such as corticosteroids), or excessive intake of alcohol.

Nonspinal Causes

Aortic Aneurysm (Dissecting)

Sudden onset of severe low or middle back pain that is not alleviated by rest in persons older than 30 years might suggest a dissecting aortic aneurysm. The patient may exhibit pallor, diaphoresis, and confusion. Pulses and blood pressure measured on each upper extremity will be asymmetrical. Emergency surgery is indicated.

Gallstones

The presence of gallbladder problems increases with age. A gallbladder attack often follows the ingestion of a fatty meal. A crampy right upper quadrant (RUQ) pain following the ingestion of a fatty meal is produced by spasms of the cystic duct that is obstructed with a stone. Gallbladder pain radiates around the trunk to the right scapula. Position does not affect the pain. Patients report belching, bloating, and an acidic stomach. Attacks may increase in frequency and severity and cause nighttime wakening. During an attack, palpation will show RUQ tenderness. Physical findings between attacks may be normal or there may be tenderness to palpation of the RUQ on inspiration (Murphy sign) if the gallbladder is inflamed. An RUQ mass may be felt if the gallbladder is obstructed. Obstruction is an emergency surgical situation.

Pyelonephritis

With pyelonephritis, the patient will appear ill and diaphoretic and may report nausea and vomiting, headache, and back or flank pain. The patient may have a fever. Severe lumbar tenderness will be found on fist percussion for costovertebral angle (CVA) tenderness. Urinalysis will show cloudy, malodorous urine, and microscopy will show the presence of casts and cells (i.e., red blood cells, white blood cells, and epithelial cells).

Pleuritis

Inflammation of the pleural lining of the lungs often follows an upper respiratory tract infection. Pleuritic pain is sharp, worsens on inspiration or with coughing, and is lessened by lying on the affected side. Physical examination of the lungs will be normal, or crackles and bronchial breath sounds will be heard on auscultation. A chest radiograph will provide information on the condition of the lungs.

Pelvic Inflammatory Disease

The symptoms of pelvic inflammatory disease (PID) depend on the extent of infection. Infection usually begins in the lower urinary tract or cervix and spreads to the endometrium, fallopian tubes, and peritoneum. The sexually active female patient may have mild to moderate dull, aching, lower abdominal, pelvic, or possibly back pain. She will report tenderness during cervical motion, uterine motion, or palpation of the adnexa. History may be positive for sexually transmitted infections (usually *Neisseria gonorrhoeae* or *Chlamydia trachomatis*), vaginal symptoms, or use of an IUD for contraception.

Psychogenic Causes
Psychological Back Pain

A careful history is needed to gain insight into the psychosocial and economic issues surrounding report of back pain. The patient may have a history of recent life stressors, be involved in a legal injury or workers' compensation action, or have a history of depression or alcohol abuse. The clinician should be aware of exaggerated signs of pain, such as moaning, grimacing, or overreaction. A patient who is a malingerer pretends to suffer, but when distracted will show inconsistent and variable results on examination, such as SLR, or will describe radiation of pain inconsistent with dermatome distribution.

DIFFERENTIAL DIAGNOSIS OF *Common Causes of Acute Low Back Pain*

CONDITION	HISTORY	PHYSICAL FINDINGS	DIAGNOSTIC STUDIES
Potentially Serious Causes			
Spinal fracture	Trauma to spine or back; pain is felt near site of injury	Palpable tenderness over site of fracture	Considered an emergency; immobilize patient and transport for radiographs
Tumor	History of cancer; progressive pain is unremitting; occurs at night and at rest	Weight loss, fever, tenderness near tumor	ESR; bone scan
Osteoblastoma	Neck or back pain not relieved by aspirin; occurs in older adolescents and young adults	Localized tenderness; may have scoliosis with muscle pain	Plain film shows an expansive osteolytic lesion surrounded by thin peripheral rim of bone; bone scan; CT scan
Osteoid osteoma	Occurs primarily in adolescents; rare in patients over age 40; well localized pain that may be more severe at night and relieved by aspirin or other prostaglandin inhibitors	Painful, well-localized scoliosis may be present	Bone scan
Infection (vertebral osteomyelitis)	History of infection, invasive procedure; continuous, dull back pain; chronic back pain	Acute onset presents with fever, diaphoresis; tenderness over affected disk; positive SLR	ESR; blood culture; bone biopsy; CT scan; MRI
Diskitis	Pain aggravated by movement; more common in children	Tenderness over affected disk	ESR
Herniated disk	LBP radiating down the buttock to below the knee, symptoms present less than one month	Positive SLR	None
Cauda equina syndrome	Constant pain in a saddle distribution; urinary retention, fecal incontinence, radiculopathy	Positive SLR, abnormal DTRs, motor weakness	MRI, surgical emergency

Continued

DIFFERENTIAL DIAGNOSIS OF *Common Causes of Acute Low Back Pain—cont'd*

CONDITION	HISTORY	PHYSICAL FINDINGS	DIAGNOSTIC STUDIES
Sciatica Problems			
Sciatica	Acute back pain with radiculopathy; history of strain or trauma, relief with sitting	Paravertebral tenderness and spasm; positive SLR; sitting knee extension, sensory findings	EMG if chronic
Nonspecific Back Problems			
Musculoskeletal strain	Pain in back, buttocks; history of new activity or exertion; relief of pain with sitting	Paravertebral tenderness, scoliosis, or loss of lumbar lordosis; no neurological signs	None
Spondylolisthesis	Young person in a sport that demands rapid movement between hyperflexion and hyperextension or requires excess loading in hyperextension	No neurological signs; pain localized to low back, just below level of iliac crest; tight hamstrings	Lumbar spine radiographs
Ankylosing spondylitis	Persons under age 40: insidious onset; progressive morning back pain relieved with exercise	Painful sacroiliac joints, reduced spine mobility; may have uveitis	ESR; spinal radiographs
Spinal stenosis	Pain worse throughout day; aggravated by standing, relieved by rest; pseudoclaudication	Signs of osteoarthritis of joints; may have neurological signs	None
Scheuermann disease	Affects mostly adolescent males; mild to moderately severe pain, worse at end of day, relieved by rest	Normal examination; may show an exaggerated thoracic kyphosis that is fixed in attempted hyperextension	Thoracic spine radiographs
Osteoporosis	Chronic, poorly localized back pain; postmenopausal; slight build; history of inactivity or endocrine disorder	Palpable tenderness over area of compression fracture; kyphosis or lordosis; loss of height	Bone densitometry; spinal radiograph to assess fracture
Nonspinal Causes			
Aortic aneurysm	Severe, acute-onset pain not related to activity or movement; increased risk in persons over age 30; pallor, diaphoresis, anxiety, confusion	Intact aneurysm will be a visible pulsatile midline upper quadrant abdominal mass; in a dissected aneurysm, upper extremity pulse and pulse pressures are asymmetrical; posterior thoracic pain may be felt	Emergency surgical referral
Gallstones	Increased incidence with age; steady, intense pain in RUQ with radiation to right scapula or shoulder; belching, bloating, fatty food intolerance	Normal physical examination or positive Murphy sign on palpation of abdomen	Surgical referral
Pyelonephritis	Ill-appearing; sweating, nausea, back or flank pain, headache	Fever: cloudy, malodorous urine; CVA tenderness on percussion	Urinalysis; urine culture

DIFFERENTIAL DIAGNOSIS OF *Common Causes of Acute Low Back Pain—cont'd*

CONDITION	HISTORY	PHYSICAL FINDINGS	DIAGNOSTIC STUDIES
Pleuritis	History of recent URI; pleuritic pain	Normal examination or crackles and bronchial breath sounds	PPD; chest radiograph
Pelvic inflammatory disease	Sexually active female; low back and abdominal pain; history of urinary or vaginal symptoms, sexually transmitted disease, IUD, multiple sex partners	Cervical and uterine motion tenderness, adnexal tenderness; cervicitis, fever	Gonorrhea, *Chlamydia* cultures; ESR
Psychogenic Causes			
Psychological back pain	History of psychosocial stressors, depression, exaggerated expressions of pain	Exaggerated or inconsistent reactions to testing; normal examination	None

CT, computed tomography; *CVA*, costovertebral angle; *DTRs*, deep tendon reflexes; *EMG*, electromyography; *ESR*, erythrocyte sedimentation rate; *IUD*, intrauterine device; *LBP*, lower back pain; *MRI*, magnetic resonance imaging; *PPD, purified protein derivative; RUQ*, right upper quadrant; *SLR*, straight leg raising; *URI*, upper respiratory tract infection.

REFERENCES AND READINGS

Balagué F, Dudler K, Nordin M: Low-back pain in children, *Lancet* 361:1403, 2003.

Bernstein R, Cozen H: Evaluation of back pain in children and adolescents, *Am Fam Physician* 76:1669, 2007.

Chou R, Qaseem A, Snow V, Casey D, Cross JT Jr, Shekelle P et al: Clinical Efficacy Assessment Subcommittee of the American College of Physicians, American College of Physicians, American Pain Society Low Back Pain Guidelines Panel. Diagnosis and treatment of low back pain: a joint clinical practice guideline from the American College of Physicians and the American Pain Society, *Ann Intern Med* 147:478, 2007.

Deyo RA, Rainville J, Kent DL: What can the history and physical examination tell us about low back pain? *JAMA* 268:760, 1992.

Deyo RA, Weinstein JN: Low back pain, *N Engl J Med* 344:363, 2001.

Koes BW, van Tulder MW, Ostelo R, Kim Burton A, Waddell G: Clinical guidelines for the management of low back pain in primary care: an international comparison, *Spine* 26:2504, 2001.

Kraft DE: Low back pain in the adolescent athlete, *Pediatr Clin North Am* 49:643, 2002.

Last AR, Hulbert K: Chronic low back pain; evaluation and management, *Am Fam Physician* 79:1067, 2009.

Manchikanti L, Singh V, Datta S, Cohen SP, Hirsch JA: American Society of Interventional Pain Physicians: Comprehensive review of epidemiology, scope, and impact of spinal pain, *Pain Physician* 12:E35, 2009.

Nasal Symptoms and Sinus Congestion

Concern about symptoms of the "common cold" accounts for a significant proportion of primary care visits by both children and adults, especially in the winter months. Symptoms include nasal congestion, rhinorrhea, postnasal drip, sneezing, itchy nose, watery and itchy eyes, and frontal headache. Severe symptoms are associated with ageusia (loss of taste) and anosmia (loss of smell).

The nose humidifies, warms, and filters inspired air. The nasal turbinates promote turbulent airflow that causes particulate matter to fall on the mucosa, where it is swept away by ciliated pseudostratified columnar cells to the nasopharynx. Rhinitis, or inflammation of the mucous membranes, is a frequent nasal symptom that is caused by bacterial or viral infection, a response to allergens, or a response to medication or extremes in environmental temperature.

Nasal polyps, septal deviation, or congenital anomaly can cause nasal obstruction. In children, nasal obstruction is very frequently unilateral and may be secondary to a foreign body inserted into the nose.

Respiratory epithelium lines the paranasal sinuses and creates drainage into the nasal cavity via the superior meatus and middle meatus. The maxillary sinus is the most frequently involved paranasal sinus because its ciliated cells carry maxillary sinus drainage against gravity. When drainage systems become impaired as a result of mucosal edema, mechanical obstruction, or impaired ciliary activity, viruses and bacteria proliferate.

The paranasal sinuses include the frontal, ethmoid, maxillary, and sphenoid (Figure 22-1). Most sinus infections are caused by bacteria common to the nasopharynx that proliferate when local or systemic defenses are impaired. The most common causative organisms producing bacterial sinusitis in both adults and children are *Streptococcus pneumoniae* and *Haemophilus influenzae*. Sinusitis may also be associated with allergies and asthmatic exacerbations or with contiguous infection of the mouth or face.

DIAGNOSTIC REASONING: FOCUSED HISTORY

What symptoms will help me narrow the possibilities?

Key Questions

- Can you describe your symptoms?
- How long have they been present?
- Do you have a history of nasal problems?
- Do the symptoms occur at any particular time of the year?
- Is there a family history of allergies or asthma?

Duration of Symptoms/History of Problems

Acute symptoms of rhinitis or sinus congestion, usually lasting 48 to 72 hours, are caused by edematous mucosa obstructing the sinus ostia. If a person has no history of similar symptoms but has systemic symptoms, such as fever, myalgias, and chills, acute infectious rhinitis caused by rhinoviruses or parainfluenza virus is likely.

Chronic rhinitis lasting weeks to years is rarely infectious; rather it is often associated with anatomical abnormalities that impair the sinus drainage system, although the mucociliary clearance mechanisms are normal.

Seasonal Occurrence of Symptoms

Suspect allergic rhinitis if a person describes seasonal occurrence of nasal symptoms associated with sneezing, wheezing, and itchy or burning eyes. A distinguishing feature of the allergic individual is the propensity to develop sustained IgE response after antigenic stimulation. IgE is an antibody capable of interacting with target cells that release mediators on contact with specific antigens. This reaction is the manifestation of an allergy.

Persons with perennial allergies have an allergen present in the environment on a year-round basis from such sources as animal dander, house dust, mold,

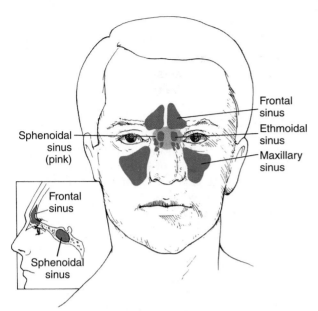

Sphenoidal sinus (pink)

Frontal sinus

Ethmoidal sinus

Maxillary sinus

Frontal sinus

Sphenoidal sinus

FIGURE 22-1 Anterior and lateral views of the paranasal sinuses. (From Barkauskas VH, Baumann L, Darling-Fisher C: *Health and physical assessment*, ed 3, St Louis, 2002, Mosby.)

feathers, and cockroaches. Seasonal allergies usually occur in early spring (tree pollens), early summer (grass pollens), and early fall (weed pollens).

Family History

Family history of asthma or allergies is frequently associated with allergic rhinitis. Other symptoms may include a sensation of head stuffiness, ear discomfort, fatigue, and a scratchy or mild sore throat.

If I suspect sinus problems, what do I need to know?

Key Questions

- How long have you had these symptoms?
- Do you have pain? Can you point to the areas of pain?
- Do your symptoms change with position changes?
- Do you have a history of sinus problems?

Acute Symptoms

Acute sinusitis is an abrupt onset of infection of one or more of the paranasal sinuses, and it occurs when the sinus ostia become obstructed, usually after an upper respiratory tract infection. Sinusitis is frequently associated with a sore throat, often irritated by postnasal discharge,

facial or tooth pain, or headache over the affected sinus, as well as morning periorbital swelling, fever, and malaise. Other less common causes include anatomical abnormality, adenoid hypertrophy, and contiguous infection, such as a dental abscess or periorbital cellulitis.

Location of Pain

An adult patient with sinusitis most often reports a prolonged cold with symptoms of nasal congestion and facial pain. Children rarely complain of headache or facial pain. The location of pain may indicate which sinus is involved. Pain of maxillary sinusitis occurs over the sinuses and is sometimes perceived as a maxillary toothache. Frontal sinusitis produces a frontal headache that is worse on morning wakening. Ethmoid sinusitis causes pain that refers to the vertex, forehead, or occipital or temporal region, whereas the pain of sphenoid sinusitis is perceived on the top of the head.

Position Change

Maxillary sinusitis produces pain that worsens with bending or leaning forward. The postnasal discharge associated with sinusitis produces a cough that worsens while lying down.

Chronic Symptoms

Chronic symptoms can be caused by prolonged obstruction of the osteomeatal complex, which leads to dysfunction of ciliary motility and movement of mucus within the sinuses. Local factors that cause mechanical obstruction include adenoid hypertrophy, conchae bullosa, nasal polyps, foreign bodies, and nasal deviations. Adults with symptoms that last more than 3 weeks experience upper molar pain or headache, postnasal drip, and rarely have a fever. In children, chronic sinusitis is defined as the presence of symptoms for longer than 30 days.

Do associated symptoms provide any clues?

Key Questions

- Do you have other acute symptoms, such as cough, fever, or muscle aches?
- Do you have other chronic symptoms, such as eye pain, bad breath, or fatigue?

Other Acute Symptoms

Acute bacterial infection of the nasal and sinus mucosa is characterized by the presence of purulent nasal discharge. Acute rhinitis caused by a bacterial or viral infection produces systemic symptoms, such as fever, myalgia, and chills. Allergic rhinitis is associated with sneezing, nasal congestion, clear and profuse rhinorrhea, and pruritus of the nose, palate, pharynx, and middle ear. Eye complaints include conjunctival irritation, itching, erythema, and tearing. Ear complaints involve a feeling of fullness in the ears with popping. Sinus complaints are pressure and/or pain of the cheeks, forehead, or behind the eyes.

Acute sinusitis in children involves the presence of symptoms for less than 30 days, a persistent cough, fever with a temperature greater than 39° C (102.2° F) for more than 3 days, and malodorous breath. The maxillary and ethmoid sinuses are most commonly affected, with the frontal sinus occasionally and the sphenoid sinus rarely affected.

Chronic Symptoms

Chronic sinusitis involves long episodes of inflammation or repeated infections that lead to anatomical destruction. The recurrent symptoms interfere with daily activities and are not relieved with nonpharmacological measures or over-the-counter medications. Patients often report a cold that does not go away, eye pain, halitosis, chronic cough, fatigue, anorexia, and malaise.

Is it viral or bacterial?

Key Questions

■ What color is your nasal drainage?
■ How long have you had these symptoms?

Acute rhinitis caused by a bacterial or viral infection produces yellow or green purulent nasal discharge. Watery or clear discharge occurs with allergic reactions. Symptoms of viral upper respiratory tract infections in children persist 5 to 10 days and then gradually subside. Many children may have up to eight colds per year.

Are symptoms unilateral or bilateral?

Key Question

■ Is the symptom on one side or both sides?
Infectious rhinitis and allergic rhinitis are usually bilateral. Unilateral symptoms are more indicative of an anatomical cause, such as nasal polyps, septal deviation, or a foreign body (typically occurs in children).

Are there risk factors that will narrow the diagnosis?

Key Questions

■ Do you smoke?
■ Are you exposed to others who smoke?
■ Do you have any other health problems?
■ Have you had a recent history of head or facial trauma?
■ Have you been diving or swimming?
■ Have you been exposed to infections in day care, school, or work settings?
■ Are you pregnant?

Smoking History

Smokers have an increased risk of sinusitis. Smoking can lead to the production of more tenacious mucus and to temporary paralysis of the nasal cilia. Exposure to passive smoke causes an increased risk of upper and lower respiratory tract infections.

Trauma History

Nasal trauma or fracture may lead to nasal congestion. A rare but serious post-trauma cerebrospinal fluid rhinorrhea can be present. Up to 80% of head injuries involve the paranasal sinuses.

Diving and Swimming

Sinusitis from diving or swimming is secondary to barotrauma, infection from contaminated water, or an allergic response to chlorine.

Exposure

Exposure to viral infections increases when children are exposed to other children. The spread of a virus occurs by direct secretion of droplets or contact with contaminated objects.

Pregnancy

The hormonal changes of pregnancy can cause nasal congestion.

Is the patient using any drugs that would cause nasal congestion?

Key Questions

■ Are you using nasal sprays or drops?
■ Do you use cocaine or other illicit drugs?
■ What other medications are you taking?

Nasal Spray

The use of topical sympathomimetic sprays or drops for more than 1 week can lead to rebound nasal congestion or vasodilation after short periods of vasoconstriction. The use of decongestants and antihistamines with low ambient humidity leads to excessive dryness and impaired ciliary function.

Drug Use

Chronic or acute cocaine use can cause rebound nasal congestion. Nasal congestion associated with conjunctivitis and irritation of the eyes may be seen in persons who abuse drugs by inhalation.

Medications

Oral contraceptives, phenothiazines, angiotensin-converting enzyme (ACE) inhibitors, and ß-blockers may cause nasal congestion.

Is there systemic disease present?

Key Questions

- Have you noticed any other body symptoms?
- Do you have any chronic health problems?

Systemic Disorders

Systemic causes of decreased mucociliary clearance include cystic fibrosis, ciliary dyskinesia syndrome, and immunoglobulin deficiency. Persons with congenital or acquired immune deficiencies, such as diabetes mellitus, leukemia, acquired immunodeficiency syndrome, and cystic fibrosis, have an increased risk of developing acute and chronic sinusitis. Hypothyroidism, acromegaly, Horner syndrome, neoplasm, and granulomatosis disorder can also cause nasal symptoms.

DIAGNOSTIC REASONING: FOCUSED PHYSICAL EXAMINATION
Perform a General Inspection

Note the patient's general appearance. Observe for signs of impaired mental status. A severe unremitting or new-onset headache, vomiting, or alteration in consciousness requires consideration for immediate referral.

Take Vital Signs

Persons with acute viral rhinitis or acute sinusitis may be afebrile or have a low-grade fever. Persons with allergic rhinitis are afebrile. The presence of mouth breathing suggests chronic nasal obstruction caused by hypertrophied pharyngeal lymphoid tissues.

Inspect the Face

Children with chronic allergic conditions have an allergic "salute"; this is a crease on the nose from continued wiping up of nasal drainage. Allergic "shiners" are dark circles under the eyes suggestive of venous congestion and stasis. Observe for facial symmetry and signs of periorbital edema. Periorbital cellulitis is the most common serious complication of severe bacterial sinusitis.

Perform a Regional Examination of the Head and Neck

Examine the eyes (including visual acuity), ears, and cervicofacial lymph nodes. Complications of severe fulminate sinusitis are rare and are caused by the direct spread of infection, secondary to destruction of the wall between the sinuses and the orbit. Symptoms can include a sudden increase in pain, acute edema of the eyelids, periorbital edema and erythema, decreased visual acuity, diplopia, and displacement of the eye laterally. The patient may experience pain on testing of extraocular muscles. These symptoms mandate immediate referral.

Observe for symptoms of coryza (acute rhinitis) as well as ear and eye drainage. Erythematous tympanic membranes are seen in acute viral rhinitis.

Examine the Mouth and Teeth

Examine the teeth for the presence of abscesses, especially the first and secondary maxillary molars and the alveolar margin of the teeth. Tenderness elicited by tapping on the maxillary teeth with a tongue blade may indicate dental root infection or maxillary sinusitis. Mouth breathing is associated with hypertrophied gingival mucosa and halitosis. Halitosis can also be a sign of dental abscess or sinusitis.

Children with acute viral rhinitis have mild erythema of the tonsils and posterior pharynx. If there is vasomotor rhinitis, mucus is present in the posterior pharynx.

Test for Smell

Severe nasal congestion or ethmoid sinusitis causes anosmia.

Inspect Condition of Nasal Mucosa and Turbinates

Use a nasal speculum and head mirror to optimally visualize the condition of the nasal mucosa and turbinates. A topical vasoconstrictive agent may be needed to shrink the swollen mucosa to visualize the middle meatus.

In infants and young children, the nares tend to open forward, and tilting the tip of the nose up with the thumb and directing the light into the nares will allow inspection of the nasal cavities.

Pale, boggy turbinates are seen with allergic rhinitis. Inflamed mucous membranes are seen with acute coryza or hay fever. Allergic rhinitis may also produce a violet-colored mucous membrane. Ulceration of the nasal mucosa may be found in persons who abuse drugs by inhalation.

Inspect for Masses

Observe for the presence of nasal polyps, which look like skinned grapes and are usually bilateral and hang from the middle turbinate into the lumen of the nose. Septal deviation or anatomical anomalies may predispose to infection. Nasal septum deviation can also lead to nasal obstruction. Squamous cell carcinoma usually occurs unilaterally. Masses that increase in size and pulsate on Valsalva maneuver may indicate an encephalocele or a meningocele.

Note the Presence and Color of Any Discharge

Pus in the ostium of the middle turbinate suggests a bacterial sinusitis. Cerebrospinal fluid (CSF) drainage will increase in a forward position. Identify CSF by testing nasal drainage for glucose and protein levels comparable to those of CSF. Foul-smelling nasal discharge is a characteristic feature of sinusitis of dental origin. Foul-smelling unilateral purulent discharge may indicate a foreign body in the nasal cavity.

Transilluminate the Sinuses

Light will pass through air-filled sinuses. Transillumination is used to assess the presence of fluid in the frontal and maxillary sinuses and cannot be used to examine the ethmoid or sphenoid sinuses. Normal transillumination of the frontal sinus rules out frontal sinusitis in 90% of cases. Complete opacity of sinuses suggests infection. However, the results of transillumination are often nonspecific, such as reduced illumination, and do not lead to a diagnosis.

Transillumination of maxillary sinuses can be done in two ways. Place a transilluminator over the infraorbital rim, blocking light from the examiner's vision with the free hand, and judge the amount of light transmission (opaque, dull, normal) through the hard palate. This should be performed in a completely darkened room. Dentures must be removed. A second method is to place the transilluminator in the patient's mouth, sealing the lips, and observe the amount of light transmitted through the maxillary sinuses. Frontal sinuses can be transilluminated by placing the instrument below the supraorbital rim.

Palpate and Percuss Frontal and Maxillary Sinuses for Tenderness

Percuss and palpate the cheeks for tenderness and swelling, indicating maxillary sinusitis of dental origin. To assess the frontal sinuses, exert pressure over the eyebrow or slightly upward pressure under the brow to assess for tenderness. Direct percussion may elicit tenderness over the affected sinus.

Test for Facial Fullness and Pressure

Bending forward from the waist (with head dropping downward) or performing a Valsalva maneuver will worsen the symptoms if a partial or complete sinus obstruction is present.

Examine the Lungs

Auscultate the lungs for signs of wheezing, rales, and loudness of breath sounds. Peak flow volume or PO_2 saturation as measured using a pulse oximeter will detect the presence of reactive upper airway disease.

Perform Neurological Testing If Indicated

To detect any complications from sinusitis, assess neurological and cranial nerve function if the patient appears severely ill. Severe complications of sinusitis are cavernous sinus thrombosis and brain abscesses.

LABORATORY AND DIAGNOSTIC STUDIES
Nasal Smear

A nasal smear performed to look for eosinophils confirms the diagnosis of allergic rhinitis. Nasal scraping of the surface epithelium along with a sample of secretions is more reliable in detecting the presence of eosinophils than is the sampling of secretions alone. Either method can be used to detect the presence of neutrophils. Specimens are graded using a semiquantitative scale of 0 to 4+, based on the concentration of cells. Table 22-1 illustrates the diagnostic classifications found with varying nasal smears.

Sinus Radiographs

Radiographs are not routinely indicated but may be obtained in patients who have severe symptoms and fail to respond to treatment. Severe symptoms may indicate complications of sinusitis, such as orbital cellulitis, brain abscess, osteomyelitis, or cavernous sinus thrombosis. A sinus radiographic series consists of four views: an anteroposterior (Caldwell) view of the ethmoid sinus, a view (Chamberlain) of the frontal sinus, a lateral view of the sphenoid and frontal sinuses, and an occipitomental (Waters) view of the maxillary sinuses.

Computed Tomography Scan

A computed tomography (CT) scan shows air, bone, and soft tissue and optimally facilitates definition of regional anatomy and the extent of disease. A CT scan is done when sinusitis becomes chronic and does not respond to symptomatic or antibiotic treatment. A CT scan may also show causes for chronic sinusitis by visualizing many disorders not detected by plain films, such as facial fractures, nasal polyps, cysts, chronic mucosal thickening, temporomandibular joint (TMJ) disorders, foreign bodies, and tumors.

Magnetic Resonance Imaging

Magnetic resonance imaging (MRI) is an excellent technique for imaging soft tissue pathology of the face and neck, especially neoplastic conditions. CT does not delineate soft tissue pathology as well as MRI.

Sinus Aspiration

Sinus aspiration is the only way to confirm the diagnosis of bacterial sinusitis and is performed by an otolaryngologist. A trocar is introduced into the maxillary sinus through the upper gingival recess.

Nasal Endoscopy

Nasal endoscopy allows direct observation of the nasal passages, larynx, pharynx, and surrounding tissue, and aids in the diagnosis of nasal polyps, chronic sinusitis, or laryngeal trauma. Before a flexible fiberoptic scope is threaded through the nasal passages, an anesthetic spray is applied to the nasal tissue while the patient is in a sitting position.

Allergy Skin Testing

Results of skin testing can confirm immunological disease and identify specific antigens responsible for allergic rhinitis, which may come from exposure to irritants in the patient's environment. The presence of serum IgE antibody suggests an allergic response.

DIFFERENTIAL DIAGNOSIS
Infectious Rhinitis

Infectious rhinitis is an acute condition frequently associated with a history of recent upper respiratory tract infection. A definitive sign of this condition is the presence of yellow or green purulent discharge and red nasal mucosa.

Allergic Rhinitis

Allergic rhinitis is distinguished by a recurrent rhinorrhea with clear watery mucus, sneezing, and pruritus. Nasal turbinates are pale and swollen. Family history

---

Table 22-1 **Diagnostic Classifications of Nasal Smear Specimens**

NASAL SMEAR	DIAGNOSTIC CLASSIFICATION
Increased eosinophils	Allergic or nonallergic eosinophilia; aspirin intolerance
Increased basophils	Same as above; nonallergic basophilia
Increased neutrophils	
With intracellular bacteria	Nasopharyngitis; sinusitis
With ciliary tophthora	Viral upper respiratory infection (URI)
With fungi	Fungal URI
With no bacteria	Irritant reaction
Bacteria (2-4+)—intracellular	Nasopharyngitis or sinusitis
No eosinophils or basophils, 2+ or fewer neutrophils, few bacteria	Normal finding

From Mygind N, Naderio R: *Allergic and non-allergic rhinitis*, Copenhagen, Denmark, 1993, Munksgaard International Publishers.

of allergies is often positive. About 25% of the population has some type of allergy. IgE-mediated reactions to aeroallergens are based on a combination of history, physical examination, and skin tests. Nasal smears can be tested for the presence of eosinophils to confirm an allergenic response.

Seasonal allergies are associated with short bursts of intense exposure to an allergen that creates symptoms consistent with a histamine-mediated response, such as pruritus, swelling, sneezing, and rhinorrhea. A common seasonal allergy is pollenosis or hay fever. A history or pattern of symptoms and exposure is critical in diagnosis.

Perennial allergies are caused by continuous exposure to allergens associated with chronic congestion. Common indoor allergens are animal dander, dust mites, and cockroaches. Outdoor allergens include grasses, trees, pollens, and weeds.

Nonallergic Rhinitis

Nonallergic rhinitis can be associated or not associated with eosinophilia on nasal smear. Nonallergic rhinitis with eosinophilia syndrome (NARES) is a diagnosis based on nasal cytology and involves symptoms similar to allergic rhinitis without an identifiable allergen cause. A history will reveal aspirin or nonsteroidal anti-inflammatory drug intolerance and rhinorrhea. Noneosinophilia is associated with any other nonallergic cause of rhinitis.

Rhinitis Medicamentosa

Drug-induced rebound congestion can follow the long-term use of topical nasal decongestants. Rhinitis medicamentosa is also used to describe nasal symptoms secondary to other medications, such as nasal congestion associated with hormone changes of pregnancy. Other drugs that have vasodilatory effects include antihypertensives that interfere with adrenergic neuronal function and hormones in oral contraceptives. Nasal vasoconstriction response is completely abolished after the administration of reserpine.

Acute Sinusitis

Acute sinusitis is characterized by purulent nasal discharge, postnasal drip, and localized facial pain over the sinus involved. It often follows a viral upper respiratory tract infection. However, symptoms such as halitosis, reduced sense of smell, or morning cough have been reported in children in the absence of facial pain. Physical examination will elicit localized tenderness to palpation or percussion over the affected sinus. Pressure and pain will increase in a forward-bending position. Purulent discharge may be visible in the posterior pharynx or may be seen emerging from the ostia of the middle turbinate. Transillumination will indicate unilateral or bilateral obstruction. Ciliary function is impaired with infection and may not be completely restored for 2 to 6 weeks. The diagnosis of sinusitis in children requires two of three major criteria (cough, purulent nasal discharge, or purulent pharyngeal drainage) or one major and two minor criteria (sore throat, wheezing, foul breath, facial pain, periorbital edema, headache, earache, fever, and toothache).

Chronic Sinusitis

An incompletely treated acute sinusitis can lead to a chronic condition. The patient presents with persistent symptoms of low-grade infection and intermittent acute exacerbations typical of acute sinusitis. Symptoms are recurrent and not controlled with over-the-counter or nonpharmacological remedies. Multiple pathogens may be causative organisms, with the most common being *Moraxella catarrhalis*, *H. influenzae*, and *S. pneumoniae*. Sinus radiographs or a CT scan will reveal mucosal thickening of 5 mm or greater. Allergy testing may reveal a perennial allergy that creates chronic inflammation.

Nasal or Sinus Obstruction

A history of aspirin intolerance or asthma with polyps is associated with obstruction. Acute obstruction suggests edema secondary to infection, allergic response, exposure to irritants, or foreign body (in children). Chronic obstruction may be secondary to congenital deformity, nasal polyps, or septal deviation. In infants, congenital choanal atresia can cause obstruction.

Nasal Polyposis

This syndrome has multiple causative factors, including a history of asthma and aspirin intolerance. The polyps are translucent grapelike growths that are mobile, rarely bleed, and prolapse into the nasal cavity. The resulting obstruction can be associated with chronic sinusitis. Any suspicious polyps should be biopsied.

Osteomyelitis of the Frontal Bone

Osteomyelitis can occur as a complication of sinusitis. Osteomyelitis occurs in children and young adults and may follow head trauma or scuba diving. *Staphylococcus pyogenes* or anaerobic streptococci are causative organisms. Patients appear severely ill and may have edema of the upper eyelid and puffy swelling over the frontal bone. Diagnosis is by radiography and blood culture.

DIFFERENTIAL DIAGNOSIS OF *Common Causes of Nasal Symptoms and Sinus Congestion*

CONDITION	HISTORY	PHYSICAL FINDINGS	DIAGNOSTIC STUDIES
Infectious rhinitis	Perennial but more common in winter months; recent URI	Red, swollen mucosa; purulent discharge	Nasal smear for neutrophils, intracellular bacteria
Allergic rhinitis	Family history of allergies; sneezing; recurrent pattern; more common in children and young adults	Pale, boggy mucosa; rhinorrhea with clear, watery mucus	Nasal smear for eosinophils; allergy testing
Nonallergic rhinitis	No allergenic cause identified	Similar to allergic rhinitis	Absence of eosinophilia on nasal cytology
Rhinitis medicamentosa	History of medication use: oral contraceptives, nasal sprays, antihypertensives; nasal congestion	Swollen mucosa; clear mucus or dry mucosa	None
Acute sinusitis	Smoker; recent URI; winter months; frontal headaches made worse with forward bending; sensation of fullness or pressure	Purulent discharge; maxillary toothache on percussion, postnasal drainage; decreased transillumination	None
Chronic sinusitis	History of previous sinus infections; dull ache or no pain; persistent symptoms	Same as in acute sinusitis; decreased or no transillumination; obstruction such as deviated septum, polyps	CT scan; nasal endoscopy; allergy testing
Obstruction	History of asthma, aspirin intolerance; foreign body in children; tumor in adults; infants with choanal atresia: difficulty feeding; cyanosis if bilateral	Increased pain with forward motion or Valsalva; pain with percussion and palpation of sinuses; no transillumination; septal deviation	Sinus radiographs; CT scan
Nasal polyposis	History of asthma, aspirin intolerance	Presence of polyps	Nasal endoscopy; may require biopsy
Osteomyelitis of frontal bone	History of head trauma, diving	Appears severely ill; periorbital and frontal edema	Sinus and skull radiographs; blood culture

CT, computed tomography; *URI,* upper respiratory infection.

REFERENCES AND READINGS

Gendo K, Larson EB: Evidence-based diagnostic strategies for evaluating suspected allergic rhinitis, *Ann Intern Med* 140:4, 2004.

Leung A, Kellner J: Acute sinusitis in children: diagnosis and management, *J Pediatr Health Care* 18:72, 2004.

Marple BF, Stankiewicz JA, Baroody FM, Chow JM, Conley DB, Corey JP et al.: Diagnosis and management of chronic rhinosinusitis in adults, *Postgrad Med* 121:121, 2009.

Nash D, Wald E: Sinusitis, *Pediatr Rev* 22:111, 2001.

Novelline RA: *Squire's fundamentals of radiology,* ed 6, Cambridge, Mass, 2004, Harvard University Press.

Rosenfeld RM, Andes D, Bhattacharyya N, Cheung D, Eisenberg S, Ganiats TG et al.: Clinical practice guideline: adult sinusitis, *Otolaryngol Head Neck Surg* 137:S1, 2007.

Skoner DP: Allergic rhinitis: definition, epidemiology, pathophysiology, detection and diagnosis, *J Allergy Clin Immunol* 108:S2, 2001.

Zacharisen M, Casper R: Pediatric sinusitis, *Immunol Allergy Clin North Am* 25:313, 2005.

CHAPTER

23

Palpitations

Palpitations are defined as an unpleasant awareness of the forceful, rapid, or irregular beating of the heart. It is a common presenting symptom that is usually benign; however, occasionally palpitations can indicate a life-threatening arrhythmia.

Palpitations are described by patients as a "thumping," "pounding," or "fluttering" sensation in the chest. This sensation can be either intermittent or sustained, and either regular or irregular. Patients often note palpitations when quietly resting, a time when other stimuli are minimal.

Causes of palpitations can be cardiac arrhythmias, psychological factors, drugs and medications, nonarrhythmic cardiac problems, and systemic (extracardiac) conditions. Arrhythmias include premature atrial and ventricular contractions, supraventricular and ventricular arrhythmias, and atrial fibrillations. Psychological causes of palpitations include panic attack or disorder, anxiety states, and somatization. Drugs and medications including alcohol, tobacco, caffeine, aminophylline, atropine, thyroxine, cocaine, and amphetamines enhance the strength of myocardial contraction and can cause the sensation of palpitations. Nonarrhythmic cardiac problems, such as mitral valve prolapse, pericarditis, congestive heart failure, valvular disease, congenital heart disease, and cardiac myopathy, can produce palpations. Systemic conditions, such as hyperthyroidism, vasovagal syncope, and hypoglycemia, can cause palpitations. Hyperdynamic cardiovascular states caused by catecholaminergic stimulation from exercise, stress, or pheochromocytoma can cause palpitations. In many cases, the cause of the palpitations is unknown.

In children, fever, anxiety, exercise, and anemia are common causes of palpitations.

Although palpitations are usually of benign etiology, the principal goal in assessing patients with palpitations is to determine if the symptom is caused by a life-threatening arrhythmia.

DIAGNOSTIC REASONING: FOCUSED HISTORY

Could this patient have a life-threatening arrhythmia?

Key Questions

- Do you have a history of coronary artery disease (CAD)?
- Are you lightheaded or have you had episodes of passing out?
- Are you having chest pain?
- Have you had difficulty breathing?
- Do you have a family history of sudden cardiac death?
- Have you had heart surgery?

Coronary Artery Disease

Patients with risk factors for or preexisting coronary artery disease (CAD) are at greater risk for ventricular arrhythmias as a cause for palpitations. Risk factors include smoking, hypertension, diabetes, a history of myocardial infarction (MI), and a family history of heart attack or stroke before age 60.

Lightheadedness/Syncope

The association of palpitations with other symptoms suggesting hemodynamic compromise, including presyncope, syncope, or lightheadedness, may signify a life-threatening cardiac arrhythmia.

Chest Pain, Dyspnea

Palpitations caused by sustained tachyarrhythmias in patients with CAD can be accompanied by angina pectoris or dyspnea. Palpitations associated with chest pain suggest ischemic heart disease or, if the chest pain is relieved by leaning forward, pericardial disease. Exertional palpitations associated with chest pain, lightheadedness, or both in the athlete may indicate an underlying cardiovascular disorder.

Sudden Cardiac Death

A family history of sudden cardiac death (SCD) may indicate an inherited cardiac problem.

Cardiac Surgery

Children and adults who have had cardiac surgery are at risk for arrhythmias and palpitations.

What else do I need to know about the palpitation?

Key Questions

- Can you describe the palpitation/sensation?
- When do the palpitations occur?
- How long do the palpitations last?
- Do the palpitations start or stop abruptly?

Description of Palpitations

Flip-flopping. Single skipped beats or a sensation of the heart stopping and then starting with a pounding, flipping, or jumping sensation, especially while sitting quietly or lying in bed and lasting only for brief periods, are typically attributed to premature contraction of the atrium or ventricle. The sensation that the heart has stopped results from the pause following the premature contraction, and the pounding or flipping sensation results from the forceful contraction following the pause.

Rapid fluttering in the chest. A feeling of rapid fluttering in the chest may result from atrial or ventricular arrhythmias, including sinus tachycardia.

Pounding in the neck. A pounding feeling in the neck is caused by the dissociation of atrial and ventricular contractions so that the atria contract against closed tricuspid and mitral valves, producing cannon A waves. The sensation of rapid and regular pounding in the neck is typical of reentrant supraventricular arrhythmias, particularly atrioventricular nodal tachycardia.

Occurrence of Palpitations

Palpitations that start during sleep or states of increased vagal tone (e.g., at termination of exercise) may be associated with vagal-mediated atrial fibrillation or certain subtypes of long QT syndromes. Palpitations that are worse at night may be caused by benign ectopy or atrial fibrillation.

Palpitations that start and stop abruptly suggest supraventricular or ventricular tachycardias. Palpitations that can be stopped using patient-initiated vagal maneuvers, such as the Valsalva maneuver, suggest supraventricular tachycardia.

Rapid palpitations during catecholamine excess, such as during exercise, suggest ventricular tachycardia, sinus tachycardia, or atrial fibrillation. Palpitations that occur regularly with exertion suggest hypertrophic cardiomyopathy or CAD.

Positional palpitations may reflect atrioventricular nodal tachycardia, pericarditis, or a structural process within the heart (e.g., atrial myxoma) or adjacent to the heart (e.g., mediastinal mass).

Could this be related to stress or a psychological condition?

Key Questions

- Have you experienced panic attacks (brief periods [seconds or minutes] of an overwhelming panic or terror accompanied by racing heartbeats, shortness of breath, or dizziness)?
- Can you describe your stress level and how you cope with stress in your life?
- Do you or does anyone in your family have a problem with panic attacks, anxiety, or depression?
- What other symptoms are you having?

Panic Disorder/Stress/Anxiety

Common psychological causes of palpitations include panic disorder and anxiety states. Patients with psychological causes for palpitations more commonly report a longer duration of the sensation (>15 min) and accompanying symptoms than do patients with other causes. Panic attacks, however, may also indicate pheochromocytoma.

Other Symptoms

Palpitations associated with hyperventilation, hand tingling, nervousness, shortness of breath, or dizziness are common when anxiety or panic disorder is the underlying cause. Children with serious arrhythmias may not report palpitations. Young infants may exhibit poor feeding or be irritable when palpitations are present.

Are drugs/medications or other substances implicated?

Key Questions

- What prescription and over-the-counter (OTC) medications are you taking?
- What recreational drugs do you use?
- Are the palpitations associated with caffeine, tobacco, or alcohol use?

Medications

Palpitations can result from OTC and prescription medications. Medications that prolong the QT interval and predispose patients to arrhythmias include antidysrhythmics, antimicrobials, antihistamines, psychotropic drugs, and other miscellaneous drugs, such as motility drugs, electrolyte-depleting diuretics, and protease inhibitors for human immunodeficiency virus. In children, cold medicines may cause palpitations.

Stimulants

Caffeine, aminophylline, ß-adrenergic agents, thyroxine, cocaine, and amphetamines enhance the strength of myocardial contraction and can cause palpitations.

Could this be secondary to a systemic condition?

Key Questions

- What other symptoms are you having?
- Have you been ill?
- Does your family have any known genetic conditions?

Symptoms/Illness

Noncardiac symptoms should also be elicited because the palpitations may be caused by a normal heart responding to a metabolic or inflammatory condition. Palpitations can be precipitated by vomiting or diarrhea that leads to electrolyte disorders and hypovolemia.

Fatigue and shortness of breath suggest anemia. Weight loss and heat intolerance may indicate hyperthyroidism. Patients with hyperthyroidism also report nervousness, emotional lability, fatigue, muscle weakness, increased sweating, menstrual changes (oligoamenorrhea), increased appetite, insomnia, thinning hair, tremors, and anxiety.

Pheochromocytoma can lead to palpitations. Patients typically report headache (usually severe, pounding, and paroxysmal), sweating, nausea and vomiting, visual problems, episodic flushing, weight loss, diarrhea, nervousness, abdominal or chest pain, panic attacks, flank pain, pallor, tremor, fatigue, anxiety, weakness, dyspnea, warmth, fever, dizziness, constipation, paresthesias, painless hematuria, and anorexia.

Genetic Disorders

Germline mutations have been identified that are the cause of familial syndromes that include a pheochromocytoma: von Hippel-Lindau syndrome, multiple endocrine neoplasia type 2, neurofibromatosis type 1 (von Recklinghausen disease), and familial paragangliomas syndromes.

DIAGNOSTIC REASONING: FOCUSED PHYSICAL EXAMINATION

Most patients with episodic palpitations are asymptomatic on physical examination. Typically, the purpose of the physical examination is to identify structural heart abnormalities to help confirm or rule out the presence of an arrhythmia (see Evidence-Based Practice box).

 EVIDENCE-BASED PRACTICE *Can History and Physical Examination Predict Arrhythmias?*

In one study, 127 patients presenting with palpitations and/or lightheadedness to 41 general practitioners (GPs) in the Netherlands underwent history and physical examination and standard electrocardiogram. The GPs' estimation of the probability of patients having an arrhythmia was compared with the diagnostic result of 30 days of continuous event recording (CER). No correlation was found between the GPs' assessment of risk and actual diagnoses. GPs were more likely to predict an arrhythmia in patients who suffer from hypertension (p = 0.049) or with a history of cardiovascular disease (p = 0.006). Vasovagal symptoms (odds ratio [OR] = 2.91, 95% confidence interval [CI] 1.1–7.6) and bradycardia (OR = 4.2, 95% CI 1.3–14.0) were significantly more common in patients with a CER diagnosis of arrhythmia. The authors concluded that physical examination and history taking alone in patients with palpitations and lightheadedness are not accurate in predicting arrhythmias and are insufficient parameters to determine the need for further diagnostic evaluation.

Data from Hoefman E, Boer KR, van Weert HC, Reitsma JB, Koster RW, Bindels PJ: Predictive value of history taking and physical examination in diagnosing arrhythmias in general practice, *Fam Pract* 24:636, 2007.

Note General Appearance

Observe the patient entering the room. Note signs of stress or anxiety. Tremors may indicate hyperthyroidism or pheochromocytoma. Flushing or sweating may occur with pheochromocytoma. Pallor suggests anemia or pheochromocytoma.

Take Vital Signs

Vital signs can provide information on cardiac function. Atrial fibrillation is suggested by an irregular pulse that has no repeating pattern (irregularly irregular). The presence of a pulse deficit (obtaining a lower pulse rate at the wrist than at the apex) or the auscultation of a variable intensity of the first heart sound suggests atrial fibrillation. These findings are due to beat-to-beat variation in stroke volume that occurs during atrial fibrillation. Hypertension may indicate underlying CAD or pheochromocytoma.

Assess Jugular Venous Pressure

The presence of cannon A waves on the jugular venous pressure (JVP) suggests an arrhythmia that is associated with atrioventricular dissociation, such as ventricular tachycardia. Cannon A waves are prominent waves in the JVP that occur with the contraction of the right atrium against a closed tricuspid valve. Cannon A waves are perceived as neck pulsations and, when rapid and regular, may be seen as a bulging in the neck, sometimes termed a frog sign.

Auscultate the Heart

A displaced and enlarged cardiac point-of-maximal impulse suggests the presence of dilated cardiomyopathy and increases the likelihood of ventricular tachycardia and atrial fibrillation. Cardiomegaly may be present with pheochromocytoma.

An irregular heartbeat, both in rhythm and strength, that begins and terminates abruptly suggests atrial fibrillation.

Listen for murmurs. The midsystolic click of mitral valve prolapse suggests a preventricular arrhythmia. The harsh holosystolic murmur of hypertrophic cardiomyopathy, which occurs along the left sternal border and increases with the Valsalva maneuver, suggests atrial fibrillation or ventricular tachycardia.

Assess Mental Status

Assess general behavior. Irritability may occur in patients with anxiety. Note body posture, movement, and facial expressions. Assess thought content for delusions that may occur with substance abuse or psychoses. Young infants may exhibit poor feeding or be irritable when palpitations are present.

Inspect the Head and Neck

Substance users may have chronic rhinorrhea, frequent nosebleeds, or lesions in the nose or around the nostrils. Pupils may be dilated secondary to substance use. The patient may have dry lips, halitosis, or an odor of alcohol or tobacco. Patients with hyperthyroidism may display exophthalmos and thinning hair. Patients with anemia may have pale mucous membranes.

Examine the Thyroid

In patients with hyperthyroidism, the thyroid may be enlarged and a bruit may be present.

Examine the Extremities

Look for onycholysis and localized myxedema (edematous skin thickening) of legs (pretibial) or dorsa of feet if you suspect hyperthyroidism.

Check Reflexes

Hyperthyroidism can produce overly brisk reflexes.

LABORATORY AND DIAGNOSTIC STUDIES
12-Lead Electrocardiogram

A standard 12-lead electrocardiogram (ECG) is the initial test in patients with palpitations and may identify the arrhythmia or provide insight into underlying structural and electrical abnormalities that may be causing the arrhythmia. Patients with electrical or structural abnormalities on 12-lead ECG require further evaluation.

ECG exercise testing is appropriate in patients who have palpitations with physical exertion and patients with suspected coronary artery disease or myocardial ischemia (see Chapter 7).

Cardiac Monitoring: Event or Continuous-Loop

These measures are used in patients with suspected cardiac arrhythmias as the cause of the palpitations. Holter monitoring or long-term (weeks, months) event monitoring is used to document ECG recordings. Holter monitoring is a continuous 24- or 48-hour ECG recording to evaluate the type and amount of irregular heartbeats during regular activities, exercise, and sleep. The patient keeps a diary to record daily activities and any symptoms experienced. At the end of the monitoring period, the data are analyzed for arrhythmias and are correlated with symptoms recorded by the patient. Cardiac event monitoring is a continuous-loop, digital memory recorder worn for extended periods of time (up to 30 days or longer) that saves and records transient events felt by the patient. These monitors are patient-activated as symptoms occur. Loop monitors save information for a predetermined period prior to the patient trigger, and can help identify the initiation sequence for arrhythmias. These stored events can be transmitted through a telephone for review.

Echocardiogram

An echocardiogram is a noninvasive ultrasound test for examining the heart that provides information about the position, size, and movements of the valves and chambers, as well as the velocity of blood flow. This test is used to determine, detect, or rule out structural abnormalities; to evaluate velocity and direction of blood flow; and to provide direction for further diagnostic evaluation.

Complete Blood Count

A complete blood count (CBC) with differential can be done to establish the presence of a systemic infection. An increase in white blood cells and bands is seen with systemic infection. Hemoglobin and hematocrit levels are useful if anemia is suspected as an underlying cause of palpitations.

Electrolytes

Evaluation of electrolytes is useful when the palpitation is from a suspected electrolyte imbalance.

Thyroid-Stimulating Hormone

Thyroid-stimulating hormone (TSH) level is used to detect hyperthyroidism. An abnormal level requires further testing. An undetectable level is diagnostic of hyperthyroidism.

Catecholamines/Metanephrines

Catecholamines and metanephrines are measured in a 24-hour urine collection to rule out pheochromocytoma. Metanephrines may also be measured in the blood. If levels are greater than two times the reference range, imaging studies are usually performed to evaluate the adrenal glands.

DIFFERENTIAL DIAGNOSIS
Cardiac Arrhythmias

Cardiac arrhythmias that result in palpitations include atrial fibrillation or flutter; supraventricular and ventricular tachycardia; premature ventricular and atrial contractions; sick sinus syndrome; and advanced atrioventricular block. The causes are primary electrical abnormality or electrical abnormality secondary to structural cardiac disease or comorbid conditions. The association of palpitations with other symptoms that indicate hemodynamic compromise, including presyncope, syncope, or lightheadedness, may signify a life-threatening cardiac arrhythmia. Chest pain and dyspnea may be the result of sustained tachyarrhythmias.

Physical findings such as a pulse deficit, irregular heartbeat, or cannon A waves on JVP measurement indicate a cardiac arrhythmia as the cause of the palpitations. ECG and cardiac monitoring may reveal the arrhythmia. Box 23-1 lists arrhythmias that can cause palpitations.

Psychological Causes

The most common psychological causes of palpitations are anxiety and panic disorder. The release of catecholamines during a panic attack or significant stress can trigger an arrhythmia. Patients with psychological causes more commonly report a longer duration of the sensation (>15 min) and accompanying symptoms than do patients with other causes. It is essential to rule out clinically significant arrhythmias before attributing palpitations to psychological causes.

Box 23-1	**Arrhythmias That Can Cause Palpitations**

Atrial fibrillation/flutter
Bradycardia caused by advanced arteriovenous block or sinus node dysfunction
Bradycardia-tachycardia syndrome (sick sinus syndrome)
Multifocal atrial tachycardia
Premature supraventricular or ventricular contractions
Sinus tachycardia or arrhythmia
Supraventricular tachycardia
Ventricular tachycardia
Wolff-Parkinson-White syndrome

From Abbott AV: Diagnostic approach to palpitations, *Am Fam Physician* 71:743, 2005.

Panic Disorder

Panic disorder is manifested by sudden attacks of fear accompanied by symptoms that may resemble a heart attack (e.g., palpitations, chest pain, dizziness). Often the symptoms develop rapidly and without an identifiable stressor. The individual may have had periods of high anxiety in the past, or may have been involved in a recent stressful situation; however, the underlying cause is typically subtle. Panic attacks subside as abruptly as they begin, typically lasting a few minutes, although they can last several hours. Asking a single question, "Have you experienced brief periods, for seconds or minutes, of an overwhelming panic or terror that was accompanied by racing heartbeats, shortness of breath, or dizziness?" can help identify patients with panic disorder.

Generalized Anxiety Disorder

Chronic anxiety, also referred to as generalized anxiety disorder (GAD), manifests as persistent worries, fears, and negative thoughts lasting at least 6 months. Excessive worry over daily activities and a tendency toward headache and nausea are seen. Typically GAD develops over a period of time and may not be noticed until it is significant enough to cause problems with functioning. Anxiety is persistent, pervasive, and occurs in many different settings.

Drugs and Medications

Palpitations that coincide with the use of a medication or drug suggest them as a probable cause. Drugs that commonly cause palpitations include alcohol, caffeine, tobacco, digitalis, phenothiazine, theophylline, ß-agonists, and cocaine.

On physical examination, look for telltale signs of stimulant use: chronic rhinorrhea, frequent nosebleeds, and lesions in the nose or around the nostrils. Pupils may be dilated secondary to substance use. Notice if the patient has an odor of alcohol or tobacco.

Nonarrhythmic Cardiac Causes

Nonarrhythmic cardiac causes of palpitations include valvular heart diseases, such as aortic insufficiency or stenosis; atrial or ventricular septal defect; cardiomyopathy; congenital heart disease; and pericarditis. Positional palpitations may reflect a structural process within the heart (e.g., atrial myxoma), adjacent to the heart (e.g., mediastinal mass), atrioventricular nodal tachycardia, or pericarditis. Echocardiogram can be useful in detecting nonarrhythmic cardiac causes of palpitations. Box 23-2 lists some nonarrhythmic cardiac causes of palpitations.

Noncardiac/Systemic Causes

Noncardiac causes of palpitations include exercise, fever, dehydration, hypoglycemia, anemia, electrolyte imbalance, hypovolemia, hyperthyroidism, and pheochromocytoma.

A CBC may identify anemia, infection, or hypovolemia as possible underlying causes. Electrolytes can identify electrolyte imbalance.

Anemia

Fatigue and pallor may indicate anemia. Hemoglobin and hematocrit levels will be low.

Pheochromocytoma

Pheochromocytomas are rare catecholamine-producing tumors of the adrenal glands. In addition to palpitations, patients with pheochromocytoma often report severe, pounding and paroxysmal headaches; sweating; nausea and vomiting; visual problems; flushing; weight loss; diarrhea; nervousness; abdominal or chest pain; panic attacks; flank pain; pallor; tremor; fatigue; anxiety; weakness; dyspnea; warmth; fever; dizziness; constipation; paresthesias; painless hematuria; and anorexia. On physical examination, patients may exhibit hypertension, tremors, postural (orthostatic) hypotension, and pallor. The heart may be enlarged.

Hyperthyroidism

Patients with hyperthyroidism may report nervousness, emotional lability, fatigue, muscle weakness, weight loss with good appetite, hyperdefecation, heat intolerance, menstrual changes (oligoamenorrhea), increased

Box 23-2	**Nonarrhythmic Cardiac Causes of Palpitations**

Atrial or ventricular septal defect
Cardiomyopathy
Congenital heart disease
Congestive heart failure
Mitral valve prolapse
Pacemaker-mediated tachycardia
Pericarditis
Valvular disease (e.g., aortic insufficiency, stenosis)

From Abbott AV: Diagnostic approach to palpitations, *Am Fam Physician* 71:743, 2005.

appetite, insomnia, and tremors. On physical examination, exophthalmos, warm skin, onycholysis, increased sweating, and thinning hair may be evident. Patients may have localized myxedema (edematous skin thickening) of the legs (pretibial) or dorsa of the feet. The thyroid may be enlarged and a bruit may be present.

Deep tendon reflexes (DTRs) may be brisk. High fever, congestive heart failure, and mental status changes suggest thyroid storm. TSH level will be low or undetectable. Elderly patients have less obvious symptoms and signs than younger patients, and a higher prevalence of cardiac manifestations, such as atrial fibrillation.

DIFFERENTIAL DIAGNOSIS OF *Common Causes of Palpitations*

CONDITION	HISTORY	PHYSICAL FINDINGS	DIAGNOSTIC STUDIES
Cardiac Arrhythmias			
	CAD, lightheadedness, syncope, chest pain, dyspnea	Pulse deficit, irregular heartbeat, cannon A waves on JVP	ECG, continuous event or loop monitoring
Psychological Causes			
Panic disorder	Panic attacks, terror	None	ECG, continuous event or loop monitoring
Stress/anxiety	Persistent worries, fears, and negative thoughts	None	ECG, continuous event or loop monitoring
Drugs and Medications			
	Use of alcohol, caffeine, tobacco, digitalis, phenothiazine, theophylline, ß-agonists, and recreational drugs such as cocaine and amphetamines	Substance users may have chronic rhinorrhea, frequent nosebleeds, or lesions in the nose or around the nostrils; pupils may be dilated secondary to substance use; dry lips, halitosis; odor of alcohol, or tobacco	ECG, continuous event or loop monitoring; toxicology screen
Nonarrhythmic Cardiac Causes			
	May have positional palpitations	Murmur may be present	ECG, continuous event or loop monitoring; echocardiogram
Noncardiac/Systemic Causes			
Anemia	Fatigue	Pallor; pale mucous membranes	ECG, continuous event or loop monitoring; Hct/Hgb
Pheochromo-cytoma	Severe pounding and paroxysmal headaches, sweating, nausea, visual problems, flushing, weight loss, diarrhea, nervousness, abdominal or chest pain, panic attacks, flank pain, pallor, tremor, fatigue, anxiety, emesis, weakness, dyspnea, warmth, fever, dizziness, constipation, paresthesias, painless hematuria, anorexia; may report familial syndrome	Sweating, tremors hypertension, postural hypotension, heart may be enlarged	ECG, continuous event or loop monitoring; 24-hour urine; catecholamines and metanephrines; plasma metanephrines; abdominal imaging

DIFFERENTIAL DIAGNOSIS OF *Common Causes of Palpitations—cont'd*

CONDITION	HISTORY	PHYSICAL FINDINGS	DIAGNOSTIC STUDIES
Hyperthyroidism	Nervousness, emotional lability, fatigue, muscle weakness, weight loss with good appetite, hyperdefecation, heat intolerance, menstrual changes (oligoamenorrhea), increased appetite, insomnia, and tremors	Exophthalmos, warm skin, onycholysis, increased sweating and thinning hair, localized myxedema of legs (pretibial) or dorsa of feet; enlarged thyroid, bruit may be present; brisk DTRs	ECG, continuous event or loop monitoring; TSH

CAD, coronary artery disease; *DTR,* deep tendon reflex; *ECG,* electrocardiogram; *JVP,* jugular venous pressure; *TSH,* thyroid-stimulating hormone.

REFERENCES AND READINGS

Abbott AV: Diagnostic approach to palpitations, *Am Fam Physician* 71:743, 2005.

Barsky AJ, Ahern DK, Delamater BA, Clancy SA, Bailey ED: Differential diagnosis of palpitations: preliminary development of a screening instrument, *Arch Fam Med* 6:241, 1997.

Batra A, Hohn A: Consultation with the specialist: palpitations, syncope, and sudden cardiac death in children: who's at risk? *Pediatr Rev* 24:269, 2003.

Dubois RW, Goodnough LT, Ershler WB, Van Winkle L, Nissenson AR: Identification, diagnosis, and management of anemia in adult ambulatory patients treated by primary care physicians: evidence-based and consensus recommendations, *Curr Med Res Opin* 22:385, 2006.

Lenders JW, Eisenhofer G, Mannelli M, Pacak K: Phaeochromocytoma, *Lancet* 366:665, 2005.

Reid ER, Wheeler SF: Hyperthyroidism: diagnosis and treatment, *Am Fam Physician* 72:623 2005.

Thavendiranathan P, Bagai A, Khoo C, Dorian P, Choudhry NK: Does this patient with palpitations have a cardiac arrhythmia? *JAMA* 302:2135, 2009.

Thiene G, Carturan E, Corrado D, Basso C: Prevention of sudden cardiac death in the young and in athletes: dream or reality? *Cardiovasc Pathol* 19:207, 2010.

Zimetbaum P, Josephson ME: Evaluation of patients with palpitations, *N Engl J Med* 19:1369, 1998.

Penile Discharge

Penile discharge results from an infectious or inflammatory process secondary to exposure or contact with organisms that enter and ascend the urethra. Males infected with *Chlamydia trachomatis* may be asymptomatic 25% of the time, and symptoms may be absent with gonorrhea infections. Coinfections with both *Neisseria gonorrhoeae* and *Chlamydia* organisms may be present in up to 25% of heterosexual males.

Urethritis in males related to a sexually transmitted infection (STI) that is acquired during unprotected sexual contact is classified as either gonococcal urethritis or nongonococcal urethritis (NGU). It is not possible to determine the causative organism based on symptoms or physical examination alone. Although patients may be tentatively classified clinically, laboratory tests are used to direct diagnosis and treatment. The most frequently identified organism (40%) in nongonococcal infection is *Chlamydia trachomatis*. Other organisms identified in NGU include *Ureaplasma urealyticum* and, less frequently, *Trichomonas*.

DIAGNOSTIC REASONING: FOCUSED HISTORY

Is this likely a sexually transmitted infection?

Key Questions

- Are you sexually active? How many sexual partners do you have?
- Do you have any new partners?
- When was the last time you had unprotected sex?
- When did you first notice the symptoms?

Sexual History

A history of multiple sexual partners signifies a risk of exposure to STIs. The incidence of *Ureaplasma urealyticum* increases with the number of sexual partners. A new partner also is a risk factor, as is a sexual partner who has other sexual partners. Sexually active

adolescents are at risk for STIs because of impetuous sexual activities, lack of barrier protection use, and use of alcohol or drugs. STIs are a serious health problem, occurring in about 25% of sexually active adolescents.

Unprotected Sex

Unprotected sex that is vaginal, oral, or anal increases the chances of STIs.

Number of Days Between Exposure and Symptom Onset

For patients with a single exposure, a shorter incubation period (2 to 6 days) is characteristic for *N. gonorrhoeae* and a longer period (2 to 3 weeks) for *C. trachomatis*. For patients with multiple or unknown exposures, the time interval may not be useful.

Are there any risk factors that point me in the right direction?

Key Question

- Have you used street or illicit drugs?

History of Drug or Substance Abuse

Substance or drug abuse is a risk factor for unprotected and indiscriminate sexual activity.

What do the characteristics of the discharge tell me?

Key Questions

- What color is the discharge?
- How much discharge are you having?
- What is the consistency of the discharge?

Color, Consistency, and Amount of Discharge

The presence of copious amounts of spontaneous yellow-greenish drainage is indicative of a gonococcal infection. A scant mucoid discharge is characteristic of a nongonococcal infection. Substance or drug abuse may produce a scant, whitish penile discharge.

Is this a local infection or process?

Key Questions

- Is the tip of your penis red and inflamed?
- Can you describe how you clean yourself?

Red, Inflamed Glans Penis

A beefy-red, inflamed glans penis is indicative of a yeast infection or a fixed drug reaction often caused by tetracycline. Lubricated condoms or spermicidal gel can cause contact dermatitis.

Hygienic Practices

Poor hygiene or aggressive hygiene with inappropriate or harsh cleansers can cause local irritation and result in inflammation.

Is this complicated urethritis?

Key Questions

- Do you have frequency, urgency, or nocturia?
- Do you have rectal, testicular, or low back pain?
- Do you have pain in any joints or muscles?
- Do you have any skin sores or lesions?

Symptoms That May Indicate Complicated Urethritis

Symptoms of urinary frequency, urgency, and nocturia may indicate complications of a urethral infection caused by spreading of the infection to other urinary tract structures, such as the prostate (see Chapter 17). Symptoms of perirectal, testicular, or low back pain indicate involvement of the vas deferens and the epididymis, which can lead to acute epididymitis and/or the involvement of the testicles and the development of orchitis.

Symptoms That May Indicate Reiter Syndrome

Reiter syndrome is a complication of NGU that follows urogenital infection and classically includes arthritis, conjunctivitis, oral mucosal ulcers, and dermatitis. More common is the joint and tendon involvement after *C. trachomatis* infection. This complication has also been reported in HIV-positive patients. It is less common in non-Caucasian populations, and the incubation period is usually 1 to 4 weeks after the onset of urethritis.

Disseminated Systemic Urethral Infection

A disseminated gonococcal infection can produce papules or petechiae that progress to pustules on the skin surfaces of the hands, arms, and legs.

Is this an upper urinary tract problem?

Key Questions

- Have you had a fever or chills?
- Have you noticed any blood in your urine?
- Are you having any acute pain?
- Where is the pain?

Fever

The presence of fever indicates an ascending infection of the upper urinary tract (e.g., pyelonephritis) or a descending infection of the lower urinary tract (e.g., prostatitis, epididymitis). A fever with a temperature of greater than 101° F (39° C) should be cause for concern and aggressive treatment.

Hematuria

Blood in the urine signifies renal involvement—specifically, pyelonephritis or lithiasis. Painless hematuria in the elderly is characteristic of bladder tumor or is a late symptom of carcinoma of the kidney.

Acute Pain

Abdominal pain, flank pain, and costovertebral angle (CVA) pain are characteristic of bladder, ureter, and kidney involvement. Urinary tract pain is usually perceived locally in the area where sensory fibers of nerves are located. However, pain can be referred to a site distant from the area that is affected because sensory nerves of the lower body are concentrated in the same segments of the spinal cord. Most pain in the urinary tract is referred pain and may not be perceived by the patient in the site where the problem actually occurs. A dull ache may be felt at the CVA or flank. Pain may be elicited by applying tension to the renal capsule, pelvis, or ureter. Ureter pain may be perceived in the bladder, penis, scrotum, or perineum. Testicular pain may be a result of renal calculi. Pain may vary in intensity from a dull ache to a sharp, stabbing, colicky pain that is unbearable.

What else could this be?

Key Questions

- Do you have scrotal pain and/or fever?
- Have you had recent instrumentation in the urethra (e.g., catheterization)?
- Have you been treated recently for an STI?
- Are you or your partner an immigrant, or have you recently engaged in foreign travel?

Scrotal Pain or Fever

Epididymitis usually presents with scrotal pain that developed over a period of several hours. The patient often is also febrile.

Recent Treatment or Instrumentation

Recent treatment or instrumentation of the urethra produces a risk of infection. Elderly males are especially at risk because they often undergo urinary tract treatment or instrumentation secondary to benign prostatic hypertrophy.

Recent Treatment for an STI

Recent treatment for an STI may indicate treatment failure, a coinfection that was not covered by the prescribed drug, or recent exposure. The appropriate laboratory test may not have been done or was not available, or treatment may have been empirically based on presenting symptoms. Infection with more than one organism or a coinfection may take place. Urethritis can also develop from a nongonococcal organism that has a longer incubation period and was not sensitive to the drug prescribed. The urethritis episode may also represent a recent exposure after treatment. Another possibility could be lack of patient compliance with treatment. The patient does not take the medication as directed or stops taking the medication when the symptoms disappear but before the causative organism is eliminated from the urethra.

Immigrant Patient/Partner or Recent Foreign Travel

Immigrants, partners of foreigners, and patients with a history of foreign travel may have exposure to STIs that are not seen frequently in the United States but have a higher incidence and prevalence in foreign countries. Resistant strains of common organisms are also prevalent in foreign countries. Referral or infectious disease consultation with urologists, infectious disease departments, or public health departments may be necessary to identify and treat patients with unusual STIs.

DIAGNOSTIC REASONING: FOCUSED PHYSICAL EXAMINATION
Note General Appearance

If the patient appears systematically ill, a more aggressive and immediate approach should be taken and an expanded examination becomes appropriate. An ascending infection is usually limited to the anterior portion of the male urethra and is most likely to cause local signs and symptoms in the male patient. The patient who appears to be in acute pain from sites other than the urethra warrants more than a focused physical examination.

Examine skin surfaces, exposed orifices, and eyes, as well as mucous membranes and bordering areas around sites that may have been exposed during sexual activity.

Note eyes for discharge or infection. Check around nares and lips for signs of infection or lesions. Inspect the chest, back, palms, and bottoms of the feet for rashes or lesions. Secondary syphilis produces typical rashes and lesions in these areas, as does Reiter syndrome. Spontaneous greenish-yellow discharge from the eyes is indicative of gonococcal infections.

Inspect the skin of the abdomen, inguinal areas, and thighs for lesions or rashes. Disseminated gonococcal infections may produce papules, petechiae, and pustules on the hands, arms, and feet. *Chlamydia* may produce hyperkeratotic lesions on skin surfaces and a rash on the penis in the uncircumcised male.

Palpate Lymph Nodes

Palpate the cervical, axillary, inguinal, and femoral lymph nodes for adenopathy. Although a nonspecific indicator of infection, lymph nodes may enlarge in response to exposure from several organisms. Virus exposure may cause lymph node enlargement, or there may be extension of bacterial organisms into adjacent lymph chains, indicating regional infections. It is important to ascertain how long the nodes have been enlarged and what symptoms have appeared during the course of enlargement. Assess the state of the nodes, such as any redness, swelling, heat, or pain, or if they are firm, mobile, or boggy. Sexually active males may have some inguinal lymph node enlargement, and the patient may or may not be aware of the enlargement. Lymph node enlargement should be documented and described.

Examine Body Hair

Examine hair on the head and in the pubic area and inspect underlying skin areas. Hair shafts can be infected with lice and nits. Hair follicles can be irritated from scratching and from secondary infection by other organisms.

Examine the Penis and Urethral Meatus

Inspect penile skin surfaces for lesions, especially the underside of the head of the penis around the area of the frenulum, where viral lesions may be found. Palpate the shaft of the penis for tenderness or for strictures of the urethra. Retract the foreskin if present and inspect the glans penis, corona, and frenulum for lesions. Inspect the meatus for redness, discharge, patency, or growths. If there is discharge, note if it is spontaneous or produced by milking or stripping the penis. Document a tender urethra and describe the character of any discharge. Note whether the discharge is profuse and yellow-green, which indicates gonococcal infection, or scant and mucoid-like, which is characteristic of *C. trachomatis* and nongonococcal infection.

Examine the Scrotum and Testicles

Inspect and palpate the scrotum for lesions. Palpate the testicles and epididymis for tenderness and any signs of inflammation. Elevating a tender testicle may alleviate pain and reduce discomfort in epididymitis. The testicle may not be defined when there is an acute infection present because of examiner-produced pain with palpation. The borders of the testicle may also be obliterated from swelling and edema.

Inspect and Examine Other Sites for Lesions and Discharge

Inspect other sites, such as the mouth and pharynx, using a tongue depressor to visualize buccal skinfolds for any lesions. The pharyngeal area may be asymptomatic. Depending on the patient's sexual practices and preferences, other sites exposed to sexual contact, such as the rectum, need to be examined. Rectal bleeding, pus, and mucus may indicate proctitis and require further anoscopic examination and special cultural and laboratory consideration (see Chapter 26). Examine any joints or tendons that are inflamed or tender or have limited range of motion.

LABORATORY AND DIAGNOSTIC STUDIES

To improve the probability of identifying the causative organism, the patient should be examined and specimens obtained at least 1 hour after the last voiding, ideally up to 4 hours after voiding. Manufacturer directions should be followed for all materials used to collect specimens, and policies and procedures should be followed to obtain valid and reliable results from laboratory and diagnostic tests.

Urine Dipstick

Urine dipstick is used as a screening test for urethritis. The leukocyte esterase (LE) strip is calibrated to turn purple in 60 seconds, indicating 5 or more white blood cells (WBCs) in the urine. LE detects esterase, an enzyme released by WBCs, and a positive LE result is indicative of urethritis (75% to 90% sensitivity, 95% specificity). The nitrite strip is calibrated to turn pink within 30 seconds and signifies nitrites produced by 105 or more organisms per milliliter. Urine that tests positive for leukocyte esterase and nitrites should be cultured for bacteria. However, note that some organisms that cause UTIs do not convert nitrate to nitrites (e.g., *Staphylococcus* and *Streptococcus*).

Urinalysis with Microscopic Examination

Look for proteinuria and glycosuria, which suggest kidney involvement. The presence of casts, red blood cells (RBCs), and bacteria is also important. Casts indicate hemorrhage or pathological conditions of the nephrons. RBCs indicate acute inflammatory or vascular disorders of the glomerulus. More than 1 or 2 RBCs/high-power field (HPF) is abnormal and can indicate renal or systemic disease or kidney trauma. Microscopic examination of the urine resulting in 20 or more organisms/HPF indicates urinary tract infection. Fewer than 20 organisms/HPF merits further study, such as culture and sensitivity.

Segmented Urine Collection for Culture and Sensitivity

Obtaining segmented urine specimens is a procedure used to identify the site along the urinary tract where the colonization of organisms is occurring and is useful in diagnosing prostatitis (see Chapter 17).

Gram Stain of Specimens

The Gram stain has 95% specificity in gonococcal urethritis. Sensitivity in urethritis is nearly 100%. Gram stain of urethral discharge should be performed to determine inflammation (WBCs) and the presence of either gram-negative or gram-positive bacteria.

If the stain is positive for polymorphonuclear neutrophils (PMNs), then the smear is examined for gram-negative intracellular diplococci (GNICDCs). If diplococci are found, the smear is considered positive for gonococcal urethritis. A smear that is equivocal or atypical indicates a mixed gonococcal and NGU. If there are no GNICDCs, then an NGU is indicated.

Culture and Sensitivity

Culture and sensitivity should be performed on specimens to confirm the identity of the causative organism and its sensitivity to antibiotics. This is especially important in populations with resistant organisms. Cultures are necessary in cases of suspected rectal or pharyngeal infection, as well as a typical urethral swab.

DNA Testing for Infectious Organisms

DNA testing using a first-void sample or a sample taken from the urethra or rectum provides rapid, sensitive, and specific results. A number of products are available. Follow manufacturer directions to collect and transport the sample. Nucleic acid amplification tests (NAATs) are available to test for *C. trachomatis* and *N. gonorrhoeae*. Single or dual organism tests are available.

Doppler Blood Flow

Doppler blood flow studies can be performed to support the diagnoses of testicular torsion and epididymitis. Testicular torsion results in a lack of blood flow to the testicle, whereas in epididymitis the blood flow is intact. Color Doppler flow studies also provide information concerning blood flow to the testicles and identify hot areas of infection.

Complete Blood Count

A complete blood count with differential can be performed to indicate a systemic response to infection.

Serology for Syphilis

Serological tests are used for screening and diagnosing syphilis and are recommended if other STIs are found or suspected. The screening tests are nontreponemal and include Venereal Disease Research Laboratory (VDRL), rapid plasma reagin (RPR), and enzyme immunoassay (EIA) tests. Diagnostic tests are *Treponema pallidum*–specific and include fluorescent treponemal antibody absorption test (FTA-ABS) and *Treponema pallidum* particle agglutination assay (TPPA).

Human Leukocyte Antigen

The human leukocyte antigen (HLA) test is done to determine antigens that are present for specific diseases. Histocompatibility locus A (HLA-B27) tissue haplotype is associated with sexually acquired reactive arthritis seen in Reiter syndrome. This test is not specific but is used to confirm the diagnosis.

DIFFERENTIAL DIAGNOSIS
Urethritis

Urethritis presents with itching, burning, or pain around the urethral opening. Symptoms vary in severity. Discharge may range from copious amounts of greenish-yellow discharge to scant mucoidlike discharge that may only be visible before the first voiding of the day. Patients commonly present with complaints of urinary frequency, urgency, and/or burning with urination, as well as penile discharge. Patients may also report a known sexual partner or that the public health department has contacted them indicating that they need to be checked for an STI. If you are unable to make a diagnosis based on history and physical findings, diagnostic testing is necessary for specific organism identification.

N. gonorrhoeae and NGU caused by *C. trachomatis* are the two most common infectious causes of urethritis. A coinfection with both organisms is found in up to 25% of the cases.

Gonococcal Urethritis

Gonococcal STIs are usually the easiest to diagnose because the patient often presents with complaints of a yellow-green discharge and burning on urination. Unprotected sexual relations increase the risk for contracting this STI. Gonococcal infection often becomes symptomatic 2 to 6 days after exposure and produces the classic yellow-green profuse spontaneous drainage. On examination, the penis will be normal in appearance except for the copious discharge. Diagnosis is established by DNA testing and is confirmed by Gram stain and urethral culture.

Nongonococcal Urethritis

NGU can produce penile discharge, although on examination, discharge may not be present. NGU typically develops over a longer incubation period of 8 to 21 days, and 75% of patients present with a clear or mucoid discharge.

Chlamydia is the most common nongonococcal causative organism. The resulting urethritis is characterized by a scant mucoid discharge visible before the first urination of the day. The patient may complain of irritation around the meatus of the urethra or have vague symptoms. On examination, stripping the penis may produce scant mucoid discharge. DNA testing is used to diagnose *Chlamydia*, and Gram stains are used to rule out and establish nongonococcal disease, of which chlamydial infection is the most frequent. Urine screening tests can be used to identify DNA chlamydial particles.

Complicated Urethritis

The examiner should recognize common complications of urethritis. Periurethritis may progress to urethral stricture in untreated cases, causing banding of the penile urethra in the shaft of the penis. Prostatitis can develop and progress to a systemic inflammatory response, causing chills and fever. Extension of inflammation to other structures of the urinary tract may result in acute infection of the epididymis and testicles. Orchitis, a testicular inflammation, presents with a swollen and tender testicle. Disseminated systemic urethral infection produces small tender papules or petechiae on the skin surfaces of the hands, arms, and legs. They may further develop into pustules and become hemorrhagic or necrotic. Joints can become involved with tenosynovitis and arthritis with synovial effusion in Reiter syndrome. Monarticular joint or tendon involvement should be investigated further.

Prostatitis

Patients with acute bacterial prostatitis are likely to look and feel sick and be febrile. They usually complain of dysuria, burning, frequency, and nocturia (see Chapter 17). Prostatic massage is contraindicated in acute bacterial prostatitis.

Patients with chronic prostatitis do not present as acutely ill but have a history of prostate problems. A causative organism may not be identified (see Chapter 17).

Epididymitis and Orchitis

The patient with epididymitis/orchitis is usually a sexually active young male, and pain is likely the presenting symptom. The patient may also have a urethral discharge. The patient may be febrile. The history usually indicates a slower onset of discomfort over hours or days compared to torsion testicle, which has a rapid onset of symptoms. Elevation of the affected testicle may reduce the discomfort. Swelling of the scrotum and testicle may be present. Doppler flow studies with color can locate hot spots and identify intact blood flow (see Chapter 17).

Reiter Syndrome

As a complication of a urethral infection, Reiter syndrome commonly includes joint or tendon involvement, but conjunctivitis and skin lesions may also be present. History includes a urethral infection within 1 to 3 weeks. HLA-B27 antigen typing may support confirmation of the diagnosis.

Balanitis

Balanitis is inflammation of the glans penis. Balanitis involving the foreskin or prepuce is called balanoposthitis. Uncircumcised men with poor personal hygiene are most affected by balanitis. Lack of aeration and irritation because of smegma and discharge surrounding the glans penis cause inflammation and edema. The most common complication of balanitis is phimosis, or inability to retract the foreskin from the glans penis.

DIFFERENTIAL DIAGNOSIS OF *Common Causes of Penile Discharge*

CONDITION	HISTORY	PHYSICAL FINDINGS	DIAGNOSTIC STUDIES
Balanitis	Not circumcised; poor hygiene practices	Localized erythema and edema; presence of smegma	None; history and physical examination
Urethritis			
Gonococcal urethritis	Unprotected sexual activity; abrupt onset of symptoms 3-5 days after exposure; yellow-green discharge; classic symptoms reported by males: frequency, urgency, dysuria; dysuria may be worse at beginning of urine flow	Yellow-green discharge; spontaneous or copious amounts with stripping of penis	Collect specimens at least 1 hr, preferably 4 hr, after last voiding; Gram stain, culture; urine DNA testing for gonococcus (NAATs)
Nongonococcal urethritis	Unprotected sexual activity; longer incubation period (8-21 days); meatal itching or irritation; scant mucoidlike discharge, if present, before first voiding of day; symptoms vary and range in severity for urgency, frequency, and dysuria	Thin mucoid discharge may be absent or minimal with penile milking or stripping	Gram stain; culture; urine DNA testing for *Chlamydia* (NAATs)
Complicated Urethritis			
Acute bacterial prostatitis	Chills, fever; 30-50 yr of age; onset of symptoms over days; pain in rectal, perianal area, low back, and abdomen	May have fever; painful prostate; do not massage	Segmental urine specimens; culture and sensitivity
Epididymitis/ orchitis	Abrupt onset over several hours; febrile, pain in scrotum and/or testicles	Tender, swollen epididymis and/or testicles; elevation of affected testicle may lessen discomfort; may have fever	Doppler flow studies with color
Reiter syndrome	Joint and tendon involvement; urethritis	Joint and tendon involvement, decreased range of motion; skin and mucous lesions; conjunctivitis	Blood, synovial fluid, HLA-B27 antigen; radiographs

NAAT, nucleic acid amplification test.

REFERENCES AND READINGS

Barth WF, Segal K: Reactive arthritis (Reiter's Syndrome), *Am Fam Physician* 60:499, 1999.

Blaivas M, Brannam L: Testicular ultrasound, *Emerg Med Clin North Am* 22:723, 2004.

Blake D: The future is here: noninvasive diagnosis of STDs, *Contemp Pediatr* 2:71, 2001.

Bremnor JD, Sadovsky R: Evaluation of dysuria in adults, *Am Fam Physician* 65:1589, 2002.

Brill J: Diagnosis and treatment of urethritis in men, *Am Fam Phys* 81:873, 2010.

Centers for Disease Control and Prevention: Sexually transmitted diseases treatment guidelines 2006, *MMWR* 55:1, 2006. [published errata appeared in *MMWR*, 55:997, 2006.].

Diaz-Parker C, Bratslavsky G: Male genitourinary disease: urethritis, epididymitis, and prostatitis, *Clin Rev* 15:40, 2005.

Luzzi GA, O'Brien TS: Acute epididymitis, *BJU Int* 87:747, 2001.

Miller KE: Diagnosis and treatment of *Neisseria gonorrhoeae* infections, *Am Fam Physician* 73:1779, 2006.

Parker CT, Thomas D: Reiter's syndrome and reactive arthritis, *J Am Osteopath Assoc* 100:101, 2000.

Richens J: Main presentations of sexually transmitted infections in men, *BMJ* 328:1251, 2004.

Simpson T, Oh MK: Urethritis and cervicitis in adolescents, *Adolesc Med Clin* 15:253, 2004.

Wren T: Penile and testicular disorders, *Nurs Clin North Am* 39:319, 2004.

Rashes and Skin Lesions

Dermatological problems result from a number of mechanisms, including inflammatory, infectious, immunological, and environmental (traumatic and exposure-induced). At times, the mechanism may be readily identified, such as the infectious bacterial etiology in impetigo. However, some dermatological lesions may be classified in more than one way. Most insect bites, for example, involve both environmental (the bite) and inflammatory (the response) mechanisms. Awareness of the potential mechanism of any skin rash or lesion is most helpful in identifying the risk a person may have for other illnesses. For example, persons with eczema are also frequently at risk for or have other atopic conditions, notably asthma and/or allergies. Thousands of skin disorders have been described, but only a small number accounts for the vast majority of patient visits.

Evaluation of rashes and skin lesions depends on a carefully focused history and physical examination. The provider needs to be familiar with the characteristics of various skin lesions; anatomy, physiology, and pathophysiology of the skin; clinical appearance of the basic lesion; arrangement and distribution of the lesion; and clinicopathological correlations. Common symptoms associated with specific lesions, such as itching or fever, are also important to know. It is necessary to quickly identify life-threatening diseases and those that are highly contagious. Ultimately, competence in dermatological assessment involves recognition through repetition.

DIAGNOSTIC REASONING: INITIAL FOCUSED PHYSICAL EXAMINATION
Initial Inspection

Dermatological assessment is similar to the assessment of most other body systems in that it depends on patient history and physical assessment. However, sometimes a brief physical assessment preceding the history can assist in the development of the initial differential diagnosis, followed by a focused history and further physical examination.

Morphological Criteria

Examination involves the classification of the lesion based on a number of morphological features (examples are listed in Tables 25-1 and 25-2 and Figures 25-1 and 25-2). Evaluation should be systematic. Generally, morphological features should be analyzed as follows:

- Identify the location of the lesion(s).
- Identify the distribution of the lesions as localized, regional, or generalized.
- Identify whether the lesion is primary (appearing initially) or secondary (resulting from change in a primary lesion).
- Identify the shape of the lesion and any arrangement if numerous lesions are present.
- Describe the margins (borders).
- Describe the pigmentation, including variations.
- Palpate to assess texture and consistency.
- Measure the size of an individual lesion or estimate size if lesions are numerous or widespread.

Examination in a systematic manner, and in part before obtaining the majority of the history, provides greater relevance to the data. Gloves are not necessary unless there are open, draining, or exudative lesions.

Table 25-1 Morphological Criteria of Rashes and Skin Lesions

NATURE OF LESION	DESCRIPTION	EXAMPLES
Primary Lesions (develop initially in response to change in internal or external environment of skin)		
Macule	Discrete flat change in color of skin; usually <1.5-cm diameter	Freckle, lentigo, purpura
Patch	Discrete flat lesion (large macule); usually >1.5-cm diameter	Pityriasis rosea, melasma, lentigo
Papule	Discrete palpable elevation of skin; <1-cm diameter; origin may be epidermal, dermal, or both	Nevi, seborrheic keratosis, dermatofibroma
Nodule	Discrete palpable elevation of skin; may evolve from papule; may involve any level of skin from epidermis to subcutis	Nevi, basal cell carcinoma, keratoacanthoma
Plaque	Slightly raised lesion, typically with flat surface; >1-cm diameter; scaling frequently present	Psoriasis, mycosis fungoides
Wheal	Transient pink/red swelling of skin; often displaying central clearing; various shapes and sizes; usually pruritic and lasts <24 hr	Urticaria
Tumor	Large papule or nodule; usually >1-cm diameter	Basal cell carcinoma, squamous cell carcinoma, malignant melanoma
Pustule	Raised lesion <0.5-cm diameter containing yellow cloudy fluid (usually infected)	Folliculitis, acne (closed comedones)
Vesicle	Raised lesion <0.5-cm diameter containing clear fluid	Herpes simplex, herpes zoster, contact (irritant) dermatitis
Bulla	Vesicle >0.5-cm diameter	Bullous pemphigoid, contact (irritant) dermatitis, blisters of second-degree sunburn
Cyst	Semi-solid lesion; varies in size from several mm to several cm; may become infected	Sebaceous cyst
Secondary Lesions (appear as result of changes in primary lesions)		
Crust	Dried exudate that may have been serous, purulent, or hemorrhagic	Impetigo, herpes zoster (late phase)
Scale	Thin plates of desquamated stratum corneum that flake off rather easily	Xerosis, ichthyosis, psoriasis
Excoriation	Shallow hemorrhagic excavation; linear or punctate; results from scratching	Contact (irritant) dermatitis
Lichenification	Thickening of skin with exaggeration of skin creases; hallmark of chronic eczematous dermatitis	Chronic eczema
Erosion	Partial break in epidermis	Herpes simplex or zoster, pemphigus vulgaris
Fissure	Linear crack in epidermis	Xerosis, angular cheilitis, severe eczema
Distribution of Lesions		
Localized	Lesion appears in one small area	Impetigo, herpes simplex (e.g., labialis), tinea corporis ("ringworm")
Regional	Lesions involve specific region of body	Acne vulgaris (pilosebaceous gland distribution), psoriasis (extensor surfaces and skinfolds)
Generalized	Lesions appear widely distributed or in numerous areas simultaneously	Urticaria, disseminated drug eruptions

Table 25-1 Morphological Criteria of Rashes and Skin Lesions—cont'd

NATURE OF LESION	DESCRIPTION	EXAMPLES
Shape/Arrangement		
Round/discoid	Coin or ring shaped (no central clearing)	Nummular eczema
Oval	Ovoid shape	Pityriasis rosea
Annular	Round, active margins with central clearing	Tinea corporis, sarcoidosis
Zosteriform (dermatomal)	Following nerve or segment of body	Herpes zoster
Polycyclic	Interlocking or coalesced circles (formed by enlargement of annular lesions)	Psoriasis, urticaria
Linear	In a line	Contact dermatitis
Iris/target lesion	Pink macules with purple central papules	Erythema multiforme
Stellate	Star shaped	Meningococcal septicemia
Serpiginous	Snakelike or wavy line track	Cutanea larva migrans
Reticulate	Netlike or lacy	Polyarteritis nodosa, lichen planus lesions of erythema infectiosum
Morbilliform	Confluent and salmon colored	Rubeola
Border/Margin		
Discrete	Well demarcated or defined; able to draw a line around it with confidence	Psoriasis
Indistinct	Poorly defined; having borders that merge into normal skin or outlying ill-defined papules	Nummular eczema
Active	Margin of lesion shows greater activity than center	Tinea species eruptions
Irregular	Nonsmooth or notched margin	Malignant melanoma
Border raised above center	Center of lesion depressed compared to edge	Basal cell carcinoma
Advancing	Expanding at margins	Cellulitis
Associated Changes Within Lesions		
Central clearing	Erythematous border surrounds lighter skin	Tinea eruptions
Desquamation	Peeling or sloughing of skin	Rash of toxic shock syndrome
Keratotic	Hypertrophic stratum corneum	Calluses, warts
Punctation	Central umbilication or dimpling	Basal cell carcinoma
Telangiectasias	Dilated blood vessels within lesion blanch completely; may be markers of systemic disease	Basal cell carcinoma, actinic keratosis
Pigmentation		
Flesh		Neurofibroma, some nevi
Pink		Eczema, pityriasis rosea
Erythematous		Tinea eruptions, psoriasis
Salmon		Psoriasis
Tan-brown		Most nevi, pityriasis versicolor
Black		Malignant melanoma
Pearly		Basal cell carcinoma
Purple		Purpura, Kaposi sarcoma
Violaceous		Erysipelas
Yellow		Lipoma
White		Lichen planus

Table 25-2 Descriptive Dermatological Terms

LESION*		CHARACTERISTICS	EXAMPLES
Annular		Ring shaped	Ringworm
Arcuate		Partial rings	Syphilis
Bizarre		Irregular or geographic pattern not related to any underlying anatomic structure	Factitial dermatitis
Circinate		Circular	
Confluent		Lesions run together	Childhood exanthems
Discoid		Disc-shaped without central clearing	Lupus erythematosus
Discrete eczematoid		Lesions remain separate Inflammation with tendency to vesiculate and crust	Eczema
Generalized grouped		Widespread Lesions clustered together	Herpes simplex
Iris		Circle within circle; bull's-eye lesion	Erythema multiforme (iris)
Keratotic		Horny thickening	Psoriasis
Linear		In lines	Poison ivy dermatitis
Multiform papulosquamous reticulated		More than one type of shape or lesion Papules or plaques associated with scaling Lacelike network	Erythema multiforme psoriasis Oral lichen planus
Serpiginous		Snakelike, creeping	Cutaneous larva migrans
Telangiectatic		Relatively permanent dilation of superficial blood vessels	Osler-Weber-Rendu disease
Universal zosteriform†		Entire body involved Linear arrangement along nerve distribution	Alopecia universalis Herpes zoster

*Examples of different configurations of skin lesions and their descriptions are contained within Table 25-1. (From Swartz MH: *Textbook of physical diagnosis: history and examination*, ed 6, Philadelphia, 2009, Saunders.)
†Also known as dermatomal.

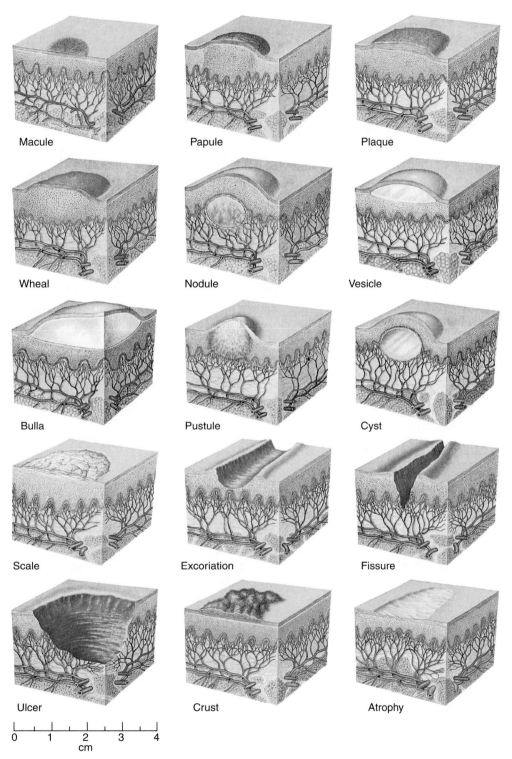

FIGURE 25-1 Types of skin lesions. (From Seidel HM, Ball JW, Dains JE, Flynn J, Solomon B, Stewart R: *Mosby's guide to physical examination*, ed 7, St Louis, 2011, Elsevier.)

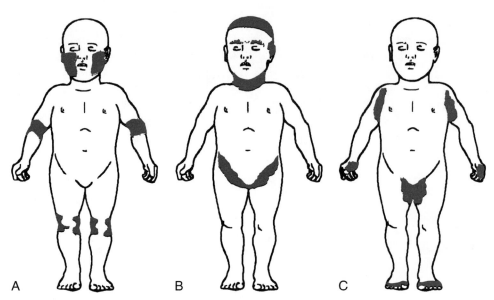

FIGURE 25-2 Typical distribution of papulosquamous eruptions in children. **A,** Atopic dermatitis: usually located on cheeks, creases of elbows, and knees. **B,** Seborrheic dermatitis: usually located on scalp, behind ears, in thigh creases, and in eyebrows. **C,** Scabies: usually located on axillae, webs of fingers and toes, and intragluteal area. (From Berkowitz C: *Pediatrics: a primary care approach*, ed 2, Philadelphia, 2000, Saunders.)

DIAGNOSTIC REASONING: FOCUSED HISTORY

Is the rash associated with an immediate life-threatening condition?

Key Questions

- Do you have a fever?
- Are you short of breath?
- Do you have difficulty swallowing?
- Is the rash tender and does it involve mucous membranes?

Fever

Fever is common in viral exanthems (rashes), and the accompanying condition is usually not life-threatening. However, fever, irritability, hypotension, and a macular or petechial rash may indicate meningococcemia. Treatment needs to be immediate to be lifesaving.

Allergic Reaction

Urticarial allergic reactions may be associated with angioedema (swelling) of the extremities, face, lips, tongue, and/or airway; cough; wheezing; shortness of breath; or heart palpitations. The sooner symptoms occur after the exposure to the allergen, the more severe is the reaction. Treatment needs to be instituted immediately.

Rash with Mucosal Involvement

Toxic epidermal necrolysis (Stevens-Johnson syndrome) is a tender, morbilliform, erythematous rash accompanied by fever, conjunctivitis, oral ulcers, and diarrhea. Immediate hospitalization is required to treat exfoliation of large areas of skin. The condition is usually drug-induced.

Is the rash acute or chronic (recurrent)?

Key Questions

- How long have you had this rash?
- Have you ever had a rash like this before?

Onset

The diagnosis of skin lesions is initially aided by categorizing the lesion as acute versus chronic or recurrent. Acute eruptions, such as urticaria or various fungal rashes (tinea), are classified as such because they have a tendency to be self-limiting or to not recur after effective treatment. Chronic rashes, such as psoriasis or eczema, may persist or be recurrent with exacerbations and remissions. Box 25-1 shows common rashes categorized by duration. Ascertain the duration of the eruption at presentation; however, the initial occurrence of a chronic rash may present acutely. Conversely, an acute eruption not optimally treated may present as a chronic problem.

Where is the rash in its evolution?

Key Questions
- What did this look like initially?
- Has the rash changed? If so, how?
- Has it spread? Where?

Initial Presentation

Most skin lesions evolve over time, although this varies from minutes with urticaria to weeks or even months with psoriasis or mycosis fungoides.

Box 25-1	**Duration of Rash**

Acute	Chronic
Allergic or contact dermatitis	Acne vulgaris
Candida dermatitis (diaper rash, intertrigo)	Bullous pemphigus
Erythema infectiosum (fifth disease)	Eczema
	Erythema nodosum
	Kaposi sarcoma
Erythema multiforme	Mycosis fungoides
Fixed drug eruptions	Polyarteritis nodosa
Folliculitis	Psoriasis
Herpes simplex virus (HSV)*	Rosacea
Herpes zoster/varicella zoster (HZ)	Seborrheic dermatitis
Impetigo	Systemic lupus erythematosus
Infestations (scabies, pediculosis)	
Insect bites	
Kawasaki disease	
Pityriasis rosea	
Septicemia (meningococcal)	
Scarlet fever	
Tinea (corporis, pedis, versicolor)	
Urticaria*	
Viral exanthems (measles)	

*Occasionally recurrent

Change in Lesion

Determining whether there has been a change from the initial appearance of a lesion provides diagnostic clues. The eruption of pityriasis rosea classically begins with a "herald patch," a single, scaly, erythematous patch usually on the trunk, followed within days by a regional outbreak of numerous smaller erythematous patches, thus providing a key diagnostic clue. The rash may look like that of ringworm, but it appears too quickly to be ringworm. Another example of evolutionary change is the eruption of herpes simplex virus (HSV), which begins with small vesicles that later umbilicate, possibly ooze, and eventually crust before healing. A rash may appear in different ways, depending on the point at which evaluation is sought.

Spread

The way in which a rash spreads is helpful in diagnosing the specific rash. There are three general ways in which a rash can spread: centripetal, or moving to the center; centrifugal, or moving away from the center; and caudal, or moving down.

What does the presence of pruritus tell me?

Key Question
- Does it itch?

Itching

All dermatoses can be classified into three groups: a small group that always itches, those that never itch, and an intermediate group in which itching is variable (Box 25-2). Pruritus is often reported to be worse at night; during the day, pruritus is less troublesome because the patient is distracted by daily routines. It is only at bedtime that the slightest sensation of pruritus becomes overwhelming; this is because the patient is focusing on trying to sleep. Once the patient scratches the area, histamine is released from the inflammatory cells (especially mast cells), and this causes more pruritus and an itch/scratch cycle is established.

Swimmer's itch occurs in areas unprotected by a swimsuit. Sea bather's itch occurs in areas under the swimsuit. Nocturnal pruritus most typically occurs in scabies infestations. Itching in the absence of rash may be an important clue to internal disease.

Box 25-2	Itching: Comparison	
Always Itch	**May Itch**	**Never Itch**
Atopic dermatitis	Psoriasis	Warts
	Impetigo	Neurofibromatosis
Urticaria	Tinea	Vitiligo
Insect bites	Pityriasis rosea	Nevi
Scabies		
Pediculosis		
Lichen planus		
Chickenpox		

What does associated pain tell me?

Key Questions

- Is it painful or sore?
- Does it burn?

Pain

Pain is a rare symptom. The classic painful rash is associated with herpes zoster (HZ), including postherpetic neuralgia, although severe psoriasis or eczema, when associated with fissures and bleeding, may be described as painful by some patients. Soreness is a more common symptom and is associated with numerous rashes. Tender erythema may be associated with toxic epidermal necrolysis.

Burning

Burning is infrequently reported. It is most notable preceding the rash in herpesvirus infections (e.g., HSV or HZ).

What do associated symptoms tell me?

Key Questions

- Do you have a fever? Sore throat? Headache?
- How are you feeling in general?

Fever, Sore Throat, and Headache

Fever is a common presenting complaint in infectious diseases accompanied by rash, such as HZ, erythema infectiosum, scarlet fever, or Kawasaki disease. Malaise, sore throat, nausea, or vomiting can occur with mononucleosis.

General Health

In a patient with a maculopapular eruption, the two most common causes are drug reaction and viral illness. Inquire about viral symptoms, such as fever, malaise, and upper respiratory tract or gastrointestinal symptoms.

Are there possible contacts or sources of contagion?

Key Questions

- Does anyone with whom you live or have close contact have something similar? If so, how long have they had it?
- Have you traveled recently? Where?
- What do you do for a living? What are your hobbies or leisure activities?
- Do you have any pets? Have you been around animals?

Living Situation

Explore the patient's living situation. The geographic details of his or her daily activities may help provide diagnostic clues, particularly for rashes caused by infectious or infestation mechanisms. Children, in particular, may contract scabies, pediculosis (lice), or impetigo by direct contact in school or daycare.

Travel

A patient may develop a rash weeks or months after travel exposure. Diseases endemic to other parts of the world may present with rash, such as erythema nodosum, which is common in Southeast Asia, or leprosy, which is common in Africa, Southeast Asia, and South America. Both eruptions may also occur secondary to tuberculosis. Camping trips to wooded areas, especially in the upper Midwestern United States, may result in a bite by a deer tick, causing Lyme disease, the leading vector-borne infectious disease. The resultant skin eruption in Lyme disease is known as erythema chronicum migrans (ECM), which begins 4 to 20 days after the bite of the tick; only a third of patients remember being bitten. Rocky mountain spotted fever (*Rickettsia rickettsii*) is transmitted by a tick bite and is common in the south Atlantic region of the U.S. Initial symptoms are nonspecific; later symptoms are rash and fever, usually requiring hospitalization.

Other Exposures

Outdoor occupations or leisure activities may expose persons to a variety of rashes and lesions, including insect bites and allergic or contact dermatitis from poison ivy or chemical substances. People exposed to animal skins contaminated with *Bacillus anthracis* can develop cutaneous anthrax, characterized by lesions that evolve from a papule, through a vesicular stage, to a depressed eschar. Sun exposure can also worsen chronic eruptions, such as rosacea or the malar butterfly rash in systemic lupus erythematosus (SLE). Ringworm is common in farmers and ranchers who work with cattle.

Pets

Fleabites produce an urticarial lesion with a central punctum. The reaction is an immunological one, making it different in each individual. Bites are usually on the legs. New lesions may appear daily, and itching is variable but sometimes intense. Fleas on a cat or dog are usually the culprits. An atypical form of scabies can be transmitted from dogs to humans and usually presents as a single lesion.

Is there anything that exacerbates or triggers the reaction?

Key Questions

- Does anything seem to make this worse?
- Do you have any known allergies?

Triggers

Patients often easily identify aggravating factors. Any rash involving vasodilation will become more vivid and likely more pruritic with heat exposure, whether via sunlight, sweating, or a hot shower. Localized eruptions, especially on the hands or forearms, prompt many patients to consider chemicals or other products as causes. Persons with eczema whose hands are frequently exposed to water are vulnerable to the development of irritant eczema on the exposed skin. Foods occasionally exacerbate skin lesions. Rosacea is a vasomotor instability disorder characterized by exacerbation with dietary consumption of vasodilators, such as coffee, tea, alcohol, or spicy foods. Stress, whether physiological (e.g., menstruation, pregnancy) or psychological, is widely believed to trigger or worsen many chronic rashes, especially eczema and psoriasis. Stress also may facilitate recurrent eruptions of HSV.

Could this rash be caused by a medication?

Key Questions

- Are you taking any medications (prescription or over-the-counter medications)?
- Do you have any medication allergies?
- Have you had a recent vaccination?

Medication

There are four types of dermatological effects of drugs: side effects (e.g., photodermatitis), allergic reactions (e.g., urticaria, fixed drug eruptions, or morbilliform eruptions), commensal skin eruptions (e.g., pityriasis versicolor in a patient on systemic corticosteroids), and worsening of existing skin eruptions (e.g., tinea eruptions mistakenly treated as eczema with topical corticosteroids). Medications used after the onset of a rash may be irritants or sensitizers and worsen the condition.

Recent Vaccination

Infants and children who have recently had a measles vaccination may display a rash 10 to 14 days after immunization.

Is there a significant dermatological family history?

Key Question

- Does anyone in your family have chronic skin problems?

Family History

A family history of dermatological problems may add insight to the diagnosis. Atopic disease (atopic dermatitis, asthma, hay fever) tends to cluster in families. Psoriasis, seborrheic dermatitis, and rosacea are also frequently noted to have a familial inheritance pattern. Multiple café au lait spots with a positive family history for neurofibromatosis can help identify children with this dominantly inherited disease.

DIAGNOSTIC REASONING: FOCUSED PHYSICAL EXAMINATION
Look at All the Skin and Mucous Membranes

A "peephole" diagnosis should be avoided; the whole organ should be examined. If the patient is not fully undressed, relevant lesions could be missed. However, it is useful to select one typical well-defined lesion to describe in detail, followed by an orderly and sequential system of examination so that no areas of the body are missed. The feet should always be examined in the presence of hand dermatitis so as not to miss a hypersensitivity reaction to a tinea infection or a concomitant hand tinea. Erythema in dark-skinned persons may be difficult to appreciate; it often is seen as postinflammatory hyperpigmentation.

Inspect for Distribution

Determine if the lesion is widespread or localized, unilateral or bilateral, symmetrical or asymmetrical. Symmetrical lesions commonly have internal causes (e.g., eczema, psoriasis, acne); asymmetrical lesions have external causes (e.g., bacterial or fungal infections, allergic contact eczema). Is the lesion predominantly on the flexor (as in atopic eczema) or extensor (as in psoriasis) surfaces? A rash on the soles or palms occurs with erythema multiforme and rickettsial infections. Determine if the distribution is confined either to protected areas or to light-exposed areas, such as in collagen-vascular diseases, photosensitive reactions to drugs, and airborne contact dermatitis. Is the lesion predominantly centrifugal (affecting the extremities, as seen in erythema multiforme, Rocky Mountain spotted fever, and insect bites) or centripetal (sparing the extremities and concentrated on the trunk)? Intertriginous distribution (neck, axilla, groin) is found in candidiasis, some inflammatory fungal infections, and some forms of psoriasis.

Inspect the Mouth

Drug eruptions from sulfonamides, penicillin, streptomycin, quinine, and atropine often have associated mucosal erosions and crusts. Mucosal involvement is common in hand and foot lesions (e.g., hand-foot-and-mouth disease), herpes, and syphilis.

Inspect the Hair

In children, a triad of hair loss, scaling, and lymphadenopathy is diagnostic of tinea capitis. A high index of suspicion is warranted in inner-city urban areas, where the condition is common.

Palpate the Skin

Palpate skin lesions to assess for tenderness, texture and consistency, firmness, fluctuance, and depth. Smooth skin has no irregularity. Uneven skin has fine scaling or some warty lesions. Rough skin feels like sandpaper and is characteristic of keratin/horn or crusts. Assessing the superficial skin for texture is done by palpation with the fingertips. Deeper palpation is done using the thumb and index fingers. Soft skin feels like the lips, normal skin like the cheeks, firm skin like the tip of the nose, and hard skin like the forehead. The depth of the lesion determines if it is on the surface or located within the dermis or the subcutaneous tissue. An indurated base is a thickening in the depths of the lesion rather than on the surface.

Palpate the Regional Lymph Glands

Many viral exanthems present with rash and lymphadenopathy. Palpation of the regional lymph glands may be of assistance in the diagnosis if neoplasm is suspected.

Perform an Abdominal Examination

The detection of hepatic or splenic enlargement may assist in the diagnosis of a systemic cause of skin disorders.

LABORATORY AND DIAGNOSTIC STUDIES
Diascopy

Diascopy is used to assess for blanching on pressure and is accomplished by pressing a glass or clear plastic slide on the lesion. Diascopy is most helpful in evaluating purpuric lesions: blood that is outside vessels (as in petechiae) will not blanch, whereas that entrapped within dilated vessels (as in telangiectasias) will demonstrate this phenomenon.

Wood's Light

Long-wave ultraviolet (UV) light is used in the diagnosis of lesions caused by fungal infections. Many, but not all, fungal rashes fluoresce. *Trichophyton*, dermatophytes that are frequently identified in tinea eruptions, do fluoresce; *Microsporum*, which can also be responsible for tinea eruptions, do not.

Skin Scraping and Potassium Hydroxide Preparation

Microscopically examine a sample of cells retrieved from a lesion, assessing for the presence of fungal or dermatophytic spores and hyphae. The lesion should be gently scraped using a scalpel (collect cells from an active area such as the border of the lesion); the cells are treated with a drop of 20% potassium hydroxide (KOH) and then warmed or allowed to stand a few minutes to soften the keratin. The addition of 40% dimethyl sulfoxide (DMSO) to the KOH solution accelerates diagnosis. Chlorazol Black E stain highlights fungal hyphae as dark blue-black against a light gray background.

Tzanck Smear

In a Tzanck smear, an indirect test for herpesvirus infections (HSV, HZ), cells are retrieved by swabbing the base of a lesion (usually a vesicle), smearing it onto a glass slide, and then staining it with Giemsa or Wright solution. Examined microscopically, the presence of multinucleated giant cells confirms the diagnosis.

Bacterial Culture

In taking a bacterial culture, exudate from a lesion is collected on a sterile swab and then cultured for growth. Gram stain may also be done. When a bacterial isolate is known, antibiotic sensitivity testing is performed.

Viral Culture

For a viral culture, cells from the base of a lesion (usually a vesicle) are collected on a Dacron swab and cultured for identification of viral infections, particularly HSV or HZ.

Punch Biopsy

In a punch biopsy, a tissue sample is assessed histopathologically for identification. Select a punch size about 2 to 3 mm larger than the lesion or sample an active area if the lesion is large. Gently swirl while exerting slight downward pressure on the punch. When well into the dermis, remove the punch and excise the sample at its base. The defect may be closed with electrocautery or suture(s) or left open to heal by second intention. Place the sample in a preservative such as formaldehyde solution.

Excisional Biopsy

In excisional biopsy, a tissue sample is assessed histopathologically for identification. Excise the entire lesion, usually making an elliptical incision around the lesion beyond its margins. Excise the base and close the defect with sutures or cauterize bleeding vessels. Place the sample in preservative.

DIFFERENTIAL DIAGNOSIS

The following conditions represent many of the most common skin eruptions observed in primary care. Consult a dermatology text for a complete review.

Follicular Eruptions
Acne Vulgaris
Acne presents as a chronic eruption of the pilosebaceous unit, with noninflammatory lesions (open or closed comedones) and/or inflammatory lesions (e.g., papules, pustules, cysts), and is most commonly a problem of adolescents. Its distribution follows that of the sebaceous glands: face, neck, chest, back, and upper arms. Neonatal acne first occurs between 2 and 4 weeks of age, lasting until 4 to 6 months of age. Persistence beyond 12 months may indicate endocrine dysfunction. African Americans and other dark-skinned persons need aggressive treatment to prevent postinflammatory hyperpigmentation.

Rosacea
Rosacea is a vasomotor instability disorder characterized by sebaceous gland hypertrophy, papules, pustules, persistent erythema, and telangiectasias. It shows a predilection for the face.

Infectious Eruptions
Impetigo
Impetigo presents as a superficial pustular, bullous, or nonbullous eruption, followed by crusting (often honey colored). The causative organism is usually *Staphylococcus* or *Streptococcus*. Contagion occurs via direct inoculation. It is typically a localized eruption that can occur anywhere on the body, with a predilection for the face and trunk.

Folliculitis
Folliculitis is a superficial pustular infection of the hair follicles. Causative organisms are usually *Staphylococcus* and occasionally *Streptococcus* or gram-negative organisms, including *Pseudomonas*, *Klebsiella*, and *Proteus*. It is typically a localized eruption that can occur anywhere on the body, with a predilection for hairy areas and flexural regions.

Furuncle
A furuncle, often referred to as a boil, is a more extensive infection secondary to a folliculitis (see Folliculitis).

Carbuncle
A carbuncle is an abscess of conjoined or adjacent furuncles (see Furuncle).

Macular and Papular Eruptions
Erythema Infectiosum (Fifth Disease)
Fifth disease, also known as slapped cheek disease, presents as a systemic illness of sudden onset characterized by a coalescing, red, maculopapular eruption on the face. A reticular eruption occurs on the extremities 2 to 3 days later. The causative organism is parvovirus B19. This is a self-limiting condition.

Children with underlying hemolytic anemia may experience an aplastic crisis.

Measles (Rubeola)

Measles are caused by a viral exanthem, and the systemic illness that results is characterized by a fine, erythematous, morbilliform eruption on the face that spreads rapidly to the trunk and becomes confluent and reticulate. Cough, purulent coryza, photophobia, and fever precede the rash. This is a self-limiting condition.

Rubella

Rubella results from a viral exanthem similar to measles and starts as fine macules and papules on the face and progresses caudally. Lymphadenopathy of postauricular nodes is characteristic of this disease.

Pityriasis Rosea

Pityriasis rosea presents with a rapidly evolving papulosquamous eruption of possible viral etiology. An initial "herald patch" is characteristic, followed within days by numerous faintly erythematous patches on the trunk and upper extremities ("T-shirt and shorts" distribution). The patches demonstrate fine scaling, and mild to severe pruritus may be present. It is more common in the spring and fall and among adolescents. In African American children, the eruption may consist only of occasional oval lesions along the cleavage lines. The remaining lesions are discrete, scattered follicular or nonfollicular papules over the trunk and proximal extremities. The face may also be involved.

Scarlet Fever

Scarlet fever is a systemic illness associated with group A ß-hemolytic *Streptococcus* (GABHS) (strep throat). It is characterized by a macular erythema of the face (flushing), except around the mouth (circumoral pallor), followed by a disseminated fine papular erythema (scarlatiniform), which may then desquamate. The rash is intensified in the flexor folds (Pastia lines). Associated symptoms are sore throat, malaise, fever, circumoral pallor, and a white or strawberry tongue.

Roseola

Roseola is a viral infection caused by human herpesvirus 6 (HHV-6). It is characterized by 2 to 3 days of sustained fever in an irritable infant who otherwise appears well. Mild edema of the eyelids and posterior cervical lymphadenopathy are occasionally seen. After the patient's temperature decreases, a pink, morbilliform, cutaneous eruption appears transiently and fades within 24 hours. This is a self-limiting condition.

Vesicular and Bullous Eruptions
Hand-Foot-and-Mouth Disease

Coxsackievirus A16 is the causative organism of this viral exanthem and systemic illness. Painful mouth ulcers followed by painful white vesicles with a surrounding erythema on the fingers, palms, toes, and soles characterize the condition. Patients usually have a low-grade fever, sore throat, and malaise for 1 to 2 days. Some develop submandibular or cervical lymphadenopathy. This is a self-limiting condition.

Insect Bites

Mosquito and horsefly bites can cause a common blistering reaction that is surrounded by faint erythema, central pallor if swollen, and usually a visible central punctum. The bites may be arranged in groups if they are multiple. The lesions are pruritic and/or sore; the condition is self-limiting. The deer tick bite causes a bull's-eye rash at the site of the bite.

Herpes Simplex Virus

HSV lesions have vesicles (solitary or grouped) that are surrounded by an erythematous base, with discrete, well-demarcated areas that later crust. The condition is associated with soreness and/or pain and may be preceded by tingling. There is a predilection for lips and genitalia. Recurrences in the same location are common and usually milder.

Herpes Zoster (Shingles)

HZ lesions present as clustered vesicles that are surrounded by an erythematous base, with discrete, well-demarcated lesions that later crust. Intense burning and pain often precede the eruption. There is a predilection for dermatomal distribution.

Varicella Zoster (Chickenpox)

Varicella lesions are discrete vesicles with a disseminated distribution; lesions develop in crops or in succession. Vesicles later crust, and occasionally secondary impetigo develops. The illness is associated with malaise and fever. This is a self-limiting condition.

Fungal Infections
Candidiasis

A yeastlike fungus that produces rashes at a variety of sites causes candidiasis; these rashes are called vulvovaginitis, thrush, intertrigo (groin, axilla, gluteal), and diaper dermatitis. The lesion is an erythematous maculopapular eruption that is well demarcated, occasionally with satellite lesions (pinpoint papules) at the periphery with maceration in moist areas. It is associated with mild to intense pruritus; the causative organism usually is *Candida albicans*.

Tinea

Tinea is a fungal eruption that causes rashes at a variety of sites: body (corporis), foot (pedis), beard (barbae), groin (cruris), and scalp (capitis). Lesions have erythematous scaling areas with a discrete border and central clearing that is often associated with pruritus or soreness. The causative organisms are *Trichophyton*, *Microsporum*, and *Epidermophyton*.

Pityriasis (Tinea) Versicolor

Pityriasis versicolor is a yeast infection characterized by a macular eruption of many colors, hypopigmentation to hyperpigmentation, and fine scaling. Macules begin insidiously, may take weeks to months to fully develop, and may coalesce. The condition is usually asymptomatic but occasionally pruritic. There is a predilection for a sebaceous gland distribution (neck, trunk). The causative organism is *Pityrosporum orbiculare* (*Malassezia furfur*). Repigmentation may take years or may never occur. Recurrences are common.

Immunological and Inflammatory Eruptions
Eczema

Eczema is a chronic relapsing inflammatory condition that can take several forms (atopic, nummular, or dyshidrotic). Eczema is characterized by erythematous macules, papules, and vesicles that occasionally weep and/or crust. When severe, eczema may be associated with fissuring and bleeding. It is associated with mild to intense pruritus. In dark-skinned persons, scaling and dryness associated with eczema give an "ashy" appearance to the skin.

Contact/Allergic Dermatitis

Contact dermatitis is an inflammatory reaction to many substances (e.g., poison ivy, nettles). Papulovesicular or bullous eruption surrounded by erythema, with weeping of exudate (noncontagious), is characteristic of the condition. It may be associated with moderate to intense pruritus.

Psoriasis

Psoriasis is a chronic, relapsing autoimmune disorder characterized by well-demarcated erythematous plaques, patches, and papules, which typically present with silvery scales. There is a predilection for the elbows, knees, hands, nails (pitting), scalp, and gluteal cleft. The condition may be pruritic or sore. The lesions may demonstrate Auspitz sign: pinpoint bleeding when the surface is scraped.

Seborrheic Dermatitis

Seborrheic dermatitis is a chronic, relapsing disorder characterized by erythematous scaling patches, which are poorly demarcated and may be pruritic. There is a predilection for the scalp, face, central chest, and genitals. The condition is aggravated by cold weather, dry skin, and stress.

Allergic Reactions
Erythema Multiforme

Erythema multiforme is an immune complex disorder involving the skin and occasionally the mucous membranes. Iris (target) lesions appear on the extremities and desquamation often follows. Common causes include medications (especially sulfonamides, penicillins, barbiturates, salicylates), histoplasmosis, mycoplasma, HSV, mononucleosis, hepatitis B, and malignancies. It is often self-limited. A severe form, Stevens-Johnson syndrome, is characterized by widespread involvement with vesicobullous lesions. It involves the mucous membranes, conjunctiva, and urethra, and also can involve the lungs, gastrointestinal tract, and kidneys.

Urticaria

Urticaria is characterized by a well-demarcated, usually disseminated, eruption that is evanescent over minutes to about 24 hours. The condition usually has an asymmetrical distribution.

Neoplastic Eruptions
Malignant Melanoma

Melanoma is an aggressive cancer with a tendency to spread rapidly and metastasize early. Characterized by asymmetry (half of a mole or lesion does not look like the other half), melanoma has an irregular, scalloped, or not clearly defined border with a color that varies or is not uniform (whether the color is tan, brown, black, white, red, or blue). The diameter is usually larger than 6 mm. However, any change in the size of a mole should be viewed with suspicion. The three most significant risk factors for the development of melanoma include history of melanoma in a first-degree relative, a large number of moles (more than 50 to 100), and atypical moles as designated by biopsy. Other factors that increase the risk of melanoma include adulthood, blond or red hair, blue or light-colored eyes, changed or persistently changing mole, Caucasian race, fair complexion, freckles, personal history of melanoma, immunosuppression, inability to tan, severe sunburns in childhood, and presence of a congenital mole.

Basal Cell Carcinoma

Basal cell carcinoma usually appears as a small, fleshy bump or nodule on the head, neck, or hands. Occasionally, these nodules may appear on the trunk of the body, usually as flat growths. These basal cell tumors do not spread quickly. It may take many months or years for one to reach a diameter of 1/2 inch. Untreated, the carcinoma will begin to bleed, crust over, and then repeat the cycle. Although this type of cancer rarely spreads to other parts of the body, it can extend below the skin to the bone and cause considerable local damage. The cure rate for basal cell carcinoma (sometimes referred to as nonmelanoma carcinoma) is 95% when properly treated.

Squamous Cell Carcinoma

Squamous cell carcinoma presents as an indurated papule, plaque, or nodule with a thick scale that is often eroded, crusted, or ulcerated. It can be found on sun-exposed skin surfaces, in areas of radiodermatitis, or on old burn scars. Although slow growing, squamous cell carcinomas arising on the lip, mouth, or ears may be associated with regional lymphadenopathy and metastasis. If promptly and properly treated, it has a cure rate of 95%.

DIFFERENTIAL DIAGNOSIS OF *Common Causes of Rashes and Skin Lesions*

CONDITION	CHARACTERISTICS	DISTRIBUTION/ PROGRESSION	ASSOCIATIONS	DIAGNOSTIC STUDIES
Follicular Eruptions				
Acne vulgaris	Comedones and/or papules, pustules, cysts	Face, neck, back, chest, upper arms	Onset of puberty, topical steroids, anabolic steroids, systemic corticosteroids, lithium, phenytoin	Usually none
Rosacea	Flushing, persistent redness, sebaceous hyperplasia, erythematous papules, telangiectasias, ocular involvement in up to 40%	Symmetrical, usually face only; may involve eyes	Topical steroids, systemic corticosteroids	Usually none
Infectious Eruptions				
Impetigo	Vesicular infection; honey-colored crusts and erosions	Face; any area of body with a minor wound, especially excoriated lesions	Scratching as a result of insect bites, atopic dermatitis, scabies	Bacterial culture
Folliculitis	Superficial perifollicular papules and pustules	Any hair-bearing body surface, but especially scalp, beard, legs, axillae	Shaving, hot tubs, contact with mineral oils, occlusive dressings	Bacterial culture
Furuncle	Very tender, deep-seated inflammatory nodule that develops from folliculitis	Same as folliculitis	May have fever	Incision and drainage for bacterial culture
Carbuncle	Multiple coalescing furuncles	Same as furuncle	Same as furuncle	Same as furuncle

DIFFERENTIAL DIAGNOSIS OF *Common Causes of Rashes and Skin Lesions—cont'd*

CONDITION	CHARACTERISTICS	DISTRIBUTION/ PROGRESSION	ASSOCIATIONS	DIAGNOSTIC STUDIES
Macular/Papular Eruptions				
Erythema infectiosum	Bright-red rash or "slapped cheeks," followed by diffuse maculopapular rash on trunk and extremities, leading to a lacy appearance as exanthem fades	Cheeks, then trunk and extremities	Aplastic anemia in children with underlying hemolytic anemias; fetal hydrops has been reported in pregnant women infected with parvovirus B19	IgM, IgG can be measured
Measles	Patient develops three Cs: cough, coryza, and conjunctivitis; Koplik spots are evident on buccal mucosa; rash begins with spike of convalescent fever; rash is centripetal in distribution, possibly becoming hemorrhagic in severe cases	Rash starts on neck and ears faintly, then covers face, arms, and chest; on second day rash covers lower torso and legs; on third day rash is on feet and face; rash begins to fade on the fourth day	Abdominal pain, otitis media, and bronchopneumonia are commonly associated; severe cases can cause encephalomyelitis	IgM can be measured for measles as well as acute and IgG titers
Rubella	Tender lymphadenopathy of postauricular, posterior occipital nodes; maculopapular and confluent rash that is lacy and not pruritic; rash lasts 3 days	Rash begins on face and spreads to trunk and extremities within first 24 hr	Infection with virus while pregnant results in congenital rubella	Confirmation by acute and convalescent IgG titers or by direct measurement of rubella IgM antibody
Pityriasis rosea	Multiple oval erythematous lesions with an inner fine circle of scale; ovals line up along skin cleavage lines on trunk, producing a Christmas tree–like pattern	Trunk, proximal extremities, rarely on face; rash is preceded by a "herald patch," appearing from a few days to 3 wk before generalized eruption	More common in spring and fall	If present on palms and/ or soles and history warrants, check RPR to rule out secondary syphilis
Scarlet fever	Fine, mildly erythematous papules and sandpaper-like rash found on trunk	Rash begins in axillae, groin, and neck; it avoids face, but there is circumoral pallor	Strawberry tongue; Pastia lines: areas of linear hyperpigmentation in deep creases	Culture for group A *Streptococcus*
Roseola	High fever for 3-4 days in infants and young children; as fever returns to normal, a diffuse maculopapular rash erupts	Rash begins on trunk and quickly spreads to arms, face, neck, and legs	Posterior cervical lymphadenopathy	None

Continued

DIFFERENTIAL DIAGNOSIS OF *Common Causes of Rashes and Skin Lesions—cont'd*

CONDITION	CHARACTERISTICS	DISTRIBUTION/ PROGRESSION	ASSOCIATIONS	DIAGNOSTIC STUDIES
Vesicular and Bullous Eruptions				
Hand-foot-and-mouth disease	Systemic illness caused by coxsackievirus A16; painful white vesicles with surrounding red halo	Painful mouth ulcers followed in 24 hr by painful vesicles on fingers, palms, toes, and soles	Low-grade fever, sore throat, and malaise; cervical and subman-dibular lymphade-nopathy possible	Tzanck smear
Insect bites	Flea, tick bites most common; intensely pruritic eruption, usually in groups of three; bull's-eye rash	Lower legs, but may appear anywhere on body if pets allowed on furniture or beds	Exposure to dogs or cats or to carpeted areas previously in contact with infected animals; outdoor exposure	Confirmatory biopsy occasionally needed
Herpes simplex virus	Primary infection with grouped vesicles on an erythematous base at site of inoculation; regional lymphadenop-athy; may be preceded by prodrome of tingling, itching, burning, or tenderness	Can occur anywhere on body, but most common areas are genitals and thighs, mouth, lips, and chin; may be disseminated in patients who are immunocompromised	Other STDs, HIV; triggered by sun, stress, fatigue, fever, trauma	Tzanck smear, viral culture; screen for other STDs, HIV if history warrants
Herpes zoster	Unilateral pain, itching, or burning preceded by 3-5 days of erup-tion of vesicles or bullae; followed by crusting and erosions	Can occur anywhere on body, but is unilateral, following a dermato-mal pattern; requires prompt referral to ophthalmologist if eye involved (Note: see lesion on tip or side of nose for indication)	Immunosuppression, older age, local trauma in children	Viral culture (not Tzanck smear)
Varicella zoster	Generalized pruritic vesicular lesions that are in different stages of healing; erythema-tous vesicles, ruptured vesicles, and crusted vesicles with scabs	Lesions usually begin on trunk and spread to face and proximal extremities	Herpes zoster occurs with reactivation of virus	ELISA titers can confirm acute infection
Fungal Infections				
Candidiasis	Beefy-red, well-demarcated plaques, often with scaling edge and satellite lesions; intertriginous areas may also show ero-sions and maceration	Diaper area in infants, body folds, mucosal surfaces, nails, and nail folds	Immunocompromised, diabetes, steroid inhalants, pregnancy, oral contraceptives, antibiotics, systemic and topical steroids	KOH, culture

DIFFERENTIAL DIAGNOSIS OF *Common Causes of Rashes and Skin Lesions—cont'd*

CONDITION	CHARACTERISTICS	DISTRIBUTION/ PROGRESSION	ASSOCIATIONS	DIAGNOSTIC STUDIES
Tinea	Variable, depending on body part affected; hair: scaling, hair loss, pustules; skin: red, scaly patch that may develop central clearing; feet: vesicles or bullae	Skin, hair, feet, nails	Immunocompromised, systemic corticosteroids, farmers and others with animal contact, hot humid weather with tight clothing or occlusive footwear	KOH, culture
Pityriasis (tinea) versicolor	Variably colored white to pink to brown scaling, round or oval macules of varying sizes; often coalescing to form large areas of discoloration	Upper trunk, axillae, neck, upper arms, abdomen, thighs, genitals	Heat, humidity, tropical climates, exercise, systemic corticosteroids, seborrheic dermatitis	KOH shows hyphae and spores in "spaghetti and meatballs" pattern
Immunological/Inflammatory Eruptions				
Eczema/ atopic dermatitis	Erythema, papules, vesicles, scaling, excoriations, crusts, pruritus always present	Symmetrical; infant: face, flexures; children: flexural creases; adults: may be discrete round patches or be regionalized to specific area	Personal or family history of asthma, seasonal allergies, and eczema; secondary colonization with *S. aureus* or HSV	Serum IgE; culture for bacteria or HSV if indicated
Contact/ allergic dermatitis	Vesicles and erosions with edema and inflammation, giving way to crusts and lichenification; pruritus	Localized, often asymmetrical; may be generalized with airborne allergens/ poison ivy; linear pattern with plant dermatitis	Occupational, recreational pursuits	Patch testing
Psoriasis	Well-demarcated, ham-colored plaques and papules with silvery scale; chronic, recurrent pruritus is common	Favors elbows and knees, scalp; intertriginous areas may involve nails	Streptococcal infection, arthritis, HIV infection, medications, alcohol, family history	ASO titer or strep culture if indicated; HIV if indicated; biopsy
Seborrheic dermatitis	Chronic scaling, flaking, erythematous dermatitis; variable pruritus	Areas where sebaceous glands are most active: face, scalp, eyebrows, eyelashes, body folds, ear folds, presternal area, mid and upper back, genitalia	Atopic history, HIV infection	HIV if indicated
Allergic Reactions				
Erythema multiforme	Hypersensitivity reaction seen as annular target or iris lesions	Begins on upper extremities and trunk	Herpesvirus, *Mycoplasma pneumoniae* infections, drugs (especially sulfonamides)	Skin biopsy may assist in diagnosis if caused by Stevens-Johnson syndrome; chest film for *Mycoplasma*

Continued

DIFFERENTIAL DIAGNOSIS OF *Common Causes of Rashes and Skin Lesions—cont'd*

CONDITION	CHARACTERISTICS	DISTRIBUTION/ PROGRESSION	ASSOCIATIONS	DIAGNOSTIC STUDIES
Urticaria	Transient wheals that may be acute or chronic (lasting >6 wk); individual lesions tend to come and go within hours; pruritic	Localized, regional, or generalized	Angioedema may also be present, may be life threatening; chronic infection, SLE, lymphoma	Biopsy; general medical workup to rule out underlying systemic disease in chronic urticaria
Neoplastic Eruptions				
Malignant melanoma	Asymmetrical border, irregular, has color variation within lesion and is >6 mm	Anywhere on body, including scalp	Usually asymptomatic, unless bleeding, ulceration, discharge present	Skin biopsy, excisional biopsy
Basal cell carcinoma	Papular or nodular lesions, with raised pearly borders and numerous superficial telangiectases	Sun-damaged areas; also seen in covered areas when there is genetic predisposition to basal cell carcinoma	Usually asymptomatic	Skin biopsy
Squamous cell carcinoma	Indurated papule, plaque, or nodule; may be eroded, crusted, or ulcerated	Sun-damaged areas, areas of radiodermatitis, old burn scars; can occur anywhere on body	Usually asymptomatic; can be associated with HPV, immunosuppression, topical nitrogen mustard, oral PUVA, chronic ulcers, industrial carcinogens, arsenic	Skin biopsy, excisional biopsy

ELISA, enzyme-linked immunosorbent assay; *HIV,* human immunodeficiency virus; *HPV,* human papillomavirus; *HSV,* herpes simplex virus; *KOH,* potassium hydroxide; *PUVA,* psoralen plus ultraviolet A (light therapy); *RPR,* rapid plasma regain; *SLE,* systemic lupus erythematosus; *STD,* sexually transmitted disease.

REFERENCES AND READINGS

Ely JW: The generalized rash part II: Diagnostic approach, *Am Fam Physician* 81:735, 2010.

Gable EK: Pediatric exanthems, *Prim Care* 27:353, 2000.

Goroll AH, Mulley AG: *Primary care medicine,* ed 6, Philadelphia, 2009, Lippincott Williams & Wilkins.

Jackson R et al: The diagnosis of skin disease, *Dermatol Nursing* 11:275, 1999.

Jaffe R: Atopic dermatitis, *Prim Care* 27:503, 2000.

McKinnon HD: Evaluating the febrile patient with a rash, *Am Fam Physician* 62:804, 2000.

Morgan-Glenn P: Scabies, *Pediatr Rev* 22:322, 2000.

Reifsnider E: Common adult infectious skin conditions, *Nurse Pract* 22:17, 23, 26, 1997.

Sanfilippo AM, Barrio V, Kulp-Shorten C, Callen JP: Common pediatric and adolescent skin conditions, *J Pediatr Adolesc Gynecol* 16:5, 2003.

Wolff TA, Tai E, Miller T: Screening for skin cancer: update of the evidence, *Ann Intern Med* 150:194, 2008.

Rectal Pain, Itching, and Bleeding

Anorectal problems can cause significant discomfort and anxiety. Because patients are often embarrassed by pain or problems in the anal area, they may delay seeking care and present with a more advanced disease or condition. Anorectal disorders can range from minor problems to those with significant morbidity. Rectal bleeding in children can be frightening for children and caretakers.

Rectal concerns include pain, irritation, discomfort, itching, soreness, and bleeding. Tenesmus is painful sphincter contraction that may be caused by anorectal infection. Rectal pain can be caused by tears, infection, or hemorrhoids. Itching can be caused by inflammation from hemorrhoids or parasites or by hypersensitivity to substances in the environment. Because colorectal cancer is common in adults and may be present with a benign condition, a high index of suspicion for cancer should be maintained when investigating all anorectal symptoms. See the Evidence-Based Practice box for screening recommendations for colorectal cancer.

The anatomy of the anorectal area is important in describing the occurrence of various disorders. The anus is the most distal portion of the gastrointestinal tract and is approximately 4 cm long. Its distal end is lined by stratified squamous epithelium, while the proximal component is lined by simple columnar epithelium. The two components are divided by the dentate line—the line where the distal end and the columns and crypts of Morgagni meet. The dentate line is also known as the anorectal junction, which also denotes the boundary between the somatic (sensory) and the visceral nerve supply. Above (proximal to) the dentate line, the rectum is supplied by stretch nerve fibers but not pain nerve fibers. Below the dentate line, the area is extremely sensitive. The columns of Morgagni are

---

⊙ EVIDENCE-BASED PRACTICE *Screening for Colorectal Cancer (CRC)*

The preferred screening for asymptomatic persons at average risk is cancer prevention testing. Patients who decline cancer prevention testing should be offered cancer detection tests. Average risk patients are those who have:
- No personal history of adenoma or CRC
- No personal history of inflammatory bowel disease (IBD)
- Negative family history (no first-degree relative or second-degree relative with CRC)

Cancer Prevention Tests
Cancer prevention tests should be offered first. The preferred CRC prevention test is colonoscopy every 10 years, beginning at age 50 (Grade 1 B). Screening should begin at age 45 years in African Americans (Grade 2 C).

Alternative CRC Prevention Tests
- Flexible sigmoidoscopy every 5-10 years (Grade 2 B)
- CT colonography every 5 years (Grade 1 C)

Cancer Detection Tests
The preferred cancer detection test is annual FIT for blood (Grade 1 B).

Alternative Cancer Detection Tests
- Annual Hemoccult Sensa (Grade 1 B)
- Fecal DNA testing every 3 years (Grade 2 B)

Grade of Recommendation/Description
1 A/Strong recommendation, high-quality evidence
1 B/Strong recommendation, moderate-quality evidence
1 C/Strong recommendation, low-quality or very low-quality evidence
2 A/Weak recommendation, high-quality evidence
2 B/Weak recommendation, moderate-quality evidence
2 C/Weak recommendation, low-quality or very low-quality evidence

Data from Rex DK, Johnson DA, Anderson JC, Schoenfeld PS, Burke CA, Inadomi JM: American College of Gastroenterology Guidelines for Colorectal Cancer Screening 2008, *Am J Gastroenterol* 104:739, 2009.

longitudinal columns of mucosa located in the proximal anus; they fuse in a ring distally to form the anal papillae at the level of the dentate line. The crypts are the invaginations of the columns of Morgagni. From four to eight anal glands drain into the crypts of Morgagni at the level of the dentate line. Most rectal abscesses and fistulas originate in these glands. Figure 26-1 shows the anatomy of the anus and rectum.

DIAGNOSTIC REASONING: FOCUSED HISTORY

Might this condition require immediate hospitalization or referral?

Key Questions

- Are you receiving anticoagulation therapy? Have you had bleeding?
- Do you have a bleeding disorder?
- Is the patient an infant?
- Do you have HIV/AIDS?
- Are you on chemotherapy?
- Is there purulent discharge?

Coagulopathy with Bleeding

Bleeding in anorectal problems is usually self-limiting and, if not a problem, resolves spontaneously or with local pressure. However, a bleeding internal hemorrhoid in a patient with a coagulopathy indicates the need for hospitalization. Newborns with melena (black, tarry stool) and/or hematemesis may have a vitamin K deficiency. Infants who present with rectal bleeding could have necrotizing enterocolitis (NEC), which is life threatening.

Immunocompromised with an Infection

Because of the acute infectious process, a perirectal abscess may require hospitalization, especially in a person who is immunocompromised because the infection is more likely to spread systematically. Individuals who are immunocompromised are at risk for the development of proctitis, especially by herpes simplex.

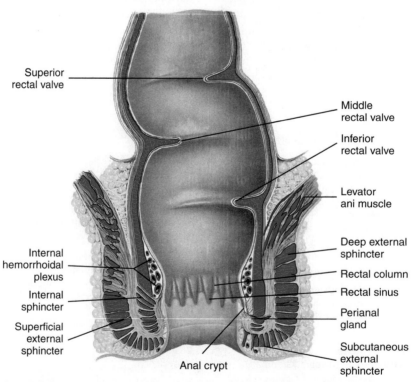

FIGURE 26-1 Anatomy of the anus and rectum. (From Seidel HM, Ball JW, Dains JE, Flynn J, Solomon B, Stewart R: *Mosby's guide to physical examination*, ed 7, St Louis, 2011, Elsevier.)

What Do the Presenting Symptoms Tell Me?

Key Questions

- Have you had any bleeding? How much bleeding has there been? When does it bleed? Describe the color of the blood.
- If a child: How old is this patient?
- Have you had pain? When does it occur? Can you describe the pain?
- Specifically, do you have pain on defecation? If a child: Does the child cry on defecation?
- Have you had itching? When does it itch?
- Can you feel a lump?
- Have you had any stains on your underwear? Can you describe the stains (e.g., blood, stool, pus)?
- Have you had diarrhea?
- Have you been constipated?

Bleeding

A patient presenting with significant passage of clots, dark blood, and loose bloody stool needs an evaluation to rule out gastrointestinal (GI) bleeding. Blood that is black and tarry and has an aroma is from the upper GI tract and is called melena. Melena stool should be differentiated in patients who have dark stool. Stool with melena will test positive for blood. When blood is bright red, the source is usually in the more distal GI tract or the rectum. Melena is seen in children with Meckel diverticulum. Bleeding from the rectum is a red flag for colorectal cancer.

Anorectal bleeding usually comes from internal hemorrhoidal veins or from a tear in the anal canal. Excoriations of the perianal skin can also cause bleeding, as can eroded skin overlying a thrombosed external hemorrhoid. Bleeding associated with defecation is characteristic of hemorrhoids and fissures. Bleeding from hemorrhoids typically occurs after defecation and is noted on the toilet paper ("wipe hematochezia") or coating the stool. The blood is bright red and may vary from a few spots on the toilet paper to a thin stream or coating on the stool. Bleeding with fissures occurs with defecation and is accompanied by pain. Spontaneous rectal bleeding can occur with proctitis. Condyloma acuminata may grow to a size sufficient to occlude the rectal opening and will bleed on defecation. Significant pathological conditions such as carcinomas and polyps can bleed intermittently.

Some foods, such as fruit juices and drinks, food coloring, and beets, affect the stool, making the stool appear reddish. Such foods as spinach, blueberries, and grape juice may cause the stool to be dark. Iron supplementation also may affect the color of the stool, making it appear dark.

A loose stool that has blood that is bright red and mixed with mucus may indicate chronic ulcerative colitis. Currant jelly–like coloring of the stool in young children often is a sign of intussusception, which is potentially life threatening.

Age of the Child with Bleeding

Premature infants. All premature infants with lower GI bleeding must be referred and evaluated for NEC.

Newborns. The most common cause of blood in the stool is from swallowing maternal blood during delivery. Newborns who have not received vitamin K and have a prolonged prothrombin time may have hemorrhagic disease of the newborn.

Neonatal stress can cause gastritis and gastroduodenal ulceration. Another cause of neonatal rectal bleeding is gastroduodenal ulceration from sepsis.

Infants younger than 6 months. Nonspecific colitis or allergic colitis due to milk allergy can cause blood-streaked stool. Bleeding can also have a bacterial etiology (see Chapter 11).

Age 6 months to 5 years. Intussusception is seen in children less than 1 year old and may cause currant jelly stool (see Chapter 2). Meckel diverticulum that ulcerates because of acid secretion onto the gastric mucosa can cause painless, sometimes significant, bleeding resulting in black or maroon stool. Henoch-Schönlein purpura may first manifest as lower GI bleeding (see Chapter 11).

Juvenile colonic polyps are seen in children ages 2 to 5 years. These are benign hamartomatous lesions. Bleeding occurs with defecation because of the sloughing of the polyps.

Anal tears resulting from constipation and stool holding can cause bleeding as well as pain. Blood may be visible on the stool or in the underwear (see Chapter 9).

Age 5 to 18 years. Ulcerative colitis presents in children as acute bloody diarrhea, cramping, and tenesmus. The child may have skin lesions, arthralgia, and growth retardation. Crohn disease may present with bloody diarrhea, abdominal pain, and fever. In mild stages, rectal bleeding may be minor with only small amounts of blood. Blood increases with proximity of the lesion to the anus (see Chapter 11).

Pain

Pain with defecation is characteristic of anal fissures. The pain may be so severe that the patient avoids defecating to avoid the pain. Children will cry with defecation. The pain may last for several hours and then subside until the next bowel movement. Patients with anal fissures complain of cutting or tearing anal pain during defecation and of gnawing, throbbing discomfort after defecation.

Hemorrhoids rarely cause severe pain unless they are ulcerated or thrombosed. Thrombosed hemorrhoids cause an inflammatory reaction by activating tissue thromboplastin within the hemorrhoidal blood vessels. Internal hemorrhoids, because they start above the dentate line, are not painful even if prolapsed or thrombosed.

Anorectal pain that begins gradually and becomes excruciating over a few days may indicate infection. A localized area of tenderness could signal an abscess. Patients with a recoil abscess or fistula complain of a throbbing, continuous, progressive pain. Pain can also occur with proctitis as a result of the infectious and inflammatory processes. The pain is not limited to defecation.

Proctalgia fugax is a unique anal pain. Patients with proctalgia fugax experience severe episodes of spasmlike pain that often occur at night. Proctalgia fugax may occur only once a year or may be experienced in waves of three or four times per week. Each episode lasts only minutes.

Tenesmus

Tenesmus is common with anal fissures, as the tear and inflammation involve the internal sphincter. On defecation, the sphincter may go into spasm. The patient experiences a tearing pain.

Itching

Itching is common with both hemorrhoids and fissures. Both external hemorrhoids that are covered by skin and fissures that involve breaks in the skin stimulate cutaneous sensation and lead to pain and itching.

Intense itching is a hallmark of pruritus ani, which occurs from hypersensitivity caused by irritating soap, lubricants, fragrance, or dyes present in toilet paper. Itching, particularly at night, can also be caused by pinworms.

Mass

The sensation of a mass or lump may indicate hemorrhoids or anal fissures. When the supportive tissues around the anal canal deteriorate, veins in the anorectal mucosa become tortuous and dilated and then bulge and descend into the anal canal. Both external and internal hemorrhoids can protrude and then regress spontaneously or be reduced manually. The patient may feel them as a bulge or lump.

With chronic anal fissures, the anal papillae hypertrophy and a skin tag ("sentinel pile") may form, which the patient may feel as a mass or lump.

Condyloma, molluscum contagiosum, and malignant lesions can also produce the sensation of a lump or mass.

Fecal Soiling

Fecal soiling is common with hemorrhoids. Mucous discharge with internal hemorrhoids is less common. Fecal soiling is also common with chronic constipation in children. Some stool discharges around the feces that is in the rectum.

Diarrhea

Explosive diarrhea can be a contributing cause of anal fissures. Diarrhea can also cause irritation and excoriation, producing symptoms of itching, bleeding, and soreness.

Constipation

Constipation can be a cause or result of anal fissures. Hard, dry stool can tear the rectal mucosa and produce an anal fissure. The pain associated with defecation because of a fissure may result in constipation because the patient avoids defecating.

Could this be caused by sexual practices?

Key Questions

- How many sexual partners do you have?
- Do your sexual practices include anal intercourse?
- Do you insert any objects into your rectum?

Multiple Sexual Partners

Multiple sexual partners place the individual at risk for the development of condyloma acuminata and viral or bacterial proctitis. HIV infection is possible and places the individual at risk for the development of proctitis.

Anal Intercourse

Anal intercourse predisposes individuals to anal fissures as a result of rectal trauma. The transmission of bacterial or viral organisms can result in condyloma acuminata or proctitis.

Foreign Bodies

The insertion of objects into the rectum can cause anal tears and fissures.

Could this be the result of sexual abuse?

Key Questions

- Have you had unwanted sexual contact? If a child: You might ask, "Has anyone touched your private parts?"
- Do you think the child has been abused?

Sexual Contact

Unwanted sexual contact that includes anal contact or intercourse may cause anal fissures as a result of rectal trauma. The transmission of bacterial or viral organisms can result in the development of condyloma acuminata or proctitis.

A Child's Reporting

Children who have been abused try to tell about the abuse in some way. Subtle indications that are not proof but may indicate abuse include a preschooler's regression to earlier safer times: for example, thumb sucking, clinging behavior, bedwetting, fear of sleeping in one's own room, and expressing feelings through art, especially drawing. Children draw what they see. Ask the child to talk about what he or she has drawn. School-age children develop physical symptoms from abuse (e.g., sore throat, stomach pains). The child's play may portray intercourse and may include violence toward animals. The child may appear to lack concentration, but in fact all energy is being focused into keeping a secret. Some children overcompensate, getting straight A's so that no one will suspect. Failure to thrive and undereating are other behaviors that may raise suspicion of abuse.

A Parent's Reporting

When a stranger sexually assaults a child, most parents bring the child into an emergency facility or clinic for immediate investigation. Abuse by a friend or family member is less overt and is often detected only when a primary care provider is alert to a suspicious history or physical findings. In some cases, a parent may voice concerns about the possibility of abuse or report that the child has told them of the incident.

A child who has been sexually abused must be referred to Child Protective Services and to a health care provider who is an expert in the area of child abuse.

Do risk factors point to a likely condition?

Key Questions

- Do you strain to have a bowel movement?
- How often do you move your bowels? How often do you experience constipation? Is your stool hard and dry?
- What is your occupation? Does it require sitting for long periods?
- Can you describe your personal hygiene practices?
- For women: How many pregnancies and deliveries have you had? Were the deliveries vaginal? How much tissue trauma did you have?
- Do you have HIV/AIDS or are you on chemotherapy?
- Do you have diabetes?
- Do you have a family history of familial adenomatous polyposis (FAP), hereditary nonpolyposis colon cancer, or Gardner syndrome?

Straining at Stool

Straining during bowel movements predisposes individuals to the development of hemorrhoids and anal fissures, especially in the presence of chronic constipation. Hemorrhoids develop secondary to the pressure. Fissures develop as a result of traumatic laceration from a hard or large stool.

Chronic Constipation

Chronic constipation predisposes an individual to hemorrhoids and anal fissures as a result of straining.

Prolonged Sitting

Occupations that require prolonged periods of sitting predispose to the development of hemorrhoids, pruritus ani, and pilonidal cysts.

Poor Hygiene

Inadequate hygiene practices are a risk factor for the development of pruritus ani and pinworms. Improper cleaning can result in excessive moisture around the canal, which causes breakdown of the epidermal layer of skin. Organisms and parasites can invade the damaged skin.

Excessive Hygiene

Another risk factor in the development of pruritus ani is overzealous cleansing. Pruritus ani can result from excessive use of chemical irritants such as soap or from excessive rubbing.

Pregnancy and Childbirth

The increased pressure and trauma from pregnancy and childbirth predispose women to the development of hemorrhoids.

Diabetes Mellitus

Diabetes mellitus places the individual at risk for the development of pruritus ani with secondary yeast infections.

Family History

FAP or hereditary nonpolyposis colon cancer places the patient at higher risk for colorectal cancer. Gardner syndrome is characterized by polyps, primarily of the colon, that are associated with benign tumors of the skin and bone. The polyps of Gardner syndrome may become malignant in individuals who also have an inherited FAP. There is genetic screening for family members of persons with FAP.

DIAGNOSTIC REASONING: FOCUSED PHYSICAL EXAMINATION
Obtain Vital Signs

Infants who present with rectal bleeding first should be assessed to determine if they are hemodynamically stable. A smaller blood volume makes blood loss more significant. Children maintain blood pressure with tachycardia and vasoconstriction, and when this compensation is exhausted, severe shock develops rapidly.

Note Gender

Many more males than females experience pruritus ani; the reason for this is not clear.

Inspect the Perirectal Area

Look for scars, warts, petechiae, bruising, and skin tags. Midline skin tags immediately anterior to the anus that have been present from birth are seen in some children. Skin tags may also develop when tears or hemorrhoidal bleeding resolves. Hemorrhoids are very uncommon in children, and their presence should heighten suspicion of sexual abuse. Perirectal erythema is common with streptococcal cellulitis, and

you may occasionally see vesicles surrounding the anus. Perianal ulceration sometimes can be seen with Crohn disease.

Perform a Digital Rectal Examination

A thorough gentle digital rectal examination is essential. Look for skin excoriation, skin tags, fissures, strictures, tears, or hemorrhoids, any of which may cause painful defecation. The knee-chest position affords the best visualization in both adults and children. A side-lying position can also be used. Spread the buttocks to reveal the mucocutaneous junction of the anus, and carefully inspect the rectum first in the resting position and then as the patient bears down. As the patient bears down, an additional 1 to 2 cm of anorectal tissue is palpable.

Look for inflammation, swelling, and erythema that characterize inflammation or infection. These signs may be present with a fissure, fistula, abscess, or proctitis.

Note any lesions or discharge. Condyloma acuminata present as warty growths that are pink or white with a papilliform surface. In anal regions, they tend to grow in radial rows around the anal orifice, forming a confluent mass that can obscure the anal opening. Examination of the entire genital region, including the anal canal, is important because they can extend 1 or 2 cm above the dentate line. Purulent discharge may be present with proctitis or an infected fissure or fistula. An external mass, verrucous growths, polyps, or ulcers may indicate malignancy.

Look carefully around the periphery to see small longitudinal ulcers or tears that characterize anal fissures. Early fissures have the appearance of superficial erosions. More advanced lesions are linear or elliptical breaks in the skin. Long-standing fissures are deep and indurated. Internal fissures are seen when the anal sphincter relaxes as the examining finger is withdrawn. A sentinel tag may be visible.

External hemorrhoids, if present, will be visible as bluish swellings. Internal hemorrhoids may or may not become visible as the patient bears down.

Palpate for tenderness. Hemorrhoids are generally not tender. Pain from an abscess, fissure, or fistula may preclude digital examination.

Palpate for the presence of a mass. Masses from anal or colorectal cancer are usually painless and may be so soft that they are easily missed on palpation.

Feel for foreign bodies, which might be present as the result of insertion of objects. Foreign bodies can also be present as a result of ingestion; for example, children may eat chicken bones or small objects.

Perform Anoscopy

Anoscopy is essential in the evaluation of all patients with rectal pain. It enables a view of the immediate internal anal canal that is not possible on manual digital rectal examination. A hand-held anoscope warmed and lubricated is eased slowly into the anus while the patient bears down to relax the external sphincter. A light source is necessary; a head lamp is preferable. Anoscopy may not be possible initially with a fissure or abscess because of the pain. However, it should be performed on a follow-up visit to detect inflammatory bowel disorder or rectal cancer.

LABORATORY AND DIAGNOSTIC STUDIES
Fecal Occult Blood Testing

Fecal occult blood testing (FOBT) should be performed on all patients with rectal pain. A positive test indicates blood in the stool that may be the result of ulcerative or malignant lesions. A stool sample is placed on a piece of filter paper, and an activating solution is applied. A positive test is indicated by the appearance of a color (usually blue or green). The sensitivity of this test in detecting colorectal cancers and adenomas ranges from 50% to 90%. It is an inexpensive and noninvasive method to screen for bleeding lesions. Serial testing (three samples) can be performed through the use of stool cards at home that are returned by mail for analysis.

Fecal Immunochemical Test

Also called immunochemical FOBT (iFOBT), fecal immunochemical test (FIT) uses antibodies to human globin to detect a specific portion of a human blood protein. FIT does not react with non-human hemoglobin or peroxidase, so food restrictions before the test are not necessary. Immunochemical FOBTs are also more specific for lower gastrointestinal tract bleeding as they target the globin portion of hemoglobin, which does not survive passage through the upper gastrointestinal tract. This test is done essentially the same way as conventional FOBT, but is more specific and reduces the number of false positive results. Vitamins and foods do not affect the fecal immunochemical test, and some forms require only one or two stool specimens.

Fecal/Stool DNA

Cells from precancerous polyps and cancerous tumors are shed in the stool and contain recognizable DNA markers. A stool DNA test can identify several of these markers, indicating the presence of precancerous polyps or colon cancer.

Abdominal X-ray

An abdominal flat plate and either upright or cross-table lateral radiography is done to screen for intestinal obstruction or pneumatosis intestinalis (see Chapter 38).

Flexible Sigmoidoscopy/Colonoscopy

Flexible sigmoidoscopy or colonoscopy should be performed when you suspect inflammatory bowel disease, polyps, or carcinoma. Colonoscopy is particularly important for adult patients older than 50 and for those with a history of familial polyposis or hereditary nonpolyposis colon cancer.

Gram Stain Rectal Discharge

Place a smear of rectal discharge on a glass slide for Gram staining. Gram-positive organisms stain purple, whereas gram-negative organisms stain red. *Neisseria gonorrhoeae*, a common cause of rectal discharge in proctitis, is a gram-negative organism.

Cultures for Infectious Organisms

When discharge or lesions are present, collect a specimen to culture for *N. gonorrhoeae* and herpes. Collect the specimen on a sterile swab and place in the medium provided. Bacterial culture confirms the identity of the causative organism and its sensitivity to antibiotics. A swab specimen of the perianal cellulitis usually yields a heavy growth of group A *Streptococcus*. Viral culture is also used for the diagnosis of herpes. Results may take from 1 to 7 days, with maximum sensitivity achieved at 5 to 7 days. The herpes culture probably will not identify the causative agent if the specimen is taken from a lesion that is 5 or more days old.

Herpesvirus Antigen Detection Test

This test detects antigens on the surface of cells infected with the herpesvirus. Cells from a fresh sore are scraped off and then smeared onto a microscope slide. This test may be done in addition to or in place of a viral culture.

Molecular Testing for Infectious Organisms

Molecular testing using a sample of the rectal discharge provides rapid, sensitive, and specific results. A number of products are available. Follow manufacturer's directions to collect and transport the sample.

DNA probes and nucleic acid amplification tests (NAATs) are available to test for *Chlamydia trachomatis* and *N. gonorrhoeae*. Single or dual organism tests are available.

Serology for Syphilis

Serological tests are used for screening and diagnosing syphilis and are recommended if other sexually transmitted infections (STIs) are found or suspected. The screening tests are nontreponemal and include VDRL (Venereal Disease Research Laboratory), RPR (rapid plasma reagin), and enzyme immunoassay (EIA) tests. Diagnostic tests are *Treponema pallidum*–specific and include FTA-ABS (fluorescent treponemal antibody absorption test) and TPPA (*Treponema pallidum* particle agglutination assay).

Alum-Precipitated Toxoid Test

The alum-precipitated toxoid (APT) test is performed to identify maternal blood ingestion in newborns. The neonate's gastric contents are mixed with 1% sodium hydroxide. A brown or rusty color indicates that the infant swallowed maternal blood.

Technetium 99m Scan

This scan is used to identify Meckel diverticulum that is bleeding.

Microscopic Examination of Stool

Stool examination should be considered in patients with symptoms of enterocolitis to rule out infection from common causes. Fecal leukocyte detection is an easy and inexpensive test that is 75% specific for bacterial diarrhea. Leukocytes are found in inflammatory diarrheal disease and are present in bacterial infections that invade the intestinal wall (*Escherichia coli*, *Shigella*, and *Salmonella*). Microscopic white blood cells and red blood cells indicate the presence of *Shigella*, enterohemorrhagic *E. coli*, enteropathogenic *E. coli*, *Campylobacter*, *Clostridium difficile*, or other inflammatory or invasive diarrhea. Leukocytes are also present in diarrhea from ulcerative colitis and Crohn disease, as well

as antibiotic-related diarrhea. They are not seen in viral gastroenteritis, parasitic diarrhea, *Salmonella* carrier states, or enterotoxigenic bacterial diarrheas. Obtain a small fleck of mucus or stool. Do not allow the specimen to dry. Place the specimen on a slide with two drops of Löffler alkaline methylene blue stain and wait 2 minutes before viewing under the microscope.

Stool for Ova and Parasites

Stool examination for ova and parasites (O & P) should also be considered in patients with symptoms of enterocolitis and in those who have been traveling and have blood in their stool. Fresh stool is required to preserve the trophozoites of some parasites. Use this test in patients with symptoms of diarrhea to rule out infection from *Campylobacter*, *Shigella*, *Giardia*, *Cryptosporidium*, and *Entamoeba histolytica*. Usually three serial samples are obtained.

Scotch Tape Test

Use this test when you suspect pinworms, which occur most commonly in children. Instruct the adult to apply adhesive cellophane tape to the perianal region early in the morning on awakening. The tape is then brought in. Place it on a glass slide and examine under a microscope for the presence of eggs. Parents may also be able to see the worms in the external anus of the child at night with a flashlight. The female worm is about 10 mm long.

DIFFERENTIAL DIAGNOSIS
Pain

Anal Fissure

Anal fissures are longitudinal ulcers that extend from just below the dentate line to the anal verge. They occur most often in the posterior midline. Acute fissures are cracks in the epithelium, but chronic fissures may result in the formation of a skin tag at the outermost edge that is visible on examination. In the chronic stage, fissures can suppurate and extend into the surrounding tissue, causing perirectal abscess.

Patients with anal fissures complain of cutting or tearing anal pain during defecation and of gnawing, throbbing discomfort after defecation. Digital and visual examinations reveal the presence of the fissure. Early fissures have the appearance of superficial erosions. More advanced lesions are linear or elliptical breaks in the skin. Long-standing fissures are deep and indurated. Internal fissures are seen when the anal sphincter relaxes as the examining finger is withdrawn. A sentinel tag may be visible at the anal verge.

Risk factors for the development of fissures include straining at stool, chronic constipation, and anal intercourse. Anal fissures are the most common cause of constipation and of rectal bleeding in children up to 2 years old.

Perirectal Abscess/Fistula

The most common source of infection is the anal glands, located at the base of the anal crypts at the level of the dentate line. Infection may also result from fissures, Crohn disease, trauma, or anal surgery.

Acute infection presents as an abscess, and chronic infection results in a fistula. The patient complains of swelling, throbbing, and continuous progressive pain. On examination, erythema and swelling in the perirectal region of ischiorectal fossa are found. Pain may preclude examination.

Proctalgia Fugax

Proctalgia fugax is fleeting pain in the anus. It is sudden and severe, lasting several seconds or minutes and then disappearing completely. The spasmlike pain often occurs at night. Proctalgia fugax may occur only once a year or may be experienced in waves of three or four times per week. Each episode is transient, but the pain is excruciating and may be accompanied by sweating, pallor, and tachycardia. Patients experience urgency to defecate, yet pass no stool. No specific cause has been found, but proctalgia fugax may be associated with spastic contractions of the rectum or the muscular pelvic floor in irritable bowel syndrome. A few patients report attacks after sexual activity. Other unproven associations are food allergies, especially to artificial sweeteners or caffeine.

Proctitis/Proctocolitis

Anorectal infection is common in individuals who engage in anal intercourse, both heterosexuals and homosexuals. Most causes of proctitis are sexually transmitted through the anal sphincter via direct invasion of the infectious agent through the mucous membrane.

Proctitis is characterized by anorectal pain, mucopurulent or bloody discharge, tenesmus, and constipation. Proctitis that is caused by an STI may be associated with intense pain. On examination, inflamed mucopurulent mucosa is present. The most common pathogens are *N. gonorrhoeae*, *Chlamydia*, *Treponema pallidum*, and herpesvirus. Herpes simplex infection can occur above or below the anal sphincter. Herpes simplex infection is common in immunocompromised individuals. Proctitis can also occur with ulcerative colitis and Crohn disease or with patients who have an intact rectum with a colostomy or ileostomy in place. Immunocompromised patients are at greater risk for proctitis.

Proctocolitis implies involvement beyond the rectum to include the sigmoid colon. The causes may include those of proctitis but are usually due to *Shigella*, *Campylobacter*, or *Giardia*. Symptoms of proctocolitis include those of proctitis but may also include diarrhea, fever, and abdominal cramping. On examination, an inflamed mucopurulent rectal mucosa is visible. Gram stain, serology to rule out syphilis, cultures, and molecular testing for infectious organisms assist in diagnosis.

Pilonidal Disease

Pilonidal disease refers to an abscess or draining sinus that occurs from subcutaneous infection in the sacrococcygeal area. Hairs penetrate the subcutaneous tissue, instigate a foreign body reaction, and produce the formation of a cyst or a sinus. Infection by skin organisms occurs, causing rupture of the sinus into the surrounding adipose tissue. The most common manifestation of pilonidal disease is a painful fluctuant mass in the sacrococcygeal region. Pilonidal disease may present as an abscess; as an acute, recurrent, or chronic pilonidal sinus; or as a perianal pilonidal sinus. Pilonidal disease occurs most often in hirsute young males. Risk factors include a sedentary lifestyle, prolonged sitting, obesity, poor hygiene, and increased sweating.

Perianal Streptococcal Cellulitis

Separation of the buttocks reveals erythema and, occasionally, vesicles surrounding the anus. The patient usually has a history of group A β-hemolytic streptococcal (GABHS) infection. Pain, erythema, proctitis, and blood-streaked stool are common.

Itching
Pruritus Ani

Pruritus ani is a symptom complex consisting of discomfort and itching. It is more common in men than women and is most often idiopathic. Discomfort is exacerbated by friction or a warm, moist, perineal environment. Poor anal hygiene or, conversely, overcleansing is often a contributing factor.

Examination may reveal mild erythema and excoriation of the perirectal skin. In later stages, the skin may be red, raw, oozing, or pale and lichenified with exaggerated skin markings.

Pinworms

Pinworms are nematodes that infect the intestine and cause perianal irritation. The pinworm eggs are ingested and migrate to the duodenum, where they hatch and mature and then travel to the cecum. The adult females emerge at night through the anus, deposit eggs in the perianal region, and die. The eggs stick to the skin and cause perianal pruritus and scratching. The worms may be visible at night, and the ova may be visible under the microscope.

Bleeding
Hemorrhoids

Hemorrhoids are dilated veins located beneath the lining of the anal canal. Internal hemorrhoids are located in the upper anal canal proximal to the dentate line and are covered by rectal mucosa and supported by longitudinal muscle fibers. External hemorrhoids are located in the lower anal canal distal to the dentate line, are covered by skin, and lack muscle support.

Internal hemorrhoids are graded by size (Table 26-1) and most often present with painless rectal bleeding; the blood is bright red and varies in quantity from a few drops coating the stool to a spattering at the end of defecation. Patients also report a dull aching and itching with prolapse. Itching occurs only with chronic prolapse.

External hemorrhoids can also cause itching but produce pain only when they become thrombosed. With thrombosis, patients report an acute onset of constant burning and throbbing pain and a new rectal lump.

External hemorrhoids are visible on examination as bluish skin-covered lumps at the anal verge. Internal hemorrhoids may become visible when the patient bears down. Risk factors for the development of hemorrhoids include pregnancy, childbirth, straining during defecation, and occupations requiring prolonged sitting.

Condyloma Acuminata

Genital warts are a common STI caused by the human papillomavirus (HPV). Patients with small lesions usually have few symptoms. When the lesions become large, patients experience bleeding, discharge, itching, and pain. On examination, warts are pink or white with a papilliform surface. They may obscure the anal opening. Examination of the entire genital region, including the anal canal, is important because they can extend 1 or 2 cm above the dentate line.

Colorectal Cancer

Anal or colorectal cancer can cause many different symptoms or be an incidental finding on rectal examination. Pain is usually absent, and rectal bleeding is inconsistent. The patient may have the sensation of a mass or lump. An external or internal mass may be palpable. Some lesions are so soft that they are missed on palpation. Anal cancer can take several forms, such as ulcers, polyps, and verrucous growths.

Ingestion of Maternal Blood

Newborns may swallow water and maternal blood, and this can appear as upper GI bleeding. To differentiate maternal blood from the newborn's blood, perform an APT test; fetal blood remains pink, whereas maternal blood turns yellow-brown. Diagnosis is best made with an APT test.

Allergic Colitis

Allergic colitis of infancy is a diagnosis of exclusion. It is seen in infants 3 weeks to 10 months old. The infant presents with loose bowel movements that are streaked with blood and mucus. The infant is otherwise healthy with normal growth. History may show early introduction of milk or a recent gastroenteritis. Laboratory studies are performed to rule out other causes such as diarrheal disease and include stool studies for leukocytes, culture, eosinophils, and complete blood cell count. All milk and soy products are eliminated from the infant's

Table 26-1	Classification of Internal Hemorrhoids	
GRADE	**DESCRIPTION**	**SYMPTOMS**
1	Do not prolapse	Minimal bleeding or discomfort
2	Prolapse with straining, reduce spontaneously	Bleeding, aching, pruritus when prolapsed
3	Prolapse with straining, require manual reduction	Bleeding, aching, pruritus when prolapsed
4	Cannot be reduced, or manual reduction ineffective	Bleeding, aching, pruritus when prolapsed

Modified from Metcalf A: Anorectal disorders. Five common causes of pain, itching, and bleeding, *Postgrad Med* 98:81, 1995.

diet. If the mother is breastfeeding, milk and soy products are eliminated from her diet. Generally the infant outgrows the problem by the age of 1 year.

Necrotizing Enterocolitis
This inflammation of the bowel may involve only the innermost lining or the entire thickness of the bowel and varying lengths of the bowel. It is seen in premature infants who have fragile and immature colons, but it may also be seen in newborns. The usual presentation may include abdominal distention, lethargy, and bloody stool; however, the signs range from feeding intolerance to sepsis. **This is a life-threatening condition and needs immediate referral.**

Meckel Diverticulum
Meckel diverticulum is a congenital abnormality that affects approximately 2% of the population, most of whom are asymptomatic. The diverticulum is thought to be what is left of the fetus's umbilical cord and intestines that were not fully reabsorbed and may contain gastric or pancreatic tissue. Painless rectal bleeding is the usual chief complaint in symptomatic cases in children younger than 2 years.

Intussusception
Intussusception is a telescoping of the intestines. It occurs most commonly in infants between 5 and 9 months of age. The infant experiences severe colicky pain. The child may become pale and limp, and then after the attack, which usually lasts for a few minutes, the child calms down and appears well. The child may vomit. The stool may contain blood and mucus typically described as currant jelly in color. **Referral is necessary to prevent strangulation of the bowel.**

Juvenile Polyps
Benign inflammatory polyps of the colon are found in children between the ages of 2 and 8 years. The patient experiences painless bleeding that occurs during or immediately after defecation. There is no risk of malignancy from these polyps. Colonoscopy is used to diagnosis the condition.

DIFFERENTIAL DIAGNOSIS OF *Common Causes of Rectal Pain, Itching, and Bleeding*

CONDITION	HISTORY	PHYSICAL FINDINGS	DIAGNOSTIC STUDIES
Pain Anal fissure	Cutting or tearing pain during defecation and gnawing, throbbing discomfort afterward	Early fissures appear as superficial erosions; more advanced lesions are linear or elliptical breaks in skin; long-standing fissures are deep and indurated; internal fissures are seen when anal sphincter relaxes as examining finger is withdrawn; sentinel tag may be visible at anal verge	Anoscopy
Perirectal abscess	Swelling, throbbing, continuous progressive pain	Erythema and swelling in perirectal area; pain may preclude examination	Anoscopy
Proctalgia fugax	Sudden, severe, transient pain in rectum often occurring at night; may be accompanied by sweating, pallor, tachycardia; may occur as 1 episode/yr or in waves of 3-4 times/wk	Normal rectal examination	Diagnosed by clinical history and negative physical examination
Proctitis/ proctocolitis	Anorectal pain; mucopurulent discharge, tenesmus, constipation with proctitis; also diarrhea, abdominal pain, and fever with proctocolitis; history of anal intercourse, immunocompromised	Purulent discharge, inflamed mucopurulent rectal mucosa	Cultures, molecular testing, Gram stain, serology for syphilis; stool examination, stool O & P

Continued

DIFFERENTIAL DIAGNOSIS OF *Common Causes of Rectal Pain, Itching, and Bleeding—cont'd*

CONDITION	HISTORY	PHYSICAL FINDINGS	DIAGNOSTIC STUDIES
Pilonidal disease	Pain in sacrum, superior to rectum; history of sedentary occupation	Erythema, swelling over sacrum, which can be fluctuant	None
Perianal streptococcal cellulitis	History of GABHS, local itching, pain	Erythema, proctitis, blood-streaked stool	Culture of perianal area
Sexual abuse	History of abuse, perianal pain, itching	Large irregular anal fissures, bruising, rectal tone decreased, warts, presence of semen	Serology for syphilis; culture (gonorrhea, *T. vaginalis*, herpes); molecular testing, (herpes, *Chlamydia*, gonorrhea)
Itching			
Pruritus ani	Discomfort and itching exacerbated by friction; history of poor anal hygiene or overcleansing	Mild erythema and excoriation over perirectal skin; in later stages: red, raw, oozing, pale lichenified perirectal skin	
Pinworms	Itching, especially at night	Visualize white-yellow worms 8-13 mm in length at night with flashlight	Scotch tape test positive for eggs
Bleeding			
Hemorrhoids	Bright red rectal bleeding with defecation or blood on stool; burning or itching; straining at stool; prolonged sitting; pregnancy and childbirth	External hemorrhoids: bluish, skin-covered lumps; internal hemorrhoids: may be visible when patient bears down	FOBT or FIT; fecal/stool DNA to exclude carcinoma
Condyloma acuminata	Few symptoms with small lesions; bleeding, discharge, itching, and pain with large lesions	Pink or white warty lesions with papilliform surface; may extend into anal canal	Serology to distinguish from condyloma lata caused by syphilis
Cancer of the colon, rectum, anus	Feeling of lump; usually painless; may or may not bleed; may have family history of polyposis syndromes	Polyp, internal or external mass, ulcers, verrucous growths	Anoscopy, flexible sigmoidoscopy, colonoscopy, fecal/stool DNA
Ingestion of maternal blood	Newborn	Hematemesis	APT test
Allergic colitis	Infant 0-6 mo, milk formula or breastfeeding mother who has intake of milk	Blood-streaked stool	None
NEC	Preterm, newborn infant	Ileus, abdominal distention, gastrointestinal bleeding, bilious vomiting	Immediate referral
Meckel diverticulum	Preschool child, painless GI bleeding	Black or maroon stool	Technetium 99m scan and referral
Intussusception	Colicky abdominal pain, vomiting, currant jelly stool	Sausage-shaped mass may be felt in abdomen	Refer
Juvenile polyps	Painless bleeding with stool, ages 2-5 yr	None	Colonoscopy

APT, alum-precipitated toxoid; *FIT*, fecal immunochemical test; *FOBT*, fecal occult blood testing; *GABHS*, group A β-hemolytic streptococcal infection; *NEC*, necrotizing enterocolitis; *O & P*, ova and parasites.

REFERENCES AND READINGS

American Gastroenterological Association: American Gastroenterological Association medical position statement: Diagnosis and care of patients with anal fissure, *Gastroenterol* 124:233, 2003.

Billingham RP, Isler JT, Kimmins MH,Nelson J,Schweitzer J, Murphy M: The diagnosis and management of common anorectal disorders, *Curr Probl Surg* 41:586, 2004.

Boyle J: Gastrointestinal bleeding in infants and children, *Pediatr Rev* 29:39, 2008.

Di Lorenzo C: Pediatric anorectal disorders, *Gastroenterol Clin North Am* 30:269, 2001.

Kong AP, Stamos MJ: Anorectal complaints: office diagnosis and treatment, part 1, *Consultant* June:731, 2005.

Lawrence W, Wright J, Cheng T: Causes of rectal bleeding in children, *Pediatr Rev* 22:11, 2001.

Mazza L, Formento E, Fronda G: Anorectal and perineal pain: new pathophysiological hypothesis, *Tech Coloproctol* 8:77, 2004.

Pfenninger JL, Zainea GG: Common anorectal conditions, part I: symptoms and complaints, *Am Fam Physician* 63:2391, 2001.

Pfenninger JL, Zainea GG: Common anorectal conditions, part II: lesions, *Am Fam Physician* 64:77, 2001.

Sneider EB, Maykel JA: Diagnosis and management of symptomatic hemorrhoids, *Surg Clin North Am* 90:17, 2010.

Wald A: Functional anorectal and pelvic pain, *Gastroenterol Clin North Am* 30:243, 2001.

Watson AJ, Loudon M: Diagnosing minor anorectal conditions, *Practitioner* 245:790, 2001.

Red Eye

The term red eye is used to denote a cardinal sign of ocular inflammation. The anatomical location in and around the eye and the probable cause of the eye disorder provide an important framework to use in assessment. General anatomical locations are the ocular adnexa, conjunctiva, cornea and anterior segment, and posterior eye (Figure 27-1).

The eye has two major defense mechanisms. The first is tears, which contain immunoglobulin A and lysozymes; these provide an important washing action. The second defense mechanism is a conjunctival immune system of lymphocytes, plasma cells, and neutrophils. Trauma or inoculation of the eye with virulent organisms disrupts these normal defense mechanisms, leading to a red eye.

Although most cases of red eye are caused by viral or bacterial conjunctivitis, other possibilities include trauma, glaucoma, systemic disease, and congenital anomalies. Determining the etiology is an important step in assessing the condition.

DIAGNOSTIC REASONING: FOCUSED HISTORY

Is this a chemical emergency?

Key Question

■ Did you get a chemical in your eye?

Chemical Injury
Chemical burns of the conjunctiva and cornea represent one of the true ocular emergencies. Alkali burns usually result in greater damage to the eye than acid burns because alkali compounds penetrate ocular tissues more rapidly.

All chemical burns require immediate and profuse irrigation and immediate referral to an ophthalmologist. Irrigate the eye with water while obtaining a history of the incident and possible chemical contact.

Could this be caused by an orbital infection?

Key Questions

■ Do you notice any swelling or tightness around the eye(s) or of the eyelid(s)?
■ Does it hurt to move your eye?
■ Do you have a fever?
■ Have you had a recent sinus infection?

Swelling, Redness, and Fever
Orbital or periorbital cellulitis can present with conjunctivitis and signal a medical emergency. They can occur as complications of sinusitis. Reports of swelling, redness, and fever should alert you to these conditions. Both conditions require immediate referral; orbital cellulitis is life threatening.

Pain with Attempted Motion of the Eye
Orbital cellulitis causes pain with movement because of the collection of pus between the periosteum and the wall of the orbit. The inflammation continues to all tissues in the orbit, and proptosis and impairment of ocular motility are seen.

Recent Sinus Infection
Sinusitis is the most common predisposing condition in patients with orbital cellulitis. The ethmoid sinuses are most commonly involved, with the maxillary sinus the next most common site of infection.

Can I rule in or rule out trauma?

Key Question

■ If trauma occurred: How was your eye injured (e.g., foreign body, chemical, blow, stab, cut)?

Blunt trauma to the ocular adnexa can cause lid swelling and/or discoloration. Rupture of the globe, fractures of the orbital bones, and internal bleeding may also be possible. Sharp trauma to the area can cause lacerations

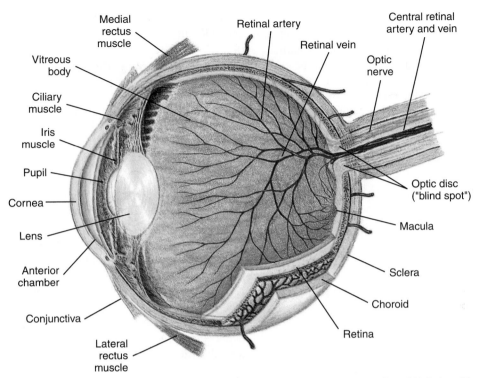

Medial rectus muscle

Vitreous body

Ciliary muscle

Iris muscle

Pupil

Cornea

Lens

Anterior chamber

Conjunctiva

Lateral rectus muscle

Retinal artery

Retinal vein

Central retinal artery and vein

Optic nerve

Optic disc ("blind spot")

Macula

Sclera

Choroid

Retina

FIGURE 27-1 Anatomical structures of the human eye. (From Seidel HM, Ball JW, Dains JE, Flynn J, Solomon B, Stewart R: *Mosby's guide to physical examination*, ed 7, St Louis, 2011, Mosby.)

of the lid and underlying lacerations of the globe. Internal bleeding may be subconjunctival (between the conjunctiva and sclera) or intraocular (hyphema). The cornea may have a foreign body and/or abrasions.

History of forceful trauma causing laceration or perforation of the globe is a surgical emergency and should be referred immediately without manipulation of the eye or eyelid.

Is this an acute or chronic condition?

Key Questions

- How long has the eye been red?
- Did the redness start abruptly or was it gradual?
- Have you had this redness before? When?

Onset

An abrupt onset of redness typifies trauma, chemical burn, foreign body, ultraviolet (UV) exposure, or contact lens problems. Onset over a few hours may indicate infection from adjacent structures (periorbital, orbital, or sinuses). Onset over a few days is characteristic of conjunctivitis. Acute redness can be caused by infection of the conjunctiva and/or eyelids. Common causative organisms include *Staphylococcus aureus*, *Streptococcus pneumoniae*, group A *Streptococcus*, *Haemophilus influenzae*, and *Neisseria gonorrhoeae*.

Recurrence

Recurrent redness is often the result of allergic conjunctivitis from a hypersensitivity reaction to a specific antigen. Iritis from systemic causes can also produce recurrent redness because of collagen destruction.

Can I narrow the problem by location?

Key Question

- Does one eye (or do both eyes) bother you?

Unilateral redness is more likely to indicate trauma or infection, whereas bilateral redness is more likely to indicate an allergy or an underlying systemic process. Blepharitis, inflammation of the eyelids, causes itching and crusting of the lash line and is usually bilateral.

A hordeolum (sty) produces redness at the base of eyelashes and is usually unilateral. A chalazion is a chronic granulomatous inflammation of the meibomian gland. It is found in the mid eyelid, often on the conjunctival side, and is usually unilateral. Some conditions can present with either unilateral or bilateral symptoms. Conjunctivitis often starts in one eye and then spreads to the other eye, sparing the limbal area of the eyes. Subconjunctival hemorrhage is often unilateral but may involve both eyes. Herpetic infection may be unilateral or bilateral.

A unilaterally painful, inflamed eye with photophobia and often a foreign body sensation and without a history of significant trauma may indicate acute glaucoma.

What does the presence or absence of pain tell me?

Key Questions

- Do you have pain in your eye?
- How severe is the pain?
- Does it feel like there is something in your eye?

Location of Pain

Decide whether the pain is coming from the eye itself or is referred from surrounding structures. The ophthalmic nerve innervates the lid, conjunctiva, cornea, and uveal tract. The retina, vitreous, and optic nerve are less well innervated and seldom are a source of pain. Referred pain can originate from contiguous structures or from inflamed structures innervated by the meningeal branches of the ophthalmic nerve.

Severity of Pain

Bacterial conjunctivitis causes minimal pain; most patients report discomfort from the discharge and matting. There may be an itching or burning pain with allergy, moderate pain with iritis, and severe pain with corneal abrasion or ulcer. Constant, boring, throbbing pain, often severe enough to interfere with sleep, can result from ocular inflammation associated with iritis, acute glaucoma, and scleritis.

Foreign Body Sensation

A foreign body in an eye is a likely cause of pain. Viral causes of conjunctivitis produce a gritty sensation in the eye. A scratchy sensation often accompanies conditions that lead to dry eye, such as Sjögren syndrome. Patients who over-wear contact lenses frequently report pain in

the eye, caused by corneal hypoxia, several hours after removing the contacts.

Do I need to worry about vision changes?

Key Questions

- Have you noticed any loss of vision?
- Have you had any blurred vision, double vision, halos, or floaters?

Vision Loss

Distinguish visual loss from blurry vision caused by the discharge associated with conjunctivitis. No decrease in vision is seen with bacterial and allergic conjunctivitis, beyond that reasonably related to blurring from the heavy discharge. Vision is mildly decreased in iritis but markedly decreased in acute glaucoma and with corneal abrasions or ulcers. Box 27-1 lists symptom patterns of pain and visual loss (also see Chapter 35).

Sudden diminution in or loss of visual acuity is an ocular emergency and may indicate corneal or uveal tract disorders, acute glaucoma, or orbital cellulitis.

Blurring

True blurring is caused by an ocular problem. When the cornea, lens, aqueous humor, or vitreous is hazy, vision blurs and often there is dazzle in bright light. Some patients describe both refractive errors and double vision as blurred vision. Heavy discharge associated with conjunctivitis can also produce perceived blurring of vision.

Box 27-1	Symptom Patterns of Pain and Visual Loss

Red Eye (No Pain or Visual Loss)	Red Eye (Painful)	
	Vision Normal	*Vision Impaired*
Conjunctivitis	Episcleritis	Iritis
Subconjunctival hemorrhage	Keratitis	Glaucoma
Episcleritis	Cluster headache	Orbital cellulitis
	Corneal abrasion	Scleritis
	Corneal ulcer	Corneal abrasion
		Keratitis
		Corneal ulcer

Double Vision

True double vision becomes single vision when one eye is covered. Sudden onset usually indicates a neurological problem. Chronic diplopia may be caused by muscular problems. Monocular diplopia usually indicates either corneal or lens changes.

Halos

Halos result from prismatic effects. They can be visual signs of corneal edema caused by an abrupt rise in corneal or intraocular pressure (acute glaucoma). Less serious causes are water drops in the cornea or lens (seen in corneal edema or cataract).

Floaters

Floaters and/or flashing lights occur with vitreoretinal traction. The traction may progress to a retinal tear or detachment. With a tear, patients may report spaghetti-like strands floating in their vision. With a detachment, patients will give a history of blurred or blackened vision over several hours that progresses to complete or partial monocular blindness.

What does the presence or characteristic of the discharge tell me?

Key Questions

- Do you have any discharge from your eye?
- Is the discharge from one eye or both eyes?
- What are the color, consistency, and characteristics of this discharge?

Presence and Characteristics of Discharge

A watery, nonpurulent discharge usually indicates allergic conjunctivitis. A mucoid (stringy or ropy) discharge is also common with allergic conjunctivitis. In allergic conjunctivitis, the discharge is usually bilateral. Discharge that is purulent or mucopurulent may indicate bacterial conjunctivitis and often affects both eyes. Copious purulent discharge may be caused by *N. gonorrhoeae* infection. Viral conjunctivitis discharge is watery and may affect only one eye. Corneal abrasions and ulcers also produce watery/purulent discharge and are usually unilateral.

In the neonate who is 24 hours old, mucoid or purulent discharge indicates chemical conjunctivitis from prophylactic instillation of silver nitrate and other medications. Severe, bilateral purulent conjunctivitis 3 to 7 days after birth may indicate gonococcal infection of the eye.

Discharge that is seen 5 to 30 days postpartum may indicate chlamydial conjunctivitis.

What does the presence of photophobia tell me?

Key Question

- Does light bother you or hurt your eye(s)?

Photophobia usually indicates ocular inflammation or irritation. Intraocular inflammation (iritis or generalized uveitis) causes pain on pupillary changes and thus leads to the avoidance of bright light. This symptom may be mild and often is not reported unless the patient is questioned specifically about this symptom. There is no photophobia with bacterial conjunctivitis. In infants and young children, photophobia signals a serious condition, such as juvenile arthritis, intraocular tumors, congenital glaucoma, herpetic keratitis, or trauma.

What other things do I need to consider?

Key Questions

- Has there been any swelling?
- Do you have excessive tearing?
- Do your eyes itch?
- Does the itching occur at different times of the year?
- Have you had a cough or fever?

Swelling

The orbital septum is a continuation of the periosteum of the bones of the orbit. It extends to the margins of both the upper and lower eyelids. Any conditions occurring in these areas can cause swelling. Secondarily, the skin of the eyelids is a very thin subcutaneous tissue that is musculofibrous and contains no fat. Thus the eyelid can allow a considerable amount of fluid to accumulate in a short period of time. Swelling and erythema under and associated with the medial canthus of the affected eye may indicate dacryocystitis. Swelling of the lids may be associated with inflammation, local infection, or trauma. Periorbital swelling may indicate cellulitis.

Tears

The lacrimal gland, which is situated in the upper lateral orbit, produces tears that are then carried across the eye to the puncta on the nasal side of the upper and lower lids. Obstruction of the passage of tears via the nasolacrimal duct to the nose causes regurgitation of fluid down the cheek (tearing). Epiphora (excessive production of tears) is common with viral conjunctivitis, corneal abrasions, infantile glaucoma, and nasal lacrimal duct stenosis.

Itching and Tearing

The hallmark of an allergic conjunctivitis is itching and tearing disproportionate to findings. Vernal conjunctivitis is seasonal, recurrent, and bilateral. Itching is intense in the spring and fall months.

Cough and Fever

Bacterial conjunctivitis is not associated with a fever. Otitis-conjunctivitis syndrome begins with a low-grade to moderate fever, mucopurulent rhinorrhea, and a cough. Three or four days after the onset of fever, the individual wakes up with the eyelashes crusted together. Ear complaints begin the same day as eye symptoms. Viral conjunctivitis, seen as slight crusting along the lid margins, may be seen with upper respiratory tract infections.

DIAGNOSTIC REASONING: FOCUSED PHYSICAL EXAMINATION
Test Visual Acuity

In adults and children older than 3½ years, use a Snellen, Tumbling E, or Lippman chart. In children, the referral standard is 20/40 or worse in both eyes or a two-line difference between eyes. Retesting before referral of children is suggested because the child may perform better (within normal limits) on the second examination.

For children younger than 3½ years, use an ophthalmoscope. Darken the room. Stay at arm's length from the child and look at the eyes at a distance of 1 m or greater. When the child looks at the light, look at both red reflexes simultaneously and compare them. They should be red and equal in coloration. This indicates that the vision and binocular alignment are good and that no major pathology of the cornea, lens, vitreous, or retina is present. If the reflexes are not equal, a referral is required to an ophthalmologist.

Test Visual Fields

Testing of visual fields assesses the function of the peripheral vision and the central retina, optic pathways, and cortex. The peripheral field is damaged in glaucoma and by tumors or vascular lesions involving the visual fibers from the chiasm to the occipital cortex.

Inspect the Lids, Lid Margins, Periorbital Tissues, and Orbital Tissues

Note redness or swelling of the lids. Look for lid lesions. Inspect the lid margins. Evert the lids and note appearance.

Unilateral inflammation of the lids and periorbital tissues without proptosis or limitation of eye movement characterizes periorbital cellulitis. If proptosis and/or limitation of eye movement are present, orbital cellulitis is the cause.

Erythematous swelling without systemic signs may be caused by contact dermatitis. All exposed skin should have the same coloring. Magenta discoloration of the eyelid is caused by *H. influenzae*.

A lid that is injected, swollen, and irritated may be so because of an underlying disease process in the conjunctiva, cornea, sclera, or intraocular area.

Examine for the presence of focal or diffuse inflammation. Blockage of the glands along the lash line may produce localized or diffuse redness or flaking of the skin as a result of staphylococcal or seborrheic causes.

With viral conjunctivitis, lids appear to have follicular changes (small aggregates of lymphocytes) in the palpebral conjunctiva. Lids that have large, flattened, cobblestone-like papillary lesions of the palpebral conjunctivae are characteristic of vernal conjunctivitis.

Inflammation of the lid margins in all four lids and with associated loss of eyelashes is common in children; this condition is known as blepharitis. The lashes are waxy, scaling, red, and irritated, and the eyes have slightly swollen lid margins.

Eye pain with no external inflammation suggests referred causes, such as sinusitis, carotid artery aneurysm, temporal arteritis, migraine or cluster headache, or trigeminal neuralgia. Optic neuritis can also cause eye pain without inflammation.

Observe for Entropion and Ectropion

Entropion occurs when the eyelid margin turns inward. The eyelashes contact the corneal and conjunctival surfaces, and the patient reports discomfort. Scarring can occur.

Ectropion occurs when the eyelid margin turns outward. A pool of stagnant tears results and does not allow proper mechanical protection of the cornea and conjunctiva. The exposed tarsal conjunctiva is also susceptible to repeated trauma.

Evert the Eyelid if Indicated by History

Eversion of the eyelid is necessary to detect a possible foreign body. This is done by first having the patient look down. Hold the upper eyelashes straightforward. Push down on the upper tarsal border with a cotton-tipped applicator. The lid everts. Hold the eyelid in this position by moving fingers to the brow. To undo, hold the lashes and pull gently forward while asking the patient to look up.

Inspect the Conjunctiva

Note bilateral or unilateral redness and the location of redness on the conjunctiva. Distinguish between peripheral or circumcorneal injection (ciliary flush). Ciliary flush is the deep conjunctival or episcleral blood vessel injection around the limbus (junction between the cornea and conjunctiva), dilating in response to corneal disease or injury. It is frequently associated with keratopathy, uveitis, and episcleritis/scleritis. Abrasions and ulcers of the cornea cause increased redness of the globe around the corneal limbus, appearing as a reddish ring surrounding the cornea. Note any discharge. Look for visible lesions or foreign bodies on the conjunctiva.

Conjunctival inflammation as a result of infection causes a red eye with peripheral injection that is maximal toward the fornix (the fold between globe and lid). Peripheral injection involves the bulbar conjunctiva without edema or exudate, and the cornea is spared.

Look for swelling of the conjunctiva (chemosis). Fluid can accumulate beneath the loosely attached bulbar conjunctiva, causing it to balloon away from the globe. Chemosis occurs most frequently and dramatically with hyperacute bacterial conjunctivitis.

Subconjunctival hemorrhage causes a bright red splash of blood that is visible on the conjunctiva and sclera. Without a history of trauma or bleeding diathesis and no presence of retinal hemorrhage, the cause may be intravascular pressure from coughing, sneezing, or straining.

Systemic autoimmune processes, such as juvenile rheumatoid arthritis, serum sickness, and Stevens-Johnson syndrome, may cause conjunctivitis. Perilimbal conjunctival injection is seen in juvenile rheumatoid arthritis.

A localized degenerative process of the substantia propriae of the conjunctiva, known as pinguecula, may invade the superficial cornea. These are yellow, elevated nodules of fibropathic material that are usually adjacent to the cornea on the nasal side.

Look at the palpebral conjunctiva and the fornices for foreign bodies and pterygia, which are neovascularized structures that can encroach on the cornea and form a pannus that interferes with vision.

Inspect the Sclera

Note the color. The sclera gives the eye its white appearance. Inflammation (scleritis) causes a dusky red color.

Examine the Cornea

Test the corneal light (red) reflex. Note if the cornea is hazy or has opacities. Look for visible foreign bodies.

The normal cornea is transparent, with blood vessels only at the limbus (the junction between cornea and conjunctiva). Illumination of the cornea tangentially may show abnormalities, such as abrasions or foreign bodies. These imperfections of the corneal surface will produce an abnormal light reflex or a break in the image as the light reflects off the cornea. The blood vessels around the limbus dilate in response to corneal disease or injury.

Topical application of fluorescein to the cornea that reveals dendrite ulcers should lead you to suspect herpes simplex virus.

Examine the Iris, Pupil, and Lens

Note pupil size and equality. Note transparency of lens. Test pupillary reaction (direct and consensual). Note any photophobia.

The anterior chamber should contain only clear aqueous humor. Trauma may cause blood to accumulate in the chamber; this is known as a hyphema. The shock wave produced by the sudden compression and decompression of the cornea is transmitted through the eye and may result in a tear in the ciliary body. Disruption of the anterior arterial circle of this structure produces bleeding that accumulates. The hyphema appears as a bright red or dark red fluid level between the cornea and iris or as a diffuse murkiness of the aqueous humor. Pus may also accumulate in this space in association with corneal infection. This is known as hypopyon. All hyphemas are abnormal and must be referred to an ophthalmologist.

The pupil is the central aperture of the iris. It floats in the aqueous humor and divides the anterior segment into anterior and posterior chambers, which communicate throughout the pupillary aperture. It slides freely on the anterior surface of the lens when dilating and contracting. Conditions that affect this anatomy cause pupil abnormalities. Inflammation of the iris (iritis) causes reduction in the reactive capacity of the iris and inequality of pupils. Acute increased intraocular pressure causes the space in the anterior chamber to become very shallow, resulting in a dilated, fixed, oval pupil.

The lens is normally transparent and not visible on inspection; however, any visible clouding of the lens as seen through the pupil is indicative of cataract formation.

Perform Ophthalmoscopy

When looking for the red reflex, note any corneal opacity as well as the depth of the opacity. Corneal opacities move in the opposite direction of the ophthalmoscope, lens opacities stay still, and vitreous opacities move in the same direction as the ophthalmoscope. Corneal clouding (edema) is seen with glaucoma.

Look for a large and deepened cup if you suspect glaucoma. Early in the course of the disease, the ophthalmoscopic examination may be normal. Do not use mydriatic agents if you suspect glaucoma.

Test Extraocular Movements

Test eye movement in all six fields of gaze. Note pain or restriction. Inflammation or underlying periostitis and impaired venous drainage as a result of reactive inflammation cause restrictive eye movement and proptosis (exophthalmos). Decreased range of motion can also occur with orbital cellulitis.

Palpate the Lid/Lacrimal Puncta

Observe for edema and note pain or tenderness on palpation. The lacrimal puncta should be turned backward slightly to catch the pool of tears in the inner canthus. Tears should not spill over the cheeks. Note if gentle palpation of each lacrimal sac produces any material that regurgitates into the eye. Unilateral swelling over the lacrimal sac on the lid margin at the side of the nose because of infection or obstruction of the lacrimal drainage system is common. Infection of the meibomian glands of the eyelids (hordeolum or internal sty) and the glands of Zeis or Moll (hordeolum or external sty) produces

pain on palpation. Internal sties are generally large and very tender and may point to the conjunctiva or epidermis portion of the lid. External sties are small and superficial and point only to the epidermis side.

Granulomatous inflammation of a meibomian gland nodule that is firm and not tender and has no inflammatory signs is a chalazion.

Examine the Tympanic Membranes

Examination of the tympanic membrane is necessary because of the frequent association with atypical *H. influenzae* acute otitis media (conjunctivitis-otitis syndrome).

Palpate Preauricular Nodes

The preauricular nodes are usually palpable with a viral infection of the eyes. Palpable adenopathy is uncommon in acute bacterial conjunctivitis but may occur in hyperacute infection caused by *N. gonorrhoeae* or *Neisseria meningitidis*.

LABORATORY AND DIAGNOSTIC STUDIES
Fluorescein Staining

Dendrite etchings on the anterior portion of the cornea are seen in herpes infection. Nodules near the limbus with surrounding hyperemia are seen in keratoconjunctivitis. Hypertrophy of the dorsal conjunctiva with elevated grayish areas near the limbus is consistent with vernal conjunctivitis. Under a blue light, a corneal abrasion and foreign body will stain bright green with fluorescein.

Culture

Cultures are not usually required in patients with mild conjunctivitis of suspected viral, bacterial, or allergic origin. However, bacterial cultures should be obtained in patients with severe, chronic, or recurrent conjunctivitis. Moisten a sterile alginate (not cotton) swab with sterile saline and wipe the lid margin or conjunctival cul-de-sac. The culture medium is then inoculated directly with the swab tip. Place on solid medium, writing R for right eye, L for left eye, and Z for another culture site. The tip of the applicator may then be broken off and dropped into the tube of liquid culture medium.

Cultures should be taken before instilling topical anesthetics because preservatives will reduce the recovery of some bacteria.

Gram Stain

Gram-positive cocci in pairs may indicate *Streptococcus pyogenes*. Gram-negative diplococci indicate *N. gonorrhoeae*. Large gram-negative diplobacilli indicate *Moraxella catarrhalis*; *H. influenzae* stains as gram-negative coccobacilli.

Complete Blood Count

A complete blood count with differential can be done to establish the presence of a systemic infection. An increase in white blood cells and bands is seen with systemic infection.

Blood Cultures

Blood cultures are obtained for any suspected orbital cellulitis or when there is reason to suspect a clinically significant bacteremia. *H. influenzae*, *Streptococcus pneumoniae*, *Staphylococcus aureus*, *Streptococcus pyogenes*, or anaerobes are possible infecting organisms.

Computed Tomography Scanning

A computed tomography scan is used to determine the presence and extent of an abscess and/or to localize the site of infection in the periorbital region as well as in the sinuses.

Intraocular Pressure

Intraocular pressure is measured with a Schiøtz tonometer. The technique is as follows: after instillation of a local anesthetic agent, the patient is placed in a supine position and asked to look directly upward. The lids are held separated, and the instrument is placed gently in a vertical position directly over the cornea with the plunger placed on the cornea. A reading on the scale is then taken. A pressure elevated greater than 21 mm Hg is seen in acute closed-angle glaucoma.

DIFFERENTIAL DIAGNOSIS
Lacrimal Sac

Dacryocystitis

Infection of the lacrimal sac occurs secondary to obstruction. In infants, it is a complication of congenital dacryostenosis. In adults, duct obstruction results from nasal trauma, deviated septum, hypertrophic rhinitis, and mucosal polyps. The patient experiences pain, swelling, and redness around the lacrimal sac with tearing. Conjunctivitis, blepharitis, and leukocytosis are associated with an acute condition; with a chronic condition, the only symptom may be slight swelling of the sac. Pus may regurgitate through the punctum.

Eyelids
Blepharitis

Blepharitis is the most common inflammation of the eyelids. It usually involves the lid margins and frequently is associated with conjunctivitis. It is bilateral and not painful, and it has no associated photophobia. The lids are inflamed, and scaling of the lid margins is seen. Loss of eyelashes occurs late. Visual acuity is unimpaired.

Hordeolum

Hordeolum is caused by infection of the glands of Zeis or Moll along the lash line. It develops acutely and manifests as a palpable indurated area along the lid margin, with a purulent center and surrounding erythema. It spontaneously drains within 1 to 2 weeks. Patients experience swelling of the eyelid and localized lid pain.

Chalazion

A chalazion is a granulomatous reaction in the meibomian gland on the tarsal plate of the lid. This is usually a chronic condition. The lesion is usually painless and indurated. When symptoms are present, they include pruritus and redness of the involved eye and eyelid.

Entropion and Ectropion

Malposition of the eyelid causes local irritation and may be a cause of red eye. In entropion the lid is turned inward; in ectropion the lid is turned outward.

Conjunctiva
Bacterial Conjunctivitis

S. aureus, *S. pneumoniae*, group A *Streptococcus*, *H. influenzae*, and *N. gonorrhoeae* most commonly cause bacterial conjunctivitis. The onset is gradual, begins unilaterally, and often becomes bilateral. The patient usually reports a scratchy sensation instead of pain. There is generally no photophobia. Examination reveals peripheral injection, purulent discharge, and matted eyelids. Visual acuity is not affected, although the presence of discharge may produce "blurring" of vision.

Viral Conjunctivitis

Occurring most commonly in young adults, viral conjunctivitis is caused by such viruses as adenovirus, picornavirus, rhinovirus, and herpesvirus. The onset is gradual and unilateral early in the course and then may become bilateral. The patient reports a scratchy, rather than painful, sensation. On examination, peripheral injection with watery discharge is apparent. Visual acuity is intact. Lids may have follicular changes (small aggregates of lymphocytes) in the palpebral conjunctiva.

Allergic Conjunctivitis

Allergic conjunctivitis is a chronic, seasonal condition caused by hypersensitivity reaction to a specific allergen. It is bilateral, itchy, and painless. The conjunctival injection is peripheral. There is ropy, mucoid discharge. The palpebral conjunctiva has a cobblestone appearance. Visual acuity is unaffected.

Neisseria gonorrhoeae Conjunctivitis

The *N. gonorrhoeae* organism can produce a bacterial conjunctivitis in newborns. It is bilateral, with very purulent discharge 48 to 72 hours after birth. Although rare in adults, it can occur through direct transmission via finger contact or via contact of the eyes in a nonchlorinated swimming pool. The infection has an abrupt onset and is characterized by copious purulent discharge that reaccumulates after being wiped away. In addition to redness and irritation, the patient has marked conjunctival injection, chemosis, lid swelling, and tender preauricular adenopathy. The condition warrants immediate ophthalmic referral.

Chemical Conjunctivitis

Chemical conjunctivitis occurs with instillation of chemical prophylaxis in the neonate. A bilateral reaction occurs within the first 24 hours.

Subconjunctival Hemorrhage

Subconjunctival hemorrhage is usually the result of a small blood vessel rupture in the conjunctival tissue and frequently develops after episodes of coughing or straining. It is painless, although often frightening to the patient. Visual acuity is not impaired.

Anterior Chamber
Hyphema

Hyphema is caused by blood in the anterior chamber of the eye, usually produced by trauma to the eye. The patient has a marked decrease in vision, with red blood cells present diffusely throughout the anterior chamber. A settled layer of blood present inferiorly or a complete filling of the anterior chamber is possible, obscuring the visual examination of the posterior chamber. The pupil is irregular and poorly reactive.

Sclera
Episcleritis

Often a benign inflammatory condition of the covering of the sclera, episcleritis is bilateral, with mild stinging. Peripheral injection is present. There is no discharge, but some lacrimation and photophobia may be present. Visual acuity is unimpaired.

Scleritis

Inflammation of the sclera can result in severe destructive disease. It is usually a unilateral inflammatory condition associated with rheumatoid arthritis, systemic immunological disease, or other autoimmune disorders. There is pain and ciliary injection. Lacrimation is present, and visual acuity is variable.

Cornea
Keratitis

Bacterial, fungal, and viral organisms can cause infection of the cornea. Moderate to severe eye pain is present, there is some discharge, and visual acuity is decreased. Pupils are equal and normal, but the cornea appears cloudy. Peripheral injection is present and diffuse. A ciliary flush is also present.

Corneal Abrasion

Corneal abrasion may be superficial, lying on top of the anterior surface of the cornea, or it may be subtarsal and become implanted on the palpebral conjunctiva, causing the cornea to become irritated when the patient blinks. The patient usually has a history of a foreign body on the anterior surface of the eye. The abrasion causes moderate to severe pain with discharge present. Visual acuity may be normal or decreased, photophobia is present, and pupil size and reaction are normal. Fluorescein stain is taken into the ulcer and can be seen under a Wood's lamp.

Herpetic Infection

Caused by the herpes simplex virus, this infection occurs unilaterally or bilaterally. The patient's presenting symptoms are pain, photophobia, and diffuse or ciliary injection. Discharge is variable, and visual acuity is markedly decreased. Dendrites are seen on fluorescein staining.

Herpes zoster can cause inflammation and scarring of the cornea, with conjunctivitis and iritis. In some cases the retina and optic nerve are involved. Severe or chronic outbreaks of herpes zoster may cause glaucoma, cataract formation, double vision, and scarring of the cornea. Patients with suspected ocular herpes infection (simplex or zoster) should be referred to an ophthalmologist.

Orbit
Periorbital Cellulitis
The patient's presenting symptoms include unilateral lid swelling, redness, fever, and hotness. The conjunctiva is clear, the eye moves freely, and vision is not impaired.

Orbital Cellulitis
The patient's symptoms include unilateral lid swelling, fever, and pain. Examination reveals proptosis, chemosis, and conjunctivitis. There is limitation of eye motion on testing of extraocular movements. The patient appears ill. This condition is life threatening and requires immediate intervention.

Uveal Tract
Iritis
Characterized by inflammation of the iris and ciliary body, iritis may be idiopathic and develop in response to coexistent conjunctivitis, keratitis, or eye trauma, or it may occur with chronic inflammatory or infectious processes. Eye pain is moderate and aching, visual acuity is decreased, and photophobia is present. There is minimal eye discharge, the affected pupil is smaller, and the cornea appears normal. There is central redness of the eye, with ciliary flush present.

Glaucoma
Acute closed-angle glaucoma. The patient's presenting symptoms include unilateral, deep eye pain and photophobia. There may be a report of halos around visualized objects. There is ciliary injection with tears and decreased visual acuity. The pupil is mid dilated and has decreased reactivity to light. The cornea is cloudy. There is diffuse redness of the eye with an intraocular pressure of greater than 21 mm Hg. This condition requires emergency referral.

DIFFERENTIAL DIAGNOSIS OF *Common Causes of Red Eye*

CONDITION	HISTORY	PHYSICAL FINDINGS	DIAGNOSTIC STUDIES
Eyelids/Lacrimal Sac			
Dacryocystitis	Unilateral, acute onset; pain	Swelling and redness around lacrimal sac; tearing; may have pus through punctum	CBC, leukocytosis
Blepharitis	Bilateral, gradual onset; no pain	Lids inflamed; scaling on visual acuity okay; loss of margins; lashes (late)	None
Hordeolum/sty	Unilateral; pain	Swelling of eyelid; indurated lesion with central pus and surrounding erythema	None initially; if repeated, screen for diabetes
Chalazion	Unilateral, chronic; painless	Indurated lesion on tarsal plate of lid; may have pruritus and redness of involved eye and eyelid	None
Entropion/ ectropion	Unilateral or bilateral	Lid turned inward or outward; local irritation and tearing; peripheral injection	None
Conjunctiva			
Bacterial conjunctivitis	Gradual onset, unilateral early, bilateral late; scratchy (no pain); photophobia	Peripheral injection; purulent discharge; matted eyelids; visual acuity okay	None initially; if not better with treatment, obtain culture and sensitivities; Gram stain
Viral conjunctivitis	Gradual onset, unilateral early, bilateral late; scratchy (no pain)	Peripheral injection; watery discharge; visual acuity okay; follicular changes (small aggregates of lymphocytes) in palpebral conjunctiva	Same as for bacterial conjunctivitis
Allergic conjunctivitis	Chronic; seasonal; bilateral; itchy (no pain)	Peripheral injection; ropy, mucoid discharge; cobblestone mucosa; visual acuity okay	Fluorescein staining; hypertrophy of dorsal conjunctiva with elevated gray areas near limbus with vernal conjunctivitis

Continued

DIFFERENTIAL DIAGNOSIS OF *Common Causes of Red Eye—cont'd*

CONDITION	HISTORY	PHYSICAL FINDINGS	DIAGNOSTIC STUDIES
N. gonorrhoeae conjunctivitis	Bilateral; newborn	Purulent discharge 48-72 hours after birth	Culture on Thayer-Martin plate; Gram stain
Chemical conjunctivitis	Bilateral	Neonate: within first 24 hours	None
Subconjunctival hemorrhage	Unilateral; painless; coughing or straining	Splash of blood in conjunctiva or sclera; visual acuity okay	None
Anterior Chamber			
Hyphema	Unilateral; trauma to eye	Red blood cells in anterior chamber; visual acuity decreased; pupil irregular and poorly reactive	Refer to ophthalmologist
Sclera			
Episcleritis	Bilateral; mild stinging	Peripheral injection; no discharge; visual acuity okay	None
Scleritis	Unilateral; deep, boring pain	Ciliary injection, teary; visual acuity variable; photophobia	Associated with systemic immunological disease
Keratitis	Bilateral; moderate to severe pain	Discharge; pupils normal; cornea cloudy; visual acuity decreased	Test for bacterial, fungal, viral infection
Corneal abrasion/ foreign body	Unilateral; pain; photophobia	Diffuse injection; tears; visual acuity variable	Fluorescein stain positive
Herpetic keratitis	Unilateral or bilateral; pain; photophobia	Ciliary flush; discharge; visual acuity markedly decreased	Fluorescein stain shows dendrites
Orbit			
Periorbital cellulitis	Unilateral	Swelling of lid; fever, redness; conjunctiva clear; eye moves freely; vision not impaired	CBC—leukocytosis, blood cultures
Orbital cellulitis	Unilateral; pain	Proptosis; lid swelling; chemosis; conjunctivitis; limitation of eye motion	CBC, blood cultures; CT scan; life threatening
Uveal Tract			
Iritis	Unilateral; moderate aching pain; photophobia	Tearing; affected pupil smaller; cornea normal; ciliary flush	Refer
Glaucoma			
Acute closed-angle glaucoma	Unilateral; deep pain; photophobia; halos	Ciliary injection; tears; visual acuity decreased	Tonometry; emergency referral

CBC, Complete blood count; *CT,* computed tomography.

REFERENCES AND READINGS

Bal SK, Hollingworth GR: Red eye, *BMJ* 331:7514, 2005.

Cronau H, Kankanala RR, Mauger T: Diagnosis and management of red eye in primary care, *Am Fam Physician* 81:145, 2010.

Greenberg MF, Pollard ZF: The red eye in childhood, *Pediatr Clin North Am* 50:105, 2003.

Jain A, Rubin PA: Orbital cellulitis in children, *Int Ophthalmol Clin* 41:71, 2001.

Leibowitz HM: The red eye, *N Engl J Med* 343:345, 2000.

Rietveld RP, ter Riet G, Bindels PJ, Sloos JH, van Weert HC: Predicting bacterial cause in infectious conjunctivitis: cohort study on informativeness of combinations of signs and symptoms, *BMJ* 329:7459, 2004.

Simon JW, Kaw P: Commonly missed diagnoses in the childhood eye examination, *Am Fam Physician* 64:623, 2001.

Wald E: Periorbital and orbital infections, *Pediatr Rev* 25:312, 2004.

Wagner RS: Pediatric ocular inflammation, *Immunol Allergy Clin North Am* 28:169, 2008.

Sleep Problems

Each year more than 10 million Americans seek medical help for sleep problems. Patients report insufficient or nonrestorative sleep, despite adequate opportunity, that results in some form of daytime impairment. Insomnia is prevalent in 30% to 40% of the adult population, with 10% to 15% reporting that it is chronic, severe, or both. More than 40% of parents report sleep problems with their children, and 20% of these are considered significant. The consequences of chronic sleep problems include difficulty with concentration, fatigue, lack of energy, and irritability. Sleep disturbances in the elderly can result in increased falls and accidents. In children, sleep disturbances can produce problems in learning and behavior, alter physical development, and affect family functioning.

Sleep has two separate stages: rapid eye movement (REM) sleep, which is linked with dreaming, and non–rapid eye movement (NREM) sleep, which is a deeper sleep state. NREM is further divided into four sleep stages. In each stage the sleep is progressively deeper. Generally an individual moves through the NREM stages from stage 1 sleep to stage 4. Stages 3 and 4 are the deepest sleep stages. At the end of stage 4, a person goes backward in the stages toward the progressively lighter sleep of stage 1. The pattern is then followed by the first REM sleep stage. Movement from stage 1 to the end of REM is termed a sleep cycle. This cycle usually lasts 90 minutes in adults and approximately 50 minutes in infants. In one night, generally five cycles are completed. As sleep cycles, the REM period increases in length from 10 minutes to occupying most of the 90-minute cycle. Also, the proportion of stage 2 increases, with stages 3 and 4 decreasing in length. The total amount and composition of sleep change throughout life. Sleep quality is often judged by the amount of time spent in stage 4 sleep. People who do not have adequate REM sleep feel they have had too little sleep.

Newborns fall directly into REM sleep. This REM sleep in infancy is thought to provide the brain stimulation for maturation. At age 5, REM sleep decreases to that of the adult, approximately 20% of total sleep. The REM portion of sleep is constant through all age ranges; however, NREM sleep stages 3 and 4 begin to decline in adolescents, and in the elderly, stages 3 and 4 disappear. The elderly may experience more frequent awakenings during the night; some need to compensate for this with rest periods during the day. Some elderly clients view their pattern of diminished sleep with frustration, whereas others accept it as an opportunity to have more time for other activities.

Sleep is regulated by two primary processes: the body's circadian rhythm, which causes an increase in sleepiness twice during a 24-hour period (usually between midnight and 7 AM and for a brief period in the mid-afternoon), and the physiological need for sleep, which is increased by sleep loss and sleep disruption.

DIAGNOSTIC REASONING: FOCUSED HISTORY

Define the nature of the problem.

Key Questions

- What kind of sleep problem are you (or the child) having?
- Are you having difficulty falling asleep?
- Are you having difficulty staying asleep?
- Are you having difficulty staying awake during the day?
- Have you taken medications for the sleep problem? If so, what are they?
- How long has the problem existed?

Nature of the Problem

Sleep disorders include sleeplessness (insomnia), episodic disturbance of behavior associated with sleep (parasomnias), and excessive sleepiness (hypersomnia). The most common childhood sleep disorders are night awakening, inability to fall asleep, problems going to bed, circadian rhythm problems, and parasomnias.

Often it is the caregiver, not the child, who perceives the sleep disturbances to be a problem.

Difficulty Falling Asleep

Difficulty in falling asleep is often related to poor sleep hygiene practices, the use of medications or stimulants, or disruption in circadian rhythms. Difficulty falling asleep also can occur as a result of pain or as a symptom of anxiety.

Difficulty Staying Asleep

Difficulty staying asleep occurs when the sleep cycle is disrupted; this may be related to physiological factors, illness, depression, pain, or use of medications or alcohol.

Daytime Sleepiness

Nighttime insomnia and daytime sleepiness are not isolated symptoms. Daytime sleepiness may be related to an increased need for sleep because of nighttime sleep loss, or it may represent narcolepsy.

Medications

All over-the-counter and prescription medications used to promote sleep can have short-term side effects, such as daytime sleepiness and headaches. Long-term use of sleep medications often produces tolerance and a need for increased doses to achieve sleep. Some of the agents, particularly the benzodiazepines, are habituating with long-term use; stopping them may cause withdrawal symptoms. Use of sleep medications by persons with sleep apnea can be dangerous.

Duration of Problem

Sleep disorders can be transient (lasting a few days), short term (lasting weeks), or chronic (lasting months to years). An acute problem, lasting a few days to a few weeks, can be caused by stress, acute illness, environmental disturbance, or jet lag. A chronic problem may be due to a specific sleep disorder, a mood disorder, or the use of medications or stimulant substances. Primary insomnia is diagnosed when no underlying cause can be identified.

Is this a specific sleep disorder?

Key Questions

- Do you have a creeping, crawling, or uncomfortable feeling in the legs that is relieved by moving the legs?
- Does your bed partner report that your arms or legs jerk during sleep?

- Do you (or the child) snore loudly, gasp, choke, or stop breathing during sleep?
- Do you (or the child) have difficulty staying awake during the day or do you fall asleep during routine tasks (for adults, especially driving)?
- Do you have episodes of muscle weakness?

Limb Sensation

Restless legs syndrome includes the sensation of crawling, pulling, and tingling with an irresistible urge to move the legs. Symptoms increase in the evening, especially when the person is lying down and remaining still. Patients often have coexisting periodic limb movements in sleep.

Limb Jerking

Periodic leg movements during sleep are common in persons older than 65 years. Bilateral, repeated, rhythmic jerking or twitching movements, primarily in the legs, characterize periodic limb movement disorder. Less frequently, movement occurs in the arms.

Snoring

Obstructive sleep apnea (OSA) is characterized by loud snoring, mouth breathing, and restless sleep patterns. The patient may report insomnia but more commonly notes excessive daytime sleepiness.

Parental smoking can be a risk factor for snoring in children. Passive smoke inhalation can provoke mucosal edema and inflammation, resulting in a narrowing of the pharynx and causing snoring.

Daytime Dozing, Excessive Sleepiness During the Day, and Muscle Weakness

Excessive daytime sleepiness may be caused by narcolepsy. Adults with narcolepsy report falling asleep while driving or while performing routine tasks. Initially, children with narcolepsy have great difficulty getting up in the mornings. When awakened, the child may appear to be confused or may be aggressive or verbally abusive. The child may fall asleep during school, in the vehicle on the way home from school, or while watching television. Cataplexy is common in adults. This disorder is identified as episodes of sudden muscular weakness and atonia generally instigated by an emotional trigger. The patient will have to lean against a wall for support because his or her legs feel rubbery.

The degree of daytime sleepiness can be quantified using the Epworth Sleepiness Scale (Box 28-1).

Could the sleep problem be secondary to a medical condition?

Key Questions

- Have you been ill recently?
- Do you have a chronic health condition?
- What medications (prescription and over-the-counter) do you take?
- Do you have depression or anxiety?

Illness: Acute or Chronic

Acute illness can be a cause of sleep disturbance. In children, otitis media and chronic serious otitis, even without acute infection, can disturb sleep. Some authors believe that middle ear pressure rises when the child is supine at night and have seen sleep improve with treatment of otitis. In children, enlarged adenoids and upper airway obstruction may cause awakening.

Gastroesophageal reflux (GERD) may cause night awakening but produce few symptoms during the day. GERD, chronic obstructive pulmonary disease (COPD), peptic ulcer disease, and congestive heart failure are associated with paroxysmal nocturnal dyspnea (PND), which frequently disturbs sleep and is often interpreted by the patient as insomnia. Prostatic hypertrophy may cause nocturia and thus disturb sleep.

Medications

Many medications can have stimulating effects and cause sleep disruption. Common offenders include antidepressants, decongestants, bronchodilators, β-blockers, thyroid preparations, phenytoin, methyldopa, and corticosteroids. The potential sedating effects of medications should also be considered in patients who report excessive daytime sleepiness. Medications such as antihistamines often cause sleep disturbances.

Pain

Pain may interfere with sleep onset or contribute to early awakenings. Patients with chronic pain may have mood and cognitive disturbances that contribute to insomnia and early morning awakening.

Box 28-1	**The Epworth Sleepiness Scale**

One tool that may be used in evaluating daytime sleepiness is the Epworth Sleepiness Scale. The scale is a simple questionnaire that measures general level of daytime sleepiness by gauging the probability of falling asleep in a variety of situations. The patient rates on a scale of 0 to 3 the likelihood that he or she would doze in each of eight different situations as part of his or her "usual way of life in recent times."

The patient's responses are added together, and the total score can range from 0 to 24. A normal range of scores is from 2 to 10, with a modal score of 6. Scores increase linearly in obstructive sleep apnea syndrome (OSAS) patients according to the severity of the apnea. Any score higher than 10 is considered significant.

The Epworth Sleepiness Scale has high test-retest reliability in normal subjects ($r = 0.82$, $p < 0.001$). It is a unitary scale with high internal consistency (Cronbach's coefficient alpha = 0.88). Strengths of the tool are that it is simple, easy to understand, and a very inexpensive measurement of daytime sleepiness.

On a scale of 0 to 3, indicate the likelihood that you would fall asleep in the following situations, taking into account your usual way of life in recent times. Using the scale below, choose the most appropriate number for each situation:

0 = would never doze
1 = slight likelihood of dozing
2 = moderate likelihood of dozing
3 = high likelihood of dozing

Situation—Likelihood of Dozing:

Situation	
Reading while seated	_____
Watching TV	_____
Sitting, inactive, in a public place such as a theater or meeting	_____
As a passenger in a car for an hour without a1 kg = 2.204 lb break	_____
Lying down to rest in the afternoon when circumstances permit	_____
Sitting and talking to someone	_____
Sitting quietly after a lunch during which you did not drink alcohol	_____
In a car, while stopped for a few minutes in traffic	_____
Total:	_____

Modified from Johns MW: Daytime sleepiness, snoring and obstructive sleep apnea, The Epworth Sleepiness Scale, *Chest* 103:30, 1993. Permission conveyed through Copyright Clearance Center, Inc.

Psychological Causes

Psychological conditions causing insomnia include depression, anxiety disorder, panic disorder, mania, and acute psychosis. People with depression tend to have early morning awakening, whereas those with anxiety disorder have trouble falling asleep (see Chapter 3).

Could this be related to sleep hygiene?

Key Questions

- What is your bedtime routine?
- What else do you do in your bedroom?
- Do you consume alcohol, nicotine, or caffeine before bedtime?
- Do you exercise before bedtime?
- How do you put your child to sleep?
- Where does your child sleep?

Bedtime Routine

Sleep hygiene is related to health practices and environmental influences on sleep. It is important to consistently go to bed at the same time and wake up at the same time.

Environment

Using the bedroom for other activities, such as work or watching television, can produce an environment that disrupts sleep. Lights and a television produce awakening cues. Routinely using the bedroom for other activities may also condition the patient to an arousal state while in the bedroom. Noise may affect sleep by leading to increasing amounts of wakefulness, increase in light sleep, and decrease in REM sleep, causing daytime sleepiness. Individual differences occur, but generally sleeping at temperatures above or below normal disrupts the ability to stay asleep.

Consumption of Stimulants

Caffeine, diet pills (with ephedrine), and nicotine are stimulants that can cause sleep disruption. Although the consumption of alcohol before bedtime promotes sleep onset, alcohol tends to shorten total sleep time and exacerbate other conditions, such as GERD and sleep apnea. Alcohol withdrawal in a heavy drinker may be associated with restlessness and sleep disturbance that can continue for a prolonged period after alcohol cessation.

Exercise

Vigorous exercise is a stimulant; it should be avoided for 1 to 2 hours before bedtime.

Child's Routine

A child who is put to bed still awake and learns to fall asleep using self-comforting measures is often able to calm himself or herself and return to sleep when he or she rouses in the middle of the night, as do most children and adults. Toddlers are fearful of separation, and routines need to be established before bedtime. This routine allows the toddler a sense of predictability and security; having a nightly routine is helpful.

Infant Sleeping Environment

The sleep environment should be quiet and dark, and the room temperature should be comfortable. Infants in waterbeds, on very soft bedding, on couches with pillows, or in any situation in which their heads may slip between the mattress and a wall or bedpost are at risk of suffocation. Sleeping with parents is done in many cultures. However, some infants who sleep with parents have sleep problems. As parents arise or move from the bed, the infant awakens because of the lighter sleep state.

Could this be related to lifestyle?

Key Questions

- Are you a shift worker?
- Do you sleep in the same bed each night?
- Do you travel frequently?

Shift Work

Shift work, particularly periodic shift work, has been a reported cause of sleep disruption. It may interrupt the usual circadian rhythm or alter usual sleeping patterns and habits.

Sleep Environment

Sleeping in unfamiliar surroundings affects the quality of sleep and increases sleep latency. It is associated with more wakefulness, an increased amount of light sleep, and a shorter REM sleep stage.

Travel

Jet lag is a common cause of sleep disruption. It may interrupt the usual circadian rhythm or alter usual sleeping patterns and habits. Even 1 to 2 hours of time zone change can disrupt the usual sleep/wake pattern.

Could this be related to age?

Key Questions

- How old is the patient (e.g., a child, adolescent, older adult)?
- What age was the child when the problem began?
- Does your child have problems going to bed?
- Does your child refuse to go to sleep?
- Does your child wake up screaming at night?

Age: Child

Newborns wake every 20 minutes to 4 hours during a 24-hour period, reflecting their sleep/wake cycle. This cycle changes between 3 and 6 months with the establishment of a diurnal sleep/wake rhythm. During this time, an initial "settling" period that typically takes 10 to 20 minutes begins to occur. Daytime sleep decreases over the next 3 years and consolidates at night. At age 4, most children no longer nap. School-age children sleep approximately 8 hours a night.

Problems going to sleep/sleep refusal. Toddlers have a strong attachment to their caregiver, and separation from this person at bedtime causes distress and sleep problems. Further, older toddlers who are in the preoperational stage are developing a sense of autonomy and use going to bed as an issue of control and/or a general pattern of oppositional behavior. Examination of the child's naptime is important. In the school-age child and adolescent, problems going to sleep may be caused by anxiety, negative conditioning, delayed sleep phase (often due to caffeine), or a bedtime that is too early. Vigorous activity before bedtime may delay sleep onset.

Waking up screaming at night. Night terrors are nocturnal episodes in which the child sits straight up in bed, screams, and is inconsolable for up to 30 minutes before relaxing and falling back to sleep. These actions occur within the first few hours of sleep. The child is not readily awakened, although he or she may seem to be awake. The child is not consolable and has no recollection of the event the next day.

Nightmares are bad dreams that awaken the dreamer. They occur later at night than night terrors. Unlike night terrors, the dream is remembered, and the child is awake and may be consoled by the caregiver.

Age: Adolescent

Adolescents have an increase in the amount of sleep required. However, a concomitant decrease in the amount of sleep obtained leaves most adolescents with a sleep debt. To recover from the debt, the adolescent usually sleeps later on the weekends.

Age: Menopausal Women

Menopause-related changes may contribute to or cause sleep disturbance. Hot flashes promote arousal from sleep. Menopause is associated with reduced total sleep time, prolonged time to initiate sleep, and reduced REM sleep.

Age: Older Adult

Older adults achieve less total nighttime sleep. They may take longer to initiate sleep, spend more time in the lighter stages of sleep, and experience increased fragmentation of the entire sleep cycle.

Older adults have more nighttime arousals and awakenings. Sleep is shorter in duration, more shallow, and more fragmented. Older adults tend to awaken earlier in the morning. If the onset of sleep is not correspondingly earlier, excessive daytime sleepiness may result. Daytime napping may compound the problem by reducing the drive for sleep at the usual bedtime hour.

Could this be conditioned insomnia?

Key Questions

- Are you able to fall asleep easily in places other than the bedroom?
- If a child: What does the child do when he or she awakens at night?
- If a child: What actions do you take to get the child back to sleep?

Sleep Location

Most cases of insomnia develop initially in response to a psychosocial stressor. As sleeplessness persists, the patient begins to associate the bed with wakefulness and heightened arousal rather than sleep. The patient may fall asleep easily outside the bedroom (e.g., while watching television or reading in another room) but feels wide awake in bed.

Child's Need for Comfort or Food

Infants who are soothed and cuddled and placed in bed when they are asleep do not learn how to settle themselves; when these infants are aroused at night, they require the same routine to fall back asleep. Children who do not have self-comforting behaviors will be unable to fall asleep on their own. These criers awaken, cry, and want to be held or rocked before they can go back to sleep. An infant older than 6 months who continues to wake during the night is considered a trained night crier.

Children who need to be fed after they are awakened at night are trained night feeders. The child does not need the additional nutrition but becomes conditioned to a feeding to go back to sleep. Caregivers often bottle-feed or breastfeed the child until the child falls back to sleep. The intake of nighttime feeding after 7 or 8 months of age may prevent the development of a more mature circadian rhythm. This rhythm is a digestive-endocrine-sleep/wake cycle that adjusts to a day/night cycle, resulting in a consolidation of sleep.

Could this be somnambulism?

Key Question
- Do you (or the child) sleepwalk?

Sleepwalking usually occurs only once a night and lasts about 15 minutes. The person gets out of bed and moves about slowly and in an automatic manner with a blank facial expression. The person may mumble. After a great deal of effort, the person can be awakened with little or no memory of the episode.

DIAGNOSTIC REASONING: FOCUSED PHYSICAL EXAMINATION
Obtain Growth Parameters and/or BMI

Children who have OSA may present with failure to thrive. In adults, obese middle-age men are most often affected by sleep apnea.

Inspect the Ears

Otitis media and serous otitis may cause wakefulness in infants and children because of the pressure of fluid accumulation in the middle ear, especially when in the supine position.

Inspect the Nose

Obstruction of the nose by secretions may cause sleep apnea in infants younger than 6 weeks. In children older than 6 weeks or in adults, nasal obstruction may cause OSA.

Inspect the Mouth, Throat, and Neck

Look for a narrow pharyngeal space, a long or edematous uvula, and enlarged tonsils and adenoids. Enlarged tonsils may cause obstruction while the person is sleeping. In adults, a heavy or thick neck is a risk factor for sleep apnea.

Auscultate the Lungs and Heart

Nighttime wheezing in patients with asthma often causes sleep disturbances. Congestive heart failure is a risk factor for sleep apnea.

Palpate the Abdomen

GERD may elicit upper abdominal pain on palpation.

LABORATORY AND DIAGNOSTIC STUDIES
Sleep Diary

A sleep diary should be kept for 1 to 2 weeks. Have the patient record bedtime, total sleep time, time until sleep onset, number of awakenings, use of sleep medications, time out of bed in the morning, a rating of quality of sleep, daytime symptoms, daytime naps, number and time of alcoholic drinks, and life stresses.

Sleep Studies

Objective assessment of sleep uses polysomnography (PSG) to assess sleep apnea, specific sleep stage abnormalities, nocturnal myoclonus, and unusual nocturnal behaviors. It is not recommended for routine evaluation of chronic insomnia. PSG includes an electroencephalogram (EEG), electro-oculogram (EOG), electromyelogram (EMG), electrocardiogram (ECG), measures of oxygen saturation, carbon dioxide values, nasal and oral airflow, thoracic and abdominal respiratory movements, and leg muscle activity. The PSG is taken during sleep, usually for the entire night. A multiple sleep latency test (MSLT) is a series of four or five nap opportunities, each separated by a 2-hour interval. The 15- to 20-minute naps are used to assess sleep disorders such as obstructive sleep apnea and narcolepsy.

Actigraphy

Actigraphy is a technique to record activity during waking and sleeping without application of any electrodes. An actigraph is worn on the wrist and is about the size of a watch. It records movement and nonmovement data plotted against time for 1 or 2 weeks. The patient wears the device continuously during sleep and daily routine activities. Actigraphy is suitable for extended examination of the sleep/wake cycle.

Ferritin Level

Serum iron stores (measured by serum ferritin) have been shown to correlate inversely with restless legs syndrome. Iron is a cofactor in tyrosine hydroxylase, the rate-limiting enzymatic step in the conversion of tyrosine to dopamine.

DIFFERENTIAL DIAGNOSIS
Restless Legs Syndrome

Restless legs syndrome includes the sensation of crawling, pulling, and tingling with an irresistible urge to move the legs. Symptoms increase in the evening, especially when the person is lying down and remaining still. The symptoms occur before sleep, causing a delay in sleep onset. Patients often have coexisting periodic limb movements in sleep. Renal failure with uremia or iron or folate deficiency sometimes underlies restless legs syndrome.

Periodic Leg Movement

Periodic leg movements during sleep are common in people older than 65 years. Bilateral repeated, rhythmic jerking or twitching movements, primarily in the legs, characterize periodic limb movement disorder. Less frequent movement can occur in the arms. The movements occur every 20 to 90 seconds and can cause brief arousal that disrupts sleep and decreases the amount of time in the deep stages of sleep. The patient may not report waking up but reports that sleep was not refreshing. The condition commonly coexists with restless legs syndrome.

Obstructive Sleep Apnea

Clinically, OSA is defined by the occurrence of daytime sleepiness, loud snoring, witnessed breathing interruptions, or awakenings due to gasping or choking, in the presence of at least five obstructive respiratory events (apneas, hypopneas, or respiratory effort–related arousals) per hour of sleep. Obstructive sleep apnea hypopnea syndrome (OSAHS) is characterized by daytime somnolence, snoring, difficult-to-control hypertension, refractory arrhythmias, angina, or heart failure.

During sleep, the normal tone of the airway muscles is relaxation, especially during REM sleep cycles. However, the diaphragm during this time is active. The activity of the diaphragm unchecked by the airway muscles leads to the collapse of the upper airway. Associated with this is any anatomical barrier, such as enlarged adenoids, with resulting obstruction. The signs, symptoms, and consequences of OSA occur as a result of repetitive collapse of the upper airway, sleep fragmentation, hypoxemia, hypercapnia, marked swings in intrathoracic pressure, and increased sympathetic activity.

Risk factors for sleep apnea include male sex and obesity (especially a heavy or thick neck). The condition may be associated with hypothyroidism, neurodegenerative disorders, and cardiovascular disorders. Generally in children, OSA is the result of enlarged tonsils and adenoids after age 6 weeks. Children ages 4 to 6 years are most prone to this condition. Most children presenting with OSA have failure to thrive and may also exhibit nocturnal enuresis, hyperactivity, learning problems, and morning headaches.

The patient may report insomnia but more commonly notes excessive daytime sleepiness. Hundreds of apneic episodes occur during the night. The frequent interruptions coupled with repeated drops in blood oxygen saturation may cause a marked decline in daytime alertness and performance. The patient should be evaluated in a sleep laboratory (see the Evidence-Based Practice box).

◎ **EVIDENCE-BASED PRACTICE** *Diagnosing Obstructive Sleep Apnea*

A recent review of the evidence indicates that questionnaires, physical examination, and clinical prediction rules estimate the pretest probability of obstructive sleep apnea hypopnea syndrome (OSAHS), but are not specific enough to make the diagnosis. The Epworth Sleepiness Scale is a reliable measure of daytime sleepiness. Physical examination offers clues—decreased visibility of the posterior pharynx when the patient opens his mouth and sticks out his tongue, truncal obesity, and a waist-to-hip ratio was >1 in men and >0.85 in women make the occurrence of OSA more likely but are not sufficient to make a diagnosis. The Institute for Clinical Systems Improvement recommends polysomnography for patients with symptoms of OSAHS and 1 or more of the following: cardiovascular disease, hypertension, coronary artery disease, obesity, sleep concern, type 2 diabetes mellitus, recurrent atrial fibrillation, and large neck circumference. Polysomnography is routinely recommended by the American Academy of Sleep Medicine for the diagnosis of sleep-related breathing disorders.

Data from Jacobs CK, Coffey J: Clinical inquiries. Sleep apnea in adults: how accurate is clinical prediction? *J Fam Pract* 58:327, 2009.

Narcolepsy

Narcolepsy is a disorder of excessive daytime sleepiness. It is characterized by sudden, irresistible attacks of daytime sleepiness that last 10 to 30 minutes. Most adults with narcolepsy also experience cataplexy, a sudden loss of muscle tone in response to sudden emotional stimuli. Although the episodes are typically brief, the person is at risk for falls or other accidents because he or she cannot move or speak. Cataplexy is not commonly seen in children. Persons with narcolepsy usually experience sleep paralysis once or twice a week at the time of sleep onset. There is a period of mental alertness, but the person is paralyzed except for respiratory and eye musculature. Hypnagogic (brief, vivid, dreamlike) hallucinations typically occur at sleep onset. Involuntary daytime sleep attacks may begin in adolescence or young adulthood. People with this problem may have symptoms for years before the disorder is diagnosed. Not all persons with the disorder experience all symptoms. Narcolepsy is fairly uncommon in children.

Delayed Sleep Phase Syndrome

This is an extreme shift in sleep-wake schedule seen in adolescents. The adolescent goes to bed but does not fall asleep for many hours, is then awakened to attend school, having had only a few hours of sleep. On the weekend, the adolescent, when allowed to sleep, will sleep at least eight hours.

Secondary to Medical Condition or Medications (Comorbid Insomnia)

GERD, COPD, peptic ulcer disease, and congestive heart failure are associated with paroxysmal nocturnal dyspnea. The sleep disturbance is often interpreted by the patient as insomnia. Prostatic hypertrophy may cause nocturia and thus disturb sleep.

Many medications can have stimulating effects and cause sleep disruption. Common offenders include antidepressants (activating selective serotonin reuptake inhibitors), decongestants, bronchodilators, β-blockers, thyroid preparations, phenytoin, methyldopa, and corticosteroids.

Pain may interfere with sleep onset or contribute to early awakenings. Patients with chronic pain may have mood and cognitive disturbances that contribute to insomnia and early morning awakening.

Psychological conditions that cause insomnia include depression, anxiety disorder, panic disorder, mania, and acute psychosis.

Poor Sleep Hygiene

Sleep hygiene is related to health practices and environmental influences on sleep. Bedtime routines, environmental distracters, and stimulants affect the ability to fall asleep. Lights and televisions produce awakening cues. Routinely using the bedroom for other activities may also condition the patient to an arousal state while in the bedroom. Noise may reduce the amount of REM sleep and lead to daytime sleepiness.

Caffeine, diet pills, and nicotine are stimulants that can cause sleep disruption. Alcohol consumed before bedtime tends to shorten total sleep time and exacerbate other conditions, such as GERD and sleep apnea.

A child who is put to bed still awake and learns to fall asleep using self-comforting measures is often able to calm himself or herself and return to sleep when he or she rouses in the middle of the night, as do most children and adults. Toddlers are fearful of separation, and bedtime routines need to be established.

Infants who sleep with parents may have sleep problems. As parents arise or move from the bed, the infant awakens because of the lighter sleep state.

The American Academy of Pediatrics recommends that all infants sleep on their backs for the first 6 months of life to decrease the risk of sudden infant death syndrome (SIDS). The sleep environment should be quiet and dark and the room temperature should be comfortable.

Lifestyle

Shift work, particularly periodic shift work, has been a reported cause of sleep disruption. It may interrupt the usual circadian rhythm or alter usual sleeping patterns and habits.

Sleeping in unfamiliar surroundings affects the quality of sleep and increases sleep latency. It is associated with more wakefulness, an increased amount of light sleep, and a shorter REM sleep stage.

Jet lag is a common cause of sleep disruption. It may interrupt the usual circadian rhythm or alter usual sleeping patterns and habits. Even 1 to 2 hours of time zone change can disrupt the usual sleep/wake pattern.

Age-Related Sleep Disorders
Night Awakening

Newborns wake every 20 minutes to 4 hours during a 24-hour period, reflecting their sleep/wake cycle. This cycle changes between 3 and 6 months with the establishment of a diurnal sleep/wake rhythm. During this time an initial "settling" period that typically takes 10 to 20 minutes begins to occur. The infant drifts from stage 1 NREM sleep into stage 3 or 4. The infant may return to stage 1 and cycle again. After one or two cycles of NREM sleep, REM is entered at about 60 to 90 minutes. The initial one third of the night is mostly deep sleep (NREM stages 3 and 4). The last half of the night is predominantly stage 2 NREM and REM. Daytime sleep decreases over the next 3 years and consolidates at night. At age 4, most children no longer nap. School-age children sleep approximately 8 hours a night. Stage 4 sleep decreases to 75 to 80 minutes. This decline is associated with an increase in stage 2 sleep. The onset of REM sleep decreases from about 140 minutes in the 6- to 7-year-old to 124 minutes in the 10- to 11-year-old.

Sleep Refusal

Toddlers are emerging from a sensory-motor period to a preoperational period. They have a strong attachment to their caregiver, and separation from this person at bedtime causes distress and sleep problems. Further, older toddlers who are in the preoperational stage are developing a sense of autonomy and use going to bed as an issue of control and/or a general pattern of oppositional behavior. Examination of the child's naptime is important. In the school-age child and adolescent, anxiety, negative conditioning, delayed sleep phase (often caused by caffeine), or a bedtime that is too early may be the cause. Also, vigorous activity before bedtime may delay sleep onset.

Night Terrors

Night terrors are nocturnal episodes in which the child sits straight up in bed, screams, and is inconsolable for up to 30 minutes before relaxing and falling back to sleep. These actions occur within the first few hours of sleep. Children at around the age of 3 years have NREM occurring more in the first part of the night; this may account for the night terror. The child is not readily awakened, although he or she seems to be awake. It is not possible to console the child, and the child has no recollection of the event the next day. Night terrors occur between the ages of 3 and 10 years.

Nightmares

Nightmares are bad dreams that awaken the dreamer. They occur later at night than night terrors and occur during REM sleep, which in children is near the end of the sleep cycle. Unlike night terrors, the dream is remembered and the child is awake and may be consoled by the caregiver. Nightmares occur at any age.

Adolescent Patterns

Adolescents have an increase in slow-wave sleep with an increase in the amount of sleep required. However, most adolescents are in a sleep debt because they tend to leave less time for sleep. Repeated changes in the sleep cycle (short sleep periods followed by occasional long sleep periods) may disrupt the circadian rhythm, causing a delayed sleep phase syndrome.

Menopausal Women

Menopause-related changes may contribute to or cause sleep disturbance. Evidence that sleep difficulties are related to the hormonal changes of menopause is mixed. Hot flashes and night sweats promote arousal from sleep.

Older Adult Patterns

Sleep in older adults is characterized by more nighttime awakenings and reduced or nonexistent deep states of NREM sleep. However, REM sleep tends to be preserved. That older adults sleep less than younger adults may reflect their ability to sleep, not their need to sleep. Although a mild deterioration in sleep quality may be normal in the aging process, significantly disrupted nighttime sleep or excessive daytime functioning is not considered part of normal aging. Older persons have a circadian rhythm disruption and tend to awaken earlier in the morning. If the onset of sleep is not correspondingly earlier, excessive daytime sleepiness may result. Daytime napping may reduce the drive for sleep at the usual bedtime hour. A night owl pattern is delayed bedtime until early morning hours, and the condition may progress to day-night reversal, where sleep does not begin until dawn and continues until midday.

Conditioned Insomnia
Trained Night Crier

Children who do not have self-comforting behaviors will be unable to fall asleep on their own. These criers awaken, cry, and want to be held or rocked before they can go back to sleep. An infant older than 6 months who continues to wake during the night is considered a trained night crier.

Trained Night Feeder

A child who needs to be fed when awakened at night is noted as a trained night feeder. The child does not need the additional nutrition but becomes conditioned to requiring a feeding to go to sleep. Caregivers often bottle-feed or breastfeed the child until the child falls back to sleep. The intake of nighttime feeding after 7 or 8 months of age may prevent the development of a more mature circadian rhythm. This rhythm is a digestive-endocrine-sleep/wake cycle that adjusts to a day/night cycle, resulting in a consolidation of sleep. Continued nocturnal feeding keeps the infant in a recurrent interruption pattern of frequent night awakening and prevents consolidation of sleep.

Somnambulism

Sleepwalking occurs during NREM stages 3 and 4, which occur in the initial one third of the night. Sleepwalking usually occurs only once a night and lasts about 15 minutes. The person gets out of bed and moves about slowly and in an automatic manner with a blank look on the face. Sometimes the person is mumbling; after a great deal of effort, the person can be awakened but will have little to no memory of the episode. Providing a safe environment is important because genuine risk of injury exists during the sleepwalking episode. Sleepwalking in an elderly person may be a sign of dementia.

DIFFERENTIAL DIAGNOSIS OF *Common Causes of Sleep Disorders*

CONDITION	HISTORY	PHYSICAL FINDINGS	DIAGNOSTIC STUDIES
Specific Disorders			
Restless legs syndrome	Irresistible urge to move legs while in bed	Normal	Sleep studies; serum ferritin
Periodic limb movement	Older than 65 years; reports of rhythmic jerking of legs or arms while asleep	Normal	Sleep studies
Obstructive sleep apnea	Apneic episodes, loud snoring, restless sleep patterns	Decreased O_2; enlarged adenoids, tonsils	Sleep studies: polysomnography
Narcolepsy	Excessive sleepiness, cataplexy	Normal	Referral to sleep specialist
Delayed sleep phase syndrome	Adolescent with extreme shift in sleep awake cycle; unable to fall asleep for many hours	Normal	Referral to sleep specialist
Secondary to medical condition or medications	GERD, COPD, PND, CHF, enlarged prostate/nocturia; depression or anxiety Medications: antidepressants, decongestants, bronchodilators, β-blockers, thyroid preparations, phenytoin, methyldopa, corticosteroids	Consistent with medical condition	Consistent with underlying medical condition; trial off or change of medication(s)
Poor sleep hygiene	Routine, habits, environment not conducive to sleep; use of alcohol, caffeine, diet pills, nicotine	Normal	Sleep diary
Lifestyle	Shift work, travel, jet lag	Normal	Sleep diary
Age-Related Sleep Disorders			
Night awakening	Single to repeated awakening at night	Initial physical examination to eliminate medical associated illness	As directed by examination
Sleep refusal	Refusal of child to go to sleep	Normal	None
Night terrors	Inconsolable awakening occurring early in sleep, lasting 15 minutes, no memory of event	Normal	None

DIFFERENTIAL DIAGNOSIS OF *Common Causes of Sleep Disorders—cont'd*

CONDITION	HISTORY	PHYSICAL FINDINGS	DIAGNOSTIC STUDIES
Nightmares	Occur later in sleep cycle; dream is remembered	Normal	None
Adolescent patterns	Decrease in amount of sleep obtained	Normal	Sleep diary
Menopausal women	Hot flashes	Consistent with menopause	Sleep diary
Older adult patterns	Nighttime arousals and awakenings; night owl pattern; early wakening; daytime napping	Physical examination to rule out underlying medical condition	Sleep diary
Conditioned insomnia	Identify initial trigger with persistent problem	Physical examination to rule out underlying medical condition	Sleep diary
Trained night crier	Child unable to soothe self	Normal	None
Trained night feeder	History of frequent feedings on awakening at night	Normal	None
Somnambulism	Sleepwalking in early sleep cycle	Normal	None

CHF, congestive heart failure; *COPD,* chronic obstructive pulmonary disease; *GERD,* gastroesophageal reflux disease; *PND,* paroxysmal nocturnal dyspnea.

REFERENCES AND READINGS

Anders T, Eiben L: Pediatric sleep disorders: a review of the past 10 years, *J Am Acad Child Adolesc Psychiatry* 36:9, 1997.

Bayard M, Avonda T, Wadzinski J: Restless legs syndrome, *Am Fam Physician* 78:235, 2008.

Bower CM: Pediatric obstructive sleep apnea syndrome, *Otolaryngol Clin North Am* 33:49, 2000.

Budur K, Rodriguez C, Foldvary-Schaefer N: Advances in treating insomnia, *Cleve Clin J Med* 74:251, 2007.

Capp P, Pearl P, Lewin D: Pediatric sleep disorders, *Prim Care Clin Office Pract* 32:549, 2005.

Culpepper L: Insomnia: a primary care perspective, *J Clin Psychiatry* 66:14, 2005.

Davis KF, Parker KP, Montgomery GL: Sleep in infants and young children: part two: common sleep problems, *J Pediatr Health Care* 18:130, 2004.

Doghramji K, Neubauer DN: Insomnia: waking up to a significant problem, *Consultant* 45:53, 2005.

Epstein LJ, Kristo D, Strollo PJ Jr, Friedman N, Malhotra A, Patil SP et al: Clinical guideline for the evaluation, management and long-term care of obstructive sleep apnea in adults, *J Clin Sleep Med* 5:263, 2009.

Hoban TF: Sleep and its disorders in childhood, *Semin Neurol* 24:327, 2004.

Kass, L: Sleep problems, *Pediatr Rev* 27:455, 2006.

Jacobs CK, Coffey J: Clinical inquiries. Sleep apnea in adults: how accurate is clinical prediction? *J Fam Pract* 58:327, 2009.

Morgenthaler T, Alessi C, Friedman L, Owens J, Kapur V, Boehlecke B et al: Practice parameters for the use of actigraphy in the assessment of sleep and sleep disorders: an update for 2007, *Sleep* 30:519, 2007. Available online at www.guideline. gov. Accessed May 30, 2010.

Schutte-Rodin S, Broch L, Buysse D, Dorsey C, Sateia M: Clinical guideline for the evaluation and management of chronic insomnia in adults, *J Clin Sleep Med* 4:487, 2008.

Shaver JL, Zenk SN: Sleep disturbance in menopause, *J Womens Health Gend Based Med* 9:109, 2000.

Thiedlke C: Sleep disorders and sleep problems in childhood, *Am Fam Physician* 63:277, 2001.

Wolkove N, Elkholy O, Baltzan M, Palayew M: Sleep and aging: 1. Sleep disorders commonly found in older people, *CMAJ* 176:1299 2007.

Zunkel GM: Insomnia: overview of assessment and treatment strategies, *Clin Rev* 15:38, 2005.

Sore Throat

Sore throat, or pharyngitis, is one of the most common concerns of patients in primary care. It is most often a transient condition of viral origin. Throat pain is the result of an inflammation of the mucosa of the oropharynx, secondary to an infectious cause (e.g., viral, bacterial, fungal, or spirochetal). Less commonly, sore throat may be a symptom of systemic illness, such as mononucleosis. The posterior pharynx is also vulnerable to irritants from the environment and drainage from the nose and sinuses. Thus pharyngitis begins as an inflammation of the mucous membranes with secondary involvement of the lymph node drainage system, rarely progressing to deep neck and mediastinal involvement. Throat pain can also be referred from other structures, most commonly the ears and thyroid gland.

Sore throats can be classified as those with pharyngeal ulcers and those without. The classification serves as a device to sort out those relatively few sore throats caused by specific viral or fungal infections that produce pharyngeal ulcers and those caused by agents and processes characterized by an absence of pharyngeal ulcers.

The goals of assessment and diagnosis are to identify those patients with group A ß-hemolytic streptococcus (GABHS) infection (because they are at risk for rheumatic fever and glomerulonephritis), to reduce the possibility of sequelae of peritonsillar and retropharyngeal abscess, and to identify epiglottitis.

DIAGNOSTIC REASONING: FOCUSED HISTORY

Is this an emergency?

Key Questions

- Have you been drooling?
- Have you been unable to swallow?
- Have you been unable to lie down?
- Have you been restless, unable to stay still?
- Have you been unable to talk?

History

The previous complaints signal acute epiglottitis. The history is usually elicited from another individual because the ill person either is a child or is too ill to talk. Acute epiglottitis is rare, with an incidence of 10:100,000 in pediatric patients younger than 15 years and 1 to 8:100,000 adult patients. The morbidity and mortality that result from airway obstruction, however, are significant.

Associated Symptoms

Symptoms of epiglottitis are sore throat, difficulty swallowing, and respiratory distress. These are characterized by drooling, dyspnea, and inspiratory stridor. *Haemophilus influenzae* type b is the most common pathogen. The incidence of *H. influenzae* type b epiglottitis is highest in children ages 2 to 5 years. Epiglottitis is a rapidly progressive illness with a potentially fatal outcome and must be recognized and referred immediately.

Peritonsillar abscess is also an acute infection that needs to be identified immediately for referral and treatment. The symptoms of peritonsillar abscess and cellulitis include a severe sore throat, odynophagia, trismus (spasm of the masticatory muscles and difficulty opening the mouth), and medial deviation of the soft palate and peritonsillar fold. These symptoms are caused by infection penetrating the tonsillar capsule and surrounding tissues. About 30% of patients with peritonsillar abscess require an emergency tonsillectomy.

Is the sore throat related to an infectious cause?

Key Questions

- Is anyone else at home sick?
- Are any of your friends or co-workers sick?
- When did the pain start?
- How severe is the pain?

Exposure

Exposure to other ill individuals increases the likelihood of viral or bacterial infection. Respiratory illness caused by GABHS is spread within families, with approximately 20% of family members becoming infected. Epstein-Barr virus (EBV) is not highly contagious and requires intimate contact between susceptible individuals and symptomatic shedders of the virus. Transmission is primarily through saliva.

Onset

The sudden onset of sore throat is often caused by GABHS. The organisms invade the pharyngeal epithelium, where they multiply and cause an intense immune response. Gradual onset is more common in infectious mononucleosis. The EBV infects B lymphocytes of the pharynx with resultant dissemination throughout the lymphoreticular system, causing an immune response that is more gradual in onset

In viral pharyngitis, a sore throat begins a day or two after the onset of other illness symptoms, reaching its peak by the second or third day.

Noninfectious causes of sore throat typically have an insidious onset. The patient often is not able to pinpoint when the sore throat started but notes that it has been persistent.

Severity

Throat pain associated with streptococcal infection is usually intense. Throat pain associated with influenza and adenovirus is severe, with prominent edema of the throat. Severe throat pain with trismus and refusal to speak indicates severe peritonsillitis, which may lead to peritonsillar abscess formation (quinsy). The throat pain produced by noninfectious causes tends to be less severe and may be described as "scratchy" or "annoying."

Young children may not be able to express the sensation of a sore throat or the severity of it. Instead, they may refuse to eat or drink. Pain in the younger child, if present, more commonly indicates the presence of epiglottitis or laryngitis, abscess, diphtheria, or scarlatina.

What does the presence of fever tell me?

Key Questions
- Have you had a fever?
- When did it start?
- How high has it been?

Patterns of Fever

Fever is almost always present with GABHS and is the most commonly occurring symptom in children. The fever is of sudden onset and the temperature rises above 38.5° C (101.5° F), with malaise, headache, and painful swallowing. Fever is also present in children and adults with epiglottitis.

Influenza is characterized by the abrupt onset of fever, with temperatures ranging from 37.8° C to 40° C (100° F to 104° F). Adenoviral infection in children typically presents with a temperature greater than 40° C (104° F). Patients with EBV have a low-grade fever.

Fever, followed by an interval of several days without fever and then recurrent fever, or a continuing fever for several days may indicate peritonsillar abscess.

The absence of fever suggests a noninfectious cause. Patients with candidiasis and aphthous stomatitis may also present without a fever.

What does the presence of upper respiratory tract symptoms tell me?

Key Questions
- Do you have a cough?
- Have you had a runny nose? If so, what color is the drainage?
- Do you have postnasal drip?
- Do you have eye redness or discomfort?
- Have your eyes been itchy or watery?
- Have you been hoarse?
- Have you been sneezing?

Cough and Rhinorrhea

Cough, rhinitis, conjunctivitis, and hoarseness rarely occur with streptococcal pharyngitis, and the presence of two or more of these signs or symptoms suggests a viral infection.

Influenza is often associated with several days of fever, cough, and rhinorrhea. Viral pharyngitis is characterized by a sore, scratchy throat, nasal congestion, rhinorrhea, and cough.

Clear nasal discharge is common in allergic pharyngitis and may produce postnasal drip that causes a sore throat.

Conjunctivitis

Conjunctivitis rarely occurs with streptococcal pharyngitis. Mild conjunctivitis is common with viral infection. Watery or itchy eyes are associated with exposure to allergens.

Sneezing

Sneezing is common with both viral infection and allergen exposure. The sneezing associated with allergic pharyngitis is more persistent and is often seasonal.

Hoarseness

Hoarseness is not uncommon in allergy-associated sore throat and may be present with viral infection as well. Inflammation produces laryngeal edema that results in hoarseness. Hoarseness is not typically associated with GABHS infection.

What do the associated symptoms tell me?

Key Questions

■ Do you have muscle aches?
■ Have you had nausea, vomiting, or diarrhea?

Systemic Complaints

Systemic complaints, such as myalgia, are common in influenza and GABHS infection. Streptococcal pharyngitis or influenza in children older than 2 years is associated with reports of headache, abdominal pain, and vomiting.

Influenza is often associated with several days of fever and systemic symptoms, such as myalgias, cough, and rhinorrhea. Common cold viruses associated with pharyngitis produce systemic symptoms, such as myalgia.

Does the presence of risk factors help me narrow the cause?

Key Questions

■ How old are you?
■ What is your smoking history?
■ What kind of work do you do?
■ Do you engage in oral sex?
■ Are you taking medications?
■ Do you have any chronic health problems?
■ Are your immunizations up to date?

Age

Group A streptococcal infection is primarily a disease in children 5 to 15 years of age. GABHS is rare in children younger than 3 years. Influenza affects all ages, whereas parainfluenza and respiratory syncytial viruses primarily affect children.

Adenoviruses, the major viral agents isolated in exudative pharyngitis in younger children, are endemic. In military populations, adenovirus type 4 and, to a lesser extent, types 3, 7, and 21 are the most common causes of pharyngitis.

Adolescents and young adults are more likely to have a sore throat associated with mononucleosis caused by EBV. Mononucleosis occurs in older adults but often without pharyngitis, adenopathy, or splenomegaly.

Irritant Exposures

Agents such as tobacco smoke, smog, dust, and allergens can irritate the throat. These agents cause mucosal irritation and set up the inflammatory process. People who work outdoors may have greater exposure to environmental allergens. Housekeepers have an increased risk of exposure to dust mites and chemical irritants.

Sexual Behavior

Pharyngitis from *Chlamydia trachomatis* or *Neisseria gonorrhoeae* is more prevalent in persons with a history of orogenital sexual activity. Gonococcal pharyngitis is present in about 10% of patients with anogenital gonorrhea.

Medications and Chronic Health Problems

Immunosuppression increases susceptibility to viral agents that produce pharyngeal ulcers (e.g., herpangina, herpes simplex). Persons with diabetes and those taking broad-spectrum antibiotics are more susceptible to candidiasis. Persons with a history of gastroesophageal reflux disease (GERD) may have a sore throat secondary to reflux of gastric contents.

Immunizations

Infants receive the DTaP and Hib vaccines as part of routine immunization. DTaP prevents diphtheria, tetanus, and pertussis. Hib prevents *Haemophilus influenzae* type b responsible for epiglottitis in children. Adults are advised to have a booster dose of Td every 10 years. Unimmunized children and adults are at higher risk for infection.

DIAGNOSTIC REASONING: FOCUSED PHYSICAL EXAMINATION

Assess Severity of Illness

Assessment of the patient begins with general observation about the severity of illness. Severe illness, with signs of upper airway obstruction, such as restlessness, stridor, difficulty breathing, drooling, inability to swallow, and high fever, signals epiglottitis and requires immediate referral. Further examination could trigger laryngospasms and lead to airway obstruction.

Inspect the Mouth

Examine the buccal mucosa, tongue, and sublingual area for the presence of ulcers. Note the location, number, size, and appearance of any lesions.

The lesions produced by the group A coxsackievirus (herpangina) first appear as small, grayish, papulovesicular lesions on the soft palate and pharynx. These progress to shallow ulcers, usually less than 5 mm in diameter.

Vincent angina (necrotizing ulcerative gingivostomatitis) is a fusospirochetal infection of the gingiva. The gingiva appears inflamed and ulcerated, often covered with a gray slough. As the infection spreads, ulcers may appear on the oral mucosa and posterior pharynx.

Aphthous stomatitis lesions affect about 20% of the general population and are associated with immunological mechanisms. They occur most often on the buccal mucosa, tongue, and soft palate. The lesions first appear as indurated papules and then progress to shallow ulcers. The ulcers have a yellow membrane and red halo. Herpes simplex lesions involve the anterior oral mucosa and the gums. Herpetic pharyngitis is manifested by vesicles, ulcers, or exudate of the oral and pharyngeal mucosa. Specifically, the lesions involve the tonsils, pharynx, uvula, and edges of the soft palate. Vesicular lesions may or may not be intact.

Streptococcal infection in children may cause enlarged papillae on the tongue, which gives the tongue a strawberry appearance.

Inspect the Posterior Pharynx and Observe Swallowing

Examine for edema, color, and exudate of the posterior pharynx, and determine the presence, size (Table 29-1), and condition of the palatine tonsils. Good visualization is critical for accurate diagnosis. Use a good light source, and ask the patient to open wide and say "ah" but not to protrude the tongue. If you cannot view the pharynx, depress the tongue firmly with a tongue blade, far enough back to have a good view but not enough to cause the patient to gag. Use two tongue depressors to retract tissues medially and laterally when examining such areas as the retromolar region, the floor of the

Table 29-1	Grading Tonsillar Size

GRADE	TONSIL LOCATION
1	Behind pillars
2	Between pillars and uvula
3	Touching uvula
4	Extending beyond midline of oropharynx

mouth, and the orifices of Wharton and Stensen ducts (Figure 29-1). The best visualization is achieved with a headlight.

Drooling may indicate peritonsillar abscess or epiglottitis partially occluding the pharynx and esophagus. Only occasionally can the red, swollen epiglottis be visualized above the base of the tongue. If you suspect epiglottitis, do not examine the pharynx because manipulation may precipitate laryngospasms and airway obstruction. Refer the patient immediately for specialist evaluation and further diagnosis, which may involve soft tissue radiography of the head and neck and laryngoscopy.

Edema of the affected tonsil, with movement of the tonsil toward midline, indicates peritonsillar abscess. Diphtheria may appear as a thick, gray tonsillar exudate or pseudomembrane, spreading to the tonsillar pillars, uvula, soft palate, posterior pharyngeal wall, and larynx. The exudate is not easily removable and bleeds easily.

Pharyngeal or tonsillar exudate can be present with either a bacterial or a viral infection. A yellowish exudate of GABHS pharyngitis is often present. Generally the exudate of viral agents tends to be whiter than that from GABHS.

A bright red uvula and the presence of petechiae on the posterior pharynx and palate indicate group A streptococcal pharyngitis. "Doughnut lesions" or red, raised hemorrhagic lesions with a yellow center, are diagnostic of streptococcal pharyngitis.

Postnasal drainage can irritate the posterior pharynx and should be observed for color. Purulent drainage that is yellow or greenish is associated with infectious sinusitis. White curdlike patches that bleed on scraping are characteristic of oral candidiasis.

When examination reveals normal findings, suspect a systemic referred cause for the sore throat, particularly acute otitis media, sinusitis, or thyroiditis.

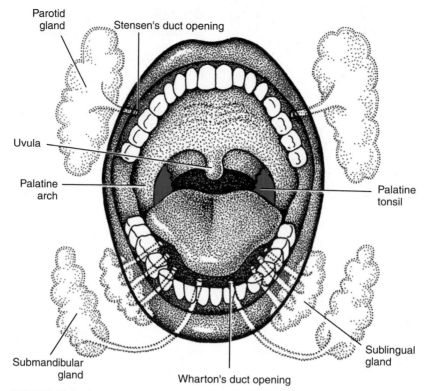

FIGURE 29-1   Anatomical structures of the mouth. (From Barkauskas VH, Baumann LC, Darling-Fisher CS: *Health and physical assessment,* ed 3, St Louis, 2002, Mosby.)

Palpate the Cervicofacial Lymph Nodes
In streptococcal pharyngitis, the anterior cervical lymph nodes are often enlarged and tender. In viral infections, the posterior cervical nodes are more often enlarged. Lymphadenopathy is a cardinal sign of infectious mononucleosis, with more than 90% of patients having enlarged posterior cervical nodes.

Inspect the Nasal Mucosa
Red, swollen turbinates indicate an infectious process, whereas pale, boggy turbinates indicate an allergic process. The presence of mucoid discharge occurs in allergic rhinitis. Purulent discharge suggests infectious sinusitis.

Inspect the Conjunctivae
Injected conjunctivae associated with a sore throat may indicate pharyngoconjunctival fever. It is caused by an adenovirus and is often associated with nonpurulent discharge, fever, and pharyngitis. It frequently occurs in epidemics. Mild conjunctivitis in the presence of

itching eyes and clear watery discharge is associated with an allergic process.

Inspect the Tympanic Membrane
Evidence of otitis media with effusion may indicate nontypical *H. influenzae* acute otitis media (conjunctivitis-otitis syndrome). Earache can be caused by referred pain, especially from the tonsils.

Palpate the Thyroid
Acute thyroiditis is associated with a sore throat in the presence of a normal throat examination but with an enlarged or tender thyroid gland.

Inspect the Skin
Evidence of a fine maculopapular erythema that has a generalized distribution with accentuation in the skinfolds, circumoral pallor, and sparing of the palms and soles indicates scarlet fever. The rash characteristically is followed by a fine desquamation, starting at the hands.

Auscultate the Lungs

Mycoplasma pneumoniae is frequently associated with sore throat in adolescents and young adults. If pneumonia is present, palpation, percussion, and auscultation of the lungs reveal an area of consolidation and adventitious breath sounds (see Chapter 13 for further discussion of the lung examination).

Palpate the Abdomen

Splenomegaly is found in about half the cases of mononucleosis, although hepatomegaly is rare. GERD may be associated with palpable upper epigastric tenderness.

LABORATORY AND DIAGNOSTIC STUDIES

The laboratory evaluation of sore throat is generally limited to the identification of GABHS. Other infectious causes, such as gonorrhea or diphtheria, are rare, and testing is conducted only if the history indicates exposure. It is important to diagnose streptococcal pharyngitis so it can be treated promptly with antibiotics, avoiding serious sequelae, such as peritonsillar abscesses or rheumatic fever.

Rapid Screening Tests

A throat swab is a rapid screen for streptococcal antigens and should be done if GABHS is suspected. If it is positive, the patient is treated without follow-up cultures. If the swab is negative, a throat culture is obtained. The test has a sensitivity of 75% to 85% and a specificity of 95% to 98%.

The Monospot is a rapid slide test that detects heterophil antibody agglutination; it is not specific for EBV. It is most sensitive 1 to 2 weeks after symptoms appear and remains positive for up to 1 year. If chronic fatigue syndrome is being considered as a differential diagnosis, specific EBV antibody tests should be considered.

Culture

A throat culture to detect GABHS is the gold standard of diagnosis, with a 10% or lower false-negative rate. When obtaining a culture, first remove crusts from lesions, taking care to touch only the throat or tonsils with the sterile swab. Avoid touching the tongue. Roll the throat swab over one tonsil, proceed across the posterior pharynx, and then swab the other tonsil. A culture for gonorrhea can confirm a diagnosis of gonococcal pharyngitis.

Antistreptolysin O Titer

GABHS produces enzymes that include streptolysin. An ASO titer is a serological test that detects the presence of a previous streptococcal infection. This titer does not increase until 1 to 6 months postinfection, so it is of no diagnostic value. It is used to aid in the diagnosis of streptococci-associated infections, such as rheumatic fever, glomerulonephritis, and pericarditis. A caution, however, is that in as many as 50% of positive streptococcal cultures, an elevated ASO titer postinfection will not be found.

Potassium Hydroxide Smear for Wet Mount

Obtain a sample of pharyngeal discharge using a cotton-tipped applicator. Look under the microscope at the KOH slide for the presence of branching and budding hyphae that are characteristic of yeast infection (see Chapter 34).

Complete Blood Count with Differential

Test results that show 50% lymphocytes and at least 10% atypical lymphocytes confirm the diagnosis of mononucleosis.

Computed Tomography Scan

Suspicion of an obstruction or swelling of the throat should be referred for further radiographic evaluation with a computed tomography scan.

Nasal Smear

Nasal cytology can be performed on nasal secretions obtained by having the patient blow the nose into a paper or by using a cotton-tipped swab to obtain secretions from the nose. The presence of eosinophils on a nasal smear stained with Wright's stain viewed under a high-power microscope suggests an allergic, inflammatory process.

DIFFERENTIAL DIAGNOSIS
Pharyngitis Without Ulcers

Epiglottitis

Epiglottitis is caused by infection with *H. influenzae* type b that produces inflammation and edema of the epiglottis and the surrounding areas, obstructing the flow of air. The edematous epiglottis may be pulled into the larynx during inspiration and can completely occlude the airway. Symptoms are respiratory distress, sore throat, difficulty with secretions, drooling, pain on swallowing, and a toxic appearance. The infection occurs in both children and adults.

Peritonsillar/Retropharyngeal Abscess

A peritonsillar abscess, also called quinsy, is a collection of pus between the tonsil and the capsule of the tonsillar pillar. This condition occurs in children but is more common in adults, especially in persons with a history of recurrent tonsillitis. The patient's presenting symptoms usually include a history of respiratory symptoms, difficulty swallowing, otalgia, malaise, fever, and cervical lymphadenopathy. On examination, there may be trismus; asymmetrical swelling of the uvula, tonsils, or posterior pharynx; or a visible abscess. Children's presenting symptoms typically include fever, toxic appearance, refusal to swallow, drooling, and stridor. Children with retropharyngeal abscess are usually under the age of 4 and need immediate referral.

Viral Pharyngitis

Most sore throats are caused by viral infections. Patients usually have symptoms of malaise, fever, headache, cough, and fatigue. The pharynx is usually erythematous, or it may be pale, boggy, and swollen. There usually is no tonsillar or pharyngeal exudate or tonsillar enlargement present, although infection with an adenovirus may produce pharyngeal exudate. The presence of concomitant upper respiratory tract symptoms such as cough and congestion makes the diagnosis of viral pharyngitis more likely than that of streptococcal pharyngitis. Common cold viruses cause sore throats most frequently during the colder months of the year.

Streptococcal Pharyngitis

The major differential diagnoses for sore throat will be viral or bacterial infection. Fewer than 10% of adults and 30% of children who seek care for sore throat symptoms have streptococcal tonsillopharyngitis. However, reliance on clinical impression to arrive at a specific diagnosis is problematic. The symptoms most likely to occur with streptococcal pharyngitis include a fever with a temperature of 38.5° C (101.5° F) or higher, tonsillar exudate, anterior cervical adenopathy, and a history of recent exposure. The incidence of streptococcal pharyngitis increases from 10% in the summer and fall to 40% during the winter and early spring. GABHS cannot be reliably diagnosed on the basis of signs and symptoms, and even when cultures are obtained, a causative agent may not be identified in 50% of patients. Table 29-2 shows the groups at risk for GABHS.

Mononucleosis

Mononucleosis causes about 5% of sore throats. It is most often a disease of young adults, and the causative agent is EBV in more than 90% of cases. History reveals a gradual onset, low-grade fever; mild sore throat; posterior cervical lymphadenopathy; and pronounced malaise and fatigue. Diagnosis can be confirmed with a positive Monospot test and a complete

Table 29-2	Groups at Risk for Group A ß-Hemolytic Streptococcus (GABHS) Pharyngitis

RISK FACTORS	DIAGNOSTIC TESTS
High Risk Tonsillar exudate Temperature >38.5° C (101.5° F) Cervical lymphadenopathy Existing valvular rheumatic heart disease	None; treat on basis of risk factors
Presumed Strep Scarlet fever Strep epidemic Antibiotics already started	None; treat
Medium Risk Exudate, nodes, or fever present Prior rheumatic fever "Low risk" by PE but <25 years old and no URI Person with diabetes Recent "strep" exposure	Rapid strep screen; if positive, treat; if negative, do culture; treat if culture positive; do not treat if culture negative
Low Risk No exudate, nodes, or fever	Rapid strep screen; if positive, treat; if negative, do not culture; do not treat if culture negative

PE, physical examination; *URI,* upper respiratory tract infection.

blood count that shows greater than 50% lymphocytosis. Splenomegaly occurs in about 50% of cases, and palatine petechiae are a less common symptom. GABHS occurs concomitantly in 10% to 20% of cases.

Gonococcal Pharyngitis

This form of pharyngitis can occur in patients with a history of orogenital sexual activity. The patient may have no symptoms. Examination shows an exudative pharyngitis with bilateral cervical lymphadenopathy. Diagnosis is confirmed through Gram staining or culture.

Inflammation

Inflammatory sore throat occurs in the presence of sinusitis or exposure to local irritants. The patient often reports a postnasal drip and allergic symptoms (itchy, watery eyes; runny nose) that may follow seasonal patterns. On examination, the patient may have sinus tenderness. The pharynx may be swollen or pale with posterior drainage present. The patient has no fever or lymphadenopathy.

Pharyngitis with Ulcers
Herpangina

Herpangina is an infection caused by the coxsackievirus. The patient reports a painful sore throat, fever, and malaise. Headache; anorexia; and neck, abdomen, and extremity pain may occur. Within 2 days of onset, small, grayish, papulovesicular lesions appear on the soft palate and pharynx. These progress to shallow ulcers, usually less than 5 mm in diameter. Outbreaks occur during the summer months. Coxsackievirus peaks in August, September, and October, although some cases occur during the winter months. It is more common in children and in immunosuppressed patients. Diagnosis is based on symptoms and characteristic oral lesions. An antibody titer can confirm diagnosis.

Vincent Angina

Vincent angina is caused by a fusospirochetal infection that results in necrotizing ulcerative gingivostomatitis. The patient's symptoms include painful ulcers, foul breath, and bleeding gums. Without secondary infection, there usually is no fever. On examination, gray, necrotic ulcers without vesicles are apparent on the gingivae and interdental papillae. Gram staining shows spirochetes and confirms the diagnosis.

Aphthous Stomatitis

Aphthous stomatitis, or "canker sores," appears as discrete ulcers without preceding vesicles. The ulcers are located on the inner lip, tongue, and buccal mucosa. Lesions last about 1 to 2 weeks. The cause of the lesions is unknown, but immunological mechanisms play a major role.

Herpes Simplex Virus Type 1

An infection from herpes simplex virus type 1 (HSV-1) is associated with fever, headache, sore throat, and lymphadenitis. Characteristic clusters of yellow vesicles appear on the palate, pharynx, and gingiva. Lesions last 2 to 3 weeks. Recurrent lesions are characterized by prodromal symptoms of burning, tingling, or itching. Active lesions are usually painful. Recent studies indicate that infections afflict about 30% to 90% of the U.S. population.

Candidiasis

Candidiasis is a yeast infection that produces white plaques over the tongue and oral mucosa with erythema; the plaques bleed when scraped. *Candida* infection occurs commonly in otherwise normal infants in the first weeks of life; in immunocompromised persons, including those with diabetes; and in persons taking antibiotics or using inhaled steroids.

DIFFERENTIAL DIAGNOSIS OF *Common Causes of Sore Throat*

CONDITION	HISTORY	PHYSICAL FINDINGS	DIAGNOSTIC STUDIES
Pharyngitis Without Ulcers			
Epiglottitis	Sore throat, difficulty with secretions, odynophagia (seen in pediatric patients <2 years), unable to lie flat, unable to talk	Respiratory distress, drooling, toxic appearance; DO NOT EXAMINE PHARYNX	Refer immediately
Peritonsillar/ retropharyngeal abscess	History of recurrent tonsillitis; sore throat, difficulty swallowing, respiratory tract symptoms, fever, malaise	Orthopnea, dyspnea, symmetrical swelling, abscess, trismus	Refer immediately: CT scan; head and neck radiographs; laryngoscopy
Viral pharyngitis	Scratchy, sore throat, malaise, myalgias, headache, chills, cough, rhinitis	Erythema, edema of throat, tender posterior cervical nodes	None
Group A ß-hemolytic streptococcal pharyngitis	Most common in persons 5-15 years; known exposure; fall/winter season; sudden onset of fever, severe sore throat, and malaise; absence of cough and upper respiratory tract symptoms	Temperature >38.5° C (101.5° F); exudate; anterior cervical lymphadenopathy	Positive rapid strep antibody screen; strep culture
Mononucleosis (Epstein-Barr virus)	Young adults; slow onset of malaise, low-grade fever, mild sore throat	Presence/absence of pharyngeal exudate, palatine petechiae, posterior cervical lymphadenopathy, splenomegaly	Positive Monospot; CBC with differential; >50% leukocytes
Gonococcal pharyngitis	History of orogenital sexual activity; may be asymptomatic	Pharyngeal exudate; bilateral cervical lymphadenopathy	Gram stain; gonorrhea culture
Inflammation	Exposure to irritants; postnasal drip; allergic symptoms	Sinus tenderness, pale or swollen pharynx, postnasal drainage visible, no fever or lymphadenopathy	Eosinophils in nasal secretions with allergies
Pharyngitis with Ulcers			
Herpangina (coxsackievirus)	More common in children; immunosuppressed; painful throat; fever, malaise	Lymphadenopathy; small grayish papulovesicular lesions on soft palate and pharynx, progressing to shallow ulcers, usually <5 mm in diameter	Serology
Fusospirochetal infection (Vincent angina)	Poor oral hygiene; painful ulcers, foul breath, bleeding gums	Gray necrotic ulcers without vesicles on gingival margins and interdental papillae	Gram stain reveals spirochetes
Aphthous stomatitis	Oral trauma, ill-fitting dentures; painful ulcers vary in size; absence of other symptoms	Shallow ulcers, no vesicles; indurated papules that progress to 1-cm ulcers; ulcer has yellow membrane and red halo; no fever or nodes	None

DIFFERENTIAL DIAGNOSIS OF *Common Causes of Sore Throat—cont'd*

CONDITION	HISTORY	PHYSICAL FINDINGS	DIAGNOSTIC STUDIES
Herpes simplex infection	History of trauma to mucosa; pain, fever, headache	Perioral lesions; lymphadenitis; vesicles on palate, pharynx, gingiva	Viral culture
Candidiasis	Immunosuppressed; persons taking antibiotics or with diabetes; sore mouth/throat	Curdlike white plaques that bleed when scraped off	KOH smear shows hyphae; culture

CBC, complete blood count; *CT,* computed tomography; *KOH,* potassium hydroxide.

REFERENCES AND READINGS

Coby BA: Diagnosis and treatment of streptococcal pharyngitis, *Am Fam Physician* 79:383, 2009.

Darrow DH, Siemens C: Indications for tonsillectomy and adenoidectomy, *Laryngoscope* 112:8, 2002.

Ebell MH, Smith MA, Barry HC, Ives K, Carey M: The rational clinical examination: does this patient have strep throat? *JAMA* 284:2912, 2000.

Gerber M: Diagnosis and treatment of pharyngitis in children, *Pediatr Clin North Am* 52:729, 2005.

Linder JA: Evaluation and management of adult pharyngitis, *Compr Ther* 34:196, 2008.

McPhee SJ, Papadakis MA: Current medical diagnosis and treatment, ed 49, New York, 2010, McGraw-Hill.

Richardson MA: Sore throat, tonsillitis, and adenoiditis, *Med Clin North Am* 83:75, 1999.

Stevens D: A sore throat or something else? *Pract Nurs* 19:83, 2008.

Vincent MT, Celstin N, Hussain AN: Pharyngitis, *Am Fam Physician* 69:1465, 2004.

30

Syncope

S yncope is the transient loss of consciousness and postural tone that results from a sudden decrease in cerebral perfusion. It is distinct from a coma, seizures, shock, vertigo, and other states of altered consciousness. It is a symptom that about 10% of adults of any age will experience at least some time during their lives and the incidence exponentially increases in people over 70 years old. It is less common in children, except when there is a seizure disorder, primary cardiac arrhythmia, or a breath-holding incident.

The causes of syncope can be difficult to determine because patients generally are seen after the event has occurred. Syncope can be quite benign, such as a vasovagal response, or it can indicate serious disease. However, even benign syncope can place the patient at risk for falls or injury. Cardiogenic syncope has high associated morbidity and mortality, and the emphasis in diagnosis is to rule out the most serious causes through a careful history and physical examination, with a few laboratory and diagnostic tests to establish a possible diagnosis. The Evidence-Based Practice box describes an evidence-based approach to the diagnosis of syncope.

DIAGNOSTIC REASONING: FOCUSED HISTORY

Is this really syncope?

Key Questions

- Did you lose consciousness?
- Did you have any prodromal symptoms?
- What were you doing when the event occurred?
- If you lost consciousness, how long did it last?
- Did your limbs jerk during the event?
- Did anyone see you faint?

Loss of Consciousness

Distinguish syncope from other symptoms. Dizziness, vertigo, and presyncope do not cause loss of consciousness or postural tone.

Prodromal Symptoms

Sweating, vertigo, nausea, and/or yawning are prodromal symptoms that are associated with syncope; seizures may be associated with an aura or tongue biting. Aura also suggests migraine etiology.

◎ EVIDENCE-BASED PRACTICE *Diagnosing Syncope*

Syncope is a common symptom with no diagnostic gold standard and a range of prognoses. The authors of this guideline undertook an extensive review of the literature to help clinicians maximize the diagnostic yield in the workup of syncope and here report the following key points that assist in the evaluation of syncope:

1. History, physical examination, and electrocardiography (ECG) are the core of syncope workup (combined diagnostic yield, 50%).
2. Neurological testing is rarely helpful unless additional neurological signs or symptoms are present (diagnostic yield of EEG, CT, and Doppler ultrasound, 2% to 6%).
3. Patients in whom heart disease is known or suspected and those with exertional syncope who are at higher risk

for adverse outcomes should have cardiac testing, including echocardiography, stress testing, Holter monitoring, or EPS, alone or in combination (diagnostic yield, 5% to 35%).
4. Syncope in the elderly often results from polypharmacy and abnormal physiological responses to daily events.
5. Long-term loop electrocardiography (diagnostic yield, 25% to 35%) and tilt-table testing (diagnostic yield, ≤60%) are most useful in patients with recurrent syncope in whom heart disease is not suspected.
6. Psychiatric evaluation can detect mental disorders associated with syncope in up to 25% of cases.
7. Hospitalization may be indicated for patients at high risk for cardiac syncope or with acute neurological signs.

Data from Linzer M, Yang EH, Estes NA III, Wang P, Vorperian VR, Kapoor WN: Diagnosing syncope. Part 1: Value of history, physical examination, and electrocardiography. Clinical Efficacy Assessment Project of the American College of Physicians, *Ann Intern Med* 126:989-996, 1997.

Pre-event Characteristics

Characterize what precipitated the episodes. Loss of consciousness precipitated by pain, exercise, urination, defecation, or stressful events is probably not a seizure. Breath-holding spells are common in children, causing syncope. They are usually precipitated by pain, anger, a sudden startle, or frustration. Syncope occurs with rest or when supine during a seizure or arrhythmia. Syncope that occurs without warning is considered cardiovascular in origin.

Event and Postevent Characteristics

Rhythmic movements of extremities during the event usually indicate a seizure, although they can occur with syncope. Disorientation after the event, slowness in returning to consciousness, and unconsciousness lasting longer than 5 minutes indicate seizure. Often children with breath-holding spells have associated cyanosis, clonic jerks, opisthotonos, and bradycardia.

Witness

The patient is unconscious when the syncopal event takes place and therefore is a poor historian. A careful history is needed from both the patient and a witness to help in the diagnosis. Adolescents who have hysterical syncope episodes generally have an audience when the event occurs and are able to describe details of the event that would not be known to an unconscious patient.

Does this require immediate referral?

Key Questions

■ Do you have a history of heart disease? What is it?
■ Do you have a congenital heart problem?
■ Are you having chest pain and/or shortness of breath?
■ Did this occur after exercise?

History of Heart Disease/Congenital Heart Problem

The presence of structural heart disease increases the risk of sudden death. Patients with a history of coronary artery disease, congestive heart failure, or ventricular arrhythmia should be hospitalized. Cardiac syncope may be either arrhythmic or mechanical in origin. Cardiac outflow obstruction from aortic or mitral stenosis or a prosthetic valve may cause syncope. Complete heart block is a leading cause of syncope, the result of interruption of atrioventricular conduction. Children who have had cardiac surgery to correct severe congenital heart disease are at risk for arrhythmias.

Chest Pain or Shortness of Breath

Obstructive mechanical blockage may be caused by pulmonary embolism, cardiac ischemia, or myocardial infarction with pump failure.

After Exercise

Syncope that accompanies exercise should be considered of cardiac origin unless proved otherwise. Syncope after exertion in a well-trained athlete who has no heart disease is likely vasovagal in origin.

What do associated symptoms tell me?

Key Questions

■ What other symptoms did you have?
■ Do you have palpitations?
■ Do you have headaches?
■ Have you experienced vertigo, dizziness, or visual changes?

Palpitations

Supraventricular or ventricular tachycardias are associated with syncope and sudden death. Ventricular tachycardia with a heart rate of 200 beats per minute may be asymptomatic or cause syncope. Chaotic ventricular activity of ventricular fibrillation is always fatal unless it is reversed with electrical defibrillation. (See Chapter 23 for more on palpitations.)

Headaches

The pain of migraine headaches and the effect of the migraine on the brainstem can cause syncope. Generally the patient has associated symptoms, such as vomiting, photophobia, severe headache (often on one side), and a strong family history of migraines. The headache continues after consciousness is regained.

Vertigo, Dizziness, and Visual Symptoms

The presence of vertigo, dizziness, diplopia, or other visual changes may accompany migraine headache. Interruption in cerebral perfusion, such as with a transient ischemic attack, also must be considered.

Is this neurocardiogenic in origin?

Key Questions

- Did this occur in response to a specific situation (e.g., stressful event, urination, defecation)?
- Were you sitting, standing, or lying flat when you fainted?
- Do you have a history of any heart problems?

Situational Fainting

Vasovagal syncope is the most common type seen in adults and healthy children. It is neurocardiogenic and tends to occur in families. It is often precipitated by emotional stress, fear, extreme fatigue, or injury. It can occur without any obvious antecedent cause. Warm temperature, anxiety, blood drawing, and crowded rooms may cause peripheral vasodilation. Lack of large muscle activity prevents the venous return that is needed for cardiac filling with consequent bradycardia and fainting. When supine, venous return to the heart occurs, awakening the patient. Rapid standing will cause recurrence of the episode. Mental alertness is present.

Situational syncope can occur in response to urination, defecation, cough, or emotional stress. Posttussive syncope follows paroxysmal coughing caused by increased intrathoracic pressure, which is then transmitted to the intracranial circulation, increasing intracranial pressure and decreasing cerebral blood flow. Postmicturition syncope, occurring during or after urination, is caused by the release of intravascular pressure on urination, which triggers vasodilation and vagally mediated bradycardia.

Is this orthostasis?

Key Questions

- What medications are you taking?
- Have you recently started blood pressure medicine or has the dose changed?
- What other health problems/conditions do you have?

Medications

About 10% of syncopal episodes are caused by prescribed medications (e.g., antidepressants, antidysrhythmics, β-blockers, diuretics), over-the-counter medications, and recreational drugs (e.g., alcohol, cocaine) that produce orthostasis, bradycardia, or prolonged QT interval. Adolescents may use drugs, such as amyl nitrite and butyl nitrite, as aphrodisiacs and euphoriants. These drugs lead to vasodilation, and syncope may occur.

Children may ingest medications that belong to family members, and a history of such activity must be investigated as a cause of the syncope.

Other Health Problems or Conditions

Diabetes may induce hypoglycemia, causing a gradual syncope. Anemias and chronic gastrointestinal bleeding from an ulcer or another source may cause syncope.

Patients who are pregnant or dehydrated or who have been on prolonged bed rest are at risk for orthostatic hypotension and syncope.

Is this explained by other factors?

Key Questions

- Have you had this before? How often?
- Did it occur with sudden head turning?
- If a child: Has the child had Kawasaki disease?
- Do you have Lyme disease?

Frequent Syncope with No Heart Disease

Psychogenic syncope is often associated with repeated episodes in which unpredictable motor reflexes appear, with a lack of pathological reflexes. Also, blood pressure and pulse rate measurements are normal, and skin and mucous membranes do not change color. Panic attacks, or hyperventilation, are often interpreted as feeling faint, but the patient does not usually appear pale, nor are the symptoms relieved when recumbent.

After Sudden Head Rotation

Carotid sinus hypersensitivity produces a cardioinhibitory response that results in a profound drop in heart rate or may induce an abrupt vasopressor response with a drop in blood pressure.

History of Kawasaki Disease

Syncope can occur in children who have had Kawasaki disease. These children are at risk for coronary heart disease, which may present as chest pain associated with exercise.

Lyme Disease

Lyme disease can cause arrhythmia in the form of heart block, which can result in syncope.

What other things do I need to consider?

Key Questions

- Do you have a family history of sudden death?
- Do you have a family history of fainting?
- If a child: Did the mother have systemic lupus erythematosus (SLE) while pregnant?

Family History of Sudden Death

A family history of idiopathic hypertrophic subaortic stenosis is a risk factor for sudden death, and referral is necessary to rule out this condition. A history of a family member who had a myocardial infarction before age 30 is a significant risk factor for sudden death.

Family History of Fainting

Neurocardiogenic syncope is common in families.

Prenatal Systemic Lupus Erythematosus

SLE in a pregnant woman may cause autoimmune injury, resulting in congenital complete atrioventicular block.

DIAGNOSTIC REASONING: FOCUSED PHYSICAL EXAMINATION
Measure Blood Pressure and Pulse Rate

Obtain blood pressure readings in standing, sitting, and supine positions. Orthostatic hypotension is either a decrease in systolic blood pressure of at least 20 mm Hg or symptoms that prevent further standing, such as fainting, weakness, or lightheadedness.

Compare blood pressure readings in the two arms. Unequal measurements may indicate a cardiac cause of the syncope.

Bradycardia of 35 to 40 beats per minute usually does not compromise cerebral blood flow. Rates below this, however, will impair cerebral circulation and function. Tachycardia up to 180 beats per minute also does not usually compromise cerebral circulation.

Observe Hydration Status

Poor hydration status secondary to diuretic use, poor nutrition, or loss of fluids from vomiting and diarrhea may be associated with syncope.

Perform Heart and Lung Examination

Observe for jugular venous distention. Palpate the precordium to assess the point of maximal impulse to estimate the size of the left ventricle. Feel for lifts. Listen for heart rate and murmurs and for radiation of murmurs. Listen for an abnormally loud S2 or the presence of an S3. Auscultate for carotid bruits and pericardial rub. Listen to the lungs to assess for rales associated with congestive heart failure.

Perform a Neurological Examination

Begin with a brief mental status examination. Assess cranial nerves, deep tendon reflexes, and motor function. Perform a Romberg test, as well as gait and proprioception evaluation. Assess pupillary asymmetry and look for nystagmus (see Chapter 12).

Perform an Abdominal Examination

Auscultate and observe for signs of aortic aneurysm.

Examine Extremities

Observe lower extremities for signs of thrombophlebitis, a source of pulmonary embolism.

LABORATORY AND DIAGNOSTIC STUDIES
Suspected or Known Cardiac Cause
Electrocardiogram

The usefulness of the electrocardiogram usually lies in identifying abnormalities that provide clues to underlying cardiac causes of syncope. These findings include evidence of conduction disorder or signs of coronary artery disease or left ventricular hypertrophy. A 12-lead ECG is used for the basic evaluation. This should be first evaluated for rhythm and rate. Hand-measured interval measurement should be made. A Q wave found in the anterolateral lead may indicate abnormal placement of the left coronary artery. A patient with a prolonged QT interval or the presence of Q waves must be referred.

Complete heart block requires immediate referral for pacemaker insertion.

Carotid Sinus Massage

Carotid sinus massage (CSM) is done to evaluate patients with suspected carotid sinus hypersensitivity. This can be performed at the bedside with the patient in a supine or upright position while under continuous ECG and blood pressure monitoring. Apply firm pressure and massage for 5 to 10 seconds one side at a time at the site of the strongest carotid pulsation. Carotid sinus hypersensitivity is diagnosed when CSM causes a ≥3 second pause, a ≥50 mm Hg fall in systolic blood pressure, or both, and associated syncope.

Event Monitoring or Continuous-Loop Monitoring

These measures are used in patients with suspected cardiac arrhythmias as the cause of the syncope. Holter (24 hours) or long-term (weeks, months) event monitoring is used to document electrocardiographic recordings. Holter monitoring is a continuous, 24-hour electrocardiographic recording to evaluate the type and amount of irregular heartbeats during regular activities, exercise, and sleep. The patient keeps a 24-hour diary to record daily activities and any symptoms experienced.

Cardiac event monitoring is a continuous-loop, digital memory recorder worn for extended periods of time (up to 30 days or longer) that saves and records transient events felt by the patient. Patients activate these monitors as symptoms occur. Loop monitors save information for a predetermined period prior to the patient trigger, and therefore can help identify the initiation sequence for arrhythmias. These stored events can be transmitted through a telephone for review.

Doppler Studies

Transcranial Doppler and carotid ultrasonography are used to detect hemodynamically significant stenoses in the major intracranial or extracranial arteries.

Exercise Stress Test

Cardiac stress testing is used to evaluate exercise-associated arrhythmias and syncope. It can confirm the presence of coronary artery disease.

Echocardiography

This is used in patients with exercise-induced symptoms to exclude left ventricular outflow tract obstruction.

Electrophysiological Studies

Electrophysiological studies (EPSs) are invasive tests that use electrical stimulation and monitoring to diagnose conduction disorders or the propensity for the development of tachyarrhythmias. Electrodes are threaded through arm or leg veins and placed at strategic positions in the ventricles, atria, or both. The electrodes record electrical signals and allow mapping of electrical impulses. The electrodes also can electrically stimulate the heart at programmed rates to trigger latent ventricular tachycardias.

Suspected Neurological Cause
Baseline Blood Testing

Routine blood tests (electrolyte levels, renal function, blood glucose level, complete blood count) rarely yield useful diagnostic information. Most patients with abnormalities in these areas have seizures rather than syncope.

Electroencephalography

Electroencephalography (EEG) may be useful in patients whose history suggests seizure.

Computed Tomography Scanning

Computed tomography (CT) may be useful if the patient has focal neurological findings.

Unexplained Syncope
Toxicology Screen

Toxicology screening may be indicated on the basis of the history.

Tilt-Table Testing

Tilt-table testing is used to provoke vasovagal syncope in susceptible persons. Provocative agents such as isoproterenol or nitroglycerin may be used. Using the table, the patient is tilted upright while continuous minute-to-minute blood pressure, heart rate, and oxygen saturation measurements are recorded. Patient symptoms are recorded in each position. Patients with neurocardiogenic syncope develop a sudden drop in heart rate and/or blood pressure after their body has been tilted up for several minutes. If symptoms of lightheadedness or fainting occur during this test, the test is considered positive for neurocardiogenic syncope.

DIFFERENTIAL DIAGNOSIS
Cardiac Causes

Cardiac causes have a higher rate of mortality than do other causes of syncope. Cardiac causes include coronary artery disease, congenital and valvular disease, cardiomyopathy, arrhythmias, and conduction system disorders. Coronary artery disease, congestive heart failure, and ventricular hypertrophy can result in arrhythmias and syncope. Patients with organic heart disease may have chest pain, dyspnea, and syncope with exertion. Patients with arrhythmias may have palpitations or sudden syncope without other physical symptoms. On physical examination, murmurs or carotid bruits may be present. Other findings might include a loud S2, precordial lift, S3, pericardial rub, or unequal blood pressure measurements in the arms. Electrocardiographic testing is indicated; other cardiac testing may be helpful.

Neurocardiogenic Causes

Vasovagal syncope is the most common type in young people, but it can occur at any age. It usually occurs in a standing position and is precipitated by fear, emotional stress, or pain. Autonomic symptoms such as nausea, sweating, blurred or fading vision, epigastric discomfort, lightheadedness, and a feeling of warmth may precede syncope by a few minutes. The syncope occurs secondary to efferent vasopressor reflexes resulting in decreased peripheral vascular resistance. Physical examination is usually negative. Tilt-table testing may be useful in establishing a diagnosis.

Situational syncope is vasovagal syncope with a known precipitant. It is commonly related to conditions that produce a Valsalva maneuver. Micturition, defecation, and cough are types of situational syncope. These stimuli result in autonomic reflexes with a vasopressor response, ultimately leading to transient cerebral hypotension. The physical examination is negative.

Carotid sinus hypersensitivity produces a cardioinhibitory response or vasopressor response that produces syncope with head turning.

Orthostasis

Orthostatic (postural) syncope indicates variable or unstable vasomotor reflexes. A drop in blood pressure when one assumes an upright position is caused by loss of vasoconstriction reflexes in the lower extremities. Sudden standing or rapid movement after assuming a standing position can trigger syncope; the prevalence of this type of syncope increases with age. The syncope is caused by hypotension that occurs as a blunted baroreceptor response and inability of the cardiovascular system to respond to hypotensive stresses. It may also occur from age-related physiological changes, volume depletion, medication, and autonomic insufficiency. Orthostatic hypotension is produced with testing.

Medication-Related Causes

Use of prescribed medications or recreational drugs can produce syncope. Medications that can cause syncope include antidepressants, antidysrhythmics, β-blockers, and diuretics. Recreational drugs (e.g., alcohol, cocaine) can produce orthostasis, bradycardia, or prolonged QT interval. Amyl nitrite and butyl nitrite cause vasodilation and syncope.

Physical findings depend on the underlying physical condition of the patient.

Neurological Causes

Neurological causes include transient ischemic attacks, migraines, and seizures. Prodromal symptoms may include vertigo, diplopia, and loss of balance. Syncope results from vertebrobasilar insufficiency. In an acute syncopal attack, circulation is briefly obstructed to the reticular activating system in the brainstem, resulting in loss of consciousness. Neurological findings, such as diplopia, pupillary asymmetry, nystagmus, ataxia, and gait instability, may be present.

Psychiatric Causes

Syncope of unexplained origin may be psychogenic. Panic and anxiety disorders, somatization, major depression, and substance abuse are the main psychiatric problems associated with syncope. Physical examination is usually negative. Psychiatric evaluation may reveal the underlying disorder.

Unknown Causes

Syncope from unknown causes accounts for about one third of all episodes of syncope. The workup is negative.

DIFFERENTIAL DIAGNOSIS OF *Common Causes of Syncope*

DISORDER	HISTORY	PHYSICAL FINDINGS	DIAGNOSTIC STUDIES
Cardiac Causes			
Organic heart disease	Shortness of breath, chest pain, palpitations, exercise-associated syncope	May have bradycardia or tachycardia, cyanosis	Refer
Arrhythmias	Palpitations; absence of other symptoms	Loud S2, S3; murmur, lift	Electrocardiogram, Holter, echocardiogram Doppler studies, cardiac stress testing
Neurocardiogenic Causes			
Vasovagal	Emotional event, standing for long periods, crowded room, warm environment	None	Tilt-table testing, CSM
Situational	Occurs with cough, micturition, defecation, swallowing	None	None
Breath holding	Children 6 mo to 5 yr; associated with anger, pain, brief cry; breath-holding LOC; may have twitching	Cyanosis or pallor	None
Hyperventilation	Anxiety- or fear-induced event, shortness of breath	None	None
Cough syncope	History of asthma; coughing paroxysm awakens child from sleep, becomes flaccid with clonic muscle spasm, LOC	Wheezes	None
Orthostasis			
Orthostatic hypotension	Position change from lying/sitting to standing, pregnancy, prolonged bed rest	Hypotension on testing orthostatic blood pressure	20 mm Hg drop in systolic pressure on standing
Medication-Related Causes			
Prescribed medications	History of antidepressants, antidysrhythmic agents, β-blockers, or diuretics	Depends on underlying condition	None
Drug-induced causes	History of use of illicit drugs	Arrhythmia may be present	Toxicology screen
Neurological Causes			
Migraine	Headache, vomiting, photophobia, positive family history	Usually none; nystagmus, photophobia	None
Seizures	Convulsions, incontinence, postictal phase	Usually none; nystagmus	Electroencephalogram
Psychiatric Causes			
Mental disorder	Symptoms consistent with depression, anxiety, panic	None	Psychiatric evaluation
Hysterical reaction	Adolescent, event occurs with audience present; gentle fall, memory of incident exact	None	None
Unknown Causes	No diagnostic characteristics	None	Workup negative

CSM, cardiac sinus massage; *LOC,* loss of consciousness.

REFERENCES AND READINGS

Batra AS, Holn AR: Palpitations, syncope and sudden cardiac death in children: who's at risk? *Pediatr Rev* 24:269, 2003.

Brignole M, Alboni P, Benditt DG, Bergfeldt L, Blanc JJ, Thomsen PE et al: Guidelines on management (diagnosis and treatment) of syncope: update 2004. Executive summary, *Eur Heart J* 25:22, 2004.

Kapoor WN: Syncope, *N Engl J Med* 343:1856, 2000.

Kenny RA: Syncope in the elderly: diagnosis, evaluation, and treatment, *J Cardiovasc Electrophysiol* 14:9, 2003.

Lewis D, Dhala A: Syncope in the pediatric patient, *Pediatr Clin North Am* 46:205, 1999.

Limmer DD, Mistovich JJ, Krost WS: Beyond the basics: syncope, *EMS Magazine* March:76, 2009.

Miller TH: Evaluation of syncope, *Am Fam Physician* 72:1492, 2005.

Narchi H: The child who passes out, *Pediatr Rev* 21:384, 2000.

Schnipper JL, Kapoor WN: Diagnostic evaluation and management of patients with syncope, *Med Clin North Am* 2:423, 2002.

Strickberger S, Benson D, Biaggioni, I, Callans D, Cohen M, Ellenbogen K et al: AHA/ACCF scientific statement on the evaluation of syncope, *J Amer Coll Cardiol* 47:474, 2006.

Taylor B, Green MS: Evaluating and managing syncope, *Clin Rev* 10:55, 2000.

Thanavaro JL: Evaluation and management of syncope, *Clin Schol Rev* 2:65, 2009.

Ungar A, Mussi C, Del Rosso A, Noro G, Abete P, Ghirelli L et al: Diagnosis and characteristics of syncope in older patients referred to geriatric departments, *J Am Geriatr Soc* 54:1531, 2006.

Willis J: Syncope, *Pediatr Rev* 21:201, 2001.

Urinary Incontinence

Urinary incontinence is any involuntary loss of urine. It occurs as a result of pathological, anatomical, psychological, or physiological factors that produce obstruction, bladder irritability, or interference with neurological functioning. Environmental factors, such as decreased mobility or inaccessibility of toilet facilities, may also produce periodic incontinence.

Urinary incontinence is a common problem, particularly in older adults. It is so common in older women that some think of it as "normal." The prevalence in U.S. women is 26% during reproductive years and 30% to 40% in postmenopausal years. In noninstitutionalized elderly women, the prevalence is 15% to 30%, and in men it is 8% to 22%. In elderly persons in nursing homes, the rate rises to almost 50%.

Urinary incontinence in adults is categorized according to the underlying anatomical or physiological impairment—specifically, stress incontinence, urge incontinence (overactive bladder), overflow incontinence, and incontinence from reversible causes.

Stress incontinence is leakage of urine during activities that increase abdominal pressure, such as coughing, sneezing, laughing, or other physical activities. It occurs most often in females and is caused by hypermotility at the base of the bladder and urethra associated with pelvic floor relaxation or intrinsic urethral weakness.

Urge incontinence is an abrupt and strong desire to void with the inability to delay urination and is caused by bladder hyperactivity or hypersensitive bladder. Detrusor muscle overactivity occurs when pathological brain disorders interfere with central inhibitory centers and fail to prevent detrusor muscle contractions.

Overflow incontinence occurs with overdistention of the bladder caused by an underactive or acontractile detrusor muscle; by sphincter-detrusor dyssynergia, which is loss of the synergistic urinary sphincter relaxation that normally occurs with bladder detrusor muscle contraction; or from bladder outlet or urethral

obstruction. Sphincter weakness can occur from damage to the urethra or its innervation or from pelvic floor muscle relaxation.

Incontinence from reversible factors originates outside of the lower urinary tract and is caused by mental status impairment, immobility, or medication. Some sources term this functional or transient incontinence.

A final category of incontinence is called mixed incontinence. This occurs when the incontinence is produced as the result of several anatomical, physiological, or functional factors. Involuntary discharge of urine in children is abnormal beyond the age of 4 years for daytime wetting and beyond the age of 6 for nighttime wetting. Daytime wetting constitutes diurnal enuresis; nighttime wetting is known as nocturnal or sleep enuresis. In children, enuresis may be organic or nonorganic; nonorganic enuresis can be primary or secondary. Primary nonorganic enuresis occurs in 75% to 90% of children. This enuresis is defined as wetting that has continued since infancy without an established pattern of dryness. Secondary nonorganic enuresis occurs in 10% to 25% of children and is defined as recurrence of wetting after continence has been established for at least 6 months. The possibility of abnormal urinary anatomy is high in young children who present with urinary tract symptoms.

DIAGNOSTIC REASONING: FOCUSED HISTORY
Adults

Could this be the result of reversible factors (see Box 31-1)?

Key Questions

- What medications are you taking?
- Do you have any of the following urinary symptoms: urgency, frequency, burning, pain, blood in the urine, flank pain?

Box 31-1	**Reversible Factors that Can Cause Urinary Incontinence in Adults**

D	Delirium, dementia, depression
I	Infection
A	Atrophic vaginitis/urethritis
P	Pharmaceuticals
E	Endocrine/excess urine production
R	Restricted mobility, retention
S	Stool impaction

Modified from Resnick NM: Initial evaluation of the incontinent patient, *J Am Geriatr Soc* 38:311, 1990.

- Do you have vaginal dryness or itching?
- Do you have pain/discomfort with sexual activity?
- Have you had changes in bowel function?
- When was your last bowel movement?
- Are you feeling depressed or "blue"?
- Are you aware of incontinence?
- How active are you?
- Are you able to get to the toilet easily?
- Do you have any chronic health problems?

Medications

Hypnotic-sedatives, diuretics, anticholinergic agents, adrenergic agents, and calcium channel blockers can cause incontinence. α-Adrenergic agonists and β-adrenergic agonists increase sphincter tone and may cause retention. Anticholinergics, prostaglandin inhibitors, calcium channel blockers, and narcotic analgesics decrease detrusor tone. Diuretics can cause incontinence because of increased production of urine. Central nervous system (CNS) depressants, such as hypnotic-sedatives, can interfere with functional ability.

Table 31-1 lists categories of medications and their mechanism of action in urinary incontinence.

Urinary Tract Infection, Vaginal Dryness, and Dyspareunia

Urinary tract infection (UTI) and atrophic vaginitis can cause incontinence through local irritation and loss of muscle tone.

Bowel Function

Fecal impaction can cause incontinence through mechanical obstruction of the urethra.

Mental Status, Mobility, and Chronic Health Problems

Excessive urine production may be a problem if mobility is restricted, health is poor, or orientation is variable. Chronic health problems, psychological factors, and restricted mobility can result in incontinence because of loss of functional ability and/or mentation.

Table 31-1	**Medications that Can Cause or Contribute to Urinary Incontinence**

MEDICATION CATEGORY	TYPE OF INCONTINENCE	MECHANISM OF ACTION
Anticholinergics	Overflow	Decreased bladder contractions with retention
Antidepressants	Overflow	Decreased bladder contractions with retention
Antipsychotics	Overflow	Decreased bladder contractions with retention
Sedative-hypnotics	Overflow	Decreased bladder contractions with retention
Antihistamines	Overflow	Decreased bladder contractions with retention
Narcotics	Overflow	Decreased bladder contractions with retention
Alcohol	Overflow	Decreased bladder contractions with retention
Calcium channel blockers	Overflow	Decreased bladder contractions with retention
β-Adrenergic agonists	Overflow	Decreased bladder contractions with retention
α-Adrenergic agonists	Overflow	Sphincter contraction with outflow obstruction
α-Adrenergic antagonists	Stress	Sphincter relaxation with urinary leakage
Diuretics	Urge	Contractions stimulated by high urine flow
Caffeine	Urge	Diuretic effect
Sedative-hypnotics	Urge	Depressed CNS inhibition of micturition
Alcohol	Urge	Diuretic effect and depressed CNS inhibition

Adapted from Weiss BD: Diagnostic evaluation of urinary incontinence in geriatric patients, *Am Fam Physician* 57:2675, 2688, 1998.

What do the presenting symptoms tell me?

Key Questions

- What is the primary symptom (e.g., urgency; dribbling; lack of sensation; nocturia; abdominal discomfort; leakage with laughing, coughing, or sneezing)?
- How frequently do you urinate?
- How much urine is voided each time?
- Do you have difficulty starting to urinate?
- Does your urine stream start and stop while you are urinating?

Primary Symptom

Urgency is the primary symptom of detrusor instability. Dribbling indicates overflow incontinence, and sphincter weakness usually increases with postural changes. Men often report nocturia and dribbling with overflow incontinence. Abdominal discomfort often occurs with overflow incontinence because of bladder distention. Incontinence with an increase in intraabdominal pressure is usually stress incontinence but can also be the result of detrusor overactivity and bladder irritability.

Frequency of Voiding

Increase in frequency of voiding occurs with detrusor instability or hyperactivity and may occur with some transient causes such as use of diuretics or large-volume fluid intake. Decreased frequency is common in overflow incontinence.

Amount of Urine Lost with Each Episode

Involuntary loss of small amounts of urine occurs with stress incontinence and overflow incontinence.

Character of Stream

Voiding a small-caliber or intermittent stream or difficulty in starting the stream indicates obstructive uropathy. In males, this may be secondary to an enlarged prostate.

Are there any other symptoms that will point me in the right direction?

Key Questions

- How much fluid do you drink in a day?
- How much caffeine and alcohol do you drink?
- What time of day do you drink fluids?
- How thirsty are you?
- Have you lost or gained weight recently?

Fluid Intake

A significant increase in the amount of fluid intake or an unusually large volume may indicate diabetes mellitus (DM). Caffeine and alcohol can act as diuretics and may be a cause of reversible incontinence. Caffeine can also be a bladder irritant and either produce or exacerbate urge incontinence. A large volume of fluid intake may produce enuresis secondary to a large urine volume, particularly if fluids are consumed in the evening before bedtime.

Thirst

Unusual thirst accompanied by an unusually large intake of fluid may indicate DM.

Weight Loss or Gain

Weight loss may indicate a chronic health problem, tumor, or dementia. Weight gain may indicate congestive heart failure, DM, or loss of mobility.

Children

Is this primary or secondary enuresis?

Key Question

- Has the child ever had consistent dryness for at least 6 months?

Primary enuresis occurs when a child has never achieved consistent dryness. Secondary enuresis is involuntary voiding of urine in a child who has had a period of dryness of more than 6 months. Secondary enuresis is often indicative of some other form of voiding dysfunction or significant underlying pathology. In children, daytime urinary incontinence beyond the age of 4 years may indicate congenital abnormalities in the urinary tract or nervous system.

Is this organic enuresis?

Key Questions

- Does the child have pain on urination?
- Does the child have intermittent daytime wetness?
- Does the child seem thirsty and urinate a lot?
- Has the child had nervous system trauma?
- Does the child have constipation or encopresis?
- Does the child have constant wetness or dribbling throughout the day?
- Does the child have an abnormal stream, such as dribbling or hesitancy?

■ Has the child had a change in gait?
■ Has the child had a recent lumbar puncture?
■ Does the child snore or have apnea at night?
■ Does the child report rectal itching at night?

Organic explanations of enuresis focus primarily on the genitourinary and nervous systems.

Genitourinary System

Fifteen percent of children with a UTI present with enuresis. It is unclear whether UTI causes the enuresis or vice versa. A wet perineum predisposes to ascending infection, and prompt treatment of the infection cures the enuresis in about one third of the cases. Asymptomatic bacteremia in school children is associated with enuresis.

Fecal retention that is chronic or intermittent is responsible for production of "functional" bladder neck obstruction. Displacement of the bladder and posterior urethra by the full rectum in the fixed and limited space of the bony pelvis causes detrusor perineal dysynergism, which is thought to be the mechanism responsible for urinary stasis and interference with micturition produced by constipation.

Abnormal daytime voiding suggests urological abnormality. Dribbling suggests the presence of an ectopic ureter, labial fusion, a deep positioned meatus or a hymen covering the meatus. Chronic leakage of urine in females may indicate an ectopic ureter that terminates in the vagina. Partial distal urethral obstruction can cause straining to urinate. Polyuria from glucose-induced osmotic diuresis can be seen in patients with DM. Renal tubules lose their ability to concentrate urine, resulting in the production of large volumes of very dilute urine.

Nervous System

Lumbosacral disorders affect bladder innervation and may cause enuresis. Head injury or brain tumor can cause polyuria and polydipsia. If the kidneys are unable to concentrate urine because of deficiency in the hypothalamic production of antidiuretic hormone (ADH), central diabetes insipidus (DI) develops, while renal unresponsiveness to ADH causes nephrogenic DI.

Interference with the nerve supply to the bladder causes a neurogenic bladder and obstruction. This can be functional, resulting from an imbalance between detrusor muscle contraction and urethral sphincter relaxation. It can also be congenital or acquired, such as with meningomyelocele or spinal cord injury.

Sleep apnea interferes with the child's ability to wake appropriately in response to stimuli to void.

Other

Pinworms (*Enterobius vermicularis*) primarily inhabit the cecum and lower bowel and are the most common cause of rectal itching in children. Pinworms have been implicated in incontinence in children, although the reason is not clear.

What risk factors does this child have for nonorganic enuresis?

Key Questions
■ Is the child a boy or a girl?
■ Is there a history of bedwetting in the family?
■ Is the child a twin?
■ What is the child's birth order?
■ Has the child been institutionalized?
■ Does the child have sickle cell disease?
■ What is the child's daily fluid intake?

Gender

Boys are more likely to have nocturnal enuresis. Girls are more likely to have diurnal enuresis related to UTI.

Family History

Children with nonorganic enuresis often have a very strong family history of fathers who had nocturnal enuresis as a child.

Twin/Birth Order

Nocturnal enuresis is most common in the firstborn and in twins.

Institutionalization

Institutionalized children have a greater tendency for enuresis because of developmental delay.

Sickle Cell Disease

Children with sickle cell anemia may have a concentrating defect and excrete low specific gravity urine in large volumes, which may make the child wet the bed.

Fluid Intake

A large volume of fluid intake may produce enuresis secondary to a large urine volume, particularly if the fluids are consumed in the evening before bedtime.

DIAGNOSTIC REASONING: FOCUSED PHYSICAL EXAMINATION
Perform Mental Status Examination

Assess orientation and cognitive function. In adults, incontinence can occur as the result of disorientation, delirium, or dementia.

In children, secondary enuresis can be caused by the presence of stress factors during the developmental period from 2 to 4 years of age. Separation from family, death of a parent, birth of a sibling, a move, marital conflict, and other stress-related causes may produce transient and intermittent enuresis.

Observe Gait

The urinary bladder receives extensive autonomic as well as somatic innervation. Lesions at all levels of the neuraxis from the cortex to peripheral nerves produce abnormalities of micturition.

Take Vital Signs

Blood pressure readings in children are important to rule out nephrotic causes of enuresis. When chronic renal failure is the result of an inadequate amount of normally functioning renal tissue, the clinical presentation may be enuresis. Fever in infants without any other signs is likely caused by UTI.

Examine the Abdomen

Palpate for masses, suprapubic tenderness, or fullness. Palpate the bladder. Abdominal distention or palpable bladder is suggestive of urinary retention and overflow incontinence.

Examine Genitalia in Males

Look for abnormalities of the foreskin, glans, meatus, penis, and perineal skin that might contribute to or produce incontinence.

Perform Pelvic Examination in Females

Note signs of pelvic prolapse (cystocele, rectocele). Palpate for pelvic mass and perivaginal muscle tone. Note condition of the vaginal mucosa and look for atrophic vaginitis. Vaginitis can cause urinary incontinence in children and adults, whereas atrophic vaginitis will produce incontinence only in adults.

Observe for evidence of sexual abuse such as abrasions, tears, or bruising. Urethral irritation, especially if discharge is present, may suggest sexual abuse in children.

Perform Provocative Stress Testing

During the pelvic examination, ask the patient to relax and then cough vigorously (or perform a Valsalva maneuver); watch for urine loss from the urethra. A positive test indicates stress incontinence.

Perform Digital Rectal Examination

Assess for perineal sensation, resting and active sphincter tone, rectal mass, fecal impaction, and fissures. A lax sphincter suggests spinal cord involvement.

In men, assess consistency and contour of the prostate. Prostate enlargement or masses suggest the possibility of overflow incontinence from obstruction.

Conduct a Neurological Examination

Assess the intactness of the neurological system. Note focal deficits, test deep tendon reflexes, and test for sensation in the perineal and perirectal areas. Assess nerve roots S2 to S4. Test for muscle tone and strength. Deficits may point to a neurological cause for the incontinence.

Examine and Palpate the Spine in Children

Look for an undetected birth defect that may be causing a neurological disturbance. A spinal dimple or hair tuft may alert you to a potential problem.

Perform Musculoskeletal Examination

Assess mobility, strength, and functional ability. In many older adults, the inability to get to a toilet causes incontinence.

An easy assessment of mobility is the timed get-up-and-go test. Time the patient getting up from a chair, walking 10 feet, and sitting back down. Although the time required to perform this test will vary, a mobile, independent, older adult can perform this activity in about 10 seconds.

Additional Procedures
Postvoid Residual

Have the patient void without straining and then catheterize. A residual volume greater than 100 mL suggests either bladder weakness (stress incontinence) or outlet obstruction (overflow incontinence).

Observe Voiding

Note hesitancy, dribbling, interrupted stream, and decreased force or caliber of stream. These symptoms suggest outlet obstruction and overflow incontinence.

LABORATORY AND DIAGNOSTIC STUDIES
Urinalysis

Dipstick urinalysis (U/A) can rule out or point to infection or systemic disease as a cause of the incontinence. Note hematuria, pyuria, bacteriuria, or the presence of leukocyte esterase or nitrites as indicators of UTI. Glycosuria or proteinuria suggests DM or renal disease.

Specific Gravity

A specific gravity greater than 1.015 rules out diabetes insipidus as the cause of incontinence.

Urine Culture

A culture can be used to determine the organism(s) producing a UTI and can confirm the diagnosis.

Urine Cytology

Urine for cytology is indicated if microscopic or gross painless hematuria is present in the absence of infection.

Bladder Diary

A 24-hour bladder diary (3-day voiding diary for children) can provide an accurate record of urine output; average voided volume; frequency of voiding; frequency and nature of incontinent episodes; and type of volume of fluid intake. Patients or parents can catch and measure urine output in a measuring cup.

Blood Urea Nitrogen and Creatinine

Use these indicators of renal function if you suspect obstruction or urinary retention.

Vaginal Specimen Microscopy, DNA Testing, or Culture

These tests can confirm vaginal infection. See Chapter 34 for the procedures for these tests.

Office Cystometrography

Have the patient void and empty the bladder. Have men lie supine and place women in the dorsal lithotomy position. Insert a sterile 12 to 14 French (nonballooned) catheter and empty the bladder. (Measure the postvoid residual and collect urine for U/A at that time.) Insert a 50-mL syringe with plunger removed into the end of the catheter and position it about 15 cm above the urethra. Fill the syringe by pouring sterile water into it in 25- to 50-mL increments. Record cumulative total fluid instillation in the bladder and note the volume at which the patient first reports the urge to void. Continue adding fluid slowly until the fluid level in the syringe rises, indicating an increase in intrabladder pressure and contraction of the detrusor muscle. The rise may be gradual or sudden. Detrusor contraction at less than 300 to 350 mL of bladder volume indicates detrusor instability (urge incontinence). Have the patient void at the end of the procedure. The amount instilled minus the amount voided will also provide a measure of postvoid residual.

Urodynamic Testing

Complete urodynamic testing includes uroflowmetry, cystometrography, perineal electromyelography, and voiding cystourethrography (VCUG). It is indicated when patient symptoms do not correlate with objective physical findings, when results may change management, after treatment failure, or if more information is needed in order to plan further therapy (see the Evidence-Based Practice box, Urodynamic Testing).

◎ EVIDENCE-BASED PRACTICE *Urodynamic Testing*

A Cochrane systematic review compared outcomes in women with urinary incontinence based on urodynamic testing. The authors concluded that women assessed using urodynamic testing in addition to clinical methods were more likely to receive medication or surgical treatment. However, there was insufficient evidence to show whether they were less likely to be incontinent after treatment than women who did not have urodynamic tests. The additional cost of testing may not be justifiable given the lack of evidence for improvement in clinical outcomes. No data were available to evaluate the use of urodynamics in other patient groups.

Data from Glazener CMA, Lapitan MCM: Urodynamic investigations for management of urinary incontinence in children and adults, *Cochrane Database of Systematic Reviews* 2002. Available online at www.cochrane.org. Accessed May 28, 2010.

Cystoscopy and Contrast Radiography

These procedures are indicated for detection of neoplasms or stones.

Ultrasound

Ultrasonography may be useful in determining the presence of an obstruction.

DIFFERENTIAL DIAGNOSIS
Incontinence from Anatomical Causes

Stress Incontinence

Stress incontinence is associated with activities that increase intraabdominal pressure, such as coughing, sneezing, running, or laughing. The underlying abnormality is typically urethral hypermotility as a result of inadequate pelvic support of the bladder neck (urethrovesical junction). Normally increased intraabdominal pressure is transmitted evenly across the bladder neck and body. When adequate support is lacking, an increase in intraabdominal pressure displaces the bladder neck outside the abdominal cavity. The subsequent disproportionate increase in bladder pressure as compared to urethral pressure results in urine loss. Poor urethral sphincter function also contributes to stress incontinence. The amount of urine lost with each episode is small. The patient usually has a history of childbirth. On examination, pelvic floor relaxation may be evident with the presence of a cystocele and/or rectocele. The urethral sphincter may appear lax, and there is loss of urine with provocative testing. Atrophic vaginitis is a common finding in postmenopausal women. U/A and culture may be performed to rule out infections or urinary tract problems. Postvoid residual is normal.

Urge Incontinence

Urge incontinence is characterized by an uncontrolled urge to void, secondary to detrusor muscle irritability or hyperactivity or to a hypersensitive bladder. Most cases result from an idiopathic inability to suppress detrusor contraction. The urine volume lost is large. Physical examination results are usually normal. Postvoid residual is normal. Diagnostic testing includes U/A and culture to rule out infection, and determination of blood urea nitrogen and creatinine levels to rule out nephropathy. On office cystometrography, the urine volume is less than 300 to 350 mL before the urge to void occurs. Complete urodynamic testing can confirm the diagnosis.

For more information, see the Evidence-Based Practice box, Determining the Type of Urinary Incontinence.

Overflow Incontinence

Overflow incontinence occurs in the presence of obstruction or interruption in the nervous system. It is a result of overdistention of the bladder from an underactive or acontractile detrusor muscle, from sphincter-detrusor dyssynergia (loss of the synergistic urinary sphincter relaxation that normally occurs with bladder detrusor muscle contraction), or from bladder outlet or urethral obstruction. Sphincter weakness can occur from damage to the urethra or its innervation or from pelvic floor muscle relaxation.

Overflow incontinence is small-volume incontinence, with symptoms of dribbling and hesitancy. In men, symptoms of an enlarged prostate may be present (i.e., nocturia, dribbling, hesitancy, and decreased force and caliber of stream). On examination, look for distended bladder, prostate hypertrophy, evidence of spinal cord disease, or diabetic neuropathy. Postvoid residual is more than 100 mL. Diagnostic testing includes

---

🎯 **EVIDENCE-BASED PRACTICE** | *Determining the Type of Urinary Incontinence*

The authors of a recent systematic review of evidence of the most accurate way to determine the type of urinary incontinence during office assessment concluded that when evaluating a woman with urinary incontinence, a systematic approach that includes a history, physical examination, and stress test increases the likelihood of correctly classifying the type of incontinence (for stress: positive LR*, 3.7; negative LR, 0.20; and for urge: positive LR, 2.2; negative LR, 0.63). The most helpful component of the assessment for determining the presence of urge incontinence is a history of urine loss associated with urinary urgency (positive LR, 4.2). A stress test (preferably a filled bladder stress test) may be helpful for diagnosing stress incontinence (filled bladder stress test: positive LR, 9.4; negative LR, 0.07). Measurement of the postvoid residual urine volume detects incomplete bladder emptying, but there are no data to support using this in women to determine incontinence type.

---

* LR = Likelihood Ratio

Data from Holroyd-Leduc JM, Tannenbaum C, Thorpe KE, Straus SE: What type of urinary incontinence does this woman have? *JAMA* 299:1446, 2008.

U/A and urine culture, as well as determination of blood urea nitrogen and creatinine levels.

Interference with the nerve supply to the bladder can result in neurogenic bladder, obstruction, and consequent overflow incontinence, caused by an imbalance between detrusor muscle contraction and urethral sphincter relaxation. Functional incontinence can also be congenital or acquired, such as with meningomyelocele or spinal cord injury, or can be a surgical complication from radical prostatectomy. On examination, the anal sphincter may be lax. Neurological testing may reveal deficits.

Incontinence from Reversible Factors
Medications
Sedatives, hypnotics, diuretics, anticholinergic agents, α-adrenergic agents, and calcium channel blockers can cause incontinence. α-Adrenergic agonists and β-adrenergic agonists increase sphincter tone and may cause retention; they can also cause urge incontinence. Anticholinergics, prostaglandin inhibitors, calcium channel blockers, and narcotic analgesics decrease detrusor tone and can produce incontinence. Diuretics can cause incontinence because of increased production of urine, and CNS depressants such as hypnotic-sedatives can interfere with functional ability.

Urinary Tract Infection
The patient with a UTI has symptoms of lower or upper tract infection, such as burning, dysuria, frequency, urgency, flank pain, and fever. The urine may have a foul odor. The patient may exhibit suprapubic or costovertebral angle (CVA) tenderness. In infants, a fever with no localizing signs frequently indicates UTI. Urine analysis and culture can confirm the diagnosis of a lower UTI (see Chapter 32).

Vaginitis
Vaginitis produces incontinence as a result of local irritation. Atrophic vaginitis indicates a loss of estrogen and a concomitant loss of the vesicourethral angle, which predisposes women to stress incontinence. Provocative stress testing can demonstrate stress incontinence. Microscopy, molecular testing, or culture can confirm vaginal infection (see Chapter 34).

Constipation and Fecal Impaction
Constipation or fecal impaction can produce obstructive overflow incontinence by mechanical pressure on the urethra. The patient may experience abdominal pain and fecal soiling. On examination, stool may be felt in the colon and/or ampulla.

Change in Mental or Functional Status
Depression, dementia, and confusion can all produce incontinence (see Chapter 8). Restricted mobility can result in incontinence because of loss of functional ability.

Diabetes Insipidus
In DI, the kidneys are unable to concentrate urine because of a deficiency in the hypothalamic production of ADH (central DI) or a renal unresponsiveness to ADH (nephrogenic DI). The result is polyuria, which may cause incontinence. The patient also exhibits polydipsia. Urine specific gravity will be less than 1.015.

Diabetes Mellitus
DM often presents with excessive fluid intake and urination. The excess fluid volume can result in incontinence, particularly in older adults with chronic health problems, restricted mobility, or compromise in mental or functional health. Urinalysis can screen for glycosuria. Follow-up testing should check fasting blood glucose levels and hemoglobin A_{1c} measurement.

Mixed Incontinence
Patients who experience incontinence as the result of several anatomical, physiological, or functional factors are considered to have mixed incontinence.

Enuresis from Organic Causes
Genitourinary Causes
Genitourinary disorders that can produce enuresis include UTI, ectopic ureter, iatrogenic damage to the external sphincter, and urethral obstruction. Physical examination is usually normal. Fever and abdominal tenderness may be present with a UTI. Anatomical genitourinary abnormalities may signal an ectopic ureter. Diagnostic testing includes urinalysis, urine culture, and specific gravity to rule out infection and DM. Referral for further evaluation may be necessary.

Neurological Causes
Nervous system involvement can also produce enuresis. Lumbosacral disorders affect bladder innervation and may cause enuresis. Head injury or brain tumor

can cause polyuria and polydipsia. Interference with the nerve supply to the bladder causes neurogenic bladder and obstruction, which can result in enuresis. Interference in innervation can occur from congenital or acquired causes. Diagnostic testing includes urinalysis, urine culture, and specific gravity to rule out infection and DM. Referral for further evaluation may be necessary. Some children with sleep apnea have been found to have an increased atrial natriuretic factor, inhibiting the renin-angiotensin-aldosterone pathway, causing enuresis.

Enuresis from Nonorganic Causes
Primary Enuresis
Primary enuresis occurs when a child has never achieved consistent dryness. The normal developmental patterns of micturition follow a characteristic pattern in children but at an individual rate. The usual progression depends on the maturation of the CNS; generally, the following stages are seen:

- **Birth to 6 months.** Bladder emptying is an uninhibited reflex action.
- **6 to 12 months.** Bladder emptying is less frequent because of CNS inhibition of reflex action.
- **1 to 2 years.** Child consciously perceives bladder fullness; CNS inhibition increases.
- **3 to 5 years.** At age 5 years, most children are aware of bladder fullness; they develop the ability to inhibit the need to void both voluntarily and unconsciously.

Primary enuresis may represent a developmental delay or maturational lag. Often there is a family history of enuresis. The enuresis usually is only nocturnal. The incidence is higher in boys than in girls and usually resolves as the child matures. Physical examination is normal. Diagnostic testing includes urinalysis, urine culture, and specific gravity to rule out other causes.

Developmental (Secondary) Enuresis
Developmental enuresis, which is secondary, may be related to changes or stresses in a child's life. It can also occur as the result of genital trauma, infection, distended colon, or fecal impaction. The enuresis occurs in a child who has had a period of dryness of more than 6 months. Diagnostic testing includes urinalysis, urine culture, and specific gravity to rule out other causes.

Small Bladder
An anatomically small bladder can also produce enuresis. The child voids frequently but not in excessive volume. Physical examination is normal. Diagnostic testing includes urinalysis, urine culture, and specific gravity to rule out other causes.

Sickle Cell Anemia
Children with sickle cell anemia have a concentrating defect and may experience enuresis because of volume excess. Physical examination findings are consistent with the sickle cell disorder. Diagnostic testing includes urinalysis, urine culture, and specific gravity.

DIFFERENTIAL DIAGNOSIS OF *Common Causes of Urinary Incontinence*

CONDITION	HISTORY	PHYSICAL FINDINGS	DIAGNOSTIC STUDIES
Incontinence from Anatomical Causes			
Stress incontinence	Small-volume incontinence with coughing, sneezing, laughing, running; history of prior pelvic surgery	Pelvic floor relaxation; cystocele, rectocele; lax urethral sphincter; loss of urine with provocative testing; atrophic vaginitis	U/A and culture; PVR normal
Urge incontinence	Uncontrolled urge to void; large-volume incontinence; history of CNS disorders, such as stroke, multiple sclerosis, parkinsonism	Normal examination	U/A and culture; PVR normal; office cystometrography: <300-350-mL volume; BUN, creatinine, urodynamic testing

DIFFERENTIAL DIAGNOSIS OF *Common Causes of Urinary Incontinence—cont'd*

CONDITION	HISTORY	PHYSICAL FINDINGS	DIAGNOSTIC STUDIES
Overflow incontinence	Small-volume incontinence, dribbling, hesitancy; in men symptoms of enlarged prostate: nocturia, dribbling, hesitancy, decreased force and caliber of stream; in neurogenic bladder: history of bowel problems, spinal cord injury, or multiple sclerosis	Distended bladder; prostate hypertrophy, stool in rectum; fecal impaction; in neurogenic bladder: evidence of spinal cord disease or diabetic neuropathy; lax sphincter; gait disturbance	U/A and culture; PVR >100 mL; BUN, creatinine; in neurogenic bladder, refer for testing
Incontinence from Reversible Factors			
Medications	Hypnotics, diuretics, anticholinergic agents, α-adrenergic agents, calcium channel blockers	Normal except for findings related to other physical conditions	U/A to rule out urinary tract problems; blood chemistry to rule out systemic problem
Urinary tract infection (UTI)	Dysuria, urgency, daytime accidents	Frequency, odor, fever	U/A and culture
Vaginitis	Itching, odor	Discharge, atrophic vaginitis, evidence of sexual abuse	Gram stain, KOH, culture
Constipation/ fecal impaction	Abdominal pain	Soiling; stool felt in colon and/or ampulla	None
Change in mental or functional status	Change in mental status; impaired mobility; new environment	Impaired mental status; impaired mobility	U/A and culture; blood chemistry
Diabetes insipidus (DI)	History of trauma to head; thirst, frequency	Weight loss	U/A specific gravity >1.015
Diabetes mellitus (DM)	Thirsty, increased frequency	Weight loss	U/A; serum glucose
Enuresis from Organic Causes			
Genitourinary causes	UTI history; dribbling; urine leakage	Fever, abdominal tenderness; anatomical abnormalities (ectopic ureter); examination may be normal	U/A and culture; specific gravity; referral for testing
Neurological causes	Head injury; spinal cord injury; polydipsia, polyuria; sleep apnea	Lax sphincter, spinal tuft, neurological deficits; altered gait; examination may be normal	U/A and culture; specific gravity; referral for evaluation
Enuresis from Nonorganic Causes			
Primary enuresis	Child has never been dry; may have family history	Normal examination; developmental delay	U/A and culture; specific gravity to rule out other causes
Developmental (secondary) enuresis	Child has been dry for 6 mo in a row; changes or stresses in child's life	Examine for genital trauma or abuse, infection, distended colon, fecal impaction	U/A and culture; specific gravity to rule out other causes; screen for glycosuria
Small bladder	Void frequently, not in excessive volume	None	Bladder capacity = child's age + 2, for children <11 yr
Sickle cell anemia	Family history	Findings related to sickle cell disease	U/A and culture; specific gravity

BUN, blood urea nitrogen; *CNS*, central nervous system; *KOH*, potassium hydroxide; *PVR*, postvoid residual; *U/A*, urinalysis.

REFERENCES AND READINGS

Abrams P, Andersson KE, Birder L, Brubaker L, Cardozo L, Chapple C et al: Fourth international consultation on incontinence recommendations of the international scientific committee: Evaluation and treatment of urinary incontinence, pelvic organ prolapse, and fecal incontinence, *Neurourol Urodyn* 29:213, 2010.

Alper B, Curry S: Urinary tract infection in children, *Am Fam Physician* 72:2483, 2005.

American College of Obstetricians and Gynecologists: Urinary incontinence in women, *Obstet Gynecol* 105:1533,2005.

Amir B, Farrell SA, Sub-Committee on Urogynaecology: SOGC Committee opinion on urodynamics testing, *J Obstet Gynaecol Can* 30:717, 2008.

Burkhart KS: Urinary incontinence in women: assessment and management in the primary care setting, *Nurse Pract Forum* 11:192, 2000.

Culligan P, Heit M: Urinary incontinence in women: evaluation and management, *Am Fam Physician* 62:2433, 2000.

Graham K, Levy J: Enuresis, *Pediatr Rev* 30:165, 2009.

Hay-Smith EJ, Bo Berghmans LC, Hendriks H, de Bie RA, van Waalwijk van Doom ES: Pelvic floor muscle training for urinary incontinence in women, *Cochrane Database Syst Rev* 1: CD001407, 2001.

Hoebeke P, Bower W, Cooms D, Dejong T, Yang S: Diagnostic evaluation of children with daytime incontinence, *J Urol* 183:699, 2010.

Holroyd-Leduc JM, Tannenbaum C, Thorpe KE, Straus SE: What type of urinary incontinence does this woman have? *JAMA* 299:1446, 2008.

Ma JF, Shortliffe LM: Urinary tract infection in children: etiology and epidemiology, *Urol Clin North Am* 31:517, 2004.

Martin JL, Williams KS, Abrams KR, Turner DA, Sutton AJ, Chapple C et al: Systematic review and evaluation of methods of assessing urinary incontinence, *Health Technol Assess* 10:1, 2006.

Rogers RG: Urinary stress incontinence in women, *N Engl J Med* 358:1029, 2008.

Vapnek JM: Urinary incontinence: screening and treatment of urinary dysfunction, *Geriatrics* 56:25, 2001.

Zorc J, Kiddoo D, Shaw K: Diagnosis and management of pediatric urinary tract infections, *Clin Microbiol Rev* 18:417, 2005.

Urinary Problems in Females and Children

Common adult female urinary concerns include changes in usual urination patterns (frequency, urgency, nocturia, incontinence), changes in urine appearance (color, cloudiness), and pain (dysuria, flank pain, or suprapubic pain).

Urinary problems in adult females can be caused by infection, inflammation, calculi (stones), congenital malformation, or trauma. The majority of urinary tract infections (UTIs) are caused by gram-negative bacteria, predominantly *Escherichia coli*. The sexually transmitted pathogens *Chlamydia trachomatis*, *Neisseria gonorrhoeae*, and herpes simplex are common causes of urethritis. Vaginitis can also cause urinary symptoms in women. Urinary stones can occur anywhere in the urinary tract and are common causes of pain, bleeding, obstruction, and secondary infection.

In children, UTI is the second most common clinical disease of childhood, following respiratory tract disorders. The symptoms of urinary tract disorder may be vague or absent, making the diagnosis easily overlooked. Infection may be present without symptoms, with symptoms that are obviously related to the urinary system, or with symptoms that may divert attention to another organ system problem. Abdominal masses in the newborn are most frequently caused by renal enlargement, specifically dysplastic kidney and/or congenital hydronephrosis. Vesicoureteral reflux (VUR) is the major structural abnormality associated with UTI and renal damage.

Trauma to the urinary tract may be caused by penetrating, blunt, or crushing injuries, or by surgery or instrumentation. Hematuria, oliguria, and pain are the most common symptoms.

DIAGNOSTIC REASONING: FOCUSED HISTORY

Are there systemic or upper urinary tract symptoms present?

Key Questions

- Have you had a fever or chills?
- Have you had nausea or vomiting?
- Have you had acute pain in the abdomen or back?
- Are you positive for HIV infection? Are you receiving chemotherapy?
- In an infant: Has the infant been irritable or had anorexia or lethargy?

Fever and Chills

The presence of fever and chills suggests a systemic inflammatory response and indicates an acute condition that should be treated aggressively. Suspect pyelonephritis or lithiasis of the upper urinary system. UTI is the most common bacterial infection in febrile infants and children who present without an obvious source of infection.

Nausea and Vomiting

Nausea and vomiting often accompany upper UTI, pyelonephritis, or lithiasis. Like fever and chills, these symptoms suggest a systemic inflammatory response and indicate that the patient may be acutely ill. In newborns and infants, nonspecific symptoms, such as vomiting, diarrhea, and feeding difficulties, may indicate UTI.

Acute Pain

Acute pain in the back or abdomen suggests upper UTI and pyelonephritis. Flank pain occurs with stretching of the renal capsule associated with parenchymal swelling, and may indicate infection, obstruction, or primary renal disease.

Urinary tract stones may produce localized back pain or excruciating pain that often radiates to the thigh.

Immunocompromised Patients

Immunocompromised patients are susceptible to overwhelming infections by both common and atypical organisms, and aggressive investigation is warranted.

Irritable Infant

UTI in neonates and infants is manifested in subtle ways, such as irritability, anorexia, and weight loss. Some infants with UTI present with bacteremia.

Is there hematuria?

Key Questions

- Have you had blood in your urine? When in the stream does it occur?
- Do you have pain with urination?
- Do you have bleeding without urination?
- Have you done any strenuous exercise recently?

Hematuria

Red-to-brown discoloration is commonly caused by infection, trauma, or urinary tract stones. It can also be caused by parenchymal renal disease, systemic disease, medications, or coagulopathies.

Pyelonephritis or urinary tract stones are common causes of gross (macroscopic) hematuria. Neoplasm, trauma, and some medications can also produce gross hematuria. Gross hematuria occurs in 60% to 90% of bladder tumors. Both bladder and renal neoplasms are less common in women than in men. Hematuria can be produced by local irritation in cystitis. Platelet disorders and hemophilia can cause both gross and microscopic bleeding. Urinary frequency or urgency, dysuria, or suprapubic pain suggests that the origin of hematuria is confined to the lower urinary tract.

Initial hematuria (at the beginning of urination) suggests the urethra is the source, whereas terminal hematuria (at the end of urination) suggests posterior urethra or bladder base involvement. Total hematuria means red blood cells are dispersed throughout the urinary stream, characterizing origination in the kidney, ureter, or bladder.

Pain

Hematuria without pain is usually caused by renal disease or tumor of the bladder or kidney. Other causes of painless hematuria include stones, polycystic kidney disease, renal cysts, sickle cell disease, and hydronephrosis. When discomfort, such as renal colic, accompanies hematuria, suspect a ureteral stone. Hematuria with dysuria suggests bladder infection or lithiasis.

Bleeding Without Urination

Bladder lesions may produce bleeding independent of micturition.

Strenuous Exercise

Transient hematuria is frequent after strenuous exercise, and the amount of bleeding is proportional to the amount of exercise and the trauma sustained by the urinary tract. Exercise-related hematuria is caused by direct trauma to the kidneys and bladder, as well as by ischemic injury. It is caused by the shifting of blood flow from the renal circulation to the heart, lungs, and skeletal muscles during periods of high oxygen demand.

Can the symptoms be localized to the lower urinary tract?

Key Questions

- What are your primary symptoms (e.g., pain, frequency, urgency, small amounts of urine, nausea, nocturia, itching)?
- Have you had any suprapubic pain?
- Do you have involuntary urination?

Primary Symptoms

Dysuria suggests inflammation of the bladder neck or urethra, usually caused by bacterial infection or irritation that injures the bladder mucosa, leading to inflammatory changes, infiltration, and edema. These changes, from mild stretching of the bladder to a loss of bladder elasticity, can result in urgency and frequency.

Dysuria is the cardinal symptom of uncomplicated lower urinary tract infection (acute bacterial cystitis). In children, it may also be the first indication of an anatomical lesion such as obstruction of the urinary tract or VUR. Other common symptoms include frequency, mild nausea, nocturia, urgency, and voiding small amounts. Fever is notably absent. Infants may have strong-smelling urine and continuously damp diapers.

Dysuria also suggests urethritis, especially if accompanied by vaginal discharge. External dysuria, a burning sensation as the urine passes the inflamed labia, suggests vulvovaginitis. Patients with vulvovaginitis may also report discharge, odor, or itching. Women who have active herpes lesions may also experience external dysuria. Young children with pinworms (*Enterobius vermicularis*) may have dysuria and vaginitis because of the abrasions that result from periurethral and perivaginal itching and scratching.

Interstitial cystitis produces diminished bladder capacity along with symptoms of frequent painful urination. Hematuria may be present. Increased frequency can also occur as a result of stones or a tumor.

Suprapubic Discomfort and Urinary Incontinence

Discomfort in the suprapubic area is indicative of bladder involvement and urinary incontinence and is characteristic of bladder neck irritability caused by inflammation. Local causes of incontinence can also include pelvic relaxation and impaired bladder muscle activity. Preschool-age children with UTIs frequently have enuresis (see Chapter 31).

Could this be the result of trauma?

Key Questions

- Have you had any recent injury?
- Have you been hit recently?
- If a child: Have you noticed the child putting foreign objects in his or her genitourinary tract?

Recent Injury

Injury or a blow to the flank area can produce hematuria, originating from the kidney. Straddle injury may result in abrasions and local inflammation, causing pain on urination. About 5% of childhood trauma involves the kidney, making it a relatively uncommon event. About 10% of the injured kidneys have underlying abnormalities, such as hydronephrosis or a horseshoe shape, making them more vulnerable to injury.

Trauma

A victim of domestic violence may present with blood in the urine secondary to trauma. Trauma may or may not be associated with pain. Active children may not remember trauma to the area.

Foreign Objects

Children have a propensity to put foreign objects in any orifice. Placing foreign objects in the vagina can cause dysuria and pyuria.

Could this be genitourinary in origin?

Key Questions

- Are you sexually active? How frequently do you engage in sexual activity?
- Have you had a new sexual partner recently?
- How many sexual partners do you have?
- Does your sexual partner have any symptoms?
- Do you use a diaphragm?
- Do you have any vaginal discharge?
- If a postmenopausal woman: Are you on hormone replacement therapy?

Sexual Activity

Factors that contribute to the development of acute bacterial cystitis include frequent sexual intercourse, use of a diaphragm, and use of spermicidal gel for contraception. Urethritis is associated with a history of a new sexual partner, a partner with urethritis, and multiple sexual partners. Masturbation may also cause dysuria in girls, as a result of either local irritation or the introduction of organisms that produce a lower UTI.

Organisms from sexually transmitted infections can cause urethritis when they are present in large numbers in the urethra. A local inflammatory response results. *C. trachomatis* is the most common pathogen, although *N. gonorrhoeae*, *Trichomonas vaginalis*, and herpes simplex can also cause urethritis. Active herpes lesions can also produce dysuria as the urine passes across the inflamed external mucosa.

Diaphragm Use

Some women who use a diaphragm experience mechanical compression of the urethra, with subsequent urine retention that predisposes them to the development of cystitis.

Vaginal Discharge and Hormone Therapy

Vaginal infections are a common cause of dysuria, particularly in college-age women. Atrophic vaginitis can also cause dysuria. Postmenopausal women who are not on hormone therapy are more likely to have atrophic vaginitis.

Are there any specific risk factors to point me in the right direction?

Key Questions

- Have you had this or similar problems before? If yes, when and how many times?
- Have you had recent catheterization or urinary tract procedures performed?
- Is there a family history of kidney or urinary problems?
- Do you have diabetes?
- How much spicy food, caffeinated beverages/food, carbonated beverages, or alcohol do you consume?
- How much water do you drink?
- Do you suppress the urge to urinate (postpone urination)?
- Do you use bubble baths, shampoos, feminine hygiene products, powders, and soaps?
- Do you have constipation?

History of Similar Problems

Patients with previous urinary problems are at risk for chronic relapsing conditions, such as unresolved infections, resistant strains of organisms, or reinfection.

Recent Instrumentation

Recent instrumentation in the urinary tract places the patient at risk for infections.

Family History of Urinary Problems

A family history of renal or urinary tract problems places the patient at increased risk for urinary tract disorders. A family history of deafness or renal insufficiency suggests hereditary nephritis or Alport syndrome.

History of Diabetes Mellitus

Diabetes mellitus is associated with recurrent bacterial cystitis.

Types of Food Consumed

Dysuria without pyuria can be caused by chemical irritants such as spicy foods, caffeine, carbonation, and alcohol.

Decreased Fluid Intake

Decreased fluid intake and concentrated urine produce an irritant effect on bladder mucosa and may cause dysuria without pyuria. It can also predispose to the development of bacterial cystitis.

Urge To Urinate

Women who ignore the urge to urinate or who postpone urination are predisposed to the development of bacterial cystitis. Urine in the bladder for a prolonged period promotes bacterial growth.

Girls who have a history of squatting or leg crossing to stop urination may have a UTI. Uncontrolled bladder contractions against a closed bladder sphincter cause the behavior. These children may develop vesicoureteral reflux and infection.

Bubble Bath and Hygiene Products

Common chemical irritants can cause dysuria without infection. The most common irritant, particularly in children, is found in bubble baths.

Constipation

Mechanical factors related to compression of the bladder and bladder neck by a hard mass of stool from constipation may cause UTI. There is also a relationship between constipation and dysfunctional voiding accompanied by incomplete bladder emptying.

What else could this be?

Key Questions

- Have you had recent treatment for a sexually transmitted infection?
- Have you been diagnosed with, but not treated for, a sexually transmitted infection?
- Have you had excessive urination?
- Have you had a sore throat or been treated for strep throat recently?

Sexually Transmitted Infections

Because vaginitis can cause urinary tract symptoms in females, a sexually transmitted vaginitis may be producing symptoms. Recent treatment for a sexually transmitted infection may indicate treatment failure, a coinfection that was not covered by the prescribed drug, or a reinfection (see Chapter 34).

Excessive Urination

The presence of polyuria suggests diabetes mellitus or diabetes insipidus. Women with diabetes mellitus are also prone to development of UTIs.

Recent Streptococcal Infection

Poststreptococcal glomerulonephritis may develop after a 1- to 3-week latency period following pharyngeal or skin infections with certain strains of group A β-hemolytic *Streptococcus*. The peak incidence is at age 7.

DIAGNOSTIC REASONING: FOCUSED PHYSICAL EXAMINATION
Note General Appearance

A patient who appears ill or who is pacing in pain is likely to have an upper urinary tract problem, such as pyelonephritis or urolithiasis. Patients with lower urinary tract problems usually do not present with signs of systemic involvement, are free of fever, and generally appear well. Neonates present with malaise, irritability, and difficulty feeding. Toddlers and preschoolers appear ill with nausea, vomiting, and diarrhea.

Obtain Vital Signs, Height, and Weight

Failure to thrive is a common presenting sign of urinary tract disease in neonates or young children. Hypertension is seen in patients with nephritis.

Examine the Skin

Neonates with UTIs may present with jaundice.

Palpate and Percuss for Flank Pain and at the Costovertebral Angle Bilaterally

Pain that is reproducible is indicative of renal capsule distention and characterizes acute pyelonephritis or acute ureteral obstruction.

Palpate and Percuss the Abdomen

Polycystic kidneys may produce abdominal distention. A flank mass may indicate a hydronephrotic kidney. Pain in the lower quadrant indicates lower ureter involvement. Suprapubic tenderness is characteristic of lower UTI. Perform deep palpation to identify kidneys or other abdominal masses. Normal kidneys are usually not easily palpated. A distended bladder rises above the symphysis pubis and is characteristic of residual urine resulting from incomplete bladder emptying. Palpation of an enlarged bladder may cause pain. In hypertensive patients, auscultate at the subcostal anterior abdomen for bruits that could indicate a renovascular cause of hypertension.

Inspect the Perirectal Area

Inspect the skin and hair for inflammation, lesions, parasites, and dermatitis. Note inflammation, presence of lesions, or vaginal discharge. Observe for the presence of labial adhesions that might predispose the child to perineal bacterial colonization. Note personal hygiene. External excoriation could be the cause of burning or pain on urination. Note if there are any abrasions, tears, or bruising present, which might indicate trauma and/or sexual abuse.

Perform a Pelvic Examination If Indicated

A pelvic examination is essential if you suspect vaginitis or vulvovaginitis as a cause of the urinary tract symptom(s). On external examination, observe for bladder or uterine prolapse. On internal examination, note vaginal color, moistness, rugation, and characteristics of discharge. Pale, dry mucosa with lack of rugation characterizes atrophic vaginitis in a mature woman. Vaginal discharge not characteristic of physiological discharge suggests a vaginal infection. (For discussion of vulvovaginitis, see Chapter 34.) Determine rectal tone. An atonic anal sphincter suggests a neurogenic bladder. Rectal examination for fecal impaction is indicated if the history suggests significant constipation or encopresis.

LABORATORY AND DIAGNOSTIC STUDIES

The extent of diagnostic investigation is determined by the history and the findings of the examination. The symptoms reported by the patient are taken into account when ordering diagnostic tests to corroborate or verify the diagnosis. General screening tests can be used to provide additional data for patients with urinary tract problems.

Urine should be freshly voided and usually taken midstream. If not examined immediately, the specimen should be refrigerated because cells begin to disintegrate after 1 to 2 hours.

Urine Dipstick

Reagent strips can be used to screen urine in the clinical setting.

Specific Gravity

Urine specific gravity depends on the patient's hydration. The urine pH also depends on the level of hydration, as well as acid-base status, time of urine collection, diet, and drugs that may affect the urine pH.

Leukocyte Esterase

The leukocyte esterase strip is calibrated to turn purple in 60 seconds, indicating 5 or more white blood cells in the urine. A positive test is indicative of urethritis (75% to 90% sensitivity, 95% specificity). Urine that tests positive for leukocyte esterase should be cultured for bacteria. Vaginal infection with *Trichomonas* can produce false positive results; diets high in vitamin C can produce false negative results.

Nitrite

The nitrite strip is calibrated to turn pink within 30 seconds and signifies nitrite produced by 105 or more organisms/mL. Urine that tests positive for nitrites should be cultured for bacteria. However, note that some organisms that cause UTIs do not convert nitrates to nitrites (e.g., *Staphylococcus* and *Streptococcus*).

Protein

The normally small amount of protein excreted by a healthy adult is usually not detectable by dipstick analysis until the patient excretes 150 to 300 mg/day. At this level, the patient will show trace amounts. In healthy persons, urine contains no protein or only trace amounts of proteins, which consists of albumin and globulins from the plasma. Glomeruli usually prevent the passage of protein from the blood to the glomerular filtrate; therefore, the persistent presence of protein in urine is a strong indication of renal disease. If more than a trace amount of protein is found, then a quantitative 24-hour evaluation is necessary. False positive results can occur with alkaline urine.

If the patient has trace levels of proteinuria, then the use of 20% sulfosalicylic acid testing for protein is appropriate. Add 8 drops of 20% sulfosalicylic acid to a sample of fresh, concentrated urine. Protein concentration is directly proportional to the degree of white turbidity produced. The absence of white turbidity indicates a false positive result by dipstick analysis.

A typical scale to indicate progressively increasing amounts of protein is 1+ (30 mg/dL), 2+ (100 mg/dL), 3+ (300 mg/dL), and 4+ (500 to 1000 mg/dL). Peripheral edema and ascites may be present in an adult who has 3+ or 4+ proteinuria, and is typically excreting 3 g or more of protein per day. Proteinuria reported for a single urinalysis is not an absolute guide in a differential diagnosis because proteinuria may be glomerular or tubular.

Glucose

Glucose in the urine is indicative of an elevated serum glucose concentration greater than 200 mg/dL. If serum glucose levels are normal while urine glucose level is elevated, then proximal renal tubular damage should be suspected.

Ketones

Ketones are detected earlier in the urine than in the blood and may indicate starvation or diabetic ketoacidosis.

Blood

Reagent strips are calibrated to detect the red blood cells (RBCs) that are present. The strip detects heme at 0.05 to 0.3 mg of hemoglobin/dL (see later paragraph titled Red Blood Cells).

Urinalysis with Microscopic Examination
Color

The urine should be clear to yellow, depending on the concentration. The precipitation of calcium phosphate or urates can turn the urine milky, especially when stored in the refrigerator. Warming the urine to body temperature causes these precipitated salts to return to solution, removing the milky appearance. Methylene blue and indigo blue can make the urine blue. Vegetable dyes and paint from toys ingested by young children can turn their urine various colors. Brown urine is often observed in glomerulonephritis. Turbidity with a foul odor indicates infection. Color changes of the urine may result from various sources: hemoglobin from systemic red blood cell lysis; myoglobin from damaged muscle cells or rhabdomyolysis; vegetable pigments from food, such as red beets; pigments from drugs, such as rifampin and phenazopyridine; or porphyrins from porphyria.

Discoloration of the urine should be investigated with microscopic examination to determine if RBCs or any foreign substances are present. Pyuria results from white blood cell (WBC) debris and leukocytes in the urine, but cloudy urine can also result from other causes.

Sediment

Sediment from casts, blood cells, and bacteria can be detected by microscopic examination. Casts indicate hemorrhage or various conditions of the nephron. RBCs indicate acute inflammatory or vascular disorders of the glomerulus. More than 1 or 2 RBCs per high-power field (HPF) is abnormal and can indicate renal or systemic disease or trauma to the kidney. Sediment is labeled as active when an abnormal number of cells, tubular casts, crystals, or infectious organisms are found.

A healthy person's urinalysis usually contains no cells, although an occasional cell per HPF is seen. More than 1 tubular epithelial and transitional epithelial cell per HPF suggests damage to the tubules or bladder wall. More than 1 RBC or WBC per HPF is considered abnormal. The more cells per HPF, the more active may be the renal disease.

Microscopic examination of the urine resulting in 20 or more organisms per HPF indicates UTI. Fewer than 20 organisms per HPF merits further study such as culture and sensitivity (C & S).

Red Blood Cells

Hematuria is the presence of more than 3 RBCs/HPF. Distorted, irregularly shaped cells suggest a glomerular problem. The major causes of hematuria include acute and chronic prostatitis or urethritis, hemorrhagic cystitis, renal stones, or tumors of the kidney, renal pelvis, ureter, bladder, and urethra. Hematuria with proteinuria usually suggests a renal origin. Isolated hematuria is usually produced by sites outside the kidneys.

White Blood Cells

Pyuria (>5 WBCs/HPF) is highly sensitive for the presence of a UTI. However, it may occur with dehydration, renal stones, appendicitis, or other extrinsic ureteral irritation in the absence of demonstrable microbial infection.

Casts

Tubular casts are formed in the distal portion of the nephron. A hyaline cast is a wispy, translucent, cylindrical replica of the tubular lumen. Red cell casts are characteristic of glomerular origin. The presence of abnormal cells, protein, hemoglobin, myoglobin, or other debris with a cast helps identify the type of renal disease.

Urine Culture and Sensitivity

Culture is indicated in children if you are uncertain of a diagnosis of uncomplicated lower tract UTI based on clinical findings and urinalysis, or if the patient has signs and symptoms of an upper UTI or complicated UTI.

Potassium Hydroxide and Wet Mount/ Preparation

Perform these procedures if you suspect vulvovaginitis as a cause of the urinary tract symptoms. See Chapter 34 for an explanation and a discussion of these procedures.

Vaginal Culture/DNA Testing for Infectious Organisms

Use these testing procedures to diagnose or confirm vaginal infection (see Chapter 34).

Ultrasonography

Ultrasonography is a noninvasive technique that can provide information about the kidneys, ureters, bladder, and vascular structures. Renal ultrasound is a good first test to determine kidney size, contour, and the presence of calculi. Urinary bladder sonogram is used to identify tumors of the bladder, thickening of the bladder wall, posterior masses behind the bladder, or obstruction of the lower urinary tract showing residual urine.

Radiography

A flat plate of the abdomen can be used to identify structures of the kidney, ureters, and bladder. Urinary calculi are usually visible on radiographs.

Computed Tomography

Noncontrast helical (spiral) CT is the gold standard for evaluating kidney stones. It has 95% sensitivity and 98% specificity.

DIFFERENTIAL DIAGNOSIS
Uncomplicated Urinary Tract Infection

Uncomplicated lower UTIs (or bacterial cystitis) are common in women. Uncomplicated UTIs occur in individuals with normal urinary tract anatomy and function. Patients present with dysuria and may have urinary frequency, hematuria, back pain, mild nausea, nocturia, urgency, and voiding of small amounts. Fever is notably absent in adults but may be present in pediatric patients. Neonates may present with prolonged jaundice and failure to thrive.

The adult patient appears well on physical examination and may or may not have costovertebral angle (CVA) tenderness. Clinical diagnosis is supported by urine dipstick findings, which may include the presence of blood, leukocyte esterase, and nitrites. However, a negative dipstick result does not rule out UTI. Microscopic analysis may show the presence of RBCs and WBCs. No casts will be present. Urine culture and sensitivity will confirm the diagnosis. See the Evidence-Based Practice boxes for evidence supporting the diagnosis of UTI in adults or children.

Urethritis

Dysuria suggests urethritis, especially if accompanied by vaginal discharge. The history often includes a new sex partner, frequent sex, a partner with urethritis, or multiple sex partners. As with uncomplicated UTI, the patient appears well and on physical examination has no CVA tenderness or fever. On urinalysis using a dipstick, findings may include the presence of blood, leukocyte esterase, and nitrites, although the patient may have urethritis in the absence of these findings. Urine culture or DNA testing confirms the presence of the offending pathogens, usually *Chlamydia*, *N. gonorrhoeae*, *Trichomonas*, and herpes.

Vulvovaginitis

Vulvovaginitis is a common cause of dysuria. The patient often describes the dysuria as "external"—a burning sensation as the urine passes inflamed labia.

◎ EVIDENCE-BASED PRACTICE   *Diagnosing Uncomplicated UTI in Adults*

In a systematic review, Bent et al (2002) report four symptoms (dysuria, frequency, hematuria, and back pain) and one sign (costovertebral angle tenderness) that significantly increase the probability of uncomplicated UTI. In women who present with one or more of these symptoms, the probability of infection is about 50%. Specific combinations of symptoms, such as dysuria and frequency without vaginal discharge and irritation, raise the probability of UTI to more than 90%. If the dipstick result is positive, the probability of UTI is high, but if the dipstick result is negative, the probability of

UTI is still high and a urine culture should be considered to rule out infection. The absence of dysuria, the absence of back pain, a history of vaginal discharge and irritation, and the presence of vaginal discharge on examination significantly decrease the probability of UTI.

Conclusion: History alone may effectively rule in the diagnosis of uncomplicated UTI. However, the history and physical examination and dipstick urinalysis cannot reliably rule out UTI in women who present with urinary tract symptoms.

Data from Bent S, Nallamothu BK, Simel DL, Fihn SD, Saint S: Does this woman have an acute uncomplicated urinary tract infection? *JAMA* 287:2701, 2002.

◎ EVIDENCE-BASED PRACTICE   *Diagnosing UTI in Infants and Children*

A meta-analysis performed by Shaihk et al (2007) offers insight into the diagnosis of UTI in infants and children based on clinical examination and urine dipstick. Although certain signs and symptoms (high fever, fever for 24 hours, history of a previous UTI, abdominal pain, nonblack race, lack of circumcision, back pain, dysuria, frequency, new-onset urinary incontinence, suprapubic tenderness, and absence of another source of fever on examination) increase the probability of UTI, no single sign or symptom has a sufficiently high likelihood ratio

to definitively diagnose UTI or sufficiently small likelihood ratio to rule out UTI. A urine dip positive for both nitrites and leukocyte esterase substantially increases the likelihood of UTI. Accordingly, a positive dipstick test should always be followed up with a confirmatory urine culture.

The bottom line: Although no sign or symptom by itself is diagnostic of UTI in children, the absence of several key signs and symptoms in combination can be used to identify infants at low risk for UTI.

Data from Shaikh N, Morone NE, Lopez J, Chianese J, Sangvai S, D'Amico F et al: Does this child have a urinary tract infection? *JAMA* 298:2895, 2007.

The patient usually has a history of vaginal discharge, odor, and/or itching. On physical examination, discharge is usually present in the vagina or from the cervix. Wet mount, KOH, and vaginal culture or molecular testing for infectious organisms can confirm the diagnosis (see Chapter 34).

In older women, atrophic vaginitis may produce urinary tract symptoms. These women may be perimenopausal or postmenopausal. Women with atrophic vaginitis may report vaginal dryness or discomfort during sexual intercourse. On physical examination, the vaginal mucosa is thin, pale, and dry, with less rugation. Diagnosis is made on the basis of clinical findings.

Interstitial Cystitis

Interstitial cystitis produces diminished bladder capacity along with symptoms of frequent, painful urination. Hematuria may be present. The cause is unknown but may be related to collagen disease, may be an autoimmune disorder or an allergic manifestation, or may occur secondary to an unidentified infectious agent. The bladder wall becomes inflamed, with mucosal ulceration and scarring that produce contraction of the smooth muscle and cause the symptoms. Middle-age women are most often affected. Typically, the patient appears well and has no physical findings. Suprapubic tenderness may be present. Urinalysis is usually negative. This is a diagnosis of exclusion, and the patient is often frustrated because no cause has been previously found for her long-standing and persistent symptoms. The patient has no evidence of urological disease on radiographic and cystometric studies. Cystoscopic evidence of interstitial disease includes focal ulceration, edema, and perivascular infiltrates.

Pyelonephritis

The patient presents with fever and chills, appears toxic, and reports back pain. Nausea and vomiting may be present. Some patients also report lower urinary tract symptoms, including frequency and dysuria. The patient feels and looks ill. On physical examination, CVA tenderness is usually present. The abdomen may also be tender. On microscopic examination, WBCs are usually present. White cell casts suggest pyelonephritis. Bacterial casts, although rare, are pathognomonic of pyelonephritis.

A urine culture and sensitivity test confirms the diagnosis and identifies the pathogen—usually *E. coli*, *Klebsiella*, *Proteus mirabilis*, or *Enterobacter*.

Urolithiasis

Urinary stones can occur anywhere in the urinary tract and may produce symptoms of acute pain, hematuria, and secondary infection. Many calculi are "silent" and may cause only hematuria, either microscopic or gross. Renal calculi may occur when a stone obstructs the urinary tract. Typical symptoms of renal colic include severe flank pain that radiates along the pathway of the ureter to the inner thigh. Chills, fever, and urinary frequency are common. The patient may have nausea, vomiting, and abdominal distention.

The clinical diagnosis is supported by urinalysis and imaging findings. The urine may be normal; however, gross or microscopic hematuria is common. Pyuria (WBCs) with or without bacteria may be present. Crystalline structures may be present. Noncontrast helical (spiral) CT is the gold standard for evaluating kidney stones.

Poststreptococcal Glomerulonephritis

This condition is an immune-mediated nephritis. It occurs most commonly in elementary school children. There is a history of recent streptococcal skin or pharyngeal infection within the past 1 to 3 weeks. Anorexia, vomiting, fever, abdominal pain, headache, and lethargy are reported. On physical examination, periorbital edema is usually present, as is hypertension. Orthopnea, dyspnea, cough, and rales may be present. Hematuria and proteinuria are present. A positive serum ASO titer confirms recent infection. A depressed serum concentration of C3 is found in the first few days of the disease.

Chemical Irritation

There is a history of the use of bubble baths, body lotions, soaps, and sprays. The patient experiences frequency, burning, and urgency with small volumes of voided urine. Children will frequently suppress voiding because of pain. Physical examination may reveal erythema of the labia and urethral outlet. Laboratory examination may reveal pyuria and bacteriuria as a result of local infection and denudation.

DIFFERENTIAL DIAGNOSIS OF *Common Causes of Urinary Problems in Females and Children*

CONDITION	HISTORY	PHYSICAL FINDINGS	DIAGNOSTIC STUDIES
Uncomplicated UTI	Dysuria, frequency, mild nausea, nocturia, urgency, voiding small amounts; neonates and young infants present with anorexia and irritability	No fever in adults; appears well; no CVA tenderness; may have suprapubic tenderness; neonates and young infants may present with failure to thrive, bacteremia and fever	Urine dipstick: + blood, + leukocyte esterase, + nitrites; microscopic analysis: RBCs, WBCs, no casts; urine C & S; in children, voiding cystourethrogram and renal ultrasound are recommended
Urethritis	Dysuria; vaginal discharge; history of new sex partner, frequent sex, partner with urethritis, multiple sex partners	Appears well; has no CVA tenderness or fever	Urine dipstick: may have + blood, + leukocyte esterase, + nitrites; urine culture; DNA testing vaginal specimen
Vulvovaginitis	History of vaginal itching, discharge, burning, dryness; postmenopausal	Inflamed or atrophic labia; vaginal or cervical discharge	Microscopic exam, vaginal cultures, molecular testing
Interstitial cystitis	Frequent painful urination; hematuria; most often middle-age women; often frustrated because no cause has been previously found for long-standing and persistent symptoms	Appears well and has no physical findings; supra-pubic tenderness may be present	Urinalysis usually negative; x-ray and cystometric studies to rule out other urological disease; cystoscopy
Pyelonephritis	Fever, chills, back pain, nausea and vomiting, toxic appearance; some patients also have fre-quency and dysuria	Feels and looks ill; fever; CVA tenderness; abdomen may be tender	Urine dipstick: + blood, + leukocyte esterase, + nitrites; microscopic examination: WBCs may have white cell casts or bacterial casts; urine C & S: *E. coli*, *Klebsiella*, *Proteus mirabilis*, *Enterobacter*; blood cultures
Urolithiasis	Pain, hematuria; may have symptoms of secondary infection; renal colic: pain that radiates to inner thigh; nausea, vomiting	May have CVA tenderness; looks ill during periods of acute pain; may have abdominal distention	Urinalysis: gross or microscopic hematuria; WBCs with or without bacteria; crystalline structures may be present; noncontrast helical CT
Poststreptococcal glomerulonephritis	History of skin or throat infection 1-3 weeks prior; lethargy, anorexia, vomiting, abdominal pain	Hypertension, periorbital edema, CVA tenderness; may have dyspnea, cough, pallor	U/A: + proteinuria, + hema-turia, + ASO titer; serum C3 low early in disease
Chemical irritation	History of bubble baths, soaps, lotions, sprays; urgency, dysuria	No fever; erythematous labia, urethral opening	Hematuria common, gross hematuria unusual and casts never seen

C & S, culture and sensitivity; *CT*, computed tomography; *CVA*, costovertebral angle; *RBC*, red blood cell; *U/A*, urinalysis; *UTI*, urinary tract infection; *WBC*, white blood cell.

REFERENCES AND READINGS

Bent S, Nallamothu BK, Simel DL, Fihn SD, Saint S: Does this woman have an acute uncomplicated urinary tract infection? *JAMA* 287:2701, 2002.

Bent S, Saint S: The optimal use of diagnostic testing in women with acute uncomplicated cystitis, *Am J Med* 113:20, 2002.

Bremnor JD, Sadovsky R: Evaluation of dysuria in adults, *Am Fam Phys* 65:1589, 2002.

Colgan R, Lindsay E, Nicolle LE, Mcglone A, Hooton TM: Asymptomatic bacteriuria in adults, *Am Fam Phys* 74:985, 2006.

Ebell MH: Treating adult women with suspected UTI, *Am Fam Phys* 73:293, 2006.

Grabe M, Bishop MC, Bjerklund-Johansen TE, Botto H, Çek M, Lobel B et al: Uncomplicated urinary tract infections in adults. In: *Guidelines on urological infections*. Arnhem, The Netherlands: European Association of Urology (EAU): 11-38, 2009. Available at www.guidelines.gov. Accessed May 28, 2010.

Graham K, Levy J: Enuresis, *Pediatr Rev* 30:165, 2009.

Grossfeld GD, Wolf JS Jr, Litwan MS, Hricak H, Shuler CL, Agerter DC et al: Asymptomatic microscopic hematuria in adults: summary of the AUA best practice policy recommendations, *Am Fam Physician* 63:1145, 2001.

Heffner V, Gorelick M: Pediatric urinary tract infection, *Clin Ped Emerg Med* 9:233, 2008.

Lindbloom EJ: What is the best test to diagnose urinary tract stones? *J Fam Pract* 50:657, 2001.

Meyers K: Evaluation of hematuria in children, *Urol Clin North Am* 31:559, 2004.

Portis AJ, Sundaram CP: Diagnosis and initial management of kidney stones, *Am Fam Physician* 63:1329, 2001.

Roberts KB: The AAP practice parameter on urinary tract infections in febrile infants and young children. American Academy of Pediatrics, *Am Fam Physician* 62:1815, 2000.

Vaginal Bleeding

The average menstrual cycle is 28 days. It is considered abnormal if the cycle occurs more often than every 21 days (polymenorrhea) or less often than every 35 days (oligomenorrhea). Bleeding at irregular intervals is known as metrorrhagia. Intermenstrual bleeding is bleeding between cycles. The average duration of menses is 4 days; a duration of longer than 7 days or blood loss heavier than 80 mL is considered excessive and is classified as menorrhagia. Hypomenorrhea occurs when the frequency of periods remains normal but the menstrual flow decreases in amount. Systemic disorders that cause an imbalance in the hypothalamic-pituitary-ovarian (HPO) axis may lead to menses that are too heavy (menorrhagia/hypermenorrhea), too often (polymenorrhea), or too heavy and irregular (menometrorrhagia).

Other systemic reasons for vaginal bleeding include blood dyscrasias, liver and kidney diseases, and medications (e.g., hormones, anticoagulants, and nonsteroidal anti-inflammatory drugs [NSAIDs]). Organic causes for aberrant menstrual cycles are multiple and include problems such as vaginitis, ectopic pregnancy, fibroids, and polyps. Vaginal bleeding in perimenopausal and postmenopausal women may indicate gynecological cancer. When organic and systemic reasons for abnormal vaginal bleeding are not found, the diagnosis of dysfunctional uterine bleeding (DUB) is warranted.

DIAGNOSTIC REASONING: FOCUSED HISTORY

Is this an acute condition that requires immediate intervention?

Key Questions

- How heavy is the bleeding?
- Do you have a bleeding disorder?
- Are you taking anticoagulants?

Patients who have profuse bleeding, have had substantial blood loss, or are hemodynamically unstable require immediate intervention.

Amount of Bleeding

More than three soaked pads or six full regular-absorbency tampons a day for 3 or more days likely equates to greater than 80 mL of blood loss (Brown, 2005). A history of flooding, clots, or leaking, especially overnight, may be associated with a clotting disorder.

Bleeding Disorder/Anticoagulants

Severe acute uterine bleeding in a nonpregnant patient usually occurs as the result of a coagulopathy or from taking anticoagulants. Women with submucous fibroids can also present with profuse bleeding.

Could this be related to pregnancy?

Key Questions

- Do you have any symptoms of pregnancy (e.g., missed period, breast tenderness, nausea, vomiting)?
- When was your last normal menstrual period?
- What are you using for birth control?
- Have you recently delivered a baby?

Pregnancy

A small amount of bleeding can occur at the time of implantation. The blastocyst burrows into the endometrium and invades the maternal blood supply; the formation and implantation of the placenta follow. If bleeding occurs from implantation, it happens about 1 week before the expected menstrual cycle. Regard women of childbearing age as pregnant until pregnancy is ruled out. It is estimated that up to 50% of all fertilized eggs die and are aborted spontaneously, usually before the woman knows she is pregnant. About 20% of pregnant women have some vaginal bleeding during the first trimester.

Recent Delivery

If the patient has recently delivered a baby, the abnormal vaginal bleeding is likely from retained placenta, infection of the uterus (endometritis), or a laceration.

If the patient is pregnant, is this a complication?

Key Questions

- How old are you?
- How many weeks pregnant are you?
- Do you have any chronic health problems?
- Are you experiencing any pain or cramping?
- Have you passed any tissue?
- Are you having any other symptoms?
- Have you ever had a sexually transmitted infection?
- Have you ever had an infection of your tubes (pelvic inflammatory disease [PID])?
- Have you ever been pregnant before this? What were the number of times and outcomes of your pregnancies?

Age

The risk for spontaneous abortion is higher in women older than age 35 years. Most ectopic pregnancies occur in women ages 25 to 34 years. However, women older than age 35 have a higher rate of death from ectopic pregnancy.

Weeks of Gestation

Among known pregnancies, the rate of spontaneous abortion is approximately 10% and usually occurs between the seventh and twelfth weeks of pregnancy. An estimated 10% to 15% of clinically recognized pregnancies result in first trimester loss. The patient experiencing an ectopic pregnancy typically presents at about 6 to 8 weeks of gestation.

Chronic Health Conditions

The risk for spontaneous abortion is higher in women with systemic diseases, such as diabetes or thyroid problems.

Pain

Low back pain or abdominal pain that is dull, sharp, or cramping may indicate spontaneous abortion or ectopic pregnancy. If there is pain associated with ectopic pregnancy, it will usually be described as "crampy," pelvic pressure, or "soreness" in the lower abdomen.

In ectopic pregnancy, the pain may lateralize to one side. Severe, sharp, and sudden pain in the lower abdominal area may indicate rupture of the ectopic pregnancy. **Ruptured ectopic pregnancy is a surgical emergency.**

Passing Tissue

The passage of tissue from the vagina suggests spontaneous abortion. Ectopic pregnancies can be accompanied by sloughing material.

Other Symptoms

Pain referred to the shoulder is suggestive of ectopic pregnancy rupture with peritoneal free fluid and significant hemorrhage. Other symptoms of rupture include feeling dizzy or faint, or actually fainting.

Sexually Transmitted Infection

Sexually transmitted infections (STIs) that have been unnoticed, untreated, or inadequately treated can cause scarring of the fallopian tubes, which is associated with greater risk for ectopic pregnancy. Ectopic pregnancy occurs in about 1 of every 200 pregnancies (Box 33-1). However, if the woman has had PID, the rate is as high as 1 of every 40 pregnancies.

Box 33-1	**Risk Factors for Ectopic Pregnancy**

History of PID
Previous ectopic pregnancy
History of tubal surgery
Infertility
In utero diethylstilbestrol exposure
Present use of IUD
Smoking

Previous Pregnancies

The risk for spontaneous abortion is higher in women older than age 35 and in women with a history of three or more prior spontaneous abortions.

Is this related to age? Where is the woman in her reproductive life cycle?

Key Questions

- How old are you?
- Are you postmenopausal?

Age

Knowing a woman's age can help focus the differential diagnosis. The majority of adolescents with abnormal bleeding experience anovulatory cycles caused when estrogen stimulates the uterine lining with no opposing progesterone. This condition leads to a thicker, more vascular, and less stable endometrium, predisposing the adolescent to dyssynchronous bleeding. A young woman's bleeding is most frequently caused by pregnancy, contraceptive methods, or infection. Women over age 40 are more likely to have problems related to polyps, fibroids, or ovarian dysfunction.

Postmenopause

If a woman is postmenopausal, the origin of bleeding irregularities is often hormone therapy (HT), endometrial hyperplasia, or endometrial cancer (see section on postmenopausal bleeding).

What does the character of the bleeding tell me?

Key Questions

- When did the bleeding begin?
- How long have you been bleeding?
- What is the flow like?
- How many pads do you use?
- Are there any accompanying problems?

Symptom Analysis

Determine the amount of flow and its duration to establish if there is menorrhagia, metrorrhagia, or menometrorrhagia. Menorrhagia is considered to be 80 mL of menses, which is estimated as saturating a sanitary pad hourly, over several hours. Metrorrhagia is defined as bleeding at irregular intervals or intermenstrual bleeding. When the menstruation has an unpredictable schedule and lasts for a prolonged time, it is termed menometrorrhagia.

Associated Complaints

Patients may experience postcoital bleeding with cervical infections, cervical polyps, or cervical cancer. Accompanying dyspareunia may indicate endometriosis. Dysmenorrhea can be caused by an intrauterine device (IUD) or adenomyosis. Pelvic pressure or pain is suspicious for persistent corpus luteum cyst. Uterine prolapse causes pelvic pressure, which

is subjectively described as "something falling out of the vagina." Fever is associated with a pelvic infection. Menorrhagia, accompanied by fatigue, weight gain, hair loss, cold intolerance, decreased libido, and constipation, is a symptom of hypothyroidism. Bleeding disorders may become apparent for the first time in the teenager, with severe menorrhagia accompanied by bruising, petechiae, and gingival bleeding.

Is this problem acute or chronic? How does it compare with usual menses?

Key Questions

- Has this kind of vaginal bleeding occurred before?
- Were your periods regular before this episode?
- How long did they last?
- What was the amount and pattern of bleeding?

Irregular Menses

In anovulatory cycles, the endometrium proliferates under the influence of high estrogen levels until it can no longer be supported—then bleeding occurs. This results in a menstrual pattern that is longer than 28 days with a very heavy flow that lasts 7 to 14 days. If the patient's estrogen levels are fluctuating, she may have two periods a month. Both of these patterns are consistent with DUB. However, organic problems with any component of the reproductive tract must be ruled out.

Acute Bleeding

One episode of acute bleeding in a woman with normally regular menstrual cycles suggests uterine fibroids or a complication of pregnancy, such as threatened abortion. In a postmenopausal woman with an intact uterus, an episode of vaginal bleeding is indicative of endometrial hyperplasia and is suspicious for endometrial cancer.

Chronic Bleeding

Chronic, irregular menstrual cycles coupled with obesity are likely to be caused by polycystic ovary syndrome (PCOS), also known as Stein-Leventhal syndrome. Chronic midcycle spotting can occur secondary to the normal midcycle drop in estrogen levels and usually is not bothersome to the patient because the amount of vaginal bleeding is very scant and the duration is short.

Could this be caused by the patient's birth control method?

Key Questions

- Do you use birth control?
- Which kind(s) of birth control do you use?
- How do you use it?

Birth Control

Menorrhagia from IUD contraception is accompanied by increased cramping and pain. If spotting or cramping is not of a usual pattern, ectopic pregnancy or infection must be considered. Displacement or perforation of the uterus by the IUD can be verified by pelvic ultrasound. Women who have recently discontinued the use of oral contraceptive (OC) pills after several years of use may experience heavier menstrual bleeding than when they were on OC pills. Breakthrough bleeding caused by OC pills may occur in the first 2 weeks of the cycle because of low estrogen level or in the last 2 weeks because of low progesterone level. Long-acting progestin contraceptives (Norplant) may cause irregular heavy menses because there is a lack of estrogen to stabilize the endometrium. Changes in bleeding patterns for progestin users necessitate ruling out pregnancy.

Is this prepubertal bleeding?

Key Questions

- How old is the child?
- Is there a family history of early sexual development?
- Is there a family history of bleeding problems or blood dyscrasias?
- Did the child ingest any birth control pills or estrogens?
- Are there any accompanying symptoms?

Pediatric Vaginal Bleeding

In the United States, the average age of menarche is 12 years old. Vaginal bleeding before age 9 is abnormal and may indicate foreign body or injury. The presence of secondary sexual characteristics indicates sexual precocity. Newborn girls may experience breast bud enlargement, galactorrhea, and a small amount of vaginal bleeding from maternal exogenous hormones. These symptoms resolve without intervention within a few weeks.

Although uncommon, malignant genital tract tumors in girls can cause vaginal bleeding. Vaginal adenosis and adenocarcinoma are the most common tumor types.

Bleeding Problems

A family history of bleeding problems or a positive review of systems and physical examination indicating the presence of petechiae or bruises suggests a bleeding tendency. Platelet counts or clotting studies are indicated.

Accompanying Symptoms

Vulvovaginitis is the most common pediatric gynecological problem. Vaginal discharge, vaginal itching, vulvar erythema, and lesions often accompany vulvovaginal bleeding. A foul-smelling discharge is noted with bacterial vaginosis, trichomoniasis, and a foreign body. Wet mounts and cultures should be taken for all vaginal discharges of a child, including cultures for gonorrhea and *Chlamydia*. If a sexually transmitted infection (STI) or sexual abuse is suspected, syphilis and human immunodeficiency virus (HIV) testing should be done. Throat and rectal cultures for gonorrhea and *Chlamydia* should also be obtained.

Trauma to the perineum is more common in children because there is less subcutaneous fat of the vulva. Large lacerations and hematomas warrant referral for examination and repair under anesthesia.

Prolapse of the urethra may cause bleeding. It is accompanied by pain at the meatus and pain with urination.

Is the patient experiencing anovulatory cycles?

Key Questions

- Have you experienced irregular menstrual cycles?
- Are you having symptoms of menopause (e.g., vaginal dryness, hot flashes, night sweats)?
- At what age did your mother or grandmother go through menopause?

Irregular Menstrual Cycles

Anovulatory cycles are the most common cause of irregular bleeding patterns among females beginning (adolescent) or ending (perimenopausal) their menstrual cycles. It is estimated that 80% of young adolescents will be anovulatory during the first year of menstruation. Regular ovulatory cycles are usually established by the second year of menses but may take up to 5 years.

Menopause Symptoms

The hot flash is the most commonly experienced symptom of menopause. It is a sensation of increased upper body warmth that begins in the chest area and progresses upward to the neck and face. Sweating, which can be so profuse as to leave clothing wet, follows the hot flash. Hot flashes often lead to disturbed sleep patterns, insomnia, and fatigue. Vaginal atrophy is experienced by the patient as vaginal dryness, dyspareunia, and atrophic vaginitis (see Chapter 34). Atrophic changes can affect the urinary system, causing urinary frequency, urgency, and exacerbation of stress incontinence.

Menopausal Syndrome

The frequency of monthly ovulation becomes irregular at about 40 years of age, and this leads to intermittent symptoms of menopause. The time frame from onset of symptoms to complete cessation of menstruation is termed the perimenopause or climacteric phase. The perimenopause phase can last up to 10 years. If menopause is completed before age 40, it is considered premature ovarian failure. The age of menopause is genetically determined and will be similar to those of the woman's mother and grandmother. Menopause is unrelated to age of menarche, pregnancies, or contraceptive methods used.

Is the patient experiencing postmenopausal bleeding?

Key Questions

- How old were you when you stopped menstruating?
- Do you still have a uterus?
- Did you have a hysterectomy? Why did you have surgery? Were your ovaries removed?
- Are you using hormones?

Age at Menopause

The average age for a woman in the United States to go through menopause is 51 years. Menopause is defined as 1 year without menstrual cycles. However, a diagnosis can be accurately made earlier by measuring the rising follicle-stimulating hormone (FSH) and the falling estradiol levels. Postmenopausal bleeding is any bleeding that occurs after the establishment of menopause. Vaginal bleeding after menopause warrants investigation to rule out endometrial cancer. Box 33-2 lists risk factors for endometrial cancer.

Intact Uterus

In postmenopausal women with an intact uterus, unexplained vaginal bleeding suggests endometrial hyperplasia with a suspicion for endometrial cancer.

Hysterectomy

Any vaginal bleeding after a hysterectomy justifies suspicion of cancer, but the bleeding will most likely be a symptom of atrophic vaginitis. If the ovaries were left in place at the time of the hysterectomy, the woman may not experience menopausal syndrome until about 8 to 10 years after the surgery. The ovaries become atrophic and nonfunctional over time, probably secondary to altered blood flow resulting from the surgery. The bleeding of atrophic vaginitis occurs from the slightest trauma; even wiping the perineum with tissue after urination can cause spotting.

Hormone Therapy

Hormone therapy for menopausal symptoms may cause vaginal bleeding in women with an intact uterus. Regimens for women with an intact uterus include the cycling of estrogen and progestin and continuous daily doses of both hormones. The cycled hormones produce a regular scheduled bleeding. However, the continuous daily combination therapy will often cause amenorrhea after 3 to 6 months of use. After a pattern of amenorrhea has been established, new bleeding should be investigated.

Unopposed estrogen therapy in a woman with an intact uterus predisposes her to endometrial cancer

Box 33-2	**Risk Factors for Endometrial Cancer**

Postmenopausal with intact uterus and abnormal vaginal bleeding
Family history of endometrial cancer
Hypertension, diabetes mellitus, liver disease
Obesity
Chronic anovulatory cycles
Unopposed estrogen therapy with intact uterus
Tamoxifen therapy

from a thick, built-up endometrium. Endometrial hyperplasia accounts for about 20% of postmenopausal women who report abnormal vaginal bleeding. Endometrial hyperplasia can be diagnosed with endometrial biopsy, ultrasonography, or dilation and curettage (D&C).

Vaginal bleeding can also be caused by a cancerous cervical lesion (diagnosed with colposcopy and biopsy), cervical polyps, or endometrial polyps. Ovarian tumors can excrete estrogens and progestins, causing vaginal bleeding. Fallopian tube cancer more commonly presents with scant vaginal bleeding or watery vaginal discharge and a pelvic mass.

Could this be from infection or inflammation?

Key Questions

- Have you noticed any sores, rashes, or lumps in the vaginal area?
- Do you have vaginal discharge or vulvar itching or burning?
- What were the results of your last Papanicolaou test?

Lesions and Lumps

Genital warts (condylomata acuminata) can cause bleeding secondary to trauma that has been induced. Typically, genital warts are located inferiorly from the fossa navicularis to the fourchette and perineal area and internally on the walls of the vagina and cervix. A painless ulcer suggests syphilis and classically appears as a solitary lesion; however, there can be more than one chancre, especially if the patient is immunocompromised. Lesions secondarily infected by bacteria may bleed. Inguinal lymphadenopathy can signal a sexually transmitted infection of the genitourinary tract.

Vaginal Discharge

Acute or chronic endometritis and PID may cause heavy menstrual bleeding. An endometrial infection disturbs the clotting properties, resulting in painful, heavy bleeding. *Chlamydia* and gonorrhea are the most frequent causes of PID.

Last Pap Test

The last Pap test result may provide clues to a chronic vaginal infection showing a predominance of coccobacilli or atrophy with inflammation; a progressive, low-grade, squamous, intraepithelial lesion; or a cancerous condition. However, the accuracy of a normal Pap test is unreliable if a cervical lesion or abnormal cervical vascular patterns are noted on physical examination.

What other causes of bleeding should I consider?

Key Questions

- Could this bleeding be from the urethra or rectum?
- Are you taking tamoxifen?
- What (other) medications are you taking?
- Do you have a history of anemia, or do you bleed easily with dental work?
- Did your mother take diethylstilbestrol (DES) when she was pregnant with you?

Urinary or Rectal Bleeding

Bleeding from the urethra or rectum can be misinterpreted as vaginal bleeding. A prolapsed cystocele or rectocele might be subject to drying, abrasion, and bleeding. These causes can be documented through physical examination, urinalysis, fecal testing for occult blood, and colonoscopy.

Tamoxifen

Tamoxifen, used for primary or secondary prevention of breast cancer, can cause endometrial hyperplasia and produce vaginal bleeding. Endometrial biopsy is required.

Other Medications

Antibiotics, phenobarbital, rifampin, phenytoin, carbamazepine, and other drugs that induce hepatic microsomal enzymes may produce lower estrogen levels and cause bleeding irregularities. Drugs containing aspirin can increase menstrual flow.

Blood Dyscrasias

Some females with a coagulation defect have excessive menstrual bleeding as the first symptom of a blood disorder; also, most platelet abnormalities will cause vaginal bleeding. If the patient has severe anemia (hemoglobin <10 g/dL) resulting from the vaginal bleeding, it is highly probable that a coagulopathy is present. If this occurs in the perimenarcheal or second or third decade of life, suspect von

Willebrand disease, which is a congenital bleeding disorder caused by deficiency in factor VIII.

DES Exposure in Utero

In utero exposure to DES has been associated with adenocarcinoma of the vagina in daughters of women who took the drug during pregnancy.

DIAGNOSTIC REASONING: FOCUSED PHYSICAL EXAMINATION
Perform a General Assessment

Determine whether the patient's general state of health includes problems of nutrition (e.g., obesity or muscle wasting), hirsutism, hypothyroidism, or hyperthyroidism, all of which may cause an endocrinopathy with consequent vaginal bleeding.

Assess Vital Signs

Determine whether a patient with profuse bleeding is hemodynamically stable. Look for orthostatic changes in blood pressure. In patients who are tachycardic and tachypneic, suspect a ruptured ectopic pregnancy. The patient will show signs of hemorrhage and shock.

Determine Patient Weight and Calculate Body Mass Index

A body mass index (BMI) of greater than 27 corresponds to being more than 20% over a healthy weight. (See nomogram in Appendix C for calculation of BMI.) Obesity causes anovulatory cycles because the adipose cell stroma converts androstenedione to estrogen (estrone) as the body fat increases. Obesity also increases sex hormone binding globulin, thereby increasing free steroid levels. Both processes can cause an imbalance in the HPO axis and increase the probability of an anovulatory cycle and heavy vaginal bleeding. Amenorrhea in anorexia nervosa may precede weight loss by many months.

Perform a Lymph Node Examination

Lymph node examination should be performed to assess for leukemia or metastatic gynecological cancer. Inguinal lymph nodes can be enlarged from an STI or a vulvar infection (e.g., bartholinitis).

Perform a Thyroid Examination

Observe and palpate the thyroid gland. Hypertrophy (enlargement) may be found in hypofunctioning glands. Hypothyroidism is known to be present in 22% of women with severe menorrhagia.

Perform a Breast Examination

The finding of spontaneous, bilateral, clear, or non-bloody nipple discharge on breast examination could indicate hyperprolactinemia, which can cause amenorrhea or irregular vaginal bleeding.

Perform a Pelvic Examination

If practitioners and patients believe bleeding to be uterine in origin, an external and internal pelvic examination can verify that etiology. Perform an examination of the external genitalia, noting whether the bleeding is coming from external hemorrhoids or a painless labial lesion, such as a squamous cell cancer or condylomata acuminata. Note bruising, lacerations on the vaginal walls, or other signs of sexual abuse. Observe the introitus for signs of a prolapsed uterus or cystocele or rectocele that might be subject to drying, abrasion, or bleeding. These signs are usually accompanied by pelvic pressure or urinary or bowel symptoms.

Observe the external genitalia for signs of estrogen deficiency: sparse hair distribution, graying or white hair color, clitoral atrophy, and thin, small labia minora. These signs strongly suggest atrophic vaginitis as the cause for bleeding.

Next perform a vaginal examination to determine if the bleeding may be caused by a vaginal infection. Note the color and condition of the vaginal walls. Pale, nonrugated vaginal walls are a sign of an atrophic vagina, which is easily abraded to cause bleeding. Pale vaginal mucosa with splotchy red patches is also a sign of vaginal atrophy. Bleeding from atrophic vaginitis most commonly follows intercourse or douching. It often is a whitish-brown discharge with no particular foul odor. The patient may also have pruritus and a burning sensation of the vagina, labia, and urinary tract because of a lack of estrogen.

Note the amount, color, consistency, and odor of the vaginal discharge. Take samples for wet mount examination from the pooled discharge in the lateral fornices. Note cervical friability and discharge from the cervical os. Take samples of the discharge and assess as noted in Chapter 34. Cervical polyps are red, glossy, nontender masses protruding from the cervical os. They are usually benign and can be removed by twisting them off with ring forceps. The specimen should be sent for pathological evaluation.

If a threatened or spontaneous abortion is suspected, check the internal cervical os to determine if it is closed or open.

Ectopic pregnancy will cause adnexal or cervical motion tenderness. However, uterine enlargement is not often appreciated. Uterine size and contour can be grossly assessed via bimanual examination. On pelvic examination, the uterus is enlarged but smaller than anticipated from dates provided. The cervix is tender to motion, and a tender adnexal mass may be palpable. Diagnosis is confirmed by positive human chorionic gonadotropin (hCG) test results and ultrasound. Serial quantitative serum hCG levels may be useful. **A ruptured ectopic pregnancy is a surgical emergency.**

Uterine leiomyomas (myomas, fibroids) typically feel firm and may make the uterus asymmetrical. These tumors can progress to a size that mimics an advanced pregnant uterus. The uterine size is measured in weeks, just as the pregnant uterus is measured. When the uterus reaches a 12- to 14-week size, referral to a gynecologist for surgery (myomectomy or hysterectomy) is appropriate. The patient may experience urinary or bowel problems (e.g., urinary frequency and constipation) because the fibroid is distorting or obstructing those systems. Carcinogenic tumors of the uterus are classically firm, hard, and rapidly growing, becoming fixed masses. Ultrasound is a valuable tool in documenting the size and growth patterns of tumors.

The average-size adult uterus measures 8 cm long, 5 cm wide, and 2.5 cm deep for the nulliparous woman. Add 1 cm to each dimension for the average size of the multiparous uterus (9 × 6 × 3.5 cm). The uterus with adenomyosis is increased in size to 2 to 3 times that of normal, may be globular, and has a uniform consistency. Adenomyosis is accompanied by worsening menorrhagia and dysmenorrhea.

The rectovaginal examination can detect lesions or nodularity of the cul-de-sac, which is present with endometriosis or the presence of a primary rectal tumor.

Pediatric Examination: Perform a Breast and Genital Examination

Assess for signs of sexual precocity by determining the presence and stage of secondary sexual characteristics of the breasts and pubic hair. Assess development using Tanner staging (see Chapter 4, Figure 4-3). Inspect the vulva, noting the hygiene status—presence of smegma in the labial folds, urine, fecal material, or erythema and lesions. Examine the urinary meatus. A prolapsed urinary meatus is noted by the presence of dark red tissue surrounding the urinary opening. This tissue is usually tender. Use an appropriate pediatric size speculum, long otoscope, or nasal speculum. It may be necessary to refer the patient for a vaginoscopy or cystoscopy under anesthesia for a complete assessment of the vagina and uterus.

Consider the possibility of infection or sexual abuse. See Chapter 34 for assessment of vaginal discharges.

LABORATORY AND DIAGNOSTIC STUDIES
Qualitative Urine/Serum hCG Tests

Qualitative urine/serum hCG tests are monoclonal antibody tests using radioimmunoassay (RIA) to determine or exclude pregnancy. The serum hCG test is more sensitive than the urine hCG test. The serum test can be performed in about 2 hours, and hCG can be detected as early as 6 days after conception. The result is reported as either negative or positive. Because the ß-subunits are measured, it is highly specific and does not cross-react with luteinizing hormone.

Depending on the specific test used, urine testing can detect pregnancy from before to several days after a missed period. The results are obtained in minutes. A positive test (usually a color change) indicates pregnancy.

Quantitative Serum hCG Test

A quantitative hCG (ß-hCG) test is the first step in determining a complication of pregnancy. The test is a fluorometric enzyme immunoassay that is highly specific for the ß-receptors of hCG, with almost no cross-reactivity with other hormones. Results are provided as values. The reference ranges for determining an abnormal pregnancy are as follows:

- Not significant: 0 to 5.0 mIU/mL
- Borderline significance: 5.0 to 25 mIU/mL
- Evaluate with serial determinations: more than 25 mIU/mL

A rapid ß-hCG test (with a sensitivity of at least 5 milliunits/mL) that measures less than 5 milliunits/mL is highly predictive in excluding ectopic pregnancy. The ß-hCG levels have a doubling time of

58 hours with pregnancy. Ectopic pregnancy causes an increase in hCG levels at the same rate as a normal pregnancy, but only up to a certain point. In ectopic pregnancy, that point is usually less than 4 to 6 weeks, at which time the hCG levels plateau or begin to fall. Therefore serial determinations are more useful than a single determination.

The ß-hCG test and ultrasound are used together to determine the possibility of ectopic pregnancy. If the discriminatory threshold of ß-hCG is 1500 milliunits/mL and a vaginal ultrasound determines the absence of a gestational sac (gestational age, 35 days) or a value of 6500 milliunits/mL and negative transabdominal ultrasound (gestational age, 42 days), the presumptive diagnosis of ectopic pregnancy can be made. A drop in serial hCG levels and an ultrasound that does not identify an intrauterine gestational sac support the diagnosis of spontaneous abortion.

Hematocrit and Hemoglobin Levels

Hematocrit and hemoglobin levels are used to determine anemia caused by blood loss from long-standing menorrhagia. Hematocrit and hemoglobin levels are not useful in evaluating acute blood loss from a single episode of heavy bleeding caused by a spontaneous abortion or ectopic pregnancy.

Complete Blood Count with Indices and Differential

Complete blood count (CBC) with indices will provide information about the degree and cause of anemia. Typically, the hematocrit and hemoglobin levels reflect the degree of anemia, with erythrocyte indices suggesting the cause. Microcytic hypochromic anemia is reflective of chronic blood loss, whereas normocytic normochromic anemia suggests acute hemorrhage. Microcytic hypochromic anemia is indicated by a mean corpuscular volume (MCV) of less than 80 μ^3 and a mean corpuscular hemoglobin (MCH) level of less than 27 pg. The MCV and MCH values are within reference range in normocytic normochromic anemia.

An increased white blood cell (WBC) count with a shift to the left (an increase in the number of bands that are immature neutrophils) points to infection as a cause of the vaginal bleeding. Additionally, the CBC can rule out leukemia and thrombocytopenia, both of which can produce abnormal vaginal bleeding.

Prothrombin Time/Partial Thromboplastin Time/Bleeding Time

If the history and/or the physical examination is suggestive of a bleeding problem, prothrombin time (PT), partial thromboplastin time (PTT), and bleeding time (BT) can differentiate between blood dyscrasias, hepatic or renal diseases, and iatrogenic causes (e.g., anticoagulants, nonsteroidal anti-inflammatory drugs).

Serum Progesterone Levels

A serum progesterone level of greater than 25 ng/mL is predictive of an intrauterine pregnancy; however, a level less than 15 ng/mL suggests an ectopic pregnancy.

Serum Follicle-Stimulating Hormone Levels

Ovarian failure, which causes a low estradiol secretion, will raise the FSH level greater than 40 mIU/mL. If both the follicle-stimulating hormone (FSH) and luteinizing hormone (LH) levels are greater than 50 mIU/mL, primary ovarian failure is established. If the patient is older than 30 years, menopause is diagnosed; if she is younger than 30 years, a chromosomal karyotype should be obtained. An FSH measurement of less than 40 milliunits/mL denotes a hypothalamic-pituitary dysfunction and secondary ovarian failure.

Serum Luteinizing Hormone Levels

A serum LH level of greater than 35 mIU/mL is frequently seen in patients with PCOS. An LH/FSH ratio higher than 2:1 is suggestive of PCOS, whereas a ratio greater than 3:1 is considered diagnostic of PCOS.

Serum Estradiol Levels

Serum estradiol levels less than 15 pg/mL are found with menopause.

Fecal Occult Blood Test or Fecal Immunochemical Test

A negative fecal occult blood test (FOBT) or fecal immunochemical test (FIT) rules out the cause of bleeding being located in the colon or rectum (see Chapter 26).

Vaginal/Lower Abdominal Ultrasound

Ultrasonography is used to determine endometrial thickness. A thickness greater than 3 mm indicates hyperplasia. In postmenopausal women, 5 mm is the cutoff for a normal unilateral stripe. It is also helpful in identifying cystic enlargement of the uterus, the presence of leiomyomas, and the presence or absence of the products of conception. Ultrasonography is used to determine complications of pregnancy such as ectopic pregnancy, placenta previa, or threatened abortion. When the intrauterine sac is identified within the uterus by ultrasound, an ectopic pregnancy is rarely the diagnosis, even though it is possible to have simultaneous intrauterine and ectopic pregnancies.

Endometrial Biopsy

Endometrial biopsy (EMB) is used to detect cancer in any perimenopausal or postmenopausal woman who is experiencing abnormal vaginal bleeding. It is used to exclude endometrial cancer in women taking tamoxifen who experience vaginal bleeding. EMB can be performed on women who are in their thirties if they are at increased risk for endometrial cancer (see Box 33-2). The sensitivity of this biopsy for endometrial carcinoma is 95% to 97%. If the test results are abnormal or inadequate in terms of amount of tissue, the next diagnostic test would be dilation and curettage (D&C). If the test is normal and abnormal bleeding continues, further workup is indicated to exclude neoplasia.

Dilation and Curettage

Dilation and curettage (D&C) is useful in determining the cause of abnormal uterine bleeding and for the removal of retained products of conception. The curetting of the entire uterus provides specimens to send to pathology to rule out carcinogenic causes for the uterine bleeding.

Hysteroscopy

Hysteroscopy allows for visualization of the uterine cavity. Endometrial biopsies, endometrial polyps, and submucosal leiomyomas can be obtained and/or removed by hysteroscopy.

DIFFERENTIAL DIAGNOSIS
Organic Causes of Vaginal Bleeding

Pregnancy

A small amount of bleeding can occur at the time of implantation. The blastocyst burrows into the endometrium and invades the maternal blood supply; the formation and implantation of the placenta follow this. If bleeding occurs from implantation, it happens about 1 week before the expected menstrual cycle. Regard women of childbearing age as pregnant until pregnancy is ruled out.

Spontaneous Abortion

A spontaneous abortion (or miscarriage) is the natural termination of a pregnancy before fetal viability (before 20 weeks). Approximately 15% of diagnosed pregnancies abort spontaneously. It is a complete spontaneous abortion if the fetus and the placenta are completely expelled and incomplete if partial tissue remains within the uterus. Most often the woman will present with persistent uterine cramping and bleeding that is increasing in severity and amount. She may have experienced passage of tissue. The typical patient experiencing a spontaneous abortion presents to the clinic at about 10 to 12 weeks of gestation. The pregnancy test may remain positive for weeks after fetal death. Serial serum hCG levels and ultrasound are useful in establishing the diagnosis.

Threatened Abortion

Threatened abortion produces menstruation-like cramping and bleeding but the cervical os remains closed. The pain is often midline or suprapubic. Perform a sterile speculum examination to inspect the external cervical os. **Only if the facility is prepared to deal with the possibility of surgical intervention** should a cotton-tipped applicator or ring forceps be passed through the os to verify its closed status. In addition to the bleeding and cramping, if the cervical os is open or if tissue is in the cervical canal, the woman is diagnosed with an inevitable abortion.

Placenta Previa

Placenta previa occurs in the third trimester of pregnancy and presents with bright red painless bleeding. The placenta is implanted in the lower segment of the uterus. When the cervix begins to dilate, the placenta is pulled away from the endometrial wall, and bleeding can occur. Any significant bleeding that leads to hemorrhage can endanger the mother and may interfere with uteroplacental sufficiency. Fetal activity is present. The uterus is nontender with a normal resting tone. Diagnosis is made by sonogram. Pelvic examination should not be performed to avoid dislodging any clot that may have formed at the cervix.

Placenta Abruptio

Placenta abruptio can occur any time after 20 weeks of gestation. As the placenta detaches from the uterine wall, the patient experiences dark red, painful bleeding. The amount of bleeding varies from scant to profuse. On physical examination, vaginal bleeding is apparent, and the uterus may be tender and demonstrate increased tone. Signs of fetal distress may be apparent. **Vaginal examination is not performed until placenta previa is ruled out as a diagnosis through the use of ultrasound.**

Ectopic Pregnancy

Ectopic pregnancy occurs in about 1 of 200 pregnancies. Ectopic pregnancy is a leading cause of maternal death in the United States. Maintain high suspicion for this life-threatening condition. A ruptured ectopic pregnancy is a surgical emergency (see Chapter 2). Ectopic pregnancy symptoms can be the same as normal pregnancy symptoms; therefore, any pregnancy accompanied by bleeding or pain must be considered high risk for ectopic pregnancy and must be evaluated to rule out the condition. Persistent one-sided pain or pain that radiates toward the midline of the abdomen is indicative of ectopic pregnancy. The patient experiencing an ectopic pregnancy typically presents at about 6 to 8 weeks of gestation. The menstrual pattern for these patients begins with a time of amenorrhea, followed by abnormal bleeding. They may have some symptoms of pregnancy (e.g., breast tenderness, nausea, and vomiting), have passed some tissue (decidual cast), or have experienced fainting or dizziness. Ninety percent of ectopic pregnancies are implanted in the fallopian tube. About half of these women will have an adnexal mass.

Leiomyomas (Myomas or Fibroids)

Fibroids are found in about 1 of 4 women over age 35. They are more frequently found in African American women than in Caucasian women, and they usually decrease in size after menopause. Depending on location, they are associated with infertility in 2% to 10% of patients. These benign tumors are estrogen dependent and may grow during HT. The most frequent symptom of leiomyomas is bleeding, which ranges from slightly heavier menstrual flow to continuous bleeding. Fibroids may occur as single or multiple tumors within the uterine layers, or they can be pedunculated. Pain is not a common complaint of women with fibroids unless there has been strangulation of a pedunculated fibroid, degeneration of a large fibroid, or compression of other organ systems.

Adenomyosis

Adenomyosis is a condition in which there are endometrial glands and stroma within the myometrium of the uterus. It is a condition, more common in multiparous women, that occurs in the later reproductive years. The uterus is 2 to 3 times its normal size, and there is often dysmenorrhea and infertility. Adenomyosis often coexists with uterine fibroids. Ultrasound may not identify this diffuse intramural lesion. Adenomyosis is found in 20% of hysterectomy specimens.

Uterine/Endometrial Cancer

Endometrial cancer is presently the most common female genital cancer in the United States. The average age at diagnosis is 61 years, but it can occur at any time during the reproductive and postmenopausal years. Uterine cancer risk factors are anovulatory states (e.g., obesity), endometrial hyperplasia (e.g., unopposed estrogen), and family history (see Box 33-2). Classic symptoms include painless vaginal bleeding and a rapidly enlarging uterus. Late symptoms, such as weight loss and weakness, are those of systemic disease.

Systemic Causes of Vaginal Bleeding

Anovulatory Cycles

Perimenopause. The perimenopausal years occur from ages 40 to 50 and last about 7 to 10 years. The perimenopausal woman experiences irregularities in her menstrual flow. Often she has spotting, followed by 1 or 2 days of heavy bleeding, or has her regular menstrual flow and a few days of spotting at the end of the cycle. These types of irregular patterns are characteristic of a degenerating corpus luteum function. A woman who has had 1 year of irregular periods and who has missed the past three cycles can be clinically diagnosed as being in perimenopause (a synonymous term is climacteric). The perimenopause progresses to menopause when the FSH level is elevated above 40 milliunits/mL or there has been an absence of periods for 1 full year. An FSH level of 30 milliunits/mL is typical of perimenopause.

Perimenarche. With perimenarche, the patient has a history of beginning her menstrual cycles and then experiencing months of amenorrhea, followed by resumption of regular cycles, due to an immature hypothalamic-pituitary-ovarian axis. The menstrual flow may be heavier, more frequent, or longer in duration than normal. The young adolescent has appropriate secondary sexual characteristics and sexual maturity ratings. These symptoms are characteristic of anovulatory cycles.

Newborn. A bloody vaginal discharge may occur normally in the female newborn because of maternal estrogen hormone withdrawal during the first few weeks of life.

Endocrinopathies

Polycystic ovary syndrome. In PCOS, the patient typically is obese and hirsute and has oligomenorrhea and large cystic ovaries. However, women with chronic anovulatory cycles and hyperandrogenemia meet the criteria for PCOS even if they are slim and without hirsutism. The LH/FSH ratio is greater than 3:1.

Thyroid dysfunction. Both hypothyroidism and hyperthyroidism are associated with abnormal menstrual bleeding. Menorrhagia can occur with hypothyroidism, whereas oligomenorrhea or scant menses may occur with hyperthyroidism.

With hypothyroidism, the patient may also experience delayed growth, weight gain, fatigue, constipation, and cold intolerance. On physical examination, you may note dry skin, coarse hair, and galactorrhea. The TSH level will be high.

With hyperthyroidism, the patient may experience weight loss, nervousness, heat intolerance, and palpitations. On physical examination, the skin may be moist and sweaty, the hair thin, and the pulse rate rapid. The thyroid gland may be enlarged or nodular. The TSH level will be low, with high triiodothyronine (T_3) and thyroxine (T_4) levels.

Hyperprolactinemia. Prolactin inhibits gonadotropin release and causes anovulatory cycles that may be associated with irregular and sometimes heavy bleeding or with amenorrhea (see Chapter 4). Galactorrhea often accompanies hyperprolactinemia. Nipple discharge will be negative for red blood cells. Prolactin levels will be elevated. Thyroid function tests can rule out hypothyroidism. Magnetic resonance imaging or computed tomography scan along with a cone view of the sella turcica assists in the diagnosis of pituitary tumor.

Vaginal Infection

Atrophic vaginitis. In atrophic vaginitis, there is a dry (shiny), pale, thin vaginal wall caused by an insufficient amount of endogenous estrogen. During menopause, the vaginal mucosa and vulva, which lack glycogen, become fragile and are susceptible to injury and infection. The patient may experience burning, dryness, irritation, dyspareunia, or atrophic vaginitis. This also occurs in the postpartum woman, the woman who is breastfeeding, or the prepubertal girl. The pH is alkaline and ranges from 6.5 to 7.0. Wet mount reveals a few WBCs and is negative for pathogens.

Endometritis. Endometritis is an infection of the endometrium, in which *Chlamydia* is the cause about 25% of the time. Group A or B *Streptococcus* produces puerperal sepsis and may lead to peritonitis, abscess, thrombophlebitis, disseminated intravascular coagulation, septic shock, and infertility. The woman has a slight vaginal discharge (lochia) that is bloody or purulent. The bleeding is accompanied by fever (temperature 39° C to 39.8° C; 102° F to 103° F) and uterine tenderness often within the first 24 hours after delivery. Endometritis should be suspected in a woman with these symptoms, especially if she has undergone an emergency cesarean section or an intrauterine manipulative procedure. Other contributing factors for endometritis are premature rupture of membranes and prolonged labor.

Pelvic inflammatory disease. Pelvic inflammatory disease (PID) is most commonly caused by *Chlamydia trachomatis* or *Neisseria gonorrhoeae* (see Chapter 2) and can produce bleeding, abdominal pain, fever, and vaginal discharge. Women with PID have an increasing amount of vaginal discharge and bleeding after intercourse. Infection begins intravaginally in most cases and then spreads upward, causing salpingitis. In the early stages, women may be asymptomatic. Patients may have a purulent discharge that originates from the endocervical columnar and transitional cells. With gonorrhea, patients often experience inflammation of Skene glands, Bartholin glands, or the urethra, which causes pain and dysuria. On examination, abdominal tenderness, CMT, and adnexal tenderness are present. As with peritonitis, patients may also have guarding and rebound tenderness. WBCs and erythrocyte sedimentation rate are usually elevated. Cultures and Gram staining can assist with the diagnosis (see Chapter 34).

Genital warts. Genital warts (condylomata acuminata) are caused by the human papillomavirus and may be precursors to genital cancer. The warts may involve the vagina, cervix, perineum, or perianal areas. Condylomata can be flat or raised verrucous lesions. The patient usually notices a bump on the genital region accompanied by itching and leukorrhea. A wet mount should be performed to rule out any co-existing vaginal infections. An acetic acid test is helpful in identifying flat warts. Refer to a dermatologist or gynecologist for treatment of warts of the urethra or anus.

Foreign body. In foreign body retention, the presenting symptom is a very malodorous, whitish discharge. In children, the foreign body is as variable as those objects found in the ears and nose. Children younger than 12 months do not have the coordination to insert anything into their vagina; suspect child abuse in those cases and inspect for bruising or excoriations. Wet mount reveals many WBCs.

Blood Dyscrasias

von Willebrand disease. von Willebrand disease is a congenital autosomal dominant bleeding disorder. Altered factor VIII activity and deficient platelet function

characterize it. The patient has a prolonged bleeding time. Hypermenorrhea may occur at menarche or may begin in women 20 to 30 years of age.

Leukemia. Hypermenorrhea may be one of the chief complaints of the woman presenting with leukemia. Other symptoms may include fatigue, bruising, and lymph node enlargement. The CBC and bleeding times will direct the workup for this diagnosis.

Other

Medications. Drugs such as rifampin, phenytoin, carbamazepine, and phenobarbital reduce the efficacy of oral contraceptives. If the woman is on a low-estrogen dose oral birth control pill, these medications are likely to be the cause of irregular vaginal bleeding. Changing the oral contraceptive to one of higher estrogenic potency will alleviate the bleeding. Tamoxifen, which acts as an anti-estrogen on breast tissue, has estrogenic effects on the endometrium and can cause endometrial hyperplasia and/or endometrial cancer. The symptom is vaginal bleeding.

DIFFERENTIAL DIAGNOSIS OF *Common Causes of Vaginal Bleeding*

CONDITION	HISTORY	PHYSICAL FINDINGS	DIAGNOSTIC STUDIES
Organic Causes of Vaginal Bleeding			
Pregnancy	Implantation bleeding; breast tenderness, nausea and vomiting	Internal cervical os closed; minimal spotting; globular, enlarged uterus; soft, bluish color cervix	Pregnancy test; ß-hCG positive
Spontaneous abortion	Vaginal bleeding following time of amenorrhea; cramping, passage of tissue; history of miscarriages	Internal cervical os open; blood from cervical os	Serial ß-hCG declining levels; ultrasound negative
Threatened abortion	Vaginal bleeding following time of amenorrhea; mild cramping	Fetal activity present; internal cervical os may be open	ß-hCG positive; ultrasound positive
Placenta previa	Late pregnancy: bright red, painless bleeding	Fetal activity present; uterus is nontender, normal resting tone	Ultrasound
Placenta abruptio	Dark red, painful bleeding; any time after 20 wk of gestation	Vaginal bleeding; uterus tender with tone; signs of fetal distress	Rule out placenta previa with ultrasound
Ectopic pregnancy	Painless vaginal bleeding; multiparity, older gravida, multiple gestation; history of PID, infertility, STIs	Internal cervical os closed; bloody discharge present	ß-hCG positive; ultrasound; laparoscopy
Leiomyomas	Heavier menstrual bleeding; menorrhagia	Enlarged uterine size; firm, spherical masses; nontender	Pelvic examination; ultrasound

DIFFERENTIAL DIAGNOSIS OF *Common Causes of Vaginal Bleeding—cont'd*

CONDITION	HISTORY	PHYSICAL FINDINGS	DIAGNOSTIC STUDIES
Adenomyosis	Worsening menorrhagia; dysmenorrhea	Pelvic enlargement (2-3 times normal size)	Pelvic examination; ultrasound not always helpful
Uterine/ endometrial cancer	Rapidly enlarging uterus; painless menorrhagia; pelvic pressure; weight loss, weakness	Enlargement of uterus, often symmetrical; fixed with advanced disease	Endometrial biopsy; D&C; ultrasound; CT or MRI
Systemic Causes of Vaginal Bleeding			
Anovulatory Cycles			
Perimenopause	Irregular menses, amenorrhea coupled with heavier and longer menstrual cycles; hot flashes, night sweats, insomnia, mood changes	Pale, dry vaginal mucosa, few rugae	FSH and LH high; estradiol low
Perimenarche	History of beginning menses within last 1-2 yr; has period of amenorrhea followed by irregular menstrual cycles that are of heavy, frequent, or long duration	Physical examination normal; secondary sexual characteristics present	History and examination
Newborn	Less than 2 months old	Small amount of vaginal spotting	History and examination
Endocrinopathies			
Polycystic ovary syndrome	Infertility; irregular menstrual cycles	Hirsute; obese; enlarged ovaries	Pelvic examination; ultrasound; enlarged ovaries with multiple fluid-filled cysts
Thyroid dysfunction	Hypothyroid: menorrhagia, delayed growth, weight gain, fatigue, constipation, cold intolerance	Hypothyroid: dry skin, fine hair, galactorrhea	TSH high
Hyperprolactinemia	Menometrorrhagia, oligomenorrhea	Bilateral, multiduct, clear-to-white nipple discharge	Serum prolactin level; MRI if indicated
Vaginal Infection			
Atrophic vaginitis	Dyspareunia; vaginal dryness	Pale, thin vaginal mucosa; brown or bloody discharge; pH >4.5	Folded, clumped epithelial cells
Endometritis	History of emergency cesarean section, PROM, prolonged labor, intrauterine manipulative procedures	Tenderness of uterus on bimanual examination; temperature 102-103° F; discharge or lochia may be purulent	WBC >10,000/mm³
Pelvic inflammatory disease	History of PID; chronic vaginitis; STIs	Bilateral abdominal pain following menses; pelvic mass; cervical motion tenderness; vaginal discharge; temperature >100.4° F	WBC, ESR; Gram staining, cultures, molecular testing

Continued

DIFFERENTIAL DIAGNOSIS OF *Common Causes of Vaginal Bleeding—cont'd*

CONDITION	HISTORY	PHYSICAL FINDINGS	DIAGNOSTIC STUDIES
Genital warts	Mild-to-moderate itching; foul vaginal discharge; child: history of sexual abuse; adult: new or multiple partners; history of warts	Moist, pale pink, verrucous projections on base; located on vulva, vagina, cervix, or perianal area; bleeding with trauma	Acetic acid test: white
Foreign body	Red and swollen vulva; vaginal discharge; history of use of tampon, condom, or diaphragm	Foreign body present (tampon, condom); bloody, foul-smelling discharge	Wet mount: many WBCs, no pathogens; history and examination
Blood Dyscrasias			
von Willebrand disease	Menorrhagia, adolescent	Bruising; petechiae; gingival bleeding	Bleeding time, factor VIII deficiency, decreased platelets
Leukemia	Menorrhagia; fatigue usually less than 3 months duration	Fever, bruising, pallor; lymph node enlargement; hepatic or splenic enlargement	WBCs: 1000-400,000/mm³ leukocytosis with immature blasts or cells; anemia, thrombocytopenia, decreased factor V or VIII
Other			
Medications	Taking rifampin, phenytoin, carbamazepine, or phenobarbital while on low-estrogen dose oral contraceptives; tamoxifen	Normal gynecological exam	Bleeding stops with higher estrogen dose oral contraceptive; endometrial biopsy

CT, computed tomography; *D&C*, dilation and curettage; *ESR*, erythrocyte sedimentation rate; *FSH*, follicle-stimulating hormone; *LH*, luteinizing hormone; *MRI*, magnetic resonance imaging; *PID*, pelvic inflammatory disease; *PROM*, premature rupture of membranes; *STI*, sexually transmitted infection; *TSH*, thyroid-stimulating hormone; *WBC*, white blood cell count.

REFERENCES AND READINGS

Albers JR, Hull SK: Abnormal uterine bleeding, *Am Fam Physician* 69:1916, 2004.

Alexander JD, Schneider FD: Vaginal bleeding associated with pregnancy, *Prim Care* 27:137, 2000.

Benjamins LJ: Practice guideline: evaluation and management of abnormal vaginal bleeding in adolescents. *J Pediatr Health Care* 23:189, 2009.

Brown DL: Congenital bleeding disorders, *Curr Probl Pediatr Adolesc Health Care* 35:38, 2005.

Casablanca Y: Management of dysfunctional uterine bleeding, *Obstet Gynecol Clin North Am* 35:219, 2008.

Ely JW, Kennedy CM, Clark EC, Bowdler NC: Abnormal uterine bleeding: a management algorithm, *J Am Board Fam Med* 19:590, 2006.

Hayden-Gray S, Emans SJ: Abnormal vaginal bleeding in adolescents, *Pediatr Rev* 28:175, 2007.

Kilbourn CL, Richards CS: Abnormal uterine bleeding: diagnostic considerations, management options, *Postgrad Med* 109:137, 2001.

Mahoney S, Parker C, Potlog-Nahari C et al: Abnormal uterine bleeding: a primary care primer, *Consultant* 46:225, 2006.

Munday PE: Pelvic inflammatory disease: an evidence-based approach to diagnosis, *J Infect* 40:31, 2000.

Rimsza M: Dysfunctional uterine bleeding, *Pediatr Rev* 23:227, 2003.

Scott LD, Hasik KJ: The similarities and differences of endometritis and pelvic inflammatory disease, *J Obstet Gynecol Neonatal Nurs* 30:332, 2001.

Strickland J, Gibson EJ, Levine SB: Dysfunctional uterine bleeding in adolescents, *J Pediatr Adolesc Gynecol* 19:49, 2006.

Vaginal Discharge and Itching

Vaginitis is an inflammation of the vagina that can cause vaginal discharge. Vaginal infections are common in postpubertal women. *Trichomonas vaginalis*, *Candida*, and bacterial vaginosis (BV) (the epithelium is not inflamed with this syndrome) account for 95% of all vaginal infections in U.S. women. Often patients have more than one infection at a given time.

Some studies suggest that pregnant women with BV have premature rupture of membranes and early delivery. The most common cervical infections are *Chlamydia trachomatis*, *Neisseria gonorrhoeae*, and herpes simplex. Postmenopausal women often have discharge related to atrophic vaginitis, caused by the deficiency of estrogen in the vaginal tissues.

Vulvar itching, burning, and a foul odor often accompany vaginal discharge. Pubic lice, scabies, pinworms, and genital warts (condylomata acuminata) can all cause itching. Common foreign bodies found in the vagina of adults are lost or forgotten tampons, which can produce a foul-smelling discharge.

Chemical vaginitis in a young girl is usually caused by sensitivity to bubble bath, whereas in the adolescent or woman it occurs because of the use of scented douches, lubricants, or hygiene sprays. Vulvovaginitis is one of the most common gynecological disorders in girls as a result of their hypoestrogenic state and their perineal hygiene, which is often poor. The vaginal mucosa is thin and less resistant to infectious organisms. The postmenopausal woman can experience these same symptoms with estrogen deficiency.

In childhood and adolescence, reports of vulvar itching, soreness, or vaginal discharge are common. The lack of estrogen stimulation; neutral pH of the vaginal secretions; lack of protective thick labia and pubic hair; and daily living habits (e.g., wiping, clothing, play equipment, environment, and baths), lead to this complaint.

DIAGNOSTIC REASONING: FOCUSED HISTORY

What kind of vaginitis might this be?

Key Questions

- What are the amount, color, and consistency of your discharge?
- Do you have itching, swelling, or redness?
- Is there an odor?

Characteristics of Discharge

Copious amounts of greenish, offensive-smelling discharge are most consistent with *T. vaginalis*. Mucopurulent or purulent discharges are associated with gonorrhea and *Chlamydia*. A moderate amount of white, curd-like discharge is consistent with *Candida* vulvovaginitis. BV typically produces a discharge that is thin and either white, green, gray, or brownish. Although characteristic symptoms associated with each type of vaginal discharge can be helpful in arriving at a diagnosis, they are not diagnostic in and of themselves. Microscopic examination of the vaginal discharge is more sensitive than the clinical picture in confirming the diagnosis (Figure 34-1).

Itching, Swelling, and Redness

Vaginitis causes inflammation of the tissues, resulting in erythema and edema. Because of the inflammatory process, the amount of discharge will produce a concomitant amount of swelling and redness of the vulva and vagina. Itching is consistently present with candidiasis. Scratching can lead to excoriations and satellite lesions. BV does not involve the inflammatory process and results in discharge with little vulvovaginal erythema and edema.

Odor

A fishy odor caused by the release of amines from organic acids is prominent with BV. It is accentuated by the addition of potassium hydroxide (KOH) to the

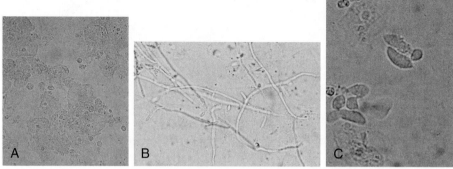

FIGURE 34-1 Microscopic differential diagnosis of vaginal infections. **A,** Clue cells (epithelial cells with clumps of bacteria) are evident in bacterial vaginosis. **B,** Budding, branching hyphae characterize candidiasis. **C,** Motile trichomonads are seen with trichomoniasis. (From Zitelli BJ, Davis HW: *Atlas of pediatric physical diagnosis,* ed 3, St Louis, 1997, Mosby-Wolfe.)

wet mount slide and is considered a positive "whiff" test. Odor commonly accompanies trichomonal infections. Retained tampons or other foreign bodies can also cause a foul odor.

Is this likely a sexually transmitted infection?

Key Questions

- Are you sexually active? Do you have multiple partners? Do you have a new partner?
- Have you had sex against your will? If a child: You might ask, "Has anyone touched your private parts?"
- What form of protection do you use? How often do you use protection?
- Have you or your partner(s) ever been tested or treated for a sexually transmitted infection (STI)?
- Do you have any rashes, blisters, sores, lumps, or bumps in the genital area?

Sexual History

Early-age onset of sexual activity, multiple partners, and nonuse of barrier contraceptives, particularly condoms, increases the risk of vaginal infection. STIs are common in women of childbearing age (12 to 50 years) who have acquired a new partner. The patient who frequently changes sexual partners or participates in risky sexual practices (e.g., rectal intercourse without a condom) is at high risk for STIs.

Do not ignore the possibility of an STI in older women or children. An older woman may be sexually active, for example, after a divorce or widowhood. Also, 50% of all children with an STI have been found to be

sexually abused. *T. vaginalis* is rare in children but can be transmitted to the neonate from an infected mother.

Recent Treatment for a Sexually Transmitted Infection

Recent treatment for an STI may indicate treatment failure, a coinfection that was not covered by the prescribed drug, or recent exposure.

Lesions

Vesicles usually indicate herpes infection. Patients typically notice them on the external labia and report that they itch or burn. Condylomata lata, condylomata acuminata, and molluscum contagiosum are all papular lesions found on the labia, perineum, and anal regions. Molluscum contagiosum, when occurring in the genital area, may extend to include the inner thighs. Typically, condylomata acuminata (genital warts) are rough, verrucous lesions that are usually located inferiorly from fossa navicularis to the fourchette and the perineal area. A painless ulcer suggests syphilis and classically appears as a solitary lesion. However, there can be more than one chancre, especially if the patient is immunocompromised.

Can this be vaginitis that is not related to an STI?

Key Questions

- Have you ever been told that you have diabetes or Cushing syndrome or that you are positive for HIV infection?
- Have you been ill recently?

- Are you taking antibiotics, hormones, or oral contraceptive pills?
- Have you received chemotherapy?
- Does the itching seem to be worse at night?
- Can you describe some of your recent activities?
- Is the patient premenarche?

Immunocompromised States

Refractory fungal vulvovaginitis may indicate undiagnosed diabetes or an immunocompromised state.

Recent Illness

Chickenpox, scarlet fever, and measles can cause vaginitis.

Medications or Chemotherapy

Birth control pills, corticosteroids, antibiotics, and chemotherapy are associated with candidal vulvovaginitis. Oral contraceptives can alter the vaginal pH, and antibiotics can alter the normal vaginal flora; both predispose to fungal infection. Corticosteroids and chemotherapy can produce an immunocompromised state and provide the opportunity for fungal infection.

Night Itching

Pinworms are intestinal parasites that inhabit the rectum or colon and emerge to lay eggs in the skinfolds of the anus. Perianal pruritus, especially at night, along with pain or itching of genitals is common (Figure 34-2).

Activities

Riding a bicycle, using pools or hot tubs, or wearing tight-fitting pants or pantyhose can lead to heat and moisture in the genital area, causing mechanical irritation and such infections as candidiasis or BV.

Premenarche

Girls who have not yet reached menarche are prone to vulvovaginal infections because of a nonestrogenized vagina and the lack of labial development and hair growth.

Is this condition acute, recurring, or chronic?

Key Questions

- How long have you had these symptoms?
- Are they getting better or worse?
- Have you ever had these symptoms before?
- How many episodes have you had in the past year?
- Are the episodes related to any particular activity or time?

Chronology of Symptoms

The occurrence of vaginal discharge after having a new sex partner suggests an acute condition, such as a sexually transmitted infection. Symptoms associated with use of condoms or spermicidal jelly suggest sensitivity to the product. If the discharge occurs monthly,

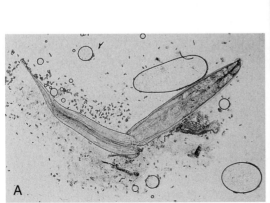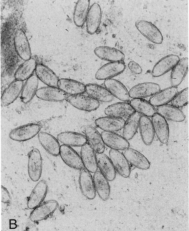

FIGURE 34-2 Pinworms (*Enterobius vermicularis*). On this wet mount, a mature worm is shown surrounded by eggs **(A)**, which are shown more clearly at higher power **(B)**. (From Zitelli BJ, Davis HW: *Atlas of pediatric physical diagnosis*, ed 3, St Louis, 1997, Mosby-Wolfe.)

becoming worse after menses, suspect a chronic condition, such as vulvovaginitis candidiasis. Recurrent episodes related to bathing activities point to chemical irritation.

If this is acute, could it be related to a previous infection?

Key Questions

- Have you been tested and treated for this condition recently?
- What medication was prescribed?
- Did you take all of the medication?
- What other prescriptions were you taking at that time?
- Have you taken any over-the-counter medications?

Adequate Diagnosis

Diagnoses made clinically on the basis of the color or appearance of discharge may be incorrect, or a concomitant vaginal infection may have been missed. However, self-diagnosis and treatment are common, especially with the over-the-counter medicines for "yeast infection."

Adequate Treatment

Most medications that are prescribed are not taken exactly as directed. Women may stop using their vaginal medications when menses begins and resume after it ends. This practice can lead to treatment failure. They may also discontinue the therapeutic agent early, as soon as relief from symptoms takes place or a drug side effect is experienced (e.g., the metallic taste of metronidazole). Drug interactions may account for inadequate therapy, or there may be the need to alter dietary regimen (e.g., abstain from alcoholic beverages).

If this is chronic, what should I suspect?

Key Questions

- Do any family members or sexual partners have recurrent vaginal or urinary tract infections? Do they have any itching, rashes, sores, lumps, or bumps?
- Do you have a new or untreated partner?
- What are your sexual practices (e.g., vaginal, oral, and/or anal sex)?
- How many yeast infections have you had in the past year?

Transmission

Caregivers, parents, and siblings can spread infections, such as candidiasis, molluscum contagiosum, herpes, lice, and pinworms to children through poor hygiene practices. Autoinoculation is also possible, especially for herpes, genital warts, and molluscum contagiosum.

New or Untreated Partner

The most common cause of reinfection is intercourse with a new or untreated partner.

Sexual Practices

Possible infection reservoirs are oral and anal cavities, which may need to be cultured for herpes or gonorrhea. Additionally, materials used during intercourse may need to be disinfected (e.g., diaphragm). Less common modes of transmission include shared intimate clothing.

Chronic Vulvovaginitis

If the patient has had more than three separate episodes of candidal vulvovaginitis in 1 year, consider diabetes or the immunocompromised state of HIV/AIDS as the underlying cause. Yeast grows best in areas that are dark, moist, warm, and high in glucose—areas where the normal flora has been compromised. The use of oral contraceptive pills or hormone replacement therapy, antibiotic (e.g., tetracycline for acne) or steroid therapy, diets high in carbohydrates or artificial sweeteners, and clothing that holds moisture against the vulva (e.g., pantyhose, tight jeans) are excellent potentiators for infection.

What are other possible causes for this vaginitis?

Key Questions

- What are your personal hygiene practices?
- Do you douche?
- Have you changed brands of contraceptive products?
- Could you have forgotten to remove your diaphragm or tampon?

Hygiene Practices

Feminine hygiene practices can contribute to vaginitis by causing a local allergic reaction, altered vaginal flora, or contamination of the vagina from the rectum. Perfumes in douches, sprays, lubricants, and bubble baths are frequent offenders in allergic vaginitis.

Once a child is out of diapers, toileting is less closely assisted, and wiping techniques may be poor, leading to contamination of the vagina with bowel flora.

Douching

Frequent douching can change the balance of normal vaginal flora by altering the pH. This allows recolonization of the vagina with enteric bacteria, leading to pruritus and discharge. Douching can cause an allergic reaction. Colored or perfumed toilet paper can irritate the perineum, causing redness and itching. Wiping with tissue after urination or defecation in the direction from the anus toward the vagina can inoculate the vagina with rectal microbes.

Contraceptive Products

Contraceptive products (e.g., spermicidal jellies, suppositories, foam, and condoms) can cause an allergic inflammation of the sensitive mucosa and produce itching, erythema, tenderness, and an increase in usual vaginal secretions.

Foreign Body

Foul-smelling vaginal discharge can be caused by a lost tampon or condom or a forgotten diaphragm. A child who puts a foreign object into her vagina may have pruritus, burning, or foul, purulent vaginal discharge. Foreign bodies in the vagina are associated with vaginal bleeding or spotting. If the object is left for some time, it can imbed and perforate the vaginal wall.

> **Are there any associated symptoms that point to a cause?**

Key Questions

- Do you have burning or pain with urination? Do you have urinary frequency or hesitation, or nocturia?
- Is intercourse painful?
- Do you have abdominal or pelvic pain?
- If an infant: Does the infant have an eye infection?
- If an infant: Does the infant have a cough?

Urinary Tract Symptoms

Atrophic vaginitis is often accompanied by dysuria, dyspareunia, and vaginal dryness. Estrogen deficiency affects the woman's entire lower genital tract and may produce symptoms that can be confused with a urinary tract infection. Low estrogen levels may exacerbate stress and urge incontinence. *Trichomonas* and *Chlamydia* may produce a coexisting urethritis that causes frequency and dysuria.

Dyspareunia and Pain

Vaginal atrophy, genital warts, or vaginal infections can cause introital dyspareunia. A more likely reason for deep vaginal dyspareunia is endometriosis, pelvic inflammatory disease (PID), or fibroids. Sexually transmitted infections like gonorrhea and *Chlamydia* can cause cervicitis, which, if left untreated, can progress to PID and produce abdominal and/or pelvic pain (see Chapter 2).

Eye Infection

Eye infections in the newborn may be associated with gonorrhea and *Chlamydia* (see Chapter 27).

Cough

Pneumonia in the newborn may be an indication of chlamydiosis (see Chapter 10).

DIAGNOSTIC REASONING: FOCUSED PHYSICAL EXAMINATION
Note Vital Signs

The presence of a fever may alert you to a serious infection, such as PID. Fever is uncommon with vaginitis.

Perform an Oral Examination

Oral thrush may accompany vulvar candidiasis, particularly in children. Look for white patches that bleed when you try to scrape them off.

Perform an External Genitalia Examination

Palpate for inguinal lymphadenopathy and tenderness, which can be present with vaginal infections. Inspect the vulva and labia, looking for erythema, excoriations, and induration. The skin is often bright red and swollen with small fissures or excoriations from candidiasis. Also, thick white curds of discharge are often noted in the labial folds. BV often produces a profuse, thin, whitish discharge that will leak out of the vagina onto the perineum. Palpate Bartholin and Skene glands and milk the urethra for discharge. Palpable Bartholin glands often coexist with STIs. If purulent discharge is seen, consider the diagnoses of gonorrhea or *Chlamydia* and obtain specimens for diagnostic tests.

Condylomata lata, condylomata acuminata, and molluscum contagiosum are all papular lesions found on the labia, perineum, and anal regions. Molluscum contagiosum, when occurring in the genital area, may extend to include the inner thighs. Herpes lesions are usually ulcerative in nature when seen clinically and need to be differentiated from other similar lesions (e.g., syphilitic chancre can be more than one lesion and tender if secondarily infected). Herpetic lesions are found in clusters and can extend from the labia into the vagina. Typically, condylomata acuminata (genital warts) are rough, verrucous lesions that are located inferiorly from the fossa navicularis to the fourchette and the perineal area.

In the overweight patient, vulvovaginitis candidiasis is frequently accompanied by intertriginous candidiasis (e.g., under the breasts and the abdominal apron).

Perform an Internal Vaginal Examination

Note the condition of the vaginal walls. A plastic speculum makes vaginal wall inspection easy and helps in the identification of a foreign body for removal. In children, the knee-chest position is very useful for inspecting the vagina. In children, an otoscope or a nasal speculum may be used; rarely is a hysteroscope (under anesthesia) needed. Pale or mottled red splotches of the vaginal mucosa are associated with atrophic vaginitis, and the sticky discharge is yellow or brown. In severe cases of atrophic vaginitis, the pale, thin mucosa may have adhered to the opposing vaginal wall, and the speculum examination often causes an oozing bloody discharge.

The appearance of the cervix should be noted. A friable or "strawberry" appearance of cervical petechiae with a frothy, foul-smelling discharge is descriptive of a *Trichomonas* infection. A mucopurulent discharge from the cervical os is an indication to obtain an endocervical sample for gonorrhea and *Chlamydia* testing. This discharge is yellowish-green when collected on an endocervical swab. The character of the discharge does not consistently identify common infectious causes of vaginitis. Treat vaginal infections before the Papanicolaou test is obtained because BV and trichomoniasis may cause inflammatory atypia results.

The wet mount is a valuable diagnostic tool, and a sample of vaginal discharge is best obtained from the lateral vaginal fornices. Three positive characteristics for any one etiology can correctly identify the causative agent (e.g., increased pH; the presence of "clue cells," which are epithelial cells full of bacteria that obscure the cell border; and a thin gray discharge seen in BV) (see Differential Diagnosis).

DNA probes and nucleic acid amplification tests (NAATs) are available to test for *Chlamydia trachomatis* and *N. gonorrhoeae*. A combination organism DNA probe is available for *Trichomonas vaginalis*, *Gardnerella vaginalis*, and *Candida* species. Cultures for BV, fungal infections, and *T. vaginalis* are not routinely recommended and are usually reserved for determining resistant organisms.

Perform a Bimanual Examination

Assess the condition of the uterus, fallopian tubes, and ovaries by checking for uterine and cervical motion tenderness (CMT), ovarian size, and presence of masses. CMT or pain on palpation of the uterus and adnexa confirms the spread of vaginitis or cervicitis to the upper genital tract and results in PID. **This warrants immediate evaluation and treatment, or referral, to prevent tubal scarring, ectopic pregnancy, and infertility.**

Perform a Vaginal-Rectal Examination

Vaginal-rectal examination is an important technique in assessing the posterior uterus and condition of the cul-de-sac as well as the rectum. Make sure that the internal examination glove is changed before rectal insertion to prevent contamination of the rectum with vaginal discharge organisms. A rectal examination is used to palpate a foreign body and to check for normal pelvic anatomy in the child.

LABORATORY AND DIAGNOSTIC STUDIES
Potassium Hydroxide and Wet Mount/Preparation

Obtain a discharge sample from the lateral fornices of the vagina, using a cotton-tipped applicator. There are several acceptable techniques for preparing a potassium hydroxide (KOH) and wet mount. One technique is to prepare two slides with a smear of vaginal discharge. To one slide, add a drop of 10% KOH and put a coverslip in place. To the other slide, add a drop of normal saline and put a coverslip in place. The whiff test is positive when the addition of the 10% KOH produces a fishy odor, which is caused by the release of amines. The whiff test has a positive predictive value of 76% for BV. Look under the microscope at the KOH slide for the presence of branching and budding hyphae that are characteristic of yeast infection. Examine the saline wet mount microscopically for motile trichomonads that signal the presence of *Trichomonas*. Clue cells are characteristic of BV (see Figure 34-1).

Test for pH

Most litmus paper reads the pH range from 3.0 to 9.0. This is a simple inexpensive test to aid in determining the cause of the vaginal discharge. Normal vaginal secretions are less than pH 4.5. A pH greater than 4.5 is consistent with BV, trichomoniasis, or atrophic vaginitis.

Fungal Culture or Sabouraud Agar Culture

Fungal culture may be needed in the diagnosis of non–*Candida albicans* (e.g., *C. glabrata*, *C. tropicalis*, *C. krusei*) that are refractory to medication regimens.

Herpes Viral Culture

Viral culture is the most specific method of diagnosing herpes. Results may take from 1 to 7 days, with maximum sensitivity achieved at 5 to 7 days. The herpes culture will probably not be able to identify the causative agent if the specimen is taken from a lesion that is 5 or more days old. It is important to document positive genital herpes infections in the pregnant woman and in skin lesions of the newborn. Collect cells or fluid from a fresh sore with a cotton swab and place them in the culture container.

Herpesvirus Antigen Detection Test

This test detects antigens on the surface of cells infected with the herpes virus. Cells from a fresh sore are scraped off and then smeared onto a microscope slide. This test may be done in addition to or in place of a viral culture.

Tzanck Smear

Tzanck smear characteristic findings are multinucleated giant cells that are likely to be found if the specimen is from an intact herpes lesion. Prepare the Tzanck smear by removing the roof of the vesicle and scraping the skin with a scalpel blade. Make sure that the base

and the margins of the vesicle are scraped; do not use the vesicular fluid for this specimen. The cellular material is spread onto a glass slide, fixed with absolute alcohol for 1 minute, and then stained with Wright's stain. Alternative staining methods are available, and guidelines can be obtained from local laboratories.

Modified Diamond Culture

Diamond culture is used to identify *Trichomonas*. However, it is seldom needed to make the diagnosis.

Thayer-Martin Culture

Thayer-Martin medium is a bacterial culture that identifies gonococcal infections. A culture is taken from the endocervical canal of the uterine cervix. First remove excess mucus from a portion of the cervix, using a cotton ball held in ring forceps or a large cotton-tipped procto-swab. Insert a sterile cotton-tipped applicator (Q-tip) into the endocervical canal and allow it to absorb the mucus for 10 to 30 seconds before inoculating the medium. Inoculate the medium bottle or plate in a zigzag manner while simultaneously rolling the small cotton-tipped applicator. When opening the Thayer-Martin culture bottle, avoid holding the bottle totally upright, which will allow for the loss of the carbon dioxide from the specimen collection bottle.

DNA Testing for Infectious Organisms

DNA testing using a sample taken from the vagina provides rapid, sensitive, and specific results. A number of products are available. Follow manufacturer directions to collect and transport the sample.

DNA probes and nucleic acid amplification tests (NAATs) are available to test for *Chlamydia trachomatis* and *N. gonorrhoeae*. Single or dual organism tests are available. For gonorrhea testing, the sample should be taken from the endocervical canal because *N. gonorrhoeae* has a predilection for the columnar and transitional cells.

A multiorganism DNA probe is available to test for *Trichomonas vaginalis*, *Gardnerella vaginalis*, and *Candida* species.

Serology for Syphilis

Serological tests are used for screening and diagnosing syphilis and are recommended if other STIs are found or suspected. The screening tests are nontreponemal and include VDRL (Venereal Disease Research Laboratory),

RPR (rapid plasma reagin), and enzyme immunoassay (EIA) tests. Diagnostic tests are *Treponema pallidum* specific and include FTA-ABS (fluorescent treponemal antibody absorption test) and TPPA (*Treponema pallidum* particle agglutination assay).

Urinalysis

Obtain a U/A if the patient has dysuria. However, external pain on urination may originate from urine on inflamed vulvar tissue, eliminating the need for urinalysis.

Microscopy and Skin Scraping

Viewing a skin scraping under the microscope is used to assist with the differential diagnosis of scabies and pubic lice (see Chapter 25).

Scotch Tape Test

Use this test when you suspect pinworms (*Enterobius vermicularis*), which occur most commonly in children. Instruct the adult to apply adhesive cellophane tape to the child's perianal region early in the morning when the child awakens. The tape is then recovered and brought in. Place it on a glass slide and examine under a microscope for the presence of eggs. Parents may also be able to see the worms by shining a flashlight on the external anus of the child at night. The female worm is about 10 mm long (see Figure 34-2).

Acetic Acid Test (Acetowhite)

The acetic acid test is best used to detect subclinical lesions caused by human papillomavirus (HPV) when a genital wart has been identified on the patient, when there has been sexual contact, or when the Pap test indicates dysplasia. The application of 5% acetic acid (vinegar) to the cervix, labia, or perianal area causes the lesion to turn white (acetowhite). Saturate a gauze pad with vinegar and place on the lesion for 5 to 10 minutes. After this soaking, the white wart will have a sharp circumscribed macular or papular border. The surface will appear verrucous. False positive results can occur with candidiasis, psoriasis, lichen planus, and sebaceous glands.

Follicle-Stimulating Hormone

Follicle-stimulating hormone (FSH) levels that are greater than 30 milliunits/mL are diagnostic of perimenopause, and levels of 40 milliunits/mL or higher represent menopause. This test is particularly helpful in establishing the hypoestrogenic status of a young woman who is experiencing premature menopause and atrophic vaginitis (see Evidence-Based Practice box).

◎ EVIDENCE-BASED PRACTICE *Clinical Diagnosis of Vaginitis*

Vaginal candidiasis, bacterial vaginosis, and trichomoniasis are the three most common causes of vaginitis.

In a systematic review of the literature, Anderson et al (2004) report that symptoms alone are not able to adequately distinguish between the causes of vaginitis and that physical findings are limited in their diagnostic power. Laboratory examination and microscopy of vaginal discharge are the most useful ways of diagnosing the three conditions.

However, the following symptoms and signs can suggest a particular diagnosis:
• Candidiasis is associated with itching, a cheesy discharge, redness, and self-diagnosis. A watery discharge makes candidiasis unlikely. Inflammatory signs are relatively specific for vaginal candidiasis but are not always present. Odor on physical examination is absent.
• Bacterial vaginosis is associated with increased discharge and a patient report of odor. An absent or mild discharge makes bacterial vaginosis unlikely. Odor is noted on physical examination.

Most diagnoses are made by microscopy and the whiff test. Anderson et al (2004) also report the following findings:
• Most studies (but not all) support that candidiasis is associated with a normal pH.
• Although the microscopic identification of yeast or trichomonads is diagnostic, negative findings do not rule out the condition.
• The presence of clue cells makes candidiasis less likely.
• A lack of lactobacilli and the presence of bacilli with corkscrew motility are highly associated with bacterial vaginosis.

The authors conclude that the likelihood ratios found in the review were not particularly robust, that the current research on vaginitis has a number of weaknesses, and that the existing diagnostic approach fails to diagnose approximately 30% of women with vaginal symptoms.

Data from Anderson MR, Klink K, Cohrssen A: Evaluation of vaginal complaints, *JAMA* 291:1368, 2004.

DIFFERENTIAL DIAGNOSIS
Discharges
Physiological Discharge

Normal vaginal discharge is produced by the cervical and vulvar glands. It is mucoid, clear, or white in color and has no foul odor. The amount varies from scant to profuse, depending on the amount of estrogen stimulation to the tissues. On occasion physiological discharge can lead to slight vulvar irritation and mild itching secondary to wetness. The vaginal pH is less than 4.5. Wet mount reveals up to 3 to 5 white blood cells (WBCs)/high-power field (HPF) and the presence of epithelial cells and lactobacilli.

Bacterial Vaginosis

BV is the most common cause of vaginal discharge and is considered a disturbance in normal vaginal flora. It is often found after intercourse with a new partner or in conjunction with other STIs. Fifty percent of women are asymptomatic; hence, treatment may not be necessary except for pregnant patients (increased preterm labor) or patients undergoing vaginal surgical procedures (increased infection). Consistent symptomatology includes a thin homogeneous white, gray, green, or brownish discharge that has a foul odor; there can be pelvic tenderness or pain but no CMT. The vaginal pH is greater than 4.5. Wet mount shows clue cells and a few lactobacilli; the "whiff" test is positive (see Figure 34-1).

Candida Vulvovaginitis

Ninety percent of women with *Candida* vulvovaginitis present with vulvar pruritus. In children, it may be accompanied by oral thrush. The discharge is often thick, white, and "curdy"; the labia are erythematous and edematous. Vaginal pH is 4.0 to 4.7. A KOH wet mount shows pseudohyphae and spores (see Figure 34-1).

Trichomoniasis

Trichomoniasis is asymptomatic in about half of the women affected and 90% of the men. It is usually transmitted via sexual contact but can also be spread by fomites. Women with chronic infections will have copious amounts of discharge and little or no inflammation of the vaginal tissues. When there is an acute infection, they will report vulvar itching, swelling, and redness. The pH is greater than 5; the discharge is white, grayish-green, or yellow and sometimes frothy; infrequently there will be a "strawberry cervix" (cervical petechiae). If the woman has douched within the past 24 hours, the sensitivity of tests will be greatly decreased. Wet mount shows "gyrating" motile protozoa and often greater than 10 WBCs/HPF (see Figure 34-1).

Atrophic Vaginitis

In atrophic vaginitis, there is a dry (shiny), pale, thin vaginal wall caused by an insufficient amount of endogenous estrogen. During menopause, the vaginal mucosa and vulva, which lack glycogen, become fragile and are susceptible to injury and infection. Patients may experience burning, dryness, irritation, or dyspareunia. This also occurs in postpartum women, those who are breastfeeding, and prepubertal girls. The pH is alkaline and ranges from 6.5 to 7.0. Wet mount shows a few WBCs and is negative for pathogens.

Allergic Vaginitis

The causes of allergic vaginitis are different for the child and the adult. In the child, the most common offending agents are bubble baths and perfumed soaps. Adult vulvovaginitis involves any harsh or caustic substance that has direct contact with the area. Often a new brand of vaginal lubricant, douche, spermicide, or condom will cause the inflammation and edema. Vinegar douches stronger than 1 to 2 tablespoons per quart of water may also irritate tissues. The wet mount is positive for WBCs and negative for pseudohyphae.

Foreign Body

The presenting symptom in foreign body retention is a very malodorous, whitish discharge. In children, the foreign body is as variable as those objects found in the ears and nose. However, children younger than 12 months do not have the coordination to insert anything into their vagina, so suspect child abuse in such cases and inspect for bruising or excoriations. Wet mount reveals many WBCs.

Chlamydia

Chlamydia is the most prevalent STI in the United States. About 30% of infected women are asymptomatic. Gonorrhea and *Chlamydia* coexist in up to 60% of patients. Women with *Chlamydia* have an increasing amount of vaginal discharge and bleeding after intercourse. Those patients at greatest risk for infection are younger than 25 years, sexually active with three or more partners, and not using barrier methods of contraception. Wet mount shows greater than 10 WBCs/HPF and few microscopic bacteria. Except for perinatal syndromes, nonsexual transmission has not been reported; therefore, suspect child abuse in children with *Chlamydia* infection.

Gonorrhea

Gonorrhea is one of the most common reportable diseases. Women are asymptomatic 50% to 80% of the time. However, the patient may have purulent discharge that originates from the endocervical columnar and transitional cells. Patients often experience inflammation of Skene glands, Bartholin glands, or the urethra, which causes pain and dysuria. Culture or DNA probe confirms the diagnosis. A finding of gonorrhea in children is considered specific evidence of sexual abuse.

Pelvic Inflammatory Disease

PID is most commonly caused by *Chlamydia trachomatis* and *N. gonorrhoeae* (see Chapter 2) and can produce bleeding, abdominal pain, fever, and vaginal discharge. Women with PID have an increasing amount of vaginal discharge and bleeding after intercourse. Infection begins intravaginally in most cases and then spreads upward, causing salpingitis. In the early stages, women may be asymptomatic. Patients may have a purulent discharge that originates from the endocervical columnar and transitional cells. With gonorrhea, patients often experience inflammation of Skene glands, Bartholin glands, or the urethra, which causes pain and dysuria. On examination, abdominal tenderness, CMT, and adnexal tenderness is present. As with peritonitis, patients may also have guarding and rebound tenderness. WBCs and erythrocyte sedimentation rate are usually elevated. Cultures and Gram staining can assist with diagnosis.

Itching and Lesions
Syphilis

The chancre of primary syphilis is an ulcerative lesion that most often develops at the site of initial inoculation. The syphilitic chancre begins as a papule and progresses to a painless to tender, hard, indurated ulcer.

The infection causes inguinal lymphadenopathy. Even without treatment, the lesion will heal in 3 to 6 weeks. Many chancres go unnoticed until the appearance of condylomata lata, the warty papule of secondary syphilis, or a maculopapular rash on the palms of the hands and soles of the feet. Diagnosis is confirmed with serological testing for syphilis.

Genital Warts

Genital warts (condylomata acuminata) are caused by the human papillomavirus and may be precursors to genital cancers. The warts may involve the vagina, cervix, perineum, or perianal areas. Condylomata can be flat or raised verrucous lesions. The patient usually notices a bump on the genital region, accompanied by itching and leukorrhea. A wet mount should be performed to rule out any coexisting vaginal infections. An acetic acid test is helpful in identifying flat warts. Referral to a dermatologist or gynecologist is indicated for treatment of warts of the urethra or anus.

Herpes

Herpetic lesions can be difficult to distinguish from ulcerative lesions. The most typical presentation is that of grouped vesicles that rupture and leave an erosion. A prodrome of tingling or itching occurs before the outbreak of the vesicles. On the vulva, the erosions are covered with a whitish, exudative layer. Herpetic outbreaks can involve the cervix, vagina, vulva, anus, or extragenital organs, like the pharynx. Culture, antigen test, or Tzanck smear confirms the diagnosis.

If the mother has an active primary herpes simplex virus infection at the time of birth, the infant has a 50% risk of becoming infected. Recurrent maternal infections impart less than a 5% risk of transmission. Clinical signs of the infant's infection become apparent in the first week of life and pose the possibility of death.

Molluscum Contagiosum

Molluscum are small (2 to 5 mm in diameter), umbilicated, flesh-tone papules. These characteristic lesions are the hallmark of the diagnosis. Scratching can spread them. Molluscum is an STI of adults and is a likely finding in HIV-infected patients. When children are found to have genital molluscum, suspect child abuse.

DIFFERENTIAL DIAGNOSIS OF *Common Causes of Vaginal Discharge and Itching*

CONDITION	HISTORY	PHYSICAL FINDINGS	DIAGNOSTIC STUDIES
Discharges			
Physiological discharge	Increase in discharge; no foul odor, itching, or edema	Clear or mucoid; pH <4.5	Up to 3-5 WBCs/HPF; epithelial cells, lactobacilli
Bacterial vaginosis	Foul-smelling discharge	Homogeneous thin white or gray discharge; pH >4.5	Presence of KOH "whiff" test; presence of clue cells; few lactobacilli (see Figure 34-1)
Candida vulvovaginitis	Pruritic discharge	White, curdy discharge; pH 4.0-5.0	KOH prep: mycelia, budding, branching yeast, pseudohyphae (see Figure 34-1)
Trichomoniasis	Watery discharge; foul odor	Profuse, frothy, greenish discharge; red friable cervix; pH 5.0-6.0	Round or pear-shaped protozoa; motile "gyrating" flagella (see Figure 34-1)
Atrophic vaginitis	Dyspareunia; vaginal dryness	Pale, thin vaginal mucosa; pH >4.5	Folded, clumped epithelial cells
Allergic vaginitis	New bubble bath, soap, douche, for example	Foul smell, erythema; "lost tampon"; pH <4.5	WBCs
Foreign body	Red and swollen vulva; vaginal discharge; history of use of tampon, condom, or diaphragm	Bloody, foul-smelling discharge	WBCs
Chlamydia	Partner with nongonococcal urethritis; asymptomatic	May or may not have purulent discharge	DNA probe; NAATs; >10 WBCs/HPF
Gonorrhea	Partner with STI; often asymptomatic	Purulent discharge; inflammation of Skene/Bartholin glands	Gram stain; culture; DNA probe; NAATs
Pelvic inflammatory disease (PID)	Bleeding, abdominal pain, fever, and vaginal discharge; increasing amount of vaginal discharge and bleeding after intercourse	CMT and adnexal tenderness; may also have guarding and rebound tenderness	WBC; culture; DNA probe; NAATs; Gram stain
Itching and Lesions			
Syphilis	History of painless ulcerative lesion; rash on palms and soles of feet; warty growth on vagina or anus	Chancre: usually 1 but can be more, painless ulceration; condylomata lata: flat, whitish papule or plaque; maculopapular rash: palm, soles, body	Serology for syphilis
Genital warts	Mild-to-moderate itching, foul vaginal discharge; child: history of sexual abuse; adult: new or multiple partners; history of warts	Moist, pale-pink, verrucous projections on base; located on vulva, vagina, cervix, or perianal area	Acetic acid test: white
Herpes	History of prodromal syndrome, paresthesias, burning, itching; may have mucoid vaginal discharge	Grouped vesicles on red base, erode to an ulcer; if on mucous membrane, exudates form; if on skin, crusts form; redness, edema, tender inguinal lymph nodes	Viral culture; Tzanck smear
Molluscum contagiosum	History of contact with infected person; if inflamed: itching	Flesh-colored, dome-shaped papules, some with umbilication; usually 2-5 mm in diameter	None

CMT, cervical motion tenderness; *HPF*, high-power field; *KOH*, potassium hydroxide; *NAAT*, nucleic acid amplification test; *WBC*, white blood cell.

REFERENCES AND READINGS

Anderson MR, Klink K, Cohrssen A: Evaluation of vaginal complaints, *JAMA* 291:1368, 2004.

Bachmann GA, Nevadunsky NS: Diagnosis and treatment of atrophic vaginitis, *Am Fam Physician* 61:3090, 2000.

Burstein G, Murray P: Diagnosis and management of sexually transmitted diseases among adolescents, *Pediatr Rev* 24:19, 2003.

Centers for Disease Control and Prevention, Workowski KA, Berman SM: Diseases characterized by urethritis and cervicitis. Sexually transmitted diseases treatment guidelines 2006 [published errata appear in MMWR Morb Mortal Wkly Rep 2006 Sep 15;55:997]. *MMWR Morb Mortal Wkly Rep* 55:35, 2006.

Coco AS, Vandenbosche M: Infectious vaginitis: an accurate diagnosis is essential and attainable, *Postgrad Med* 107:63, 2000.

Eckert LO: Clinical practice. Acute vulvovaginitis, *N Engl J Med* 355:1244, 2006.

Egan ME, Lipsky MS: Diagnosis of vaginitis, *Am Fam Physician* 62:3090, 2000.

French L, Horton J, Matousek M: Abnormal vaginal discharge: using office diagnostic testing more effectively, *J Fam Pract* 53:805, 2004.

Jasper J: Vulvovaginitis in the prepubertal child, *Clin Ped Emerg Med* 10:10, 2009.

Mitchell H: ABC of sexually transmitted infections: vaginal discharge—causes, diagnosis, and treatment, *BMJ* 328:1306, 2004.

Nyirjesy P: Chronic vulvovaginal candidiasis, *Am Fam Physician* 63:697, 2001.

Owen MK, Timothy L, Clenney TL: Management of vaginitis, *Am Fam Physician* 70:2125, 2004.

Parks D, Yetman R: Diagnosis and management of pelvic inflammatory disease in adolescents, *J Pediatr Health Care* 17:145, 2003.

Teran S, Walsh C, Irwin KL: *Chlamydia trachomatis* infection in women: bad news, good news, and next steps in prevention, *J Am Med Womens Assoc* 56:100, 2001.

Vision Loss

Vision loss is a condition that ranges from visual impairment to total blindness. For vision to occur, light is transmitted through the eye to photoreceptors in the retina that collect light and send neural impulses to the brain. These impulses are then processed to give information on what is being seen. Vision loss occurs with any interruption in this visual pathway, such as opacification of the cornea, lens, or vitreous body (see Figure 27-1 for the anatomical structures of the eye). Vision loss also occurs when light energy cannot be converted into neural impulses, such as in glaucoma, retinal detachment, ischemic optic nerve atrophy, and pituitary or occipital tumors. Because vision loss is a self-reported condition, functional causes, formerly called malingering or hysteria, can be considered.

The most common causes of vision loss in adults are cataracts, glaucoma, age-related macular degeneration, and diabetic retinopathy. In all cases, impaired vision requires evaluation by an ophthalmologist. However, knowledge of the causes of vision loss can provide important clues to the diagnosis of these conditions.

DIAGNOSTIC REASONING: FOCUSED HISTORY

What is the extent of vision loss?

Key Questions
- What can you see? Can you detect light?
- Is your vision blurred?
- To self: Does the patient look at me?
- If a child: Does the child's eye wander?

Total Absence of Vision
Disease that affects the optic nerve or retina, such as retinal detachment, leads to total loss of vision. Blindness is a complete lack of form and visual light perception.

Blurring of Vision
Distinguish between loss of vision and loss of visual acuity. Vision loss is the absence of vision, completely or partially, in one or both eyes. Blurriness refers to a change in the acuity of vision. The most common cause of visual acuity change is refractive error.

Ability to Focus
Patients who are without sight have no ocular alignment and commonly manifest a gross searching and wandering nystagmus. Nystagmus in the first year of life suggests bilateral vision loss until proved otherwise. In infancy, vision loss is a common cause of nystagmus.

Visual Fixation
Even though the visual system is incompletely developed at birth, most infants can see and will demonstrate visual interest when stimulated by a human face. At birth the infant will have visual fixation present, and by 2 months of age fixation will be well developed. Any parental concern about a child's visual functioning is an important history finding.

Is this an emergency that requires immediate intervention?

Key Questions
- Was the loss of vision sudden?
- Is the loss in one or both eyes?
- Is the loss complete or partial?
- Is there any pain with the loss of vision?
- Are there other symptoms associated with the loss, such as a flash of light?
- Was the loss momentary or persistent?

Onset
Sudden loss of vision suggests a vascular etiology, specifically occlusion of the central retinal artery until proved otherwise. In occlusion of the central

retinal artery, the patient notes that vision is lost suddenly, and light cannot be distinguished from dark. Loss of vision in one eye indicates that the problem is anterior to the chiasm; hemianopic field defects in both eyes suggest a postchiasmal lesion (Figure 35-1).

Occlusion of the artery is an emergency and requires immediate treatment.

Pain

Sudden loss of vision with eye pain and photophobia indicates pathology of the cornea, iris, and ciliary body. Sudden loss of vision with a red painful eye may indicate acute-angle glaucoma (see Chapter 27). Inflammation, demyelinization, or degeneration of the optic nerve causes pain on movement of the eye and is thought to be the result of general inflammation of the

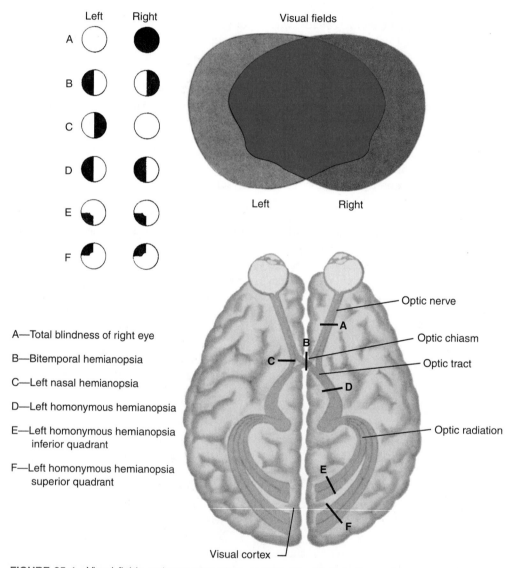

A—Total blindness of right eye

B—Bitemporal hemianopsia

C—Left nasal hemianopsia

D—Left homonymous hemianopsia

E—Left homonymous hemianopsia inferior quadrant

F—Left homonymous hemianopsia superior quadrant

FIGURE 35-1   Visual fields and examples of visual field defects along the optic nerve, optic chiasm, optic tracts, and optic radiations in the cortex. (From Rudy EB: *Advanced neurological and neurosurgical nursing,* St Louis, 1984, Mosby.)

posterior portion of the orbit or inflammation of the optic nerve (cranial nerve II). Retrobulbar neuritis is the most common disease in this category.

A common cause of sudden loss of vision without pain is vitreous hemorrhage. The patient describes floaters that begin to drift in front of the eye, followed by a red glow. The vision gradually fades until only light and dark are distinguished. Painless vision loss is also associated with macular degeneration, retinal detachment, diabetic retinopathy, and anterior ischemic optic neuropathy.

Other Symptoms
In children, acute optic neuritis rarely occurs as an isolated condition and is usually a manifestation of a neurological or systemic disease such as meningitis, viral infection, or demyelinating diseases. It may also be associated with lead poisoning and long-term use of certain drugs, most notably chloramphenicol or vincristine.

Flash of Light with Loss of Vision
Patients who have retinal detachment describe a flash of light shortly before loss of vision. Some patients describe a veil over the eye either just before or immediately after the flash. The reason for the flashes is that detachment of the retina causes mechanical stimulation of the rods and cones as it tears away from the pigment epithelium and floats free.

Patients whose retinae pull away or tear but do not detach experience the same flash of light as those with retinal detachment. They may also experience momentary total or partial loss of vision in the affected eye.

Transient Loss of Vision
Some patients with migraine headache experience a scotoma, or an area of impaired vision within the visual field, before the onset of the headache. The scotoma may be either positive (the patient sees a light spot or scintillating flashes [e.g., scintillating scotoma]) or negative (the patient experiences a blind spot). Scotoma may be prodromal to a migraine headache. Profound anxiety can produce a transient loss of vision or a perceived loss of vision.

Can I rule out trauma?

Key Questions
- Is there a history of head trauma?
- Is there a history of eye trauma?
- Has there been a chemical or thermal injury?

Head Trauma
Loss of vision is most likely to occur after trauma to the occiput. The vision loss is sudden and complete, but vision usually returns in a matter of hours. Severe head trauma with skull fracture but without direct damage to the eyeball can result in loss of vision that occurs immediately or shortly thereafter. Occasionally a patient can have good vision in the affected eye after the accident and subsequently loses vision as a result of severe retrobulbar hemorrhage. In children, trauma is the most common cause of retinal detachment. Shaken baby syndrome may result in retinal and vitreous hemorrhage.

Eye Trauma
Blunt trauma occurs when an object impacts the bony orbit of the eye. High-velocity injuries to the eye are not always immediately obvious. Small perforations or penetrations of the cornea may appear similar to corneal abrasions. Sharp trauma includes impact from a sharp object that may perforate the cornea, leaking fluid from the eye.

Cataract formation is a result of major trauma to the eye in children. Opacification of the lens can result from a blunt or penetrating injury.

Chemical or Thermal Trauma
Alkaline burns from household cleaners and lawn and garden products can cause irreversible vision loss. Exposure to extreme heat or flames can damage the cornea and eyelids.

Minutes make a difference with chemical trauma to the eye—treat first and examine later. Wash the eye with water or normal saline solution immediately.

Is the vision loss because of a chronic problem?

Key Questions
- How long has vision loss been present?
- Has vision decreased over time?

Progression of Vision Loss
Slowly progressive degenerative disease of any part of the eye can cause progressive vision loss. Progressive loss of visual acuity and color vision can be seen with optic gliomas, the most frequently occurring tumor of the optic nerve in childhood. A history of neurofibromatosis can be found in 25% of

patients. Children who have surgery for cataracts are especially at risk for glaucoma. Glaucoma may cause chronic loss of vision. Age-related macular degeneration is associated with decreased reading vision (see Chapter 27).

Is this related to a genetic, familial, or intrauterine risk?

Key Questions

- Is there a family history of vision or eye problems?
- Is there a history of maternal, intrapartum, or neonatal conditions?

Family History

A family history of retinoblastoma, congenital cataracts, or metabolic or genetic disease is a risk factor for visual and ocular abnormalities. Retinoblastoma occurs in 12% of children with a family history. Hereditary congenital cataracts occur in 10% to 25% of children with a family history. Autosomal dominant inheritance is the most common cause.

Maternal, Intrapartum, and Neonatal Risks

Infants at risk for vision problems are those who are premature; have been on oxygen therapy; are low birth weight; or have mothers who have had infections related to HIV/AIDS and toxoplasmosis, rubella, cytomegalovirus, and herpes simplex—known as the TORCH complex of infections. These conditions during pregnancy may produce blindness at birth or vision loss later in life. Down syndrome is associated with cataracts. Children with galactosemia develop cataracts in infancy. Children with galactokinase deficiency develop cataracts in the first decade of life.

Is the loss because of a systemic disease?

Key Question

- Do you have a chronic disease?

Chronic Disease

Diabetic retinopathy is a leading cause of vision loss. It is a progressive condition resulting from incompetent arterioles or microinfarctions and allowing hard exudates to leak into the retina. The risk of retinopathy increases with the duration of diabetes. Neurodegenerative disease

and juvenile rheumatoid arthritis can cause visual changes. Prolonged treatment with systemic steroids almost invariably results in the formation of posterior subcapsular cataracts. Marfan syndrome may cause dislocated lens.

Could this be an anatomical problem?

Key Questions (to self)

- Do the eyes cross?
- If a child: Does the child squint, especially in the sun?
- Do the eyes appear symmetrical?
- Are the eyes bulging or sunken?

Eye Alignment

Amblyopia is impaired vision in an eye that appears to be structurally normal. It is defined in one of the following three ways:

1. Strabismic amblyopia occurs when one eye is out of alignment and the fovea of that eye receives an image that is different from that received in the opposite eye. The brain suppresses the image in the deviating eye to avoid diplopia and visual confusion.
2. Refractive amblyopia occurs when the refraction of each eye is so different that the child uses the eye that focuses the best, resulting in poor development of the other eye.
3. Deprivation amblyopia is anything that prevents an image from being received clearly by the retina. Conditions such as severe ptosis, congenital cataracts, or vitreous opacity may cause this.

Squinting

Squinting blocks out the outer rays from the object, resulting in a smaller amount of distortion, and increases the chance of being able to more clearly perceive the image on the retina. This often occurs with strabismus. Excessive squinting in bright light may indicate glaucoma.

Exophthalmos

Bilateral exophthalmos is protrusion of the eyeballs that occurs with hyperthyroidism. Lid lag is observed on downward gaze as a lag in the falling of the lid with the globe as it moves downward. Unilateral exophthalmos may indicate a tumor located behind the eye.

Enophthalmos

Enophthalmos is the backward displacement of the eyeball in the eye socket, leading to a sunken appearance. It is caused by starvation, dehydration, or trauma.

Ptosis

With ptosis, the eyelid margin is at or below the pupil. The eyelid appears to be drooping and interferes with vision. Ptosis may indicate a lesion of the oculomotor nerve (cranial nerve III), a neuromuscular weakness, or a congenital condition.

Is there a pattern to the vision loss?

Key Question

■ When does the vision loss occur?

Pattern of Vision Loss

Retinitis pigmentosa is characterized by progressive disorganization of the pigment of the retina, usually accompanied by a decrease in the number of retinal vessels and some degree of optic atrophy. Night blindness is often the first symptom of vision loss. A progressive loss of vision may occur over decades. Dimming of vision upon standing can occur in someone with low blood pressure or impending shock.

Individuals who are extremely myopic often experience a reduction in vision at nighttime and may refer to that condition as "night blindness." Vitamin A deficiency or the result of retinotoxic drugs, such as quinine, can cause night blindness.

Can I associate the vision loss with the age of the patient?

Key Questions

■ What is your age?
■ If a child: Is there a history of developmental delay?
■ If a child: Is there a change in school performance?

Vision Loss with Aging

Age-related macular degeneration is the leading cause of permanent blindness in older adults. The prevalence increases with each decade over 50 years to almost 35% by the age of 75. The majority of adults over 50 years have some degree of visual impairment.

Developmental Delay

Decreased vision can result in developmental delays. Motor development requires good visual cues and depth perception. Poor school performance may be the first indication of vision loss related to refractory errors and progressive myopia in some children. Craniopharyngiomas can compress the optic nerve system, causing a decrease in visual acuity and a decrease in school performance (Box 35-1).

Box 35-1	Normal Development of Vision and Eye Movements

Age	Normal Vision and Eye Movements
Birth (term)	Fixation
	Poor following
	Intermittent strabismus frequently present
	Visual acuity 20/400 to 20/600
1 mo	Horizontal following to midline
	Normal alignment
	Visual acuity 20/300
2 mo	Vertical following begins
	Normal alignment
	Visual acuity 20/200
3 mo	Good horizontal and vertical following
	Normal alignment
	Visual acuity 20/100
	Accommodation begins
	Binocularity detectable
6 mo	Visual acuity 20/20 to 20/30
	Binocularity well developed
8 to 10 yr	End of sensitive period for amblyopia

From Monte M: The eye in childhood, *Am Fam Physician* 60:907, 1999.

DIAGNOSTIC REASONING: FOCUSED PHYSICAL EXAMINATION

Children become increasingly threatened the closer the examiner comes to the face. The least-threatening assessment should be done first.

Assess for Visual Acuity

Visual acuity for distance vision in adults and children older than 4 years is tested using the Snellen or Tumbling E charts. Test each eye separately, with and without corrective lenses. Normal visual acuity tested using a Snellen chart is 20/20 in the best eye without correction. A Snellen of 20/70 indicates visual impairment, and vision that cannot be corrected to better than

20/200 is legal blindness. A Rosenbaum pocket card held 15 inches from the eyes is used to test near or reading vision.

To test for central vision in infants, observe the infants' eyes as they follow large objects, such as the face or hand of the examiner, in various gazes. In children ages 1 to 3 years, use the cover/uncover test and observe the corneal light reflex.

Any child who has a difference of one line between the two eyes must be referred. Vision of 20/50 for 5 year olds and 20/40 for children 6 years and older requires referral. Retest using the Snellen chart before referring because children tend to do better on a second examination (Table 35-1).

Assess Lids, Pupils, and Orbits

Note the position of the eyelids. Eyelids that droop (ptosis) may cause vision loss. Assess for the symmetry of each eye, and observe for a transparent cornea.

The appearance of a white pupil (leukokoria) may indicate a cataract, retinoblastoma, persistent hyperplastic primary vitreous (PHPV) retinal detachment, vitreous hemorrhage, or intraocular inflammation, such as by *Toxocara canis*, which is a roundworm that is contracted from dogs and invades the liver, abdomen, and eyes.

Pupil size is smaller in infants and older adults. Five percent of people will have noticeable differences in

Table 35-1	**Pediatric Eye Evaluation Screening Recommendations for Primary Care Providers, Nurses, Physician's Assistants, and Trained Lay Personnel**	
RECOMMENDED AGE FOR SCREENING*	**SCREENING METHOD**	**CRITERIA FOR REFERRAL TO AN OPHTHALMOLOGIST**
Newborn to 3 mo	Red reflex†	Abnormal or asymmetrical
	Inspection	Structural abnormality
6 mo to 1 yr	Fix and follow with each eye	Failure to fix and follow in cooperative infant
	Alternate occlusion	Failure to object equally to covering each eye
	Corneal light reflex	Asymmetrical
	Red reflex†	Abnormal or asymmetrical
	Inspection	Structural abnormality
3 yr (approximately)	Visual acuity‡	20/50 or worse or two lines of difference between eyes
	Corneal light reflex/cover-uncover	Asymmetrical ocular refixation movements
	Red reflex†	Abnormal or asymmetrical
	Inspection	Structural abnormality
5 yr (approximately)	Visual acuity‡	20/40 or worse or two lines of difference between eyes
	Corneal light reflex/cover-uncover	Asymmetrical/ocular refixation movements
	Stereoacuity§	Failure to appreciate stereopsis
	Red reflex†	Abnormal or asymmetrical
	Inspection	Structural abnormality
Older than 5 yr	Visual acuity‡	20/30 or worse or two lines of difference between eyes
	Corneal light reflex/cover-uncover	Asymmetrical/ocular refixation movements
	Stereoacuity§	Failure to appreciate stereopsis
	Red reflex†	Abnormal or asymmetrical
	Inspection	Structural abnormality

Reprinted with permission from the American Academy of Ophthalmology: *Pediatric Eye Evaluations Preferred Practice Pattern*, ©1997, American Academy of Ophthalmology, Inc.

*Note: These recommendations are based on expert opinion.
†Physician or nurse responsibility.
‡Figures, letters, "tumbling E," or optotypes.
§Optional: Random Dot E Game (RDE), Titmus Stereograms (Titmus Optical, Inc., Petersburg, VA), Randot Stereograms (Stereo Optical Company, Inc., Chicago).

pupil size (physiological anisocoria). However, many types of central nervous system diseases also cause differences in pupil size.

Enlargement of the pupil may be caused by ocular injury, acute glaucoma, systemic parasympatholytic drugs, and dilating drops. Constriction of the pupil is seen in iris inflammation and patients with glaucoma who are treated with pilocarpine. Irregularity of the pupil contour is invariably abnormal, occurring in iritis, syphilis of the central nervous system, trauma, and congenital defects.

Inspect for Nystagmus

On far lateral gaze, some eyes will develop a rhythmic twitching motion (nystagmus) in the direction of gaze followed by a drift back. This is a normal finding. However, nystagmus is a neurological sign that may indicate disease or structural changes in the vestibular-cerebellar-oculomotor system. Pathological nystagmus is seen when the movement is in the same direction, regardless of the direction of gaze. Nystagmus in the first year of life suggests bilateral vision loss until proved otherwise.

Assess Visual Fields

Testing of the visual fields assesses the function of the peripheral vision and central retina, the optic pathways, and the cortex. The peripheral field is damaged in glaucoma and by tumors or vascular lesions involving the visual fibers from the chiasm to the occipital cortex. A central vision loss is decreased visual function surrounded by normal function. Hemianopsia is a visual defect in the right and left halves of the visual field; this is due to a lesion involving the chiasm. In homonymous hemianopsia, the same half of the visual field of each eye is affected by a lesion posterior to the chiasm (see Figure 35-1).

Test Corneal Light Reflex

The corneal light reflex test is used to detect strabismus. Alignment of the eyes is most easily demonstrated by observing the reflection of a light on the cornea. The light should fall in each eye at the same point. An asymmetrical light reflex will be present in a deviating eye or in an eye with an asymmetrical contour.

Perform a Cover/Uncover Test

Have the patient look with both eyes at a specific point. With one eye covered, watch the uncovered eye. If this eye moves to fix on the point, it was not aligned before the other eye was covered and a heteropia, or deviation of an eye, is present. If the uncovered eye does not move, alignment is present and this is referred to as orthophoria. Repeat the test for the other eye.

Perform an Alternating Cover/Uncover Test

Alternate the cover rapidly on each eye and note any movement of the eyes. Perform this test to discover a latent tendency for misalignment of the two eyes, a condition referred to as heterophoria.

Use the Amsler Grid

An Amsler grid is used to test for distortion of central vision. The patient is asked to wear reading glasses, and the chart is held 15 inches from the eyes. Ask the patient to stare at the dot and tell you if the lines around the dot are curved or bent. Distortion, called metamorphopsia, is found in age-related macular degeneration or central vision loss (Figure 35-2).

Test for Extraocular Movements

Extraocular movements test six pairs of ocular muscles and three cranial nerves (III, IV, and VI). Strabismus is any condition in which the normal binocular alignment of the eyes to a single point in any and all fields of gaze is disturbed; there is an imbalance in neuromuscular sensory and motor control of the extraocular muscles. Half of patients with strabismus also have amblyopia.

RIGHT

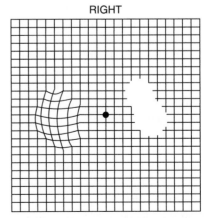

FIGURE 35-2 Example of metamorphopsia and a scotoma projected on an Amsler grid. (From Hampton GR, Nelson PT: *Age-related macular degeneration principles and practice,* New York, 1992, Raven Press.)

Paralytic strabismus is a deviation in the direction opposite the muscle involved. Double vision is usually a symptom but may not be present if the condition occurred at an early age and the child suppressed the vision in one eye or developed a compensatory head malposition.

Nonparalytic strabismus is present when the angle of deviation is the same in all cardinal fields of gaze.

Obtain a Direct and Consensual Pupillary Response

In monocular blindness, the affected eye will have no direct pupil response but will react consensually to stimulation of the opposite eye. Stimulation of the blind eye, however, will not cause consensual reaction of the opposite normal eye.

Perform an Ophthalmoscopic Examination

Examination of the optic disc can rule out optic atrophy, papilledema, and glaucoma. Death of the fibers of the optic nerve results in disappearance of the vessels of the disc, leading to pallor or whiteness of the disc.

Observe for a red light reflex, especially in the early days and months of life. If the red reflexes are not equal, refer to an ophthalmologist. To obtain a red reflex in a newborn or young infant, swaddle and then hold the child. Position the ophthalmoscope diopter at 0, direct it to the eye, and gently swing or slightly parachute the infant. The vestibular system usually triggers the infant's eyes to open because of the maneuver.

In older children and adults, darken the room and instruct the patient to stare at an object or a glow sticker in the distance. When the patient looks at the ophthalmoscope light, look at both red reflexes simultaneously and compare them. A uniform red glow equal in color is normal. Absence of a red reflex indicates that some abnormality is blocking the transmission of light through the eye.

The earliest sign of papilledema is a hyperemic disc caused by increased venous pressure. The dilated vessels leak their contents. The fluid leak causes elevation of the disc, which may spread beyond the disc margins, making the edges of the disc appear swollen or indistinct. In glaucoma, one sees a glaucomatous cup. The disc edge appears to be displaced slightly backward, causing a cup shape.

Hemorrhages scattered in the vitreous cavity tend to disperse and absorb light. A red reflex is not seen; only darkness will be seen. This is a common finding in advanced diabetic retinopathy.

LABORATORY AND DIAGNOSTIC STUDIES
Ophthalmoscopy with Pupillary Dilation

Direct ophthalmoscopy allows a view into the retina and optic nerve. More of the peripheral posterior segment is seen when the eye is dilated with a mydriatic drug.

If the iris seems abnormally close to the cornea, dilation is contraindicated because of the risk of inducing acute-angle closure glaucoma.

Tonometry

A tonometer is a device that measures intraocular pressure. Intraocular pressure greater than 21 mm Hg is considered a high-risk factor for glaucoma.

Fluorescein Dye

Fluorescein dye is used to detect the presence of abrasions or a foreign body on the corneal surface. If the corneal epithelium has been disturbed, fluorescein will pool within these areas and stain the hydrophilic stoma. A stain showing a dendritic pattern indicates herpes infection.

DIFFERENTIAL DIAGNOSIS

Early detection and treatment of vision and eye diseases yield immense benefits.

Strabismus and Amblyopia

The most common causes of vision loss in children are amblyopia and strabismus. Amblyopia, or lazy eye, is reduced visual acuity in one eye that is not correctable with lenses. It is caused by incomplete visual system development when a refractive error is not corrected in childhood. Strabismus is a condition in which the two eyes do not point in the same direction when the patient is looking at a distant object. These conditions cause vision loss in 2 out of every 100 children. The risk of the development of amblyopia is greatest during the first 2 to 3 years of life, but the potential for recurrence exists until visual development is complete at 9 years of age.

Refractive Errors

Refractive errors are a common visual disorder of childhood, occurring in 20% of children by 16 years of age. Permanent visual impairment may result if optical correction is not provided at an appropriate age.

Myopia (nearsightedness) is when the cornea and lens of the eye focus the image in front of the retina. Hyperopia (farsightedness) is a refractive error in which the focus of an image is behind the retina. Hyperopia can be corrected to some degree by adjustment of the natural lens (accommodation) normally done for near-focusing. The use of accommodation can cause visual fatigue, discomfort, and headache.

Astigmatism

Astigmatism is an irregularity in the refractive system of the eye that prevents light from being focused onto the retina. It can be secondary to the shape of the cornea or lens and is usually correctable with lenses.

Cataracts

A cataract is any opacity of the crystalline lens of the eye. There are many causes of cataracts, and they can be defined by onset, cause, or anatomy.

Congenital cataracts are inherited in an autosomal dominant form and are associated with intrauterine infections by the TORCH complex of organisms. Cataracts of infancy and childhood occur in 1 per 1000 live births, and congenital glaucoma occurs in 1 per 10,000 live births.

Adult cataracts are a major cause of visual impairment in the elderly because with time, the human lens begins to develop opacities. Cataracts can be caused by galactosemia, metabolic disorders (e.g., diabetic cataracts), and trauma (e.g., from heat or blunt trauma); steroid-induced cataract formation is also possible. The first signs of opacity are the inability to focus on near objects (presbyopia) and altered color vision.

Optic Neuritis

Optic neuritis occurs more often in younger adults, 20 to 50 years old, and in women; it is typically monocular. It is often idiopathic and may be associated with multiple sclerosis, post viral infection, and granulomatous inflammatory conditions. Vision loss occurs over a few hours to days and is extremely variable. Visual field loss includes central scotoma in 90% of patients. In the majority of patients, pain precedes the vision loss and is worse with eye movement.

Optic Nerve Hypoplasia

This visual disorder affects the optic nerve, the bundle of fibers that transmits signals from the retina to the brain. It is a nonprogressive disorder in which the optic nerve is 25% smaller than the normal size. Some children have a loss of peripheral vision while others lose central vision.

Injury

More than 100,000 eye injuries occur annually in the general population, of which 90% are preventable with the use of protective eyewear. Exposure to long periods of high heat or blunt trauma to the eye globe can result in cataracts.

Retinoblastoma

This is the most common intraocular tumor of childhood; it occurs bilaterally in 30% of cases. A common symptom is strabismus. Retinoblastoma is inherited in an autosomal dominant manner. Early lesions are flat, transparent, or white masses in the retina. The tumor can spread to the brain through the optic nerve or into the bone marrow.

Retinopathy of Prematurity

This condition is seen in premature infants and refers to the changes of ischemia, blood vessel growth, and fibrosis that occur because of inadequate oxygen delivery to the peripheral retina. The vessels of the retina normally complete vascularization by 40 weeks of gestation. Infants who are born before this time may have incomplete vascularization with subsequent poor vessel development and visual impairments. Infants smaller than 1500 grams (g) are at greatest risk.

Central Retinal Artery Occlusion

Patients with this condition have a sudden onset of severe vision loss in one eye. There is no associated pain. The loss is caused by plaque lodging at the level of the lamina cribrosa. On physical examination a few hours after occlusion, the retina becomes edematous and white or opaque. There is a reddish-orange reflex from the intact choroidal vascular and foveola that creates a "cherry red spot" that contrasts with the surrounding white retina. With time, the retinal artery opens and the retinal edema clears.

Glaucoma

Glaucoma is loss of vision because of increased pressure in the eye; it is characterized by defects in the visual field and optic nerve damage. It is the second leading cause of blindness in the United States. The condition is painless, and symptoms appear in late stages. Ophthalmic examination reveals pathological cupping of the optic disc that may be asymmetrical. Patients with intraocular pressures above 21 mm Hg should be referred to an ophthalmologist (Box 35-2).

Retinal Detachment

This condition occurs when the neurosensory retina is separated from the retinal pigment epithelium. About half of patients will have brief flashes of light (photopsia) or floaters (entopsia). It is caused by a collection of fluid beneath the neurosensory retina, traction from fibrovascular elements associated with diabetic retinopathy, or trauma. Nearly 95% of detachments are treatable.

Macular Degeneration

Age-related macular degeneration is the leading cause of blindness in the United States. It may be asymptomatic or associated with gradual loss of central vision. Risk factors include advanced age, family history, cigarette smoking, hyperopia, and hypertension. There are two forms of pathological macular degeneration. The exudative form results in rapid vision loss caused by the development of a subretinal pigment epithelial neovascular membrane. The nonexudative form is associated with gradual loss of central vision. Distortion upon testing with the Amsler grid is found in macular degeneration.

Diabetic Retinopathy

Diabetic retinopathy is a retinovascular disease that occurs in two forms. Nonproliferative retinopathy is characterized by microaneurysms, macular edema, lipid exudates, and intraretinal hemorrhages. In proliferative retinopathy, blood vessels regenerate on the retina. The patient may be asymptomatic or have decreased vision or floaters. Diabetic retinopathy progresses with the duration of diabetes.

Box 35-2   **Adult Vision Screening**

Visual acuity should be assessed intermittently after age 40 with no optimal interval recommended. Routine screening for glaucoma by primary care providers is not recommended.

Uveitis

Uveitis is a general term used to describe inflammatory activity of the iris, ciliary body, and choroid. Symptoms vary according to cause and severity, but most patients experience some decrease in vision, light sensitivity, and tearing. Pain may be variable. Acute uveitis lasts less than 3 months, but the condition may have a chronic recurrent pattern.

Optic Nerve Glioma

Optic nerve gliomas are present in two forms. In the adult, they are malignant glioblastomas; in the child, they are benign pilocytic astrocytomas. They appear in children younger than age 10 and are highly associated with neurofibromatosis, a condition associated with café au lait lesions of the skin. In children, gliomas may appear as the rapid onset of vision loss with headache. Of the malignant optic nerve gliomas, nearly 75% present with unilateral, rapidly progressive vision loss with pain.

Craniopharyngioma

Craniopharyngiomas are tumors that arise from squamous epithelial cells of the brain. They are most common in the first two decades of life but also may occur in adults 50 to 70 years old. Children's presenting symptoms include headache and visual disturbance caused by increased intracranial pressure. Nystagmus and bitemporal hemianopsia are pathognomonic for this tumor. In the older patient, visual deficit is common in the presence of normal optic discs.

Chemical or Thermal Trauma

A chemical burn is an ophthalmic emergency. Alkaline solutions denature eye proteins and lyse cell membranes, allowing the chemical to penetrate the eye. Acid burns can also cause severe damage, but the acid solution precipitates proteins, decreasing the amount of penetration damage.

Congenital Infection

Congenital TORCH infections can cause vision problems in infants. Postnatal screening is performed to diagnose a TORCH infection.

DIFFERENTIAL DIAGNOSIS OF *Common Causes of Vision Loss*

CONDITION	HISTORY	PHYSICAL FINDINGS	DIAGNOSTIC STUDIES
Strabismus	Family reports child's eyes cross, family history	Extraocular movements abnormal, cover/uncover test positive	Refer
Amblyopia	May have history of premature birth, Down syndrome, cerebral palsy, hydrocephalus	Vision decreased in one eye	Refer
Refractive errors	Sitting close to television, squinting	Loss of visual acuity	Screen with Snellen, Tumbling E, or figures; refer
Cataracts	Blurred vision, glare, distortion and change in color perception, increased age, history of infection, trauma, or chronic disease	Whitish appearance of pupil, bilateral or unilateral	Refer
Optic neuritis	History of multiple sclerosis, viral infection, pain with eye movement, rapid vision loss	Decreased visual acuity, reduced color perception, afferent pupil defect and central scotoma	Refer
Optic nerve hypoplasia	History of vision loss, may have central vision but no peripheral vision	Optic nerve is one half to one third normal size, pale to gray in color, surrounded by yellow halo	Refer
Injury, penetrating injury	History suggesting head or eye trauma (blunt or sharp)	Directed by history	Refer because of high incidence of penetrating injury
Retinoblastoma	Family history, child 2 years old or younger	Partial or absent red reflex, strabismus	Refer
Nystagmus	History of eyes moving repetitively, searching	Rhythmic, repetitive oscillation of eyes	Refer
Retinopathy of prematurity	Premature birth <36 weeks, 1500 g, oxygen administered, may be a twin	Abnormalities of retinal vessels	Refer
Central retinal artery occlusion	Sudden onset of painless vision loss, may come and go	Macular edema, cherry red spot; may see vessel narrowing	Refer
Glaucoma	Most often painless, gradual vision loss, blurring, and halos; more common in older adults; history of systemic disease	Decreased visual acuity; may have increased intraocular pressure on palpation of eye globe	Refer for tonometry
Retinal detachment	Sensation of flashing light accompanied by shower of floaters; history of trauma to head or face	Retina markedly elevated; appears gray with dark blood vessels; may lie in folds	Refer
Macular degeneration	Older than 60 years, decreased central vision, blue eyes, image larger in one eye	Hyaline (drusen) deposits on retina near macula, gray-green areas of pigment under retina, decreased visual acuity	Amsler grid
Diabetic retinopathy	History of diabetes, floaters, gradual vision loss	Venous dilation, retinal hemorrhages	Refer
Uveitis	History of infection or chronic inflammation, mild to moderate pain, photophobia, tearing	Findings vary according to cause and severity	Refer

Continued

DIFFERENTIAL DIAGNOSIS OF *Common Causes of Vision Loss—cont'd*

CONDITION	HISTORY	PHYSICAL FINDINGS	DIAGNOSTIC STUDIES
Optic nerve glioma	Dimness of vision with loss of fields; may be unilateral rapid vision loss with pain	Visual field defects, optic atrophy	Refer
Craniopharyngioma	Unilateral vision loss, headache, child or adult	Funduscopic examination may be normal	Refer
Chemical burn	History of acid or alkaline exposure	Treat first, then examine	Immediate eye irrigation and referral
Thermal burns	History of exposure to high heat, occupational risk	Corneal opacities	Refer
Congenital infections	TORCH, maternal exposure to measles	Retinitis, optic nerve hypoplasia	Screen for TORCH, refer

TORCH, toxoplasmosis, rubella, cytomegalovirus, and herpes simplex.

REFERENCES AND READINGS

Anonymous: Glaucoma: early detection can minimize vision loss, *Mayo Clin Health Lett* 23:7, 2005.

Coles WH: *Ophthalmology: a diagnostic text*, Baltimore, Md, 1989, Williams & Wilkins.

Harvey PT: Common eye diseases of elderly people: identifying and treating causes of vision loss, *Gerontology* 49:1, 2003.

McPhee SJ, Papadakis MA: *Current medical diagnosis and treatment*, ed 49, New York, 2010, McGraw-Hill.

Norton I: Practical ophthalmology—a survival guide for doctors and optometrists, *Emerg Med Australia* 17:5, 2005.

Quillen DA: Common causes of vision loss in elderly patients, *Am Fam Physician* 60:99, 1999.

Thompson L, Kauffman L: The visually impaired child, *Pediatr Clin North Am* 50:225, 2003.

Tingley DV: Vision screening essentials: screening today for eye disorders in the pediatric patient, *Pediatr Rev* 28:54, 2007.

World Health Organization: Visual impairment and blindness, *Fact Sheet* 282, May 2009. Available online at http://www.who.int/mediacentre/factsheets/fs282/en/print.html. Accessed June 23, 2010.

Weight Loss/Gain (Unintentional)

Unintentional weight loss is a decrease in body weight that is not voluntary. Weight loss in the adult is clinically significant when it exceeds 5% of usual body weight over a 6 to 12 month period. Weight loss in the newborn may occur immediately after birth but weight should begin to increase by 2 weeks of age. Weight loss will occur with reduced energy (food) intake and increased metabolism or energy output. Every day individuals adjust energy balance to maintain a healthy weight through healthy eating and regular physical activity. Malignancy and endocrine disorders are at the top of the list of causes of unintentional weight loss, followed by gastrointestinal, cognitive, behavioral, and functional disorders, as well as age-related changes.

Weight gain occurs when caloric intake exceeds body requirements, causing the body to store fat. Most adults do not intentionally gain weight, but as we age, a decrease in physical abilities leads to a decrease in metabolic rate (amount of energy used in a given period), which in turn contributes to weight gain. Unexplained weight gain may be more difficult to identify, especially in the U.S., where the prevalence of obesity is 32.2% among adult men and 35.5% among adult women. The prevalence of childhood obesity is increasing. Unexplained weight gain may be endocrine-related, age-related, or associated with cognitive impairments.

DIAGNOSTIC REASONING: FOCUSED HISTORY
Unexplained Weight Loss

Has the patient lost weight? Is the weight loss really unexplained?

Key Questions

- How do you know that you (or the child) have lost weight?
- How old are you?

- How is your appetite?
- Can you describe your typical diet and activity patterns?
- If an infant: If breastfeeding, how is breastfeeding going?
- If an infant: If feeding formula, what kind is it and how do you prepare it?

Measuring Weight

Individuals might note that their clothes are too loose or too tight. Weight is usually measured by asking the patient to step on a balance or electric scale clothed and without shoes. Height is measured by asking the patient to stand with the back against a wall with heels touching the wall. There are several ways to classify and measure body weight, but the most commonly used method is the body mass index (BMI) formula, which is BMI = weight (kg)/height (m^2) (see Appendix C). To enhance the reliability of measurement of weight changes, ask the patient to weigh himself or herself at the same time each day using the same scale.

Weight and height in infants and children is measured by a scale and plotted on a National Center for Health Statistics growth chart. Infants and children should be measured in a supine position until the age of 2 years. Head circumference is also measured and plotted.

Age

Aging can be associated with both weight loss and weight gain. Normally with aging there is less lean muscle tissue, fat is deposited in the trunk and less in the limbs, and metabolism slows. In the elderly it is especially important to assess what medications are being taken that could suppress appetite, cognitive status, and memory. Functional limitations that may impact nutrition include the ability to chew and swallow, prepare meals, and shop for food. Social isolation can also contribute to eating less.

Appetite

Appetite can be suppressed due to the presence of acute or chronic illness. Cachexia will result from inadequate energy intake and pathologic wasting of muscle or fat tissue. The key symptom in cachexia is anorexia, or loss of appetite. Psychosocial factors, such as anxiety or depression, can contribute to a loss of appetite or lifestyle habits that include skipping meals or eating foods of poor nutritional value.

Eating Habits/Nutritional Adequacy and Physical Activity

Weight maintenance is a balance of energy expended and energy consumed. General healthy dietary guidelines can be found in the Dietary Guidelines for Americans (Box 36-1) and on MyPyramid (http://mypyramid.gov). Daily caloric needs vary by age, gender, pregnancy, and level of physical activity. Athletes in training may underestimate their caloric needs (Box 36-2).

Excess intake of fruit juices may decrease a child's appetite and cause weight loss. Conversely, excess intake of fruit juices with high caloric content may cause weight gain.

Breastfeeding

Observing and discussing issues regarding breast-feeding with the mother may reveal important information. Infants should be breastfed 8 to 12 times in a 24-hour period. Breastfeeding requires more energy expenditure from the infant, and occasionally infants fall asleep while feeding and thus do not receive an adequate amount of breast milk. Nipple soreness is usually caused by improper positioning and/or poor latching or unlatching and can lead to a diminished milk supply. Maternal hydration is important for adequate milk supply.

Formula-Fed Infant

Investigating what formula the infant is being fed and how the formula is prepared is important. Formulas come in powder and liquid forms. Powder formula requires reconstitution with water. Liquid formula comes in two forms: concentrated (requiring the addition of water) and ready-to-feed. Taking a history of how the formula is prepared is important to determine whether incorrect preparation is causing weight loss.

Are emotional issues contributing to weight loss?

Key Questions

- Have you recently had a stressful event in your life? How are you coping?
- Do you or anyone in your family have a problem with anxiety or depression?
- How are you doing in school or at work?
- If a child: Is the child gaining weight appropriately?

Psychosocial Factors

Emotions have a big impact on appetite and eating behavior. One reaction to extreme stress or depression may be a loss of appetite. Individuals may have

---

Box 36-1	**Key Recommendations for Maintaining A Healthy Weight**

- To maintain body weight in a healthy range, balance calories from foods and beverages with calories expended.
- To prevent gradual weight gain over time, make small decreases in food and beverage calories and increase physical activity.

Key Recommendations for Specific Population Groups

- *Those who need to lose weight.* Aim for a slow, steady weight loss by decreasing calorie intake while maintaining an adequate nutrient intake and increasing physical activity.
- *Overweight children.* Reduce the rate of body weight gain while allowing growth and development. Consult a healthcare provider before placing a child on a weight-reduction diet.
- *Pregnant women.* Ensure appropriate weight gain as specified by a healthcare provider.
- *Breastfeeding women.* Moderate weight reduction is safe and does not compromise weight gain of the nursing infant.
- *Overweight adults and overweight children with chronic diseases and/or on medication.* Consult a healthcare provider about weight loss strategies prior to starting a weight-reduction program to ensure appropriate management of other health conditions.

From U.S. Department of Health and Human Services, U.S. Department of Agriculture: *Dietary guidelines for Americans, 2005.* Available online at www.healthierus.gov/dietaryguidelines. Accessed August 5, 2010.

Box 36-2	**Key Recommendations for Physical Activity**

Engage in regular physical activity and reduce sedentary activities to promote health, psychological wellbeing, and a healthy body weight.
- To reduce the risk of chronic disease in adulthood: Engage in at least 30 minutes of moderate-intensity physical activity, above usual activity, at work or home on most days of the week.
- For most people, greater health benefits can be obtained by engaging in physical activity of more vigorous intensity or longer duration.
- To help manage body weight and prevent gradual, unhealthy body weight gain in adulthood: Engage in approximately 60 minutes of moderate- to vigorous-intensity activity on most days of the week while not exceeding caloric intake requirements.
- To sustain weight loss in adulthood: Participate in at least 60 to 90 minutes of daily moderate-intensity physical activity while not exceeding caloric intake requirements. Some people may need to consult with a healthcare provider before participating in this level of activity.

Achieve physical fitness by including cardiovascular conditioning, stretching exercises for flexibility, and resistance exercises or calisthenics for muscle strength and endurance.

Key Recommendations for Specific Population Groups
- *Children and adolescents.* Engage in at least 60 minutes of physical activity on most, preferably all, days of the week.
- *Pregnant women.* In the absence of medical or obstetric complications, incorporate 30 minutes or more of moderate-intensity physical activity on most, if not all, days of the week. Avoid activities with a high risk of falling or abdominal trauma.
- *Breastfeeding women.* Be aware that neither acute nor regular exercise adversely affects the mother's ability to successfully breastfeed.
- *Older adults.* Participate in regular physical activity to reduce functional declines associated with aging and to achieve the other benefits of physical activity identified for all adults.

From U.S. Department of Health and Human Services, U.S. Department of Agriculture: *Dietary guidelines for Americans, 2005.* Available online at www.healthierus.gov/dietaryguidelines. Accessed August 5, 2010.

patterns of coping with stress by controlling food intake. Anorexia nervosa and bulimia are eating disorders most often diagnosed in young females. With these two disorders, despite the low or normal weight, the individual perceives herself or himself as overweight. Anorexia nervosa carries a high risk of complications due to electrolyte imbalances.

Failure To Thrive

Failure to thrive in infants may have a nonorganic etiology. Causes include but are not limited to caretaker's employment status, social isolation, family stress, substance abuse, postpartum depression, and poor parenting skills.

What cues indicate a pathologic process?

Key Questions

- Have you had a fever or any signs of illness?
- Have you ever been diagnosed with cancer?
- Have you had a change in urinary or bowel habits?
- Do you experience fatigue?
- In a room where others are comfortable, are you often too cold or too warm?

- Have you had a change in appetite or thirst?
- If a child: Has your child's appetite changed?
- If a child: Has your child's activity level changed?

Acute or Chronic Conditions

Fever associated fatigue and lymphadenopathy may indicate an infection. Chronic conditions, such as cough, shortness of breath, nausea, vomiting, anemia, fatigue, weakness, change in moles, pain, abnormal menstrual bleeding, breast discharge, or chronic headaches, can contribute to unintentional weight loss. Crohn disease is an inflammatory bowel disease that can be associated with a reduced appetite.

Unintentional weight loss is a red flag for cancer occurrence or reoccurrence. Weight loss can occur from loss of appetite and decreased caloric intake, or from the body's inability to absorb nutrients because of the cancer.

Diabetes

Diabetes is a disease caused by insulin secretion deficiency and insulin resistance resulting in elevated blood glucose levels that do not allow nutrients to enter cells. Along with weight loss, untreated diabetes is often associated with increased hunger, excessive thirst, and frequent urination.

Endocrine Disorders

Hyperthyroidism is a condition that speeds up metabolism, thus burning more calories. It is the most common thyroid function disorder. Symptoms include trembling, insomnia, and hair loss.

Hypothyroidism is when thyroid hormones are insufficient. In less developed countries, it is most often due to is iodine deficiency; however, in the U.S., autoimmune processes are the major cause. Onset of symptoms is insidious and involves every organ system. A history will reveal symptoms of lethargy, dry skin, cold intolerance, deepening of voice, and facial puffiness. Cushing syndrome is a result of prolonged exposure to excessive levels of glucocorticoid cortisol, which has a catabolic effect on most tissues. Muscle wasting and weakness is due to generalized protein catabolism.

Appetite/Activity Level Change

A change in an infant or child's appetite and activity level is a good indicator of illness. Appetite can decrease with an inactive lifestyle or the presence of chronic pain, irritable bowel syndrome, or other conditions that might be exacerbated by eating.

What other symptoms might help narrow the possibilities?

Key Questions

- When was your last cancer screening?
- If a child: Has your child recently switched to solid food?
- Do you have a family history of cystic fibrosis?
- Does anyone in your household have a history of tuberculosis?

Cancer Screening

Routine cancer screening recommendations vary by gender and age and include colon cancer screening, skin exams, and, for women, periodic screening mammography for breast cancer and Pap smears for cervical cancer screening. Additional screening for cancer, especially the use of computed tomography, will depend on associated symptoms and history of risk factors. The United States Preventive Services Task Force (USPSTF) conducts rigorous assessments of the scientific evidence for the effectiveness of a range of clinical preventive services, including screening, counseling, and preventive medications. The USPSTF recommendations are considered the gold standard for clinical preventive services (http://www.ahrq.gov/clinic/uspstfix.htm). Lack of regular screening places patients at an increased risk for undetected cancer.

Diet Change

Infants who were on formula or breast milk but switched to solid food may exhibit malabsorption conditions (such as lactose intolerance or celiac disease) that can cause weight loss or slowed weight gain.

Family History

The cystic fibrosis (CF) gene is autosomal recessive. Four percent of white persons in the U.S. are estimated to be carriers (heterozygous) of the CF gene. CF may present as lack of weight gain between the first and sixth months.

Tuberculosis is often associated with reduced appetite and weight loss and is contracted among individuals who are exposed to an active infection, especially within a family or household.

What self-treatment was used? Did it help?

Key Questions

- Are you taking any prescribed or over-the-counter (OTC) preparations to lose weight?
- How would you describe your eating habits and dietary practices?

Medication History

There are numerous weight loss drugs on the market and many of them contain ephedrine, a stimulant that suppresses appetite. These drugs can be associated with cardiac arrhythmia and an elevation in blood pressure. In general, drugs to lose weight are not commonly prescribed but are readily available over the counter. Individuals may use fasting or purging as a method of rapid weight loss; fasting also is often done as an observance of religious or spiritual practice.

Some drugs cause an altered taste sensation and decease in appetite. Maternal ingestion of drugs while nursing may affect breast milk supply. Dopamine agonists, such as cabergoline, reduce prolactin and are sometimes used therapeutically to stop lactation. Dopamine antagonists, such as metoclopramide and most antipsychotics, may increase prolactin and milk production. Other drugs that have been associated with hyperprolactinemia include selective serotonin reuptake inhibitors (SSRIs) and opioids.

How serious is this situation? Is this a recent change?

Key Questions

- How long have you been concerned about your weight loss?
- Is anyone else concerned about your weight loss?
- What is your ideal or usual weight?

Validate Weight Change
A careful history may document changes in activity level or a precipitating incident before weight loss was noticed as a problem.

Concern about Weight Loss
Anorexic patients do not believe they have a weight loss problem and have a morbid fear of weight gain. Often family members or friends become concerned and refer the patient to be evaluated.

Ideal or Usual Weight
Normal or ideal weight for age and gender can be checked against actuarial tables, such as the 1999 Metropolitan Height and Weight Tables for Men and Women (http://www.bcbst.com/mpmanual/hw.htm). Continued unintended weight loss noted for more than 6 months should be evaluated. Weight can be verified by using a reliable weight scale. Note if the person was weighed with or without shoes. Clothing worn should be lightweight.

Unexplained Weight Gain

Is the weight gain explained by diet and exercise habits?

Key Questions

- Can you describe what you eat in a typical day?
- Has your eating pattern changed?
- Can you describe your level of physical activity?

Balance of Energy Intake and Expenditure
Maintaining an ideal body weight depends on achieving a balance of energy intake and energy expenditure (Table 36-1). Calorie intake can exceed expenditure when a person consumes large quantities of food and food with high calorie content but gets little aerobic exercise. Factors that contribute to inactivity are sedentary jobs, TV watching, and reliance on the automobile. Environmental and genetic factors contribute to a small percentage of cases of obesity.

Is the weight gain associated with aging?

Key Questions

- What is your age?
- For females: When was your last menstrual period?

Aging
Normal aging is associated with slower metabolism and reduced energy requirements.

Menopause
Menopause is defined as the absence of a menstrual period for one year. About 90% of menopausal women gain some weight between the ages of 35 and 55. Hormones have a direct impact on appetite, metabolism, and fat storage. Lower levels of progesterone, androgen, and testosterone contribute to lower metabolism and weight gain.

Could weight gain be related to other behaviors?

Key Questions

- How much alcohol do you consume in a week or a day?
- Do you smoke? If so, how much do you smoke? How long have you smoked? At what age did you start smoking? Have you recently quit?
- Do you take any medications?

Alcohol and Smoking
Drinking multiple glasses or bottles of alcohol daily or weekly will increase calorie intake. Many adults will gain 5 to 10 pounds in the first few months after quitting smoking.

Medications
Such drugs as corticosteroids, lithium, tranquilizers, phenothiazines, and tricyclic antidepressants may lead to fluid retention.

Table 36-1	Estimated Calorie Requirements (In Kilocalories) for Each Gender and Age Group at Three Levels of Physical Activity[a]

Estimated amounts of calories needed to maintain energy balance for various gender and age groups at three different levels of physical activity. The estimates are rounded to the nearest 200 calories and were determined using the Institute of Medicine equation.

GENDER	AGE (YEARS)	SEDENTARY[b]	Activity Level[b,c,d] MODERATELY ACTIVE[c]	ACTIVE[d]
Child	2-3	1,000	1,000-1,400[e]	1,000-1,400[e]
Female	4-8	1,200	1,400-1,600	1,400-1,800
	9-13	1,600	1,600-2,000	1,800-2,200
	14-18	1,800	2,000	2,400
	19-30	2,000	2,000-2,200	2,400
	31-50	1,800	2,000	2,200
	51+	1,600	1,800	2,000-2,200
Male	4-8	1,400	1,400-1,600	1,600-2,000
	9-13	1,800	1,800-2,200	2,000-2,600
	14-18	2,200	2,400-2,800	2,800-3,200
	19-30	2,400	2,600-2,800	3,000
	31-50	2,200	2,400-2,800	2,800-3,200
	51+	2,000	2,200-2,400	2,400-2,800

[a]These levels are based on Estimated Energy Requirements (EER) from the Institute of Medicine Dietary Reference Intakes macronutrients report, 2002, calculated by gender, age, and activity level for reference-sized individuals. "Reference size," as determined by IOM, is based on median height and weight for ages up to age 18 years and median height and weight for that height to give a BMI of 21.5 for adult females and 22.5 for adult males.
[b]Sedentary means a lifestyle that includes only the light physical activity associated with typical day-to-day life.
[c]Moderately active means a lifestyle that includes physical activity equivalent to walking about 1.5 to 3 miles per day at 3 to 4 miles per hour, in addition to the light physical activity associated with typical day-to-day life.
[d]Active means a lifestyle that includes physical activity equivalent to walking more than 3 miles per day at 3 to 4 miles per hour, in addition to the light physical activity associated with typical day-to-day life.
[e]The calorie ranges shown are to accommodate needs of different ages within the group. For children and adolescents, more calories are needed at older ages. For adults, fewer calories are needed at older ages.
From U.S. Department of Health and Human Services, U.S. Department of Agriculture: *Dietary guidelines for Americans, 2005.* Available online at www.healthierus.gov/dietaryguidelines. Accessed August 5, 2010.

Could this be caused by an endocrine disorder?

Key Questions

- Has the weight gain been sudden or gradual?
- How much do you weigh now compared to a year ago?
- Have you noticed any other symptoms or changes in your appearance?

Acuity of Weight Gain

Women who are premenopausal may note gradual weight gain over a few years. Some medications, such as ß-blockers, corticosteroids, and antidepressants, are associated with weight gain. Edema from congestive heart failure or renal failure can cause weight gain in a few days or weeks.

Endocrine Symptoms

Hypothyroidism is associated with fatigue, constipation, and the inability to tolerate cold temperatures. Cushing syndrome is associated with truncal weight gain, moon facies, and a "buffalo hump." Both of these disorders may develop over an extended period of time. Polycystic ovary syndrome is associated with obesity and hirsutism.

DIAGNOSTIC REASONING: FOCUSED PHYSICAL EXAMINATION

A thorough health history and general physical examination, including screening for psychosocial causes (see Chapter 3), will help to identify behavioral risk factors or a pattern of associated symptoms that suggest a systemic disorder.

Note General Appearance

Observe the patient entering the room. Especially note the fit of clothing as well as general hygiene and signs of stress or anxiety.

When examining an infant, observe interaction with the caregiver. Failure-to-thrive infants may avoid eye contact, show a lack of smiling or sounds, and have poor interaction with their environment. The infant may also prefer not to be cuddled and be difficult to comfort, and may appear withdrawn even from the caregiver.

Take Vital Signs

Vital signs will provide information on cardiovascular and respiratory function. Height and weight can be compared to actuarial tables to see norms for weight by age and gender. Calculate BMI. Bradycardia may indicate hypothyroidism; tachycardia may indicate anemia, dehydration, or hyperthyroidism. Fever may indicate infection.

Weigh and Measure Newborn

A decrease in weight of more than 8% necessitates followup within 48 hours, and a bilirubin level should be drawn to assess for hyperbilirubinemia. A loss of more than 10% of birth weight warrants careful assessment of possible causes and consideration of admission to the hospital.

Assess Mental Status

The major cognitive changes to detect as related to weight loss or gain are dementia and depression (see Chapter 8). Dementia can be assessed using the mini-MMSE (see Figure 8-1) and distinguished from depression (see Box 8-1). Screen for the presence of an eating disorder.

Conduct a Comprehensive Physical Examination
Assess the Skin

Examine the skin for intactness, turgor, and presence of lesions to determine hydration status and overall nutrition status. Hypothyroidism is associated with dry, flaky skin; skin darkening occurs with Addison disease.

Assess the Heart

Palpate the anterior thorax for the point of maximal impulse (PMI), lifts, and heaves. Auscultate for adventitious sounds (see Chapter 7).

Examine the Head and Neck

Assess the head and neck for presence of lymphadenopathy. Moon facies indicates Cushing syndrome. Palpate the thyroid for masses or asymmetry.

Assess the condition of the teeth and gums. Test the patient's ability to swallow using water or test for the gag reflex. Patients with diabetes may have xanthomas associated with hyperlipidemia.

Examine the Abdomen

Observe for contour. Patients with diabetes tend to have truncal obesity. Redistribution of fat in older patients may also cause them to have truncal obesity. Palpate for tenderness or lumps, auscultate for bowel sounds, and check for rebound tenderness. Patients with malabsorption may have ascites.

Examine the Extremities

Conduct a musculoskeletal exam to assess strength, mobility, and balance (see Chapter 20). Assess for loss of muscle mass and subcutaneous fat associated with cachexia, malabsorption, and aging. Patients with hypothyroidism may have generalized edema and delayed recovery of deep tendon reflexes. Patients with hyperthyroidism may have overly brisk deep tendon reflexes. Patients with diabetes may have peripheral neuropathy.

Complete Blood Count with Indices and Differential

A complete blood count (CBC) with indices will provide information about the degree and cause of anemia; microcytic hypochromic anemia reflects chronic blood loss and normocytic normochromic anemia suggests acute blood loss. The white blood cell (WBC) count indicates the presence of inflammation or infection (see Chapter 34).

Fasting Blood Glucose

A fasting blood glucose (FBG) is a blood specimen taken at least 2 hours after a meal. The normal value for fasting FBG is below 100 mg/dL of glucose; an FBG of 100 to 125 mg/dL of glucose indicates pre-diabetes. If a random blood glucose is obtained within 2 hours after a meal, a normal value is 140 mg/dL or below.

Glycosylated Hemoglobin (A_{1c})

Glycosylated hemoglobin (A_{1c}) reflects the average blood glucose over a 3-month period. A normal value is below 7%. The A_{1c} result is not dependent on when the most recent meal was consumed, but the results may be affected by the presence of anemia or sickle cell disease. The A_{1c} result may be a poor reflection of blood glucose when severe anemia or sickle cell disease is present.

Thyroid-Stimulating Hormone

An elevated serum thyroid-stimulating hormone (TSH) level identifies hypothyroidism. A low or indetectable level indicates hyperthyroidism.

Bilirubin

Bilirubin values are usually reported as two fractions: conjugated (direct) and unconjugated (indirect). Conjugated hyperbilirubinemia is present if >50% of elevated total bilirubin is the conjugated form. Normal total conjugated bilirubin in newborns is <2 mg/dL; the level peaks to 12.9 mg/dL at 3 to 4 days of life and then decreases. A tool designed to help clinicians assess the risks of the development of hyperbilirubinemia in newborns over 35 weeks gestational age can be found at http://www.bilitool.com. Cystic fibrosis can lead to liver failure and hyperbilirubinemia.

Total Serum Protein

A total serum protein measures the amount of total protein and albumin (from the liver) and globulin (from the liver and immune system) in the blood. Normally there is more albumin than globulin with a ratio of >1. Albumin checks kidney function and reflects dietary protein. Elevated globulin may indicate infection.

Sweat Chloride Test

The quantitative pilocarpine iontophoresis test measures the amount of chloride and sodium in the sweat of patients with cystic fibrosis. Normal sweat contains <60 mEq/L of chloride and sodium. Two tests on different occasions are needed for accurate diagnosis of cystic fibrosis.

Urinalysis

The extent of diagnostic investigation of urine will depend on history and physical examination findings. Dipstick urinalysis can point out infection, proteinuria, and glycosuria (see Chapter 32).

Fecal Occult Blood Testing

The fecal occult blood test (FOBT) is an initial screening method to detect gastrointestinal bleeding (see Chapter 26).

Chest Radiograph

A chest x-ray can reveal the presence of consolidation, lesions of the lung, and heart contour.

Tests of the Gastrointestinal Tract

A barium upper gastrointestinal (GI) series is used to examine the upper GI region, but small lesions may not be detected. Any abnormality needs to be evaluated by endoscopy. The lower GI tract is evaluated using sigmoidoscopy or colonoscopy. A colonoscopy will detect the presence of polyps and lesions along the entire large intestine (see Chapter 2).

Computed Tomography

Computed tomography (CT) scanning can be done on different body regions. Abdominal CT examines the uterus, pancreas, GI tract, and other abdominal organs.

Mammography

Screening mammograms consist of two views—craniocaudal (CC) and medial lateral oblique (MLO)—to detect nonpalpable breast lesions. Compare results to previous screening mammograms (see Chapter 5).

Pap Test

The Pap test is designed to detect cancer cells in the cervix and vagina. A Pap test is generally recommended by age 18 years or in sexually active females, and is repeated every 3 to 5 years depending on the patient's age and history.

Metabolic Rate

Estimated energy needs should be based on resting or basal metabolic rate (BMR). BMR decreases with age and with the loss of lean body mass. An equation using actual weight, height, gender, and age is the most accurate for estimating BMR and calculating daily caloric requirements (Box 36-3).

DIFFERENTIAL DIAGNOSIS
Unintentional Weight Loss

Cancer

Cancer alters the body's appetite signals and metabolism resulting in cachexia, a condition in which body fat stores are depleted and muscle mass decreases. The most common malignancies that cause weight loss are gastrointestinal, lung, hematologic, and musculoskeletal. As many as 40% of people with cancer reported unexplained

Box 36-3	**Basal Metabolic Rate (BMR) Formula**

Women

$$BMR = 655 + (4.35 \times \text{weight in pounds}) + (4.7 \times \text{height in inches}) - (4.7 \times \text{age in years})$$

Men

$$BMR = 66 + (6.23 \times \text{weight in pounds}) + (12.7 \times \text{height in inches}) - (6.8 \times \text{age in years})$$

weight loss at the time of diagnosis. Some people notice weight loss despite a good appetite. Others lose their appetite and may even become nauseated by food or have difficulty swallowing.

Nutritional Status

Nutritional status is assessed by obtaining a history of dietary habits and physical activity patterns, as well as anthropometric measures (such as height and weight to calculate BMI, and waist and hip circumference to determine distribution of body fat). Poor or inadequate nutrition in severe forms is most often found in developing countries and is manifested in two forms: kwashiorkor, which is a protein deficiency, and marasmus, which is caused by inadequate food intake. Weight loss not explained by dietary intake is most likely due to systemic disease.

Endocrine Disorders

Diabetes mellitus. In the U.S. and worldwide, more than 90% of cases of diabetes are type 2. Type 1 diabetes is more often associated with weight loss despite increased appetite. Persons with type 2 diabetes may experience increased thirst and urinary frequency but often are asymptomatic. Some symptoms, such as blurred vision or peripheral neuropathy, may reflect long term manifestations of an undiagnosed disease. Despite weight loss, patients tend to exhibit central obesity.

Hyperthyroidism. Patients with hyperthyroidism may report palpitations, nervousness, emotional lability, fatigue, muscle weakness, weight loss despite good appetite, hyperdefecation, heat intolerance, menstrual changes (oligo-amenorrhea), increased appetite, insomnia, and tremors. On physical examination, exophthalmos, warm skin, onycholysis, increased sweating, and thinning hair may be evident. Patients may have localized myxedema (edematous skin thickening) of legs (pretibial) or dorsa of feet. The thyroid may be enlarged and a bruit may be present. Deep tendon reflexes (DTRs) may be brisk. High fever, congestive heart failure, and mental status changes suggest thyroid storm. TSH level will be low or indetectable.

Addison disease. Addison disease is a disorder that occurs when the adrenal glands do not produce enough of their hormones. Associated symptoms may include changes in blood pressure or heart rate, darkening of the skin, weakness, salt craving, and loss of appetite.

Malabsorption

Malabsorption is a condition where absorption and digestion of nutrients is disrupted. The disorder is caused by an insufficiency of a variety of digestive enzymes. In celiac disease, there is an immunologic response to gluten. The degree of weight loss varies and is accompanied by chronic diarrhea and growth retardation. Patients exhibit muscle wasting and loss of subcutaneous fat. In the presence of severe hypoproteinemia, ascites may be present.

Anorexia Nervosa

Anorexia most often affects young females who, despite weight loss, have a self-image of being overweight and an intense fear of gaining weight. Diagnosis is based on a body weight 15% below what is expected, a distorted body image, and the absence of at least three menstrual periods. Examination demonstrates loss of body fat, and dry, scaly skin.

Depression or Anxiety

Mood regulation through eating is a way some individuals cope with depression or anxiety (see Chapter 3). Major depression is diagnosed by the presence of a depressed mood or loss of interest or pleasure in usual activities. Bipolar disorder involves episodes of mania or hypomania, often followed by depression. In mania, the patient experiences an elevated or irritable mood, often described as a "high" (see Chapter 3).

Cognitive Impairment

Dementia or compromised cognitive function can disrupt normal self-regulation of appetite and hunger (see Chapter 8). Dementia is a nonspecific syndrome in which affected areas of cognition may include memory, attention, language, and problem solving. When it occurs early in life it is labeled as organic brain syndrome. In the elderly, dementia has a rate of memory and cognitive loss that exceeds that of normal aging (see Chapter 8).

Psychosocial Factors (Alcohol Use, Social Isolation, Economic Status)

Excessive alcohol intake may reduce appetite, which can lead to poor nutrition. Individuals are generally social beings and social isolation may reduce any motivation to prepare balanced meals or to eat when alone. Older adults and young families may have financial constraints in purchasing healthy foods, since fresh fruits and vegetables cost more than fast foods and snack foods (see Chapter 3).

HIV/AIDS

Acquired immune deficiency syndrome (AIDS) is a disease of the immune system caused by the human immunodeficiency virus (HIV). This condition progressively reduces the effectiveness of the immune system and leaves individuals susceptible to opportunistic infections and tumors. HIV is transmitted through direct contact of a mucous membrane or the bloodstream with a bodily fluid containing HIV, such as blood, semen, vaginal fluid, preseminal fluid, and breast milk. Persons with HIV infection develop opportunistic infections due to their impaired immune response, and often have systemic symptoms of infection such as fevers, sweats (particularly at night), swollen glands, chills, weakness, and weight loss.

Gastroesophageal Reflux in Infants

Regurgitation is commonly seen in newborns and young infants while feeding. Immature upper gastrointestinal motility is thought to be the cause. Excessive reflux may cause caloric deprivation resulting in weight loss.

Crohn Disease

Crohn disease is an inflammatory bowel disease that presents with abdominal cramping, rectal bleeding, and bloody diarrhea. Weight loss is common because of malabsorption. There is a genetic link in families with a two- to four-fold increase in risk when a first-degree relative has the disease. The disease can affect any part of the tract from the mouth to the anus. Disease affecting the small bowel affects nutritional status and weight loss.

Tuberculosis

Tuberculosis is caused by *Mycobacterium tuberculosis* and is spread by droplets through the respiratory tract (see Chapter 10). Weight loss is a common symptom of tuberculosis. Diagnosis is based on a positive sputum culture.

Cystic Fibrosis

Cystic fibrosis is an exocrine gland disorder that produces mucus blockage in major organs and is associated with an autosomal recessive trait (see Chapter 10). Growth retardation and weight loss are common symptoms of cystic fibrosis.

Unintentional Weight Gain
Energy Balance

A 24-hour food intake history is the first approach to assessing nutritional and caloric intake. A history of physical activity or energy expenditure is done to assess the balance between calories consumed and energy expended.

Aging

In women, cessation of estrogen secretion during menopause is associated with lower levels of progesterone, androgen, and testosterone, which can lead to weight gain and greater truncal fat deposition.

Endocrine Disorders

Hypothyroidism. Hypothyroidism (myxedema) is associated with weight gain and symptoms of cold intolerance, constipation, hoarseness, depression, and fatigue. Physical examination reveals bradycardia, dry skin, and delayed recovery of deep tendon reflexes. A TSH is elevated in primary hypothyroidism.

Cushing syndrome. Cushing syndrome is associated with weight gain. Diagnosis is made through the presence of associated symptoms, glucose tolerance tests, and the dexamethasone suppression test. Cushing syndrome is associated with central truncal obesity, moon facies, supraclavicular fat pads and thin extremities.

DIFFERENTIAL DIAGNOSIS OF *Common Causes of Unintentional Weight Loss/Gain*

CONDITION	HISTORY	PHYSICAL FINDINGS	DIAGNOSTIC STUDIES
Weight Loss			
Cancer	Loss of appetite	None or may look cachectic	Diagnostic imaging studies, CT, MRI, x-ray, CBC
Undernutrition	Poor calorie/nutrient intake, error in formula preparation	Loss of body mass	Total serum protein
Diabetes mellitus	Polyuria, polyphagia, polydipsia	Truncal obesity; xanthomas	FBG, hemoglobin A$_{1c}$, glucose tolerance test
Gastroesophage-al reflux (infants)	History of regurgitation	None	Upper GI, barium swallow
Addison disease	Salt craving, fatigue	Darkening of the skin	Serum electrolytes, 24 hour urine for aldosterone
Hyperthyroidism	Tachycardia, heat intolerance, sweating	Exophthalmos, warm skin, onycholysis, thinning hair, pretibial myxedema, enlarged thyroid, brisk DTRs	TSH, T$_4$
Malabsorption	Intolerance to gluten; chronic diarrhea, growth retardation	Muscle wasting, loss of subcutaneous fat; may have ascites	Colonoscopy, stool culture, fecal fat
Depression	Loss of appetite and/or interest in food	None or may have poor personal hygiene	Thyroid function tests, refer for psychological evaluation
Dementia	Disorientation to person, time, or place	None or loss of body mass; poor personal hygiene	MMSE
Anorexia nervosa	Female to male 10:1, perfectionist, high achiever, amenorrhea	Cachexia, hair loss, dry skin, orthostatic hypotension	Thyroid function tests, serum electrolytes
Psychosocial factors	Alcohol consumption, social isolation, financial resources	None or poor personal hygiene with chronic alcoholism	Liver function tests
Infection	Fever, fatigue	Redness or swelling of tissues or lymph nodes	Blood or tissue culture, CBC
Crohn disease	Weight loss, fever, diarrhea, family history	Perirectal fissure, anal skin tag	CBC, colonoscopy, barium enema, small bowel follow-through
Cystic fibrosis	Weight loss, cough, chronic diarrhea, positive family history	Digital clubbing, growth retardation, weight loss	Sweat test
Nonorganic failure to thrive	Weight loss, maternal isolation, maternal depression	Decreased skin fold thickness, decrease subcutaneous fat	Normal labs in 98%
Tuberculosis (TB)	Contact with person who has TB, travel to endemic area, HIV	Cough, weight loss	PPD, HIV, chest x-ray
Weight Gain			
Intake/energy balance	Excessive calorie intake; inactivity	Generalized excess of subcutaneous fat	None
Aging	Menopause history; metabo-lism change	Truncal obesity; loss of peripheral subcutaneous fat; loss of muscle mass	Serum estrogen level

Continued

DIFFERENTIAL DIAGNOSIS OF *Common Causes of Unintentional Weight Loss/Gain—cont'd*			
CONDITION	**HISTORY**	**PHYSICAL FINDINGS**	**DIAGNOSTIC STUDIES**
Hypothyroidism	Cold intolerance, weight gain, constipation; medication history	Bradycardia, dry skin, generalized edema, delayed recovery of DTRs	TSH, T_4
Cushing syndrome	Thirst, polyuria	Moon facies, truncal obesity, thin extremities	FBG, dexamethasone suppression test

CBC, complete blood count; *CT,* computed tomography; *DTR,* deep tendon reflex; *FBG,* fasting blood glucose; *GI,* gastrointestinal; *HIV,* human immunodeficiency virus; *MMSE,* Mini Mental State Examination; *MRI,* magnetic resonance imaging; *PPD,* purified protein derivative; T_4, thyroxine; *TSH,* thyroid-stimulating hormone.

REFERENCES AND READINGS

American Congress of Obstetricians and Gynecologists: *ACOG announces new pap smear and cancer screening guidelines, 2010.* Available online at http://www.acog.org/acog_districts/dist_notice.cfm?recno=13&bulletin=3161. Accessed July 28, 2010.

Austin J, Marks D: Hormonal regulators of appetite. *Int J Pediatr Endocrinol* Epub, 2009.

Flegal KM, Carroll MD, Ogden CL, Curtin LR: Prevalence and trends in obesity among US adults, 1999-2008, *JAMA* 303:235, 2010.

Maciosek MV, Coffield AB, Edwards NM, Flottemesch TJ, Goodman MJ, Solberg LI: Priorities among effective clinical preventive services: Results of a systematic review and analysis, *Am J Prev Med* Jul 31:52, 2006.

Healthallrefer.com: Symptoms guide: weight gain—unintentional. Available online at http://health.allrefer.com/health/weight-gain-unintentional-info.html#. Accessed January 6, 2010.

McPhee SJ, Papadakis MA: *Current medical diagnosis & treatment,* ed 49. New York, 2010, Appleton & Lange.

Metalidis C, Knockaert DC, Bobbaers H, Vanderschueren S: Involuntary weight loss. Does a negative baseline evaluation provide adequate reassurance? *Eur J Intern Med* 19:345, 2008.

Reife CM: Involuntary weight loss, *Med Clin North Am* 79:299, 1995.

U.S. Department of Health and Human Services, U.S. Department of Agriculture: *Dietary guidelines for Americans, 2005.* Available online at http://www.health.gov/dietaryguidelines/dga2005/document/default.htm. Accessed March 26, 2010.

III

Diagnostic Imaging

An x-ray is a stream of high energy photons produced by an x-ray tube used for their penetrating power in radiography. The short wavelength produced by this light energy is unique in that it penetrates opaque objects. Releasing the beam onto a photosensitive surface causes a photochemical reaction, which results in an image on the x-ray film in conventional systems or on an image receptor in digital systems. For ease of reference, the term "image" will be used throughout the chapter. The density of the material determines the penetration of the light energy. The image is a result of the amount of x-rays being absorbed by the density of the tissue/organ as it passes to the receptor. Two terms are used to describe this absorption. The first is radiolucent, which means there is no interference with the flow of the x-ray particles. The result is a black or very dark image. The second term is radiopaque; in this instance, something lies between the beam and the cassette that causes the beam to absorb or disperse, thereby not allowing the beam to reach the cassette and making the image appear white.

Decreasing density (black) Increasing density (white)

$\longrightarrow$

Radiolucent Radiopaque

Gradations of gray result from variations in density of the tissue or organ. There are four basic roentgen densities, and all images include one or more of these densities (see Table 37-1). A chest image demonstrates all four densities: from the black of the air in the lung tissue to the full white density of the rib bones. The densities of the objects result in the shadows on the image.

The radiograph image is a two-dimensional shadow picture of a three-dimensional object. Because the image is two-dimensional, it is important that the clinician think three-dimensionally when viewing the image. This thinking requires knowledge of the normal anatomy of the area being x-rayed and transference of this knowledge to the shadows on the image.

Chapters 37 and 38 address specific x-rays commonly used for diagnosis.

The Chest X-ray

The chest x-ray is the most commonly performed diagnostic x-ray examination. It is performed to evaluate the lungs, heart, and chest wall. A chest image is typically the first imaging test used to help diagnose symptoms such as shortness of breath, persistent cough, trauma, chest pain, and fever. Chest images are also used to diagnose and monitor conditions such as pneumonia, lung cancer, and congestive heart failure.

DIAGNOSTIC REASONING: VIEWING THE CHEST IMAGE

What are the first steps in reviewing an image?

Key Questions (to self)

■ Do the images being examined belong to the correct patient?
■ Do I have two views of the area being examined?
■ Is the image correctly displayed on the view box?
■ Are the images of good quality?
■ Do I know the anatomy of the chest?

TABLE 37-1   Chest Image Densities

DENSITY	DESCRIPTION	EXAMPLES
Gas (air)	Black, radiolucent	Lung tissue, trachea, bronchi, gas in stomach or intestine
Fat	Gray, less radiolucent	Soft tissue around muscle
Water	Whitish, slightly radiopaque	Heart, blood vessels, muscle, diaphragm
Metal	All white, radiopaque	Calcium of ribs, vertebrae, scapulae, clavicles, other bones, prostheses, contrast media

From Kersten L: *Comprehensive respiratory nursing,* Philadelphia, 1989, Saunders.

Identification of Image and Patient

Before viewing an image it is important to verify that the image being viewed is from the patient being evaluated. Pertinent information about the patient should be found on the image in the upper corner and should be verified.

Views

Frontal and lateral views. Generally, two images are taken when examination of the chest is requested. One is a frontal view; it is usually a posteroanterior (PA) view, where the patient is standing 6 feet from the cassette and the image is taken from back (posterior) to front (anterior) (Figure 37-1, A). A second image is the lateral view (Figure 37-1, B). In a lateral view, the patient is standing with the hands held above the head and the lateral thorax is against the cassette. A left lateral view (where the left thorax is against the image cassette) is usually ordered instead of a right lateral view because it provides a better view of the area behind the heart and the bases of the lower lungs. Additional views are occasionally ordered for specific reasons.

Anteroposterior (AP) chest image. This view is created when the beam passes from the anterior to the posterior surface of the chest and then onto the image. Patients who are in bed or who cannot stand usually have these images ordered. When viewing the AP images the heart and mediastinum appear larger because they are located in the anterior chest, and in this position the chest is farther from the image cassette.

Expiration image. This type of image is ordered when a pneumothorax is suspected. A maximum expiration by the patient will cause the lung tissue to compress. The lung tissue is then compared to the pleural air. With a pneumothorax, the pleural air will occupy more space.

Lateral decubitus image. This view is used to assess fluid and air levels in the pleural spaces. The patient is lying on his or her side with the image cassette

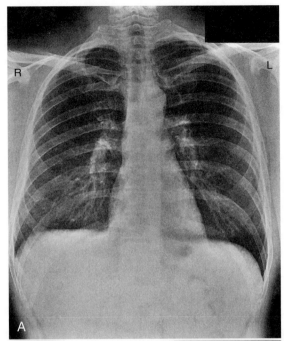

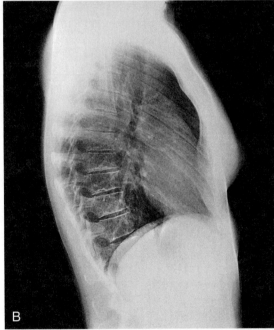

FIGURE 37-1 Patient positioning for AP and left lateral chest images. **A,** A patient positioned for a posteroanterior projection of the chest. **B,** Proper patient position for a left lateral chest view. Note the left side of the patient is placed against the image receptor. (From Ballinger PW, Frank ED: *Merrill's atlas of radiographic positions and radiographic procedures*, ed 10, Vol 1, St Louis, 2003, Mosby.)

upright against the patient's chest. The beam is sent perpendicular to the image cassette. Air rises and fluid falls to the dependent area.

Oblique image. The oblique image is used to distinguish anterior from posterior lesions by avoiding bony structures. It is also used for examining the trachea. Oblique images can be right or left obliques. In a right oblique, the patient's anterior right side is against the image cassette.

Lordotic image. The lordotic image identifies right and left middle lung fields. The x-ray machine is tilted to a 45-degree angle. This position offers a better view of lung apices that can otherwise be obscured by clavicles and upper ribs on the PA view.

Image Box Placement

Place the PA image on the lightened view box with the patient's left side facing the reader's right side. The image is labeled with an R or L. If there is no labeling, look for the aortic arch. The arch is the first bump seen on the image and is on the patient's left or the viewing clinician's right. In the rare patient with dextrocardia, the reverse is true.

The left lateral image should be placed on the view box such that the left side of the patient is facing the reader.

Image Quality

The number of x-rays beamed through the patient onto the image affects the details seen on the image. If not enough beams were delivered, the image will be underexposed and appear lighter than normal. If too many beams were delivered, the image will become overexposed and will be darker than normal. On the PA view, thoracic vertebral bodies should be barely visible through the heart shadow; on the lateral view, the spinal bodies should be visible.

To obtain a good chest image, the x-ray is taken with the patient in full inspiration. If the image is taken on expiration or poor inspiration, the heart appears larger and the lungs look cloudy. The 10 posterior ribs above the diaphragm should be evident in a good quality image.

The angle of the beam should be direct and the patient should be positioned properly. If the patient is at an improper angle, the beam will be more scattered and details will be lost. To determine if the patient is positioned correctly, note the clavicles. The medial heads of the clavicles should be positioned over the spine. If the heads are not centered, alignment may not be correct, causing the image to be slightly oblique. The costophrenic angle and the lateral lung fields should be visible.

Reviewing Anatomy

Reviewing the normal anatomy of the structures of the chest is helpful when learning how to interpret a chest image.

Superimposing the anatomy onto a chest image will help to correlate the normal structures to the shadows (Figure 37-2).

What approach should be used when viewing an image?

Key Questions (to self)

- What is your initial impression?
- Are you using a systematic examination technique?

Initial Impression

Most clinicians view images initially by standing 6 to 8 feet from the image and giving the image a once-over glance. The purpose of this activity is to observe for any obvious abnormality as well as to obtain an overall impression of the thorax for size, shape, and symmetry.

Systematic examination of the image after an initial overview is mandatory. All parts of the chest anatomy are evaluated at 2 to 4 feet from the image, concentrating on one part of the image at a time, to observe any abnormalities. A suggested systematic examination follows.

DIAGNOSTIC REASONING: SYSTEMATIC EXAMINATION

How do I assess the PA view?

Soft Tissue

Examine the periphery of the image to evaluate the amount of soft tissue present (for obesity or cachexia), calcifications, or gas collections indicating subcutaneous emphysema. Note the presence of breasts in female patients. Be aware that breast tissue may cover the lower lung fields.

Trachea

Located in the anterior mediastinum, the trachea should be checked for size and position. The trachea will appear deviated in a rotated patient. Abnormal pathological deviations may be a result of pressure on the mediastinum, including tumors, pneumothorax, or emphysema. A mass will push the trachea away from midline. The trachea will deviate toward a large pneumothorax and

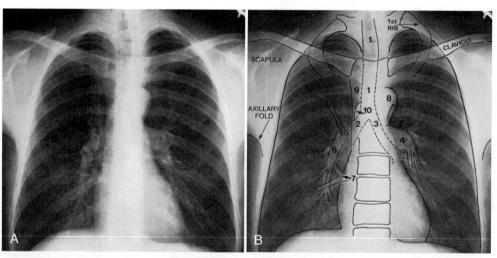

FIGURE 37-2   Normal PA image. **A,** Unlabeled. **B,** A diagrammatic overlay showing the normal anatomic structures numbered or labeled: *1,* trachea; *2,* right main brochus; *3,* left main bronchus; *4,* left pulmonary artery; *5,* right upper lobe pulmonary artery; *6,* right interlobar artery; *7,* right lower and middle lobe vein; *8,* aortic arch; *9,* superior vena cava; *10,* azygos vein. (From Fraser R (ed): *Fraser and Paré's diagnosis of diseases of the chest,* ed 4, Vol 1, Philadelphia, 1999, Saunders.)

away from a tension pneumothorax. Thickening of the trachea may indicate lymph node enlargement or an upper mediastinal tumor.

Clavicles

The clavicles should be present and symmetrical and located at the second and third intercostal spaces. Scrutinize for fracture lines, which appear black on the image because of air space surrounded by white bone and tissue.

Bony Thorax

Note the size and shape of the thorax. Scoliosis is visible on the frontal image, whereas kyphosis and funnel chest are best seen on the lateral view. Examine individual shoulder girdles for shape, size, and contour. Bony structures are evaluated for deformity, mineralization, density, and cortical thickness, as well as for fractures.

Scapulae

The distance between the scapulae is increased when the shoulders are rotated forward in the PA image. This position also ensures that the scapulae will be out of the lung fields. Observe for fractures and symmetry.

Thoracic Spine

Look through the mediastinum and lungs to view the spine and observe for symmetry of the rib cage. Vertebral evaluation is best done on the lateral image. Look for compression fractures, height of vertebral bodies, disk spaces, and density of bones.

Ribs and Intracostal Spaces

Count the posterior ribs; 10 should be visible. If eight or fewer ribs are visible, this is either a poor image or an expiratory image. Be careful to begin the rib count at the first thoracic vertebra. Locate the anterior end of the first rib just below the medial end of the clavicles, follow it back to its posterior end, and start counting ribs (Figure 37-3). The posterior ribs are more superior than the anterior ribs. Check ribs side to side and completely to the lateral end. Most fractures occur on the lateral parts of the ribs. Normal ribs appear sloped at the edges; ribs that are horizontal or flattened indicate emphysema or chronic obstructive pulmonary disease (COPD).

Describe abnormalities using ribs or interspaces as location markers horizontally and chest lines as

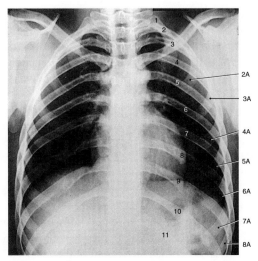

FIGURE 37-3 Respiratory lung movement. Full expiration with the ribs numbered. The anterior ribs are labeled with a suffix. (From Ballinger PW, Frank ED: *Merrill's atlas of radiographic positions & radiologic procedures,* ed 10, St Louis, 2003, Mosby.)

vertical markers. Interspaces are numbered using the posterior rib and according to the rib above. Observe the widths of the intracostal spaces, which should be equal bilaterally.

Decreased lung volume narrows the intracostal spaces. Conditions that cause this include interstitial fibrosis (bilateral) or a foreign body (unilateral). Increased lung volume increases the intracostal spaces in such conditions as asthma and COPD.

Diaphragm

The diaphragm separates the abdominal contents from the pleural cavity. Any changes in these areas can be seen radiographically to affect the diaphragm. Count down the posterior ribs near the spine; the diaphragm should be at the tenth or eleventh rib. The diaphragm should have a curve that is shaped upward. The right side is usually higher (1 to 2 cm) than the left because the liver is located under the right hemidiaphragm; this will be more visible on a lateral image of the diaphragm. Note if the diaphragm is elevated or flattened.

Suspect hepatomegaly in patients who have marked asymmetry of the right diaphragm. A unilateral elevation of the diaphragm is seen with a pneumothorax.

Patients who do not take a deep breath, who have ascites or intestinal obstruction, or who are in the third trimester of pregnancy will have elevated diaphragms. A diaphragm that is low and flat indicates structures within the thorax are enlarged, as seen in COPD.

Note any free air in the peritoneum visible below the right lower diaphragm edge. The air appears as lucency (decreased opacity) under the crescent of the hemidiaphragm, typically as result of a perforated viscus.

Costophrenic Angle

The edge of the diaphragm curves downward at the costophrenic junction, meeting the ribs and forming an angle that is sometimes referred to as the letter "V" on its side. This angle should be sharp. Blunting of the angle is caused by pleural effusion, pneumonia, neoplasm, or fibrosis (Figure 37-4).

Gastric Air Bubble

The gastric air bubble should always be on the examiner's right side as the image is viewed (the patient's left side). The stomach lies close beneath the left diaphragm. The liver, spleen, and kidneys are occasionally visible and should be noted for size.

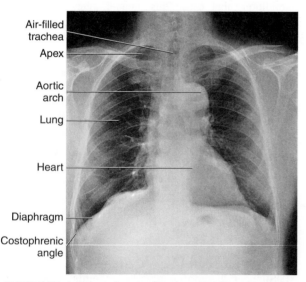

Air-filled trachea
Apex
Aortic arch
Lung
Heart
Diaphragm
Costophrenic angle

FIGURE 37-4   Normal costophrenic angle. (From Ballinger PW, Frank ED: *Merrill's atlas of radiographic positions and radiologic procedures,* ed 10, Vol 1, St Louis, 2003, Mosby.)

Mediastinum

The mediastinum is located between the sternum anteriorly, the vertebral bodies posteriorly, and the lungs laterally. It encompasses a number of structures including the heart and its large vessels, as well as the trachea, thymus, and lymph nodes.

A prominent structure is the aortic arch (see Figure 37-4). The arch is the first prominent bulge along the left mediastinal border. Assess for size and length. As patients age, the aorta increases in thickness and length. An increase in size is also seen in an aortic aneurysm.

The ascending aorta is the small bulge on the right.

Hilar Area

The hilar area contains the roots of the lungs and is where the major bronchi and pulmonary vessels project outward.

Note the size of the hilar area. Increased fullness or size generally indicates lymphoma, metastatic carcinoma, tuberculosis, or fungal (*Histoplasma*) adenopathy.

Pulmonary Vasculature

Pulmonary arteries become smaller as they progress out to the chest periphery, ending approximately 1.5 cm from the pleural surface. Normal markings extend approximately one third of the way into the lung fields.

Increased pulmonary pressure causes engorgement of the pulmonary vessels, and increased markings are seen that resemble a branching tree. When engorgement occurs, a butterfly appearance is seen. Pulmonary edema causes blurred borders and hilar clouding.

Heart

Measure the size of the heart using a ruler. The heart should be less than 50% of the transverse diameter of the thorax. The measurement should be compared to the widest thoracic diameter (found below the diaphragm and between the ribs), resulting in the cardiac/thoracic (C-T) ratio. The normal ratio is 1:2 (Figure 37-5).

Left ventricular hypertrophy extends the heart border to the left, increasing the size of the heart and decreasing the C-T ratio.

Look for the silhouette sign, which occurs when two structures have the same density and are in contact with each other, resulting in a loss of borders on the x-ray. Because the right and left borders of the heart are air-filled, lesions in the lung cause the differentiation of the heart border to be lost.

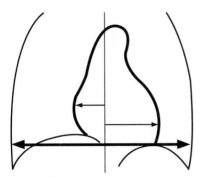

FIGURE 37-5 The normal cardiac-thoracic ratio is 1:2.

Pleura

Follow the pleura around the lungs and note any thickening, calcification, effusion, or pneumothorax.

Pleural thickening is seen as increased soft tissue around the periphery of the lung. An effusion will blunt the costophrenic angle. A pneumothorax will pull the visceral pleura into the lung field, away from the chest wall.

Lungs

Examine the lungs from central to peripheral. The lungs will appear whiter when looking from top to bottom because of the increasing thickness of the chest areas. The lung markings will decrease by thirds as the viewer goes from central to peripheral. The markings are also more prominent in the bases of the lungs than in the upper lung fields.

Compare right and left lung fields, starting at the top and continuing across and down. Do this in small segments, evaluating each area carefully. Look for lesions, lung markings, and density changes such as areas of opacity (seen in white), which represent consolidation, nodules, and calcifications. Note the lung volume. Decreased volume is seen with atelectasis. Large-volume lungs with a narrow mediastinum and a flat diaphragm are typically viewed in the patient with emphysema.

Final Look

Research has shown that there are three high-risk locations where pathology is often missed. They are the following: the upper lobes of the lungs, costophrenic areas, and peripheral lung margins. Take one more look at each of these areas.

How do I assess the lateral view?

Key Questions (to self)

- In what position is the patient?
- How do I know the image quality is good?
- What are the indications for a lateral image?
- Am I using a systematic approach to reviewing the image?

The common position for the lateral view is with the patient's left chest against the image cassette. The beam passes from right to left through the patient. Remember that the right side of the patient is closer to the beam and therefore structures are magnified on the right side as compared to the left. The left lateral position is preferred because the heart is less magnified and the bases of the lungs are more easily seen.

A right lateral image is ordered when the right side of the lung needs to be less magnified and sharper, such as when a tumor is suspected. In the lateral position, the ribs will seem to be superimposed on each other and the sternum will appear thin.

A good quality lateral image shows lung markings, fissures (the septa that divide the lobes of the lung), and good visualization of the spine.

A lateral image can help localize a lesion seen on the PA view or it may verify lobar consolidation. In addition, the lateral image allows the viewer to see behind the sternum and cardiac shadow.

Use a systemic approach when viewing the lateral image, similar to the PA review.

Anatomy

Review the anatomy of the lateral chest (Figure 37-6).

Vertebral Bodies

The amount of soft tissue is greater at the lung apices than at the lung bases; therefore, the vertebral bodies appear darker as they approach the diaphragm. Kyphosis is noticeable on the lateral image. Examine each vertebra for fractures, and scrutinize the intervertebral disk spaces.

Diaphragm

The right diaphragm is visible and is higher than the left because of the heart. On the left, the latter two thirds of the diaphragm should be visible. The gastric bubble is below the left diaphragm.

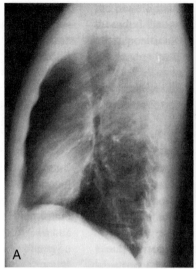
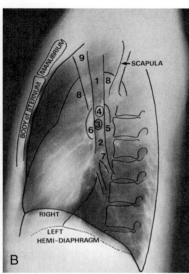

FIGURE 37-6 Lateral chest image. **A,** unlabeled **B,** A diagrammatic overlay showing the normal anatomic structures numbered or labeled: *1,* tracheal air column; *2,* right intermediate brochus; *3,* left upper lobe bronchus; *4,* right upper lobe bronchus; *5,* left interlobar artery; *6,* right interlobar artery; *7,* confluence of pulmonary veins; *8,* aortic arch; *9,* brachiocephalic vessels. (From Fraser R (ed): *Fraser and Paré's diagnosis of diseases of the chest,* ed 4, Vol 1, Philadelphia, 1999, Saunders.)

Costophrenic Angle

The angle is seen in the most dependent part of the lung. Both angles should be visible and sharp.

Fissures

Fissures are septa that divide the lobes of lungs. The major oblique fissure separates the left upper lobe from the left lower lobe. The right major fissure separates the right upper and middle lobes from the right lower lobe. The right minor fissure separates the right upper lobe from the right lower lobe. Fissures are generally not seen on plain images because their small surface provides no shadow or interface. However, these fissures may be seen when pathology occurs in the lung.

Pleura

Follow the pleura around the lungs from the posterior costophrenic area to the posterior sternal margin and posterior ribs.

Retrosternal Area

The retrosternal space is usually dark because of the presence of air. It is the lower one third of the sternum and appears in contact with the right ventricle. When this area is seen as opaque, air has been replaced with solid material, and anterior mediastinal disease should be considered. The area is enlarged when pulmonary overinflation occurs, as in emphysema. The retrosternal space will not be visible with an enlarged heart.

Heart/Retrocardiac Area

Identify the right ventricle, left ventricle, and left atrium. The retrocardiac area of the lateral chest image is normally dark due to air. If the space is opaque, then the air has been replaced with an effusion, consolidation, or mass.

Lungs

The scapulae make visualizing the upper lobe difficult in the lateral image. Lung lesions are often hidden by the heart on the PA view. Localizing a lesion in the left lung is best accomplished with the lateral image.

Final Look

Take a last look at each of the areas where lesions are often missed: the upper lobes, peripheral lung margins, retrocardiac area, and costophrenic area.

What other imaging studies should I consider?

Key Questions (to self)

- What other common imaging studies are available for the chest?
- What imaging studies would give me the best information for a particular complaint?

Computed Tomography

Computed tomography (CT), sometimes called computed axial tomography (CAT), provides a cross-sectional slice of the area examined. Unlike plain images, which superimpose structures onto an image, a CT scan gives only one slice. The beams of x-rays pass through the body in an axial plane as the x-ray tube moves in a continuous arc around the patient. Detectors are placed opposite the beam to catch the electrical pulses. The image is the result of the x-rays that are not absorbed by the tissues between the beam and the detectors. Detectors pick up the electrical impulses that are fed into a computer that provides the "picture." CT is used to distinguish overlapping shadows from the chest image. It is also very useful in showing fine details of the pulmonary parenchyma and hilum.

MRI

Magnetic resonance imaging (MRI) produces a computer-based sectional image that does not use ionizing radiation. MRI uses the hydrogen molecules in the body to produce the image. A radio frequency pulse transmitted through coils causes some of the hydrogen molecules to absorb energy and spin in a different direction from the other hydrogen ions (resonance). When the radio frequency pulse stops, the hydrogen molecules stop spinning and release their excess stored energy. A gradient magnet located inside the main magnet, which provides the slicing capability of the image, picks up the change. The results are sent to the computer system, providing a two-dimensional image. MRI of the chest is used to view lesions of the chest wall and is less useful for examining the lungs.

PET Scan

Positron emission tomography (PET) scans provide information on the biochemical metabolism of an organ or tissue. Positrons come from the nucleus of a proton as it decays to a neutron. When released, the positron eventually collides with an electron, resulting in the release of two high-energy gamma photons. These gamma photons are released at 180 degrees from each other. The PET scan patient is given a radiotracer that follows the destruction of the positron and the resulting gamma photons. PET scans are built with hundreds of detectors on circular rings that are located directly across from each other. The detectors allow the localization, in three-dimensional space, of the decay of the gamma photons. PET scans show the chemical function of an organ or tissue rather than its structure; very highly active metabolism is seen with cancer cells. PET scans are ordered for evaluating the effects of lung cancer therapy.

Echocardiogram

High-frequency sound waves are directed into the body, which are then recorded as they deflect off organs and structures. These deflections are transmitted back to a transducer that records the difference in acoustic impedance. This recording is changed into an electrical signal, which is then analyzed by a computer to produce an image. Echocardiograms are useful to evaluate heart size and valvular function.

DIFFERENTIAL DIAGNOSIS OF *the Chest Image*

WHAT TO LOOK AT	NORMAL FINDING	ABNORMAL FINDING	SUGGESTED CAUSE
Clavicles	Midline, symmetrical, intact	Dark lines; clavicles not centered	Fracture; patient rotated; image taken off center
Chest wall	Chest wall has rounded contour	Sternum pushed outward (lateral image)	Pectus carinatum
		Sternum pushed inward (lateral image)	Pectus excavatum
Inspiration	Adequate inspiration	Less than 10 ribs identified	Inadequate inspiration
Vertebral column	Straight, equal disk spaces	Curved	Kyphoscoliosis (lateral view); scoliosis (PA view)
		Collapsed disk spaces	Degenerative disk disease
Ribs	All ribs intact	Rib fractures present	Trauma
	Able to count 10 ribs	Less than 10 ribs identified	Inadequate inspiration
	Ribs sloped at edges	Ribs horizontal or flattened	Hyperinflated lungs, acute asthma, COPD

Continued

DIFFERENTIAL DIAGNOSIS OF *the Chest Image—cont'd*

WHAT TO LOOK AT	NORMAL FINDING	ABNORMAL FINDING	SUGGESTED CAUSE
Trachea	Midline	Deviation from midline	Atelectasis: trachea deviated toward area of atelectasis; pneumothorax: air, fluid, tumor, lymph node enlargement push trachea away from center; rotated image
Hilar region	Normal size, centrally located	Area enlarged	Pulmonary artery congestion; lymph node enlargement
	Vascular markings extend <1/3 out into lung field	Vascular markings >1/3 into lung field	Bronchopneumonia or pulmonary congestion
	Bronchi invisible because air-filled bronchi have same density as air in lungs	Bronchograms present (bronchi become visible when lung tissue filled with fluid is contrasted with air-filled bronchi)	Infiltration; pulmonary edema
		Infiltrates or consolidation of lung tissue	Pneumonia
Gastric air bubble	Present on right	Not visible	Image placement error; image label error
Diaphragm	Right higher than left; right at level of sixth rib	Elevated	Collapsed lobe or multisegmental collapse; pleural effusion
		Radiolucent line present that follows curvature of diaphragm	Free air present
		Flattened diaphragm	Emphysema, asthma, tension pneumothorax
		Elevation on left	Perforated ulcer or gas distention of stomach
		Bilateral elevation	Pregnancy, obesity, peritoneal fluid
Costophrenic angle	Present, sharp edges	Blunted edges or absent	Pneumonia, pleural effusion
Visceral pleura	Traced around chest wall	Hairline shadow, dark black with no lung markings	Pneumothorax
Heart size	Cardiac ratio <50%	Cardiac ratio >50%	Enlarged heart, patient rotated
Heart borders	Presence of heart borders	Loss of border	Infiltrates
Lungs	Translucent	Fluffy appearance	Engorged vasculature
		Honeycomb appearance	Acute respiratory distress syndrome
		Butterfly appearance	Pulmonary edema
		Density changes to consolidation	Bacterial pneumonia
		Web-shaped density	Pulmonary embolism

COPD, chronic obstructive pulmonary disease.

REFERENCES AND READINGS

Dettenmeier P: *Pulmonary nursing care*, St Louis, 1992, Mosby.

Fraser R, (ed): *Fraser and Paré's diagnosis of diseases of the chest*, ed 4, Vol 1, Philadelphia, 1999, Saunders.

Gaber KA, McGavin CR, Wells IP: Lateral chest x-ray for physicians, *J Royal Soc Med* 98:310, 2005.

Kersten L: *Comprehensive respiratory nursing: a decision making approach*, Philadelphia, 1989, Saunders.

Landay M: *Interpretation of the chest roentgenogram*, Boston, 1987, Little Brown and Co.

Novelline R: *Squire's fundamentals of radiology*, ed 5, Cambridge, Mass, 1997, Harvard University Press.

Tarrac SE: A systematic approach to chest x-ray interpretation in the perianesthesia unit, *J Perianesth Nurs* 24:41, 2009.

Wilson S, Thompson J: *Respiratory disorders*, St Louis, 1990, Mosby.

The Abdominal X-ray

Unlike the chest x-ray, the abdominal x-ray is used primarily for acute conditions and has a more limited use than the chest x-ray. Often the abdominal x-ray will require additional imaging and the use of contrast radiographic substances to make structures more visible. Generally abdominal images are taken to help in diagnosing pain, vomiting, and lack of or abnormal bowel sounds. They are also useful in finding stones in the kidneys, ureter, bladder, and gallbladder; ingested foreign objects; and air distribution. Frequently a chest image is done at the same time. Every female patient should be asked if she is pregnant before an image is performed.

DIAGNOSTIC REASONING: VIEWING THE ABDOMINAL IMAGE

What are the first steps in reviewing the image?

Key Questions (to self)

- Does the image being examined belong to the correct patient?
- Do I have all views of the area being examined?
- Is the image correctly displayed on the view box or screen?
- Is the image of good quality?
- Do I know the anatomy of the abdomen?

Image and Patient Identification
As with the chest x-ray, it is important to determine that the image being viewed is from the patient being evaluated. Pertinent information about the patient should be found on the image in the upper corner and should be verified.

Views
Flat plate or anteroposterior (AP) view. For an AP view, the patient lies in a supine position on the x-ray table. A cassette is placed beneath the patient, with the x-ray machine above the patient. The beam passes from front to back. The patient is asked to exhale and the x-ray is taken. Due to the size of the cassette, a second image may be needed while the patient is in this position to see the entire abdomen from diaphragm to groin.

Left lateral decubitus view. In a left lateral decubitus image, the x-ray machine moves to a position where the beam is horizontal to the patient and the left chest is closest to the image. This view is obtained when an obstruction or perforation may have occurred, resulting in free air in the abdomen.

Erect view. For an erect view, an x-ray of the abdomen is taken as the patient is standing. A standing erect x-ray is used to assess for free air; however, this is seen only when an excessive amount of air is present.

Chest x-ray. A chest x-ray may be ordered to rule out free air collection beneath the diaphragm, a pneumonia that may be causing abdominal symptoms, a pleural effusion, or a subphrenic abscess.

Kidneys, ureter, bladder (KUB). The term KUB is often used to indicate a flat plate of the abdomen. An x-ray of the kidneys, ureter, and bladder is done to look for stones or abnormalities.

Image Box Placement
The image, or x-ray film, is placed on the lightened view box with the patient's left side facing the reader's right side. The image is labeled with an "R" or "L" on the bottom. Digital imaging is common where the x-ray image is viewed on a computer screen.

Image Quality
The amount of x-ray beamed through the patient affects the details seen on the image. If too few beams were delivered, the image will be underexposed and appear lighter than normal. If too many beams were delivered, the image will become overexposed and will be darker than normal. An underexposed

abdominal image is not usually a problem. However, an overexposed image (darker than normal) requires a high density spotlight looking for any free air. If the spine is visible, most other structures should be seen.

Reviewing Anatomy

Reviewing the normal anatomy of the structures of the abdomen is helpful when learning how to interpret an abdominal image. Superimposing the anatomy onto the image will help to correlate the normal structures to the shadows. The abdomen, unlike the chest image, is more difficult to read due to soft tissue organs. A review of the principles of radiology will help explain this. Radiodense objects, like bone and calcium, are easy to see (white). Radiolucent objects, such as air and fat, are also easy to see (dark). Structures of intermediate density are more difficult to see because they appear gray (such as solid organs of the abdomen) and gray densities next to each other are invisible. Organs that have varying densities next to each other (such as the liver border next to fat) assists in identification. Careful viewing and knowledge of anatomy is important (Figure 38-1).

What approach should be used when viewing the image?

Key Questions (to self)

- What is my initial impression?
- Am I using a systematic examination technique?

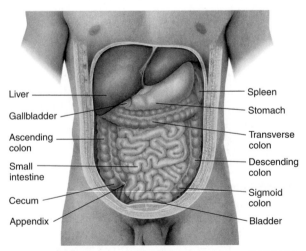

FIGURE 38-1   Normal abdominal anatomy. (From Seidel HM, Ball JW, Dains JE, Flynn J, Solomon B, Stewart R: *Mosby's guide to physical examination,* ed 7, St Louis, 2011, Mosby.)

Initial Impression

When beginning to view the image, it is helpful to ask why you ordered the image, what you expect to see based on the history and physical examination, and if you see it. Initially, view the gas pattern and look for any extraluminal air, soft tissue masses, or calcifications.

Systematic Examination

Systematic examination of the image after an initial overview is mandatory. All parts of the abdominal anatomy are evaluated at 2 to 4 feet from the image, concentrating on one part of the image at a time to observe any abnormalities. A suggested systematic examination follows.

DIAGNOSTIC REASONING: SYSTEMATIC EXAMINATION

How do I assess the AP view?

Bones

Identify the lower rib cage, lumbar spine, sacrum, pelvis, and hip joints. In each instance, look for fracture, cortical density, and joint and disc space.

Bladder

The inferior aspect of the bladder projects 5-10 mm above the symphysis pubis. If the bladder is full, it will appear as a soft tissue density in the pelvis (Figure 38-2).

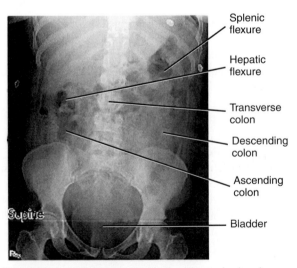

FIGURE 38-2   Supine abdominal radiograph showing colon, bladder, and flexures. (Modified from Johns Hopkins University, Piccini J, Nilsson K [eds]: *The Osler medical handbook,* ed 2, Philadelphia, 2006, Saunders.)

Uterus

The uterus sits on top of the bladder, possibly indenting the bladder, and is often not seen on plain x-ray.

Liver

Observe for homogeneous density in the right upper abdominal quadrant. The lower border of the liver is found in the right flank near the right costal margin. The adjacent fat provides the contrast showing the liver edge (Figure 38-3).

Spleen

The spleen is found in the left upper quadrant between the diaphragm and fundus of the stomach. It is the size of the adult fist and is usually not seen. Because the spleen must be very enlarged to be seen, ultrasound may be more beneficial (see Figure 38-3).

Psoas Muscle

The psoas muscle shadows are visible as diverging lines on both sides of the spine starting from the first lumbar vertebra towards the pelvis (see Figure 38-3).

Kidneys

The kidneys are retroperitoneal organs that are visualized on the x-ray due to the presence of perirenal fat. Visualization may be obscured by bowel loops. The left kidney is higher than the right. The shadow should appear smooth with the superior pole closest to the midline. Kidneys are located on either side of the lower thoracic and upper lumbar spine between the upper border of the eleventh thoracic vertebra and the lower border of the third lumbar vertebra (see Figure 38-3).

Stomach

The stomach can be identified in its location above the transverse colon by the bandlike shadows of the gastric rugae in the supine view, and by the gas fluid level beneath the left hemidiaphragm in the erect view. When supine, air in the stomach will rise anteriorly and fluid will pool posteriorly (Figure 38-4).

Colon

The colon often has a bubbly appearance representing a mixture of gas and fecal material. It lies on the periphery of the abdomen and may be filled with air or feces. The colon begins at the hepatic flexure and goes to the rectum. Fecal matter in the bowel gives a "mottled" appearance. This is seen as a mixture of grey densities representing a gas liquid-solid mixture (Figure 38-5). A mechanical obstruction causes the large bowel to become dilated >6 cm. The dilated colon is above the

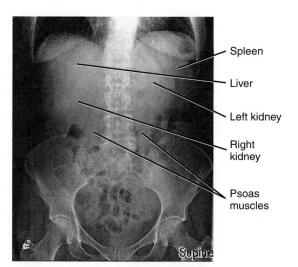

FIGURE 38-3 Supine abdominal radiograph showing kidneys, spleen, liver, and psoas muscle. (Modified from Johns Hopkins University, Piccini J, Nilsson K [eds]: *The Osler medical handbook*, ed 2, Philadelphia, 2006, Saunders.)

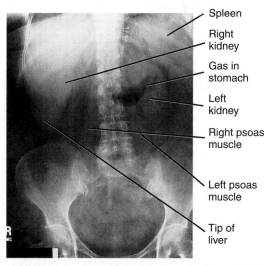

FIGURE 38-4 Normal gas in the stomach. (From Mettler F: *Essentials of radiology*, ed 2, Philadelphia, 2005, Elsevier.)

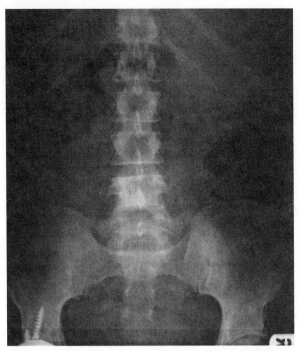

FIGURE 38-5   Constipation. (From Walsh T, Caraceni A, Fainsinger R, Foley K, Glare P, Goh C et al: *Palliative medicine*, Philadelphia, 2009, Elsevier.)

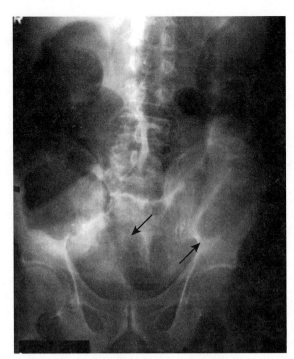

FIGURE 38-6   Mechanical large bowel obstruction. (From Herring W: *Learning radiology: recognizing the basics*, St Louis, 2007, Elsevier.)

obstruction and no air in the colon appears below the point of obstruction (Figure 38-6). A paralytic ileus (post surgery) shows a bowel that is dilated but has gas throughout the small and large intestine with no delineation.

Small Bowel

The small bowel lies in the center of the abdomen within the "frame" of the large bowel; often little small bowel is seen on the image. The normal small bowel diameter should not exceed 3 cm. A small bowel obstruction presents as multiple dilated loops in the central abdomen with no air in the large bowel (Figure 38-7).

Calcifications

Whiteness of calcifications is due to the absorption of the x-rays. Calcifications seen in the pancreas, kidney (Figure 38-8), gallbladder, and aorta are abnormal. Occasionally one may see a calcification in the area of the appendix called an appendicolith. In women, fibroids may become calcified and visible.

Gas Patterns/Extraluminal Air

Air is naturally swallowed and can be seen in the stomach. When a patient is in the supine position, the gas will rise to the anterior portion of the stomach. Gas in the small bowel is located in the left midabdomen and the lower central abdomen. Gas in the colon often has a bubbly appearance representing a mixture of gas and fecal material. Gas within the peritoneal cavity outside the sealed gastrointestinal tract is abnormal and is termed pneumoperitoneum (Figure 38-9).

Artifacts

Artifacts may be immediately obvious. Piercing of the umbilicus is very popular, especially in young women; genital piercing is not infrequent. Metallic objects are obvious. There may be clips or materials from previous surgeries.

If my patient has abdominal pain, what other x-ray should I consider?

Key Question (to self)

▪ What are the indications for ordering other x-rays?

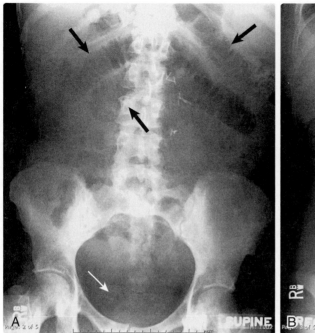
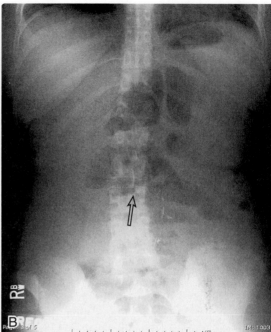

FIGURE 38-7 **A,** Supine view of the abdomen showing mechanical small bowel obstruction (*black arrows*) and no air in the rectum (*white arrow*). **B,** Erect view of the abdomen showing small bowel obstruction. (From Herring W: *Learning radiology: recognizing the basics,* St Louis, 2007, Elsevier.)

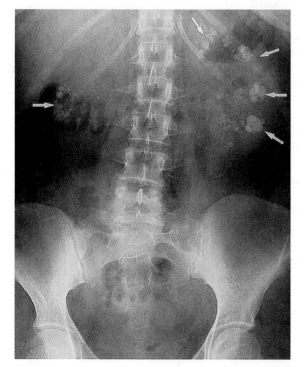

FIGURE 38-8 Nephrocalcinosis. (From Mettler F: *Essentials of radiology,* ed 2, Philadelphia, 2005, Saunders.)

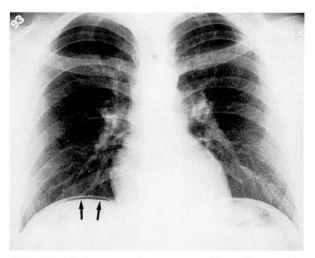

FIGURE 38-9 Pneumoperitoneum. (From Mettler F: *Essentials of radiology,* ed 2, Philadelphia, 2005, Saunders.)

Upright Abdominal X-ray and Standing Chest X-ray

If an obstruction or ileus is suspected, an upright abdominal film and a standing chest x-ray are ordered. The upright abdominal film provides a view of the air/fluid levels within the bowel to differentiate between an obstruction and an ileus. Additionally, if free air in the abdomen is a concern, the standing image will demonstrate free air underneath the hemidiaphragm, which is unable to be seen on the plain abdominal x-ray. A standing chest image should be viewed using the procedure outlined in Chapter 37. When looking for free air in the abdomen, pay particular attention to the area under the right diaphragm. Extraluminal free air appears as a crescent of radiolucent gas between the diaphragm and the liver, and usually indicates a perforated viscus (see Figure 38-9).

Left Lateral X-ray

If the patient is too ill to stand, a left lateral x-ray will be useful in finding free air in the abdomen. In the left lateral decubitus image, the patient is lying on the left side for 10 to 15 minutes and a horizontal beam is used. In this image, small amounts of free air can be seen over the lateral aspect of the right lobe of the liver. Often the free air is seen as a dark shadow between the white of the abdominal wall and the liver (Figure 38-10).

Additional Causes of Abdominal Pain

Abdominal pain may also be caused by chest pathology mimicking abdominal pain, for example, pleurisy, pneumonia, and pleural effusion. A chest x-ray should be ordered.

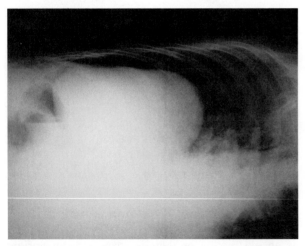

FIGURE 38-10 Left lateral free air. (From Adam A, Dixon A: *Grainger & Allison's diagnostic radiology*, ed 5, Philadelphia, 2008, Churchill Livingstone, Elsevier.)

What other imaging studies should I consider?

Key Questions (to self)

- What other common imaging studies are available for the abdomen?
- What imaging studies would give me the best information for a particular patient concern?

Upper GI Series

For an upper GI series, the patient drinks a barium solution that passes through the digestive tract and fills and coats the esophagus, stomach, and first part of the small intestine, making them more visible with the x-ray. A fluoroscope is held over the body part being examined and transmits continuous images to a video monitor. This test is used to diagnose hiatal hernia, reflux, narrowing of upper GI tract, and esophageal conditions.

Small Bowel Series

For a small bowel series, the barium ingested for the upper GI series is allowed to pass through the stomach into the small bowel and images are taken. This test is used to detect tumors, and malabsorption syndrome.

Lower GI Series

In a lower GI series, barium enemas are used to examine the large intestine and the rectum. For this test, barium or an iodine-containing liquid is introduced gradually into the colon through a tube inserted into the rectum. As the barium passes through the lower intestines, it fills the colon. As in the upper GI series, a fluoroscope transmits continuous images to the video monitor. A lower GI series is used to diagnose colon polyps, tumors, diverticular disease, narrowing or obstructions, ulcerative colitis, or Crohn disease.

Colonoscopy

In a colonoscopy, a colonoscope is inserted into the rectum and advanced through the large intestine and part of the small bowel. The scope has a fibrotic light and camera projecting images onto a monitor. Polyps can be identified, biopsied, and/or entirely removed. Colonoscopy is used to evaluate intestinal bleeding, inflammatory bowel disease, colorectal polyps, or cancer.

Sigmoidoscopy

In a sigmoidoscopy, a flexible sigmoidoscope is passed through the rectum to view the last 2 feet of the colon. The scope transmits images of the inside of the rectum and colon. Biopsies may be taken of polyps or suspicious tissue on the intestinal wall. This test is useful for viewing inflammatory conditions in the rectum and lower colon, polyps, bleeding, and ulcerations.

Computed Tomography

Computed tomography (CT), or computed axial tomography (CAT), provides a cross-sectional slice of the area examined (see Chapter 37). A CT is useful for diagnosing sigmoid diverticulitis, appendicitis, bowel obstruction, and extracolonic causes of abdominal pain.

Endoscopy

A flexible fiberoptic tube called an endoscope is equipped with a camera at the end. The camera is connected to either an eyepiece for direct viewing or a video screen that displays the images on a monitor. The endoscope is inserted into the mouth and threaded down the esophagus to the stomach and small intestine. Endoscopy is useful for diagnosing gastric bleeding, hiatal hernia, and swallowing difficulties; for removing stuck objects such as food; and for biopsy.

Ultrasound

Ultrasound is a noninvasive test that uses high frequency sound waves to produce images. The ultrasound images are captured in real time. They can show the size, structure, and movement of the body's internal organs, as well as blood flowing through blood vessels and pathologic lesions. It is useful for evaluating the size of the spleen, gallstones, aortic aneurysm, kidney stones, and abdominal masses.

DIFFERENTIAL DIAGNOSIS OF *the Abdominal Image*

WHAT TO LOOK AT	NORMAL FINDING	ABNORMAL FINDING	SUGGESTED CAUSE
Visible spine	Image of good quality	Spine not visible	Poor quality image
Metallic objects	History of piercing	Present without history	Foreign object ingested
Gastric air bubble	Present on the right	Not visible	Image placement error, label error
Liver	Right upper quadrant	Enlarged	Many causes: CHF, ETOH abuse, hepatitis
Spleen	Left upper quadrant, usually not seen	Must be very enlarged to be visualized	Many causes: infectious, anemia, trauma, cancers
Kidneys	Left higher than right, 3 vertebrae in size	Enlarged, calcifications	Renal calculi, hydrosis
Small bowel	Central portion of image, loops normally 2-3 cm, little air	Dilated more than 3 cm, multiple distended loops	Constipation, ileus, small bowel obstruction
Large bowel	Periphery of image, slight air in rectum	Dilated more than 5 cm, multiple dilated loops	Large bowel obstruction
		Mottled appearance	Constipation
Fluid	In erect image, present in stomach, 2-3 levels in small bowel, never in large bowel	Fluid present in small bowel	Small bowel obstruction

Continued

DIFFERENTIAL DIAGNOSIS OF *the Abdominal Image—cont'd*

WHAT TO LOOK AT	NORMAL FINDING	ABNORMAL FINDING	SUGGESTED CAUSE
Free air	Normally not seen	Free air in abdomen	Rupture of hollow viscus
Diaphragm	Right higher than left; right at level of 6th rib	Elevated	Collapsed lobe or multi-segmental collapse; pleural effusion
		Radiolucent line present that follows the curvature of the diaphragm	Free air present
		Flattened diaphragm	Emphysema, asthma, tension pneumothorax
		Elevation on left	Perforated ulcer, or gas distention of stomach
		Bilateral elevation	Pregnancy, obesity, peritoneal fluid
Bladder	Usually not visible	Visible when full	Full bladder, bladder stone
Uterus	Sits on top of bladder, usually not visible	Visible with uterine fibroids	Possible fibroids
Aorta	Usually not visible	Calcifications in abdominal aorta	Abdominal aortic aneurysm
			Ultrasound often used for diagnosis of size

CHF, congestive heart failure; *ETOH,* ethyl alcohol.

REFERENCES AND READINGS

Adam A, Dixon A (eds): *Grainger & Allison's diagnostic radiology,* ed 5, Philadelphia, 2008, Churchill Livingstone, Elsevier.

Brickel I, Kelly B: Abdominal x rays made easy: normal radiographs, *Student BMJ* 10:103, 2002.

Herring W: *Learning radiology: recognizing the basics,* St Louis, 2007, Mosby.

Mettler F: *Essentials of radiology,* ed 2, Philadelphia, 2005, Saunders.

Novelline RA: *Squire's fundamentals of radiology,* ed 6, Cambridge, Mass, 2004, Harvard University Press.

Walsh T, Caraceni A, Fainsinger R, Foley K, Glare P, Goh C et al: *Palliative medicine,* Philadelphia, 2009, Saunders.

Conversion Tables

LENGTH				WEIGHT			
in	**cm**	**cm**	**in**	**lb**	**kg**	**kg**	**lb**
1	2.54	1	0.4	1	0.5	1	2.2
2	5.08	2	0.8	2	0.9	2	4.4
4	10.16	3	1.2	4	1.8	3	6.6
6	15.24	4	1.6	6	2.7	4	8.8
8	20.32	5	2.0	8	3.6	5	11.0
10	25.40	6	2.4	10	4.5	6	13.2
20	50.50	8	3.1	20	9.1	8	17.6
30	76.20	10	3.9	30	13.6	10	22
40	101.60	20	7.9	40	18.2	20	44
50	127.00	30	11.8	50	22.7	30	66
60	152.40	40	15.7	60	27.3	40	88
70	177.80	50	19.7	70	31.8	50	110
80	203.20	60	23.6	80	36.4	60	132
90	228.60	70	27.6	90	40.9	70	154
100	254.00	80	31.5	100	45.4	80	176
150	381.00	90	35.4	150	66.2	90	198
200	508.00	100	39.4	200	90.8	100	220

1 in = 2.54 cm
1 cm = 0.3937 in

1 lb = 0.454 kg
1 kg = 2.204 lb

From Seidel HM, Ball JW, Dains JE, Flynn J, Solomon B, Stewart R: *Mosby's guide to physical examination*, ed 7, St Louis, 2011, Mosby.

Temperature Equivalents

Celsius*	Fahrenheit†	Celsius*	Fahrenheit†
34.0	93.2	38.6	101.4
34.2	93.6	38.8	101.8
34.4	93.9	39.0	102.2
34.6	94.3	39.2	102.5
34.8	94.6	39.4	102.9
35.0	95.0	39.6	103.2
35.2	95.4	39.8	103.6
35.4	95.7	40.0	104.0
35.6	96.1	40.2	104.3
35.8	96.4	40.4	104.7
36.0	96.8	40.6	105.1
36.2	97.1	40.8	105.4
36.4	97.5	41.0	105.8
36.6	97.8	41.2	106.1
36.8	98.2	41.4	106.5
37.0	98.6	41.6	106.8
37.2	98.9	41.8	107.2
37.4	99.3	42.0	107.6
37.6	99.6	42.2	108.0
37.8	100.0	42.4	108.3
38.0	100.4	42.6	108.7
38.2	100.7	42.8	109.0
38.4	101.1	43.0	109.4

*To convert Celsius to Fahrenheit: $(\frac{9}{5} \times$ Temperature$) + 32$
†To convert Fahrenheit to Celsius: $(\frac{5}{9} \times$ Temperature$) - 32$

Body Mass Index Chart

Are you at a healthy weight?

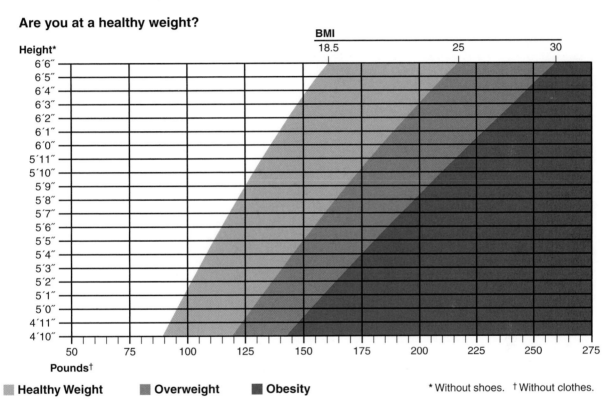

Healthy Weight   **Overweight**   **Obesity**   * Without shoes. † Without clothes.

The BMI (weight-for-height) ranges shown above are for adults. They are not exact ranges of healthy and unhealthy weights. However, they show that health risk increases at higher levels of overweight and obesity. Even within the healthy BMI range, weight gains carry health risks for adults.

Directions: Find your weight on the bottom of the graph. Go straight up from that point until you come to the line that matches your height. Then look to find your weight group.

➤ BMI of 25 defines the upper boundary of healthy weight.
➤ BMI of 25 to 30 defines overweight.
➤ BMI of higher than 30 defines obesity.

From Dietary Guidelines Advisory Committee: The report of the dietary guidelines advisory committee on dietary guidelines for Americans, 2000.

INDEX

A

Abdomen
  anatomic diagram and review of, 458, 458f
  examination of
    in chest pain evaluation, 89
    in constipation evaluation, 115
    in cough evaluation, 126
    in diarrhea evaluation, 140-141
    in fatigue evaluation, 188
    in male genitourinary evaluation, 213
    in skin rash/lesion evaluation, 312
    in syncope evaluation, 369
    in urinary incontinence evaluation, 378
  muscles, 16
  pain (*See* abdominal pain)
  quadrants, 9b
Abdominal aortic aneurysm, 9
Abdominal distention, 16, 213
Abdominal emergencies
  indicators of, 21b
Abdominal masses, 17
Abdominal pain
  acute conditions that cause
    acute pancreatitis, 22, 25-29b
    appendicitis, 21-23, 25-29b
    cholecystitis/lithiasis, 22, 25-29b
    dissection of aortic aneurysm, 22, 25-29b
    ectopic pregnancy, 21, 25-29b
    Henoch-Schönlein purpura, 23, 25-29b
    ileus, 23, 25-29b
    incarcerated hernia, 23, 25-29b
    intussusception, 23, 25-29b
    malrotation, 23, 25-29b
    mesenteric adenitis, 22, 25-29b
    myocardial infarction, 22, 25-29b
    obstruction, 23, 25-29b
    pelvic inflammatory disease, 22-23, 25-29b
    peptic ulcer perforation, 21, 25-29b
    peritonitis, 22, 25-29b
    pneumonia, 23, 25-29b
    pyelonephritis, 22, 25-29b
    salpingitis, 22-23, 25-29b
    ureterolithiasis, 22, 25-29b
    urinary tract infections (UTIs), 22, 25-29b
    volvulus, 23, 25-29b
  characteristics and severity of, 8
  in children, 8-9
  chronic conditions that cause lower
    abdominal wall disorders, 24, 25-29b
    diverticular disease, 24, 25-29b
    dysmenorrhea, 24, 25-29b
    habitual constipation, 24, 25-29b
    hernia, 24, 25-29b
    irritable bowel syndrome (IBS), 23-24, 25-29b
    lactose intolerance, 24, 25-29b
    ovarian cysts, 24, 25-29b

Abdominal pain *(Continued)*
    simple constipation, 24, 25-29b
    uterine fibroids, 24, 25-29b
  chronic conditions that cause upper
    esophagitis, 24-25, 25-29b
    functional dyspepsia, 25, 25-29b
    gastritis, 25, 25-29b
    gastroenteritis, 25, 25-29b
    gastroesophageal reflux disease (GERD), 24-25, 25-29b
    peptic ulcer, 25, 25-29b
    recurrent abdominal pain (RAP), 25-29, 25-29b
  classification of, 8-9
  diagnostic reasoning/key patient history questions, 9-15
    character of pain, 12
    last bowel movement, 10
    onset/duration, 9-10
    organ system signs, 14-15
    pain location, 10-11, 12t
    precipitating or aggravating factors, 12-13
    previous pain, 10
    radiation of, 11-12, 13
    relieving factors, 12-13, 14
    severity and progression, 10
    stool characteristics, 13-15
    vomiting, 13
  and fatigue, 186
  laboratory and diagnostic studies, 18-20
  with male genitourinary problems, 211-212
  with penile discharge, 297-298
  physical examination procedures, 15-18
  referred pain to breast, 76
  types and causes of, 8, 9b, 25-29b
  vaginal bleeding with, 397
  x-rays to evaluate, 460 (*See also* abdominal x-rays)
Abdominal ultrasound
  for abdominal pain evaluation, 20
  during chest pain evaluation, 90
  definition and procedures for performing, 463
Abdominal wall disorders
  causing lower abdominal pain, 24, 25-29b
Abdominal x-rays
  and colonoscopy, 462
  and computed tomography (CT scans), 463
  diagnostic reasoning/viewing the image
    anatomy review, 458, 458f
    image box placement, 457
    image quality, 457-458
    verifying image with patient, 457
    views, 457
  endoscopy, 463
  lower GI series, 462
  sigmoidoscopy, 463
  small bowel series, 462
  ultrasound, 463
  upper GI series, 462
  upright and standing, 461-462, 461f

Page numbers followed by *f*, *t*, and *b* indicate figures, tables, and boxes, respectively.

Abscesses
  brain, 231, 232-233b
  breast, 70-71, 72-73b
  perirectal, 322-323, 328-329, 331-332b
  peritonsillar, 362, 364-365b
  retropharyngeal, 362, 364-365b
Abstract reasoning problems, 102
Accommodation
  eye lens, 431
Acetic acid test
  for detect human papillomavirus (HPV), 418
Achilles tendinitis, 258, 262-265b
Acne vulgaris, 313, 316-320b
Acoustic nerves
  examining for hearing acuity, 179
Acoustic neuroma
  causing peripheral vertigo, 156
Acquired immunodeficiency syndrome (AIDS)
  fatigue symptoms with, 185
  increased risk of headaches with, 223-224
  questions during anorectal evaluation, 322-323, 324
  as risk factor for confusional states, 101
  and weight loss (unintentional), 444, 445-446b
Acromioclavicular joint injuries, 255, 262-265b
Actigraphy, 350
Activated partial thromboplastin time (aPTT), 90
Active range-of-motion tests
  during limb evaluation, 252
Activities
  assessing during HEEADSSS interview, 34-35, 36t
  and chest pain, 84
  causing dizziness and vertigo, 150
  physical causing infections, 413
Activities of daily living
  and fatigue, 185
Activity levels
  and calorie balance, 435, 436b, 437b, 439, 440t
  and weight gain (unintentional), 439, 440t, 444, 445-446b
  and weight loss (unintentional), 436, 437b, 438
Acute abdominal pain
  life-threatening conditions associated with, 9
Acute bacterial prostatitis
  description and diagnosis of, 217, 219-220b
Acute bronchitis, 129, 131-132b
Acute closed-angle glaucoma, 343, 424-425, 431-432, 432b, 433-434b
Acute coronary insufficiency, 91, 95b
Acute epiglottis
  and dyspnea, 169, 171-172b
  as possible cause of hoarseness, 239-240, 241-242b
  and sore throat, 356
Acute laryngotracheobronchitis, 129, 131-132b
Acute leukemia, 259, 262-265b
Acute low back pain (ALBP)
  AHRQ causative guidelines, 267
  definition of, 267
  diagnostic reasoning/key patient history questions
    age, 268
    aggravating factors, 270
    alleviating factors, 270
    bowel and bladder symptoms, 269
    current illness, 271
    family history of, 271
    fever, 267
    medication use, 269
    night pain, 270

Acute low back pain *(Continued)*
    numbness or tingling, 271
    pain location, 269
    pain onset and characteristics, 269-270
    pain radiation, 270-271
    recurring pain, 270
    stumbling or movement problems, 271
    systemic diseases, 268-269
    trauma, 268
  differential diagnoses of
    ankylosing spondylitis, 275-276, 277-279b
    aortic aneurysm, 276-277, 277-279b
    cauda equina syndrome, 275, 277-279b
    diskitis, 275, 277-279b
    gallstones, 276, 277-279b
    herniated disk, 275, 277-279b
    musculoskeletal strains, 275, 277-279b
    nonspinal causes of, 276-277, 277-279b
    osteoblastoma, 275, 277-279b
    osteoid osteoma, 275, 277-279b
    osteomyelitis, 275, 277-279b
    osteoporosis, 276, 277-279b
    overuse strains, 275, 277-279b
    pelvic inflammatory disease (PID), 277, 277-279b
    pleuritis, 276-277, 277-279b
    postural strains, 275, 277-279b
    psychological back pain, 277, 277-279b
    pyelonephritis, 276, 277-279b
    Scheuermann disease, 276, 277-279b
    sciatica, 275, 277-279b
    spinal fracture, 268, 274, 277-279b
    spinal metastasis, 275, 277-279b
    spinal stenosis, 276, 277-279b
    spondylolisthesis, 275, 277-279b
  laboratory and diagnostic studies, 274
  lumbar nerve root compromise testing, 267, 268f
  overview of, 267
  physical examination procedures, 271-274
    back and spine inspection and palpation, 272, 272f, 274
    deep tendon reflex tests, 273-274
    FABER test, 272, 272f
    gait assessment, 271
    hip mobility test, 273
    range-of-motion tests, 272
    rectal sphincter tone, 274
    sensory function test, 273
    straight leg raising (SLR) test, 272-273
Acute myocardial infarction (MI), 91, 95b
Acute optic neuritis, 425
Acute otitis media (AOM)
  and bottle propping, 175
  definition of, 174
  symptoms and earaches caused by, 181, 182-183b
Acute pancreatitis, 22, 25-29b, 94, 95b
Acute sinusitis, 281, 286, 287b
Addison disease
  and weight loss (unintentional), 443, 445-446b
Adenomyosis, 406, 408-410b
Adequacy
  as hypothesis testing characteristic, 3
Adolescents
  activity and weight recommendations for, 436b, 437b
  constipation from milk consumption, 112-113
  "growing pains," 247

Adolescents *(Continued)*
  increased sleep needs in, 189
  psychological diagnostic questioning of, 34-35, 34b
  RAFFT questionnaire, 34b
  sleep problems in, 349, 353, 354-355b
  sore throats in, 358
  tiredness in, 184
Adventitious sounds auscultation
  during chest pain evaluation, 87-88
Affective changes; *See also* psychological disorders
  diagnostic evaluation of, 30-45
Age
  and acute low back pain (ALBP), 268
  and breast lumps, 63
  of constipation onset, 112
  earache prevalence according to, 174
  as male genitourinary system diagnoses variable, 211-212
  and reproductive life cycle
    affecting vaginal bleeding, 397-398
  and sore throats, 358
Age at menarche
  and amenorrhea, 50-51
  affecting vaginal bleeding, 400
Agency for Healthcare Research and Quality (AHRQ), 5b, 267
Aging
  macular degeneration with, 432
  as pulmonary embolus risk factor, 160-161
  as risk factor for confusional states, 101
  and sleep problems, 349, 352-353, 354-355b
  vision loss with, 427
  and weight gain (unintentional), 439, 444, 445-446b
  and weight loss (unintentional), 435
Agitation
  as clue to psychological disorders, 30
Agnosia, 104
Airplane travel
  and earaches, 175-176
Airway obstruction
  causing dyspnea, 165
Alanine aminotransferase (ALT) levels, 189
Alcohol
  aggravating gastritis, 12
  as trigger for migraines and cluster headaches, 225
Alcohol abuse
  assessing during HEEADSSS interview, 34-35, 36t
  blood alcohol level tests, 39, 105
  CAGE questionnaire, 33, 33b
  and confusion, 98, 101b
  description and symptoms of, 33, 33b, 34b, 40, 42-45b
  diagnostic questioning to detect, 33, 33b, 34b
  and fatigue, 185
  causing female urinary dysfunction, 388
  affecting mental state, 100
  causing palpitations, 293, 294-295b
  RAFFT adolescent questionnaire, 34b
  causing sleep problems/shortening, 346-347, 348
  T-ACE prenatal questionnaire, 33b
  causing urinary incontinence, 375, 375t, 381, 382-383b
  and weight gain (unintentional), 439
  and weight loss (unintentional), 444, 445-446b
Alcohol withdrawal
  in older adults, 104
  causing sleep disturbances, 348

Alcoholism
  causing acute fatigue, 185, 190, 191-192b
  CAGE questionnaire, 33, 33b
  associated with confusional states, 101b
Alkaloid atropine plant exposure, 198
Allergic colitis, 323, 330-331, 331-332b
Allergic conjunctivitis
  itching and tearing with, 338
  causing red eye, 342, 343-344b
Allergic dermatitis
  characteristics, associations and diagnosis of, 316-320b
  definition and mechanisms of, 315
Allergic rhinitis, 130, 132-133b, 280-281, 285-286, 287b
Allergic vaginitis, 419, 421b
Allergies
  and dyspnea, 161-162
  history of
    and coughs, 123
    and dyspnea, 160, 162
  and hoarseness, 237, 235
  nasal symptoms with, 280-281
  skin rashes and lesions due to, 308
    erythema multiforme, 315
    urticaria, 315
Allergy skin testing, 285
Alpha-adrenergic agonists
  causing urinary incontinence, 375, 375t, 381, 382-383b
Alternating cover/uncover eye tests, 429
Alum-precipitated toxoid test (APT), 328
Alzheimer disease
  stages of, 108b
Alzheimer-type dementia, 107b
Amblyopia, 426, 430, 433-434b
Amenorrhea
  congenial or chronic disorders that may cause
    Cushing syndrome, 57, 58-59t
    polycystic ovary syndrome, 57, 58-59t
    thyroid dysfunction, 57, 58-59t
    Turner syndrome, 57, 58-59t
  constitutional problems that may cause
    anorexia nervosa and bulimia, 57, 58-59t
    delayed puberty, 57, 58-59t
    exercise-induced amenorrhea, 57, 58-59t
  definition of, 46
  diagnostic reasoning/key history questions
    age of menarche, 50-51
    androgen excess, 53
    and athletic training intensity, 51
    body mass index (BMI), 51, 54, 54b
    breast development stages, 47, 49, 49f, 50f
    cervical procedures, 53
    chest wall stimulation, 52
    congenital or chronic, 51
    contraceptive use, 47
    emotional state, 51
    endometriosis, 53
    estrogen deficiency, 53
    galactorrhea, 52
    gynecological problems, 53
    hemorrhages at childbirth, 53
    HPO axis problems, 52
    hyperprolactinemia, 52, 52b
    infertility, 52-53
    medications that may cause, 52, 52b
    menstrual history, 51

Amenorrhea *(Continued)*
  nipple stimulation, 52
  onset of menstruation, 47
  pituitary tumors, 52
  pregnancies, 46
  primary *versus* secondary, 46-47
  pubertal development stages, 47, 49, 49f, 50f
  thyroid dysfunction, 51
  uterus-related, 53
  weight changes, 51, 53-54
  drugs that may cause, 52b
  hypothalamic-pituitary-ovarian axis problems causing
    ovarian failure, 57-58, 58-59t
  laboratory and diagnostic studies, 55-57
  normal menstrual cycle, 46, 47f, 48t
  ovarian and endometrial cycle correlation, 46, 48t
  physical examination procedures, 53-55
    breast exam, 54-55
    lymph node palpation, 54
    pelvic examination, 55
    sexual maturity assessment, 49f, 50f, 54
    thyroid gland palpation, 54
  pregnancy as most common cause of, 57
  primary *versus* secondary, 46-47
  uterine and outflow tract problems causing
    Asherman syndrome, 57, 58-59t
    cervical os stenosis, 57, 58-59t
    chest wall stimulation, 58, 58-59t
    imperforate hymen, 57, 58-59t
    medications, 58, 58-59t
    nipple stimulation, 58, 58-59t
    pituitary adenoma, 58-59t, 58-59
    Sheehan syndrome, 58, 58-59t
American Urological Association Symptom Index, 209, 210t
Amsler grid, 429, 429f, 432
Amyotrophic lateral sclerosis, 238
Anal fissures
  detection of, 115
  pain associated with, 328-329, 331-332b
  pain causing constipation, 111
  tenesmus with, 324
Anal sphincter
  anal fissures and tears, 321, 328-329, 331-332b
  anatomy of, 322f
  relaxation and defecation problems, 111
  sphincter contraction tenesmus, 321
Anaphylaxis
  and dyspnea, 160, 169, 171-172b
Androgen excess
  and amenorrhea, 53
Anemia
  associated with confusional states, 101b
  and dyspnea, 170, 172-173b
  and fatigue, 184, 190, 191-192b
  from heavy menstrual flow, 186
  causing palpitations, 293, 294-295b
Angina pectoris, 288
Anginal pain, 81-82
Angiotensin-converting enzyme (ACE) inhibitors, 130,
  132-133b, 161
Anhedonia, 34b
Animal exposure
  and diarrhea, 137
  and fever, 198
  and flea bites causing skin rashes/lesions, 311

Ankles
  Achilles tendinitis, 258, 262-265b
  anatomical diagram of, 249f
  ankle sprain, 258, 262-265b
  medial tibial stress syndrome, 258, 262-265b
  pain diagnostic questions, 245-248
  shin splints, 258, 262-265b
Ankylosing spondylitis
  causing acute low back pain (ALBP), 275-276,
    277-279b
Anorectal area; *See also* rectum
  anal soreness, 321
  anatomy of, 321-322, 322f
  bleeding differential diagnoses
    allergic colitis, 330-331, 331-332b
    bowel inflammation, 331, 331-332b
    colorectal cancer, 330, 331-332b
    condyloma acuminata, 330, 331-332b
    hemorrhoids, 330, 330t, 331-332b
    intussusception, 331, 331-332b
    juvenile polyps, 331, 331-332b
    maternal blood ingestion, 330, 331-332b
    Meckel diverticulum, 331, 331-332b
    necrotizing enterocolitis, 331, 331-332b
  and constipation, 118, 118-119b
  itching differential diagnoses
    pinworms, 330, 331-332b
    pruritus ani, 329-330, 331-332b
  pain differential diagnoses, 328-329, 331-332b
    anal fissure, 328-329, 331-332b
    perianal streptococcal cellulitis, 329, 331-332b
    perirectal abscess, 328-329, 331-332b
    perirectal fistula, 328-329, 331-332b
    pilonidal disease, 329, 331-332b
    proctalgia fugax, 329, 331-332b
    proctitis/proctocolitis, 329, 331-332b
  questions regarding bleeding, 322
  tears and fissures, 321
  tenesmus, 321, 324
Anorectal manometry
  during abdominal pain evaluation, 20
  during constipation evaluation, 117
Anorexia nervosa
  and amenorrhea, 54, 57, 58-59t
  and weight loss (unintentional), 439, 443, 445-446b
Anoscopy
  anorectal examination with, 327
  during constipation evaluation, 116-117
Anovulatory cycles
  irregular menstrual cycles, 399-400
  menopause, 400
  and vaginal bleeding, 406-407, 408-410b
    in newborns, 407, 408-410b
    perimenarche, 406-407, 408-410b
    perimenopause, 406, 408-410b
Antacids, 12-13
Anterior chamber (eye)
  anatomical illustration of, 335f
  hyphema, 342, 343-344b
Anterior cruciate ligament (ACL) tear, 258, 262-265b
Anterior ischemic optic neuropathy, 425
Anterior posterior (AP) image
  of abdomen, 457
  assessment of chest x-ray, 448-449, 449f, 450-455,
    450f

Antibiotics
    causing diarrhea, 138, 144, 146-147b
    causing serum sickness, 247
Anticholinergic agents
    fever from, 199
    causing urinary incontinence, 375, 375t, 381, 382-383b
Anticoagulants
    as pulmonary embolus risk factor, 161
    and vaginal bleeding, 396
Antinuclear antibodies (ANA)
    tests during limb pain evaluation, 253
Antipyretics
    for lowering hypothalamic set point, 194
Antistreptolysin titer (ASO), 202, 361
Anuria
    and male genitourinary evaluation, 209
Anus; *See also* anorectal area
    anal soreness, 321
    anatomy of, 321-322, 322f
    bleeding conditions affecting, 330-331
    disorders causing pain, 328-329
    itching around, 329-330
Anxiety
    as clue to psychological disorders, 30
    diagnostic questions, 34
    causing dizziness and vertigo, 150
    and fatigue, 187, 190, 191-192b
    history of and dyspnea, 161
    medications that can cause, 31, 32b
    and palpitations, 289
    as pulmonary embolus risk factor, 160-161
    causing sleep problems, 346, 348
    symptoms of, 34, 41, 42-45b
    and weight loss/gain (unintentional), 443, 445-446b
Aorta
    normal vs abnormal x-ray findings, 463-464b
Aortic aneurysm
    causing acute low back pain (ALBP), 268, 276-277, 277-279b
Aortic dissection, 91, 95b
Aortic stenosis, 92-93, 95b
Aphonia, 236
Aphthous stomatitis, 363, 364-365b
Appendicitis, 8, 15-18, 21-23, 21b, 25-29b
Appetite
    and fatigue, 185
    and weight loss (unintentional), 436, 438
Apraxia, 102, 104
Arrhythmias, 92, 95b
    history information regarding, 290b
    causing palpitations, 292, 292b, 294-295b
    predictions, 290b
    causing syncope, 370-371, 372b
Arterial blood gases (ABGs), 90, 168-169
Artifacts
    on x-rays, 460, 463-464b
Aryepiglottic fold, 236f
Asherman syndrome, 53, 57, 58-59t
Aspartate aminotransferase (AST) levels, 189
Aspirin, 198
Assessments
    overview of advanced health, 2
    overview of basic health, 2
Assistive devices
    and limb pain, 245
Asterixis, 104

Asthma
    and coughs, 120-121, 129, 132-133b
    and dyspnea, 160, 161-162, 170-171, 172-173b
    and hoarseness, 237
Astigmatism, 431, 433-434b
Asymptomatic inflammatory prostatitis, 218, 219-220b
Ataxic gait, 226
Athletes
    calorie needs of, 436, 437b
    exercise-induced amenorrhea, 51, 57, 58-59t
    overuse injuries, 244-245
Atopic dermatitis, 163, 309-310, 310b
Atrophic vaginitis
    assessing in urinary incontinence patients, 375
    description and causes of, 407, 408-410b
    urinary problems with, 392-393, 394b
    vaginal discharge with, 419, 421b
Atrophy
    skin, 307f
Audiometry
    during dizziness and vertigo evaluation, 154
    to evaluate earaches, 180-181
Aura
    migraine with, 224
    seizures and syncope, 366
Autism
    CHAT screen, 40b
Autism spectrum disorder, 40, 40b, 42-45b
Autonomic defecation control, 111
Avian influenza, 184b

B
Babinski sign, 104
Bacillus aureus food poisoning
    causing diarrhea, 143, 146-147b
Back pain; *See* acute low back pain (ALBP)
Bacteremia
    with high fever, 195-196
Bacterial conjunctivitis
    and red eye, 338, 341, 343-344b
Bacterial cystitis
    urinary problems with, 391-392, 392b, 394b
Bacterial infections
    nasal symptoms with, 282
    causing urinary tract infections, 385
Bacterial pneumonia, 128, 131-132b
Bacterial tracheitis, 169, 171-172b
Bacterial vaginosis
    description and vaginal discharge with, 419, 421b
    microscopic illustration of, 412f
    symptoms and diagnosis of, 418b
    vaginal bleeding and discharge due to, 399
Baker cyst, 258, 262-265b
Balance
    assessment during headache evaluation, 228
    and dizziness, 149-158
    as indicator of psychological or substance abuse disorders, 39
    sensations of imbalance, 149-150
    systems affecting, 149
    testing in older adults, 104
    visual, vestibular and sensory systems controlling, 149
Balanitis, 301, 302b
Bárány maneuvers
    for vertigo and dizziness evaluation, 153

Barium enema, 117
Barium esophagography, 239
Barotrauma
  and earaches, 175-176, 181-182, 182-183b
Basal body temperature
  charting during amenorrhea evaluation, 56
Basal metabolic rate (BMR) test, 442, 443b
BATHE model, 32-34
Bed wetting, 374; *See also* enuresis
Behaviors
  analysis of, 30
  changes in children with fever, 197
  changes with delirium, 100
Benign exertional headaches, 229, 232-233b
Benign paroxysmal positional vertigo (BPPV), 155-156
Benign paroxysmal vertigo (BPV) of childhood, 155
Benign prostatic hyperplasia
  description and diagnosis of male, 208, 218, 219-220b
Beta-adrenergic agonists
  causing urinary incontinence, 375, 375t, 381, 382-383b
B-hemolytic streptococcus (GABHS) infections
  ASO titer to detect, 361
  groups at risk for Group A, 362t
  sore throat indications of, 356-357, 358
Bicipital tendinitis, 255, 262-265b
Biliary colic pain, 11-12
Bilious vomiting, 114
Bilirubin test, 442
Biopsies
  history of breast, 75
  male genitourinary system, 217
Bipolar disorder
  definition and symptoms of, 34-35, 35b, 41-45, 42-45b
  diagnostic questions, 34-35, 35b
  DIG FAST symptoms of, 35b
Bird flu, 184b
Birth control methods
  and amenorrhea, 47
  and vaginal bleeding, 399
Bitemporal hemianopsia, 424f
Bladder
  anatomic diagram and x-ray view of, 458, 458f
  detrusor muscle
    and urinary incontinence, 374
  normal vs abnormal x-ray findings, 463-464b
  problems and acute low back pain (ALBP), 269
  small and urinary incontinence, 382
  tumors, 219, 219-220b
  and urinary incontinence, 374-382, 382-383b
Bladder diary
  for urinary incontinence evaluation, 379
Bleeding
  with anorectal disorders, 322-323
  causes of rectal
    allergic colitis, 330-331, 331-332b
    bowel inflammation, 331, 331-332b
    colorectal cancer, 330, 331-332b
    condyloma acuminata, 330, 331-332b
    hemorrhoids, 330, 330t, 331-332b
    intussusception, 331, 331-332b
    juvenile polyps, 331, 331-332b
    maternal blood ingestion, 330, 331-332b
    Meckel diverticulum, 331, 331-332b
    necrotizing enterocolitis, 331, 331-332b

Bleeding *(Continued)*
  with constipation, 112, 114
  causing fatigue, 186
  with pain and itching in anorectal area, 321-333
  prepubertal vaginal, 399
  vaginal *(See* vaginal bleeding)
Bleeding time (BT), 404
Blepharitis, 335-336, 341, 343-344b
"Blind spot"
  anatomical illustration of, 335f
Blindness; *See also* vision loss
  description of, 423
  illustration of total, 424f
Blood
  loss with menstrual bleeding, 396
  menstrual cycle, 396, 398
  in stools with diarrhea, 136
  in urine, 297
Blood alcohol level tests, 39, 105
Blood chemistry tests, 105
Blood clots
  as pulmonary embolus risk factor, 160-161
Blood dyscrasias
  and vaginal bleeding, 401-402
    leukemia, 408, 408-410b
    von Willebrand disease, 408, 408-410b
Blood glucose levels, 437-438
Blood pressure
  measurement of
    during chest pain evaluation, 86-87
    during dizziness and vertigo evaluation, 152
    during dyspnea evaluation, 165-166
    during syncope evaluation, 368-369
Blood reagent strips
  for female/child urinary problem evaluation, 390
Blood urea nitrogen (BUN) and creatinine test
  to evaluate diarrhea, 142
  in male genitourinary evaluation, 215
  for urinary incontinence evaluation, 379
Blurring of vision, 336, 423
Body mass index (BMI)
  and amenorrhea, 51, 54, 54b
  chart, 467f
  and fatigue, 185, 187
  measurement of, 467f, 435
  and vaginal bleeding, 402
Body temperature
  charting during amenorrhea evaluation, 56
  during dyspnea evaluation, 165-166
  examining in diarrhea cases, 140
  hypothalamus regulation of, 194
  measurement for fever evaluation, 194-195, 200
Body weight; *See* weight gain; weight loss
  ideal, 439, 440t
Bones
  assessing in abdominal x-ray, 458
  fractures, 244
  infections, 205, 206-207b
  and ligaments of elbow, 248f
  and ligaments of shoulder, 248f
Bony thorax
  as seen on chest x-rays, 451, 455b
Bordetella pertussis infection, 128, 131-132b

Bottle propping
  and earaches, 175
Botulism, 170, 171-172b
Bouchard (PIP) joint nodes, 250
Bowel movements/habits
  and constipation, 111, 113
  "normal" frequency, 111
  straining, 325
  taking history of
    during abdominal pain assessment, 10
Bowel obstruction
  acute abdominal pain from, 9, 23, 25-29b
  and blood in stool, 13-15
Bowel sounds, 16, 140-141
Bowels
  and acute low back pain (ALBP), 269
  assessing in urinary incontinence patients, 375-376
  changes with thyroid dysfunction, 51-52
  inflammation causing anorectal bleeding, 331, 331-332b
Brain abscesses, 231, 232-233b
Brainstem dysfunction
  causing central vertigo, 155
Breakfast habits
  and constipation, 113
Breast cancer, 70, 72-73b
  clinical breast examination to detect, 66b
  risks factors, 62, 62b
Breast cysts, 70, 72-73b
Breast development stages
  and amenorrhea, 47, 49, 49f, 50f
Breast implants
  ruptured, 63, 71, 72-73b
Breast lumps; *See also* nipple discharge
  diagnostic reasoning/key history questions
    age, 63
    childbirth, 63
    duration and growth, 61
    fever, 63
    hot or painful breasts, 63
    infections, 62
    mastitis and lactation, 63
    nipple discharge, 62
    nipple soreness/cracks, 63
    post menopausal, 62
    previous mammograms or biopsies, 63
    risks, 62, 62b
    timing, consistency and duration, 63
    unilateral *versus* bilateral, 61
  differential diagnoses
    abscesses, 70-71, 72-73b
    breast cancer, 70, 72-73b
    breast cysts, 70, 72-73b
    duct ectasia, 71, 72-73b
    fat necrosis, 70, 72-73b
    fibroadenoma, 70, 72-73b
    fibrocystic breast changes, 71, 72-73b
    hyperprolactinemia, 71, 72-73b
    inflammatory breast cancer, 71, 72-73b
    intraductal papilloma, 71, 72-73b
    lipoma, 70, 72-73b
    male acute mastitis, 71, 72-73b
    male breast cancer, 71-73, 72-73b
    mastitis, 71, 72-73b
    multiple or bilateral, 71, 72-73b

Breast lumps *(Continued)*
    neonatal discharge, 71, 72-73b
    nipple discharge conditions, 71, 72-73b
    ruptured implants, 71, 72-73b
    tuberculosis, 70, 72-73b
    Witch's milk, 71, 72-73b
  fluctuation and mobility of, 76
  laboratory and diagnostic studies, 68-69
  pain associated with, 75, 79-80, 79-80b
  physical examination procedures, 65-68
  single mass differential diagnoses, 70-71
  statistics, 61
  three most common types of
    breast carcinoma, 61
    fibroadenomas, 61
    fibrocystic, 61
Breast pain
  diagnostic reasoning/key history questions, 74-76
    abdominal pain, 76
    age of patient, 74
    chest pain or shortness of breath, 76
    chest trauma, 75
    chicken pox, 75
    hot or red breast, 75
    localization and radiation, 75
    lumps or discharge, 75
    medications, 75
    menstrual cycle relationship, 74
    missed periods or pregnancy, 75
    patient description of pain, 74
    pre- or postmenopausal, 74
    previous mammograms or biopsies, 75
  differential diagnoses
    abscesses, 78, 79-80b
    costochondritis, 78, 79-80b
    cyclic mastalgia, 78, 79-80b
    herpes zoster, 79, 79-80b
    Klinefelter syndrome, 79, 79-80b
    mammary duct ectasia, 78, 79-80b
    mastitis, 78, 79-80b
    menstrual cyclic mastalgia, 78, 79-80b
    noncyclic mastalgia, 78, 79-80b
    pregnancy, 78, 79-80b
    shingles, 79, 79-80b
  with gynecomastia in men, 74
  with Klinefelter syndrome, 74
  laboratory and diagnostic studies, 76-78
  lumps associated with (*See* breast lumps)
  overview of, 74
  physical examination procedures, 76
Breastfeeding
  activity and weight recommendations for, 436b, 437b
  and weight loss (unintentional), 436
Breasts
  clinical examination of, 65-68, 66b, 76
    during amenorrhea evaluation, 54-55
    breast and nipple inspection, 65-66
    breast palpation, 66-68
    lymph node palpation, 66, 67f
    nipple well assessment, 68
    previous mammograms or biopsies, 63
  fine-needle aspiration (FNA) biopsy, 69
  hot or painful, 63
  lymphatic drainage of, 66, 67f

Breath sounds
  during chest pain evaluation, 87, 88t
  during cough evaluation, 126
  during dyspnea evaluation, 167
Breath-holding
  causing syncope, 372b
Breathing
  abnormal patterns of, 164, 165b
  observations during cough evaluation, 125
British Medical Journal, 5b
Bronchiolitis, 129, 131-132b
Bronchogenic carcinoma, 130, 132-133b
Bronchoscopy
  during chest pain evaluation, 90
Brudzinski sign, 202, 204-205
Bubble baths
  causing female and child urinary dysfunction, 388, 393, 394b
Bulge sign, 258, 261t
Bulimia, 54, 57, 58-59t
Bulla, 304-305t, 307f
Burning
  of skin rashes and lesions, 310
Burns
  fever from, 199
  causing vision loss, 425
Burping
  pain relieved by, 14
Bursitis, 253, 262-265b
Buttocks
  patient locating pain in, 250

C

C. difficile
  causing diarrhea, 144, 146-147b
C. difficile toxin assay, 142
C. trachomatis
  incubation period of, 296
  causing penile discharge, 300, 302b
  causing urethritis, 300-301
Caffeine
  causing female and child urinary dysfunction, 388
  causing sleep disruption, 348
CAGE questionnaire
  for alcoholism, 33, 33b
Calcifications
  anatomic diagram and x-ray view of, 459-460, 461f
Calories/activity levels
  guidelines for, 435, 436b, 437b, 440t
  and weight gain (unintentional), 439, 440t, 444, 445-446b
Camping; *See* outdoor activities
Cancer
  breast, 70, 72-73b
  cervical, 398
  causing chronic fatigue, 191, 191-192b
  colon, 116b
  colorectal, 118-119, 118-119b, 321-322, 321b, 330, 331-332b
  endometrial, 400, 400b, 406, 408-410b
  laryngeal, 237, 240, 241-242b
  prostate, 216, 216b
  as pulmonary embolus risk factor, 160-161
  and weight loss (unintentional), 438, 442-443, 445-446b
Candida infections
  DNA probe testing for, 19
  microscopic illustration of, 412f

Candida vulvovaginitis
  description and vaginal discharge with, 419, 421b
Candidiasis
  characteristics, associations and diagnosis of, 316-320b
  definition and mechanisms of, 314-315
  causing sore throat, 363, 364-365b
  symptoms and diagnosis of, 418b
Canker sores, 363, 364-365b
Capillary refill, 166
Carbon dioxide poisoning, 226
Carbon monoxide poisoning, 230-231, 232-233b
Carbuncle, 313, 316-320b
Cardiac disorders
  causing syncope, 370-371, 372b
Cardiac enzyme tests, 19
  during abdominal pain evaluation, 19
  during chest pain evaluation, 89
Cardiac ischemia, 367
Cardiac monitoring
  during dizziness and vertigo evaluation, 154
  of palpitations, 291-292
Cardiac syncope, 367
Cardiovascular system
  assessment during fatigue evaluation, 187
  causes of vertigo, 156
  conditions associated with confusional states, 101b
  considering during abdominal pain evaluation, 14
  problems causing vertigo, 150
  testing during dizziness and vertigo evaluation, 154
Carotid sinus hypersensitivity
  causing syncope, 371, 372b
Carotid sinus massage (CSM), 369-370
Carotid ultrasonography, 370
Carpal tunnel syndrome, 260, 261t, 262-265b
Cataplexy, 346-347, 352
Cataracts
  definition and vision loss from, 431, 433-434b
  formation from trauma, 425
  indications of, 428-429
Cat-scratch disease, 198
Cauda equina syndrome, 267, 275, 277-279b
Celiac sprue, 139
Central retinal artery occlusion, 431, 433-434b
Central vertigo
  definition of, 149
  and headaches, 150
  neurological symptoms with, 150
  and nystagmus, 152-153, 153t
Centrifugal/centripetal skin lesions, 309, 312
Cerebellar dysfunction
  causing central vertigo, 155
Cerebellar function tests, 104
Cerebral perfusion
  decrease and syncope, 366
  transient ischemic attacks (TIAs), 367-368
Cerebrovascular accidents
  and transient ischemic attacks (TIAs), 367-368
Cerebrovascular system
  conditions associated with confusional states, 98, 101b
Cerumen
  impaction and earaches, 177, 181, 182-183b
  lavage of obstructions, 177-178
Cervical cancer, 398
Cervical lymphadenitis, 182, 182-183b
Cervical os stenosis, 57, 58-59t

Cervical spine disorders
    causing headaches, 222f, 230, 232-233b
    causing referred pain earaches, 174
Cervicitis, 415
Cervix
    and amenorrhea, 53
    cervical cancer, 398
    polyps, 398
Chalazion, 341, 343-344b
CHAT screen
    for autism, 40b
Chemical conjunctivitis, 342, 343-344b
Chemicals
    trauma to eyes
        emergency treatment of, 334
        causing vision loss, 425, 432, 433-434b
    urinary problems due to, 393, 394b
Chest
    asymmetrical movement, 165b
    examination of
        during dyspnea evaluation, 164, 166-167
    imaging studies of, 448 (See chest x-rays)
        computed tomography (CT scans), 454-455
        echocardiogram, 455
        magnetic resonance imaging (MRIs), 455
        positron emission tomography (PET), 455
    shape, symmetry and muscle inspection, 125
Chest pain
    and breast pain, 76
    in children, 81, 86
    diagnostic reasoning/key patient history questions
        acute versus chronic determination, 83
        awakening with or awakening from pain, 84
        chest trauma history, 84
        cough and sputum production, 84
        duration of, 82
        emotional state, 86
        family history, 86
        fever, 84
        food association, 85
        gastrointestinal origin questions, 85
        lightheadedness, dizziness or fainting, 84
        location and character of pain, 83-84
        onset of, 82
        pain characteristics, 81-82, 85
        palpitations, 84
        panic disorder history, 86
        pattern of, 84
        recent activities or exercise, 84
        risk factor assessment, 82-83
        skin symptoms, 85
        associated symptoms, 82
        systemic conditions that may cause, 85-86
    emergent pain differential diagnoses
        acute coronary insufficiency, 91, 95b
        acute myocardial infarction (MI), 91, 95b
        aortic dissection, 91, 95b
        arrhythmias, 92, 95b
        congenital coronary anomalies, 92, 95b
        pneumothorax, 92, 95b
        pulmonary embolus, 91-92, 95b
    laboratory and diagnostic studies, 89 (See also chest x-rays)
    life-threatening assessment, 81
    nonemergent pain differential diagnoses
        acute pancreatitis, 94, 95b

Chest pain (Continued)
        aortic stenosis, 92-93, 95b
        chest trauma, 93, 95b
        cholecystitis, 94, 95b
        cocaine use, 94, 95b
        costochondritis, 93, 95b
        esophagitis, 93, 95b
        herpes zoster, 93-94, 95b
        lung and mediastinal tumors, 94, 95b
        mitral regurgitation, 93, 95b
        mitral valve prolapse, 93, 95b
        myocarditis, 92, 95b
        peptic ulcer disease, 94, 95b
        pericarditis, 92, 95b
        pleuritis, 93, 95b
        pleurodynia, 94, 95b
        pneumonia, 93, 95b
        precordial catch syndrome, 94, 95b
        psychogenic origins, 94, 95b
        shingles, 93-94, 95b
        stable angina, 92, 95b
        Tietze syndrome, 93, 95b
    overview of, 81
    with palpitations, 288
    physical examination procedures, 369
    and syncope, 367
Chest percussion
    during chest pain evaluation, 87
    during cough evaluation, 125-126
Chest radiography; See chest x-rays
Chest trauma
    causing breast pain, 75
    causing chest pain, 93, 95b
    history questions regarding, 84
Chest wall stimulation, 52, 58, 58-59t
Chest x-rays
    during cough evaluation, 127
    diagnostic reasoning/systematic examination
        bony thorax, 451, 455-456b
        clavicles, 451, 455-456b
        costophrenic angle, 452, 452f, 455-456b
        diaphragm, 451-452, 455-456b
        gastric air bubbles, 452, 455-456b
        heart, 452, 453f, 455-456b
        hilar area, 452, 455-456b
        lungs, 453, 455-456b
        mediastinum, 452, 455-456b
        pleura, 452, 455-456b
        pulmonary vasculature, 452, 455-456b
        ribs and intracostal spaces, 451, 451f,
            455-456b
        scapulae, 451, 455-456b
        soft tissue, 450, 455-456b
        thoracic spine, 451, 455-456b
        trachea, 450-451, 455-456b
    for dyspnea evaluation, 168
    for fatigue cases, 189
    image box placement, 449
    image quality, 449-450
    lateral view assessment, 453, 454f
        anatomy, 453, 454f, 455-456b
        costophrenic angle, 454, 454f, 455-456b
        diaphragm, 453, 454f, 455-456b
        fissures, 454, 454f, 455-456b
        heart, 454, 454f, 455-456b

Chest x-rays *(Continued)*
  lungs, 454, 454f, 455-456b
  pleura, 454, 454f, 455-456b
  retrosternal area, 454, 454f, 455-456b
  vertebral bodies, 453, 454f, 455-456b
  reviewing procedures, 448-450
  verifying image with patient, 448
  views and examples of, 448-449, 449f
    anteroposterior (AP) image, 448-449, 449f, 450f
    expiration image, 448
    lateral decubitus image, 448
    lordotic images, 449
    oblique images, 449
Cheyne-Stokes respirations, 165b
Chicken pox
  causing breast pain, 75
  itching of, 310b
  skin rashes and lesions, 314, 316-320b
Childbirth
  and anorectal disorders, 326
  and breast lumps, 63
  hemorrhages and amenorrhea, 53
  recent and vaginal bleeding, 397
  and stress incontinence, 380
Children
  abdominal pain, 8-9
  activity and weight recommendations for, 436b, 437b
  acute optic neuritis in, 425
  anorectal disorders in, 323
  back pain, 267
  behavior and psychosocial concerns, 30
  bowel movement frequency, 111
  brain tumors, 223
  breath-holding precipitating syncope, 367
  chest pain, 81, 86
  constipation in, 113-114
  coughing *(See* cough)
  daytime wetting by, 374
  earaches, 174, 177-178
  enuresis, 376-377, 382
  eye movements and development, 427, 427b
  eye tests and screens, 427-428, 428t
  fatigue signals, 184
  fecal soiling of underpants, 114
  fevers, 184b, 199
  foreign body aspiration
    and coughing, 121, 130, 132-133b
    and dyspnea, 160
  "growing pains," 247
  headaches, 228
  hearing loss, 177
  with heart disease and dyspnea, 165
  Kawasaki disease and syncope, 368
  optic gliomas in, 425-426, 432
  Oucher Pain Scale, 10, 11f
  overweight, 436b
  palpitations in, 288
  papulosquamous eruptions in, 308f
  prepubertal vaginal bleeding, 399
  retinoblastomas in, 431
  sleep and night terror problems, 346-347, 348-350, 352-353, 354-355b
  stool characteristics in, 13-15
  toilet training and constipation, 114
  trained night crier or feeder, 353-354, 354-355b

Children *(Continued)*
  urinary dysfunction *(See* urinary dysfunction)
  urinary incontinence in, 376-377, 382
  vaginal bleeding, 399
  Yale Observation Scale Predictive Model
    for quantifying fever and illness in, 199, 200t
Chlamydia infections
  description and vaginal discharge with, 419-420, 421b
  DNA probe testing for, 19, 215, 417
  lesions with, 298
  causing penile discharge, 296, 301, 302b
  causing urethritis, 385
  vaginal bleeding and discharge due to, 399
Chlamydia trachomatis
  description and vaginal discharge with, 420, 421b
  causing pelvic inflammatory disease (PID), 407
  causing prostatitis, 208, 219-220b
  causing urethritis, 385
Chlamydial pneumonia, 129, 131-132b
Choking
  on foreign bodies, 121, 130, 132-133b
  history during cough evaluation, 122
Cholecystitis
  abdominal pain from, 14, 22, 25-29b
  causing chest pain, 94, 95b
Cholesteatoma
  causing dizziness and vertigo, 152, 156
  symptoms and earaches from, 181, 182-183b
Cholesterol levels
  and coronary artery disease (CAD), 82-83
Chondromalacia patellae, 257, 262-265b
Chorea
  with Huntington disease, 104
Choroid
  anatomical illustration of, 335f
Chromosomal disorders
  Klinefelter syndrome, 74, 79
Chromosome analysis (karyotyping), 56
Chronic bacterial prostatitis, 208, 217-218, 219-220b
Chronic bronchitis, 130, 132-133b
Chronic diarrhea
  versus acute adult diarrhea, 135
  versus acute in children, 135-136
Chronic fatigue syndrome, 184, 191, 191-192b
Chronic leakage
  assessing in urinary incontinence patients, 377
Chronic obstructive pulmonary disease (COPD), 128, 131-132b
  breath sounds with, 168
  and dyspnea, 161-162, 168, 170, 172-173b
  respiration characteristics of, 164-165, 165b
  sleep problems due to, 347, 352
Chronic pelvic pain syndrome, 218, 219-220b
Chronic prostatitis, 218, 219-220b
Chronic sinusitis, 130, 132-133b
Circadian rhythms
  and difficulty staying asleep, 346
  and sleep problems, 345-346
Clavicles
  as seen on chest x-rays, 451, 455b
Clinical decision-making
  and diagnostic process, 2-3
  goals of, 3
  process of, 2
  summary of, 5

Clinical judgment
  development of, 4
Clostridium perfringens
  causing diarrhea, 143, 146-147b
Clotting disorders
  and anorectal bleeding, 322-323
  and vaginal bleeding, 396, 401-402
Clue cells
  microscopic illustration of, 412f
Cluster headaches, 224, 229, 232-233b
Cocaine use
  causing chest pains, 94, 95b
  nasal symptoms with, 283
Cochlea
  anatomic diagram of, 175f
Cochrane Collaboration web source, 4-5
Cognitive impairment
  conditions associated with, 100
  with confusional states, 100
  and weight loss/gain (unintentional), 443,
      445-446b
Coherence
  as hypothesis testing characteristic, 3
COLDSPA mnemonic
  in diagnostic process, 2-4
Colic, 8
Collateral ligament test, 258, 261t
Colon
  anatomic diagram and x-ray view of, 458f, 459-460,
      459f
  symptoms with diarrhea, 135
Colon cancer
  screening techniques, 116b
Colon transit studies, 117
Colonic motility, 111, 113
Colonoscopy
  for abdominal pain evaluation, 20
  for anorectal disorder diagnosis, 327
  for colon cancer screening, 116b, 117
  for constipation evaluation, 116b, 117
  for diarrhea evaluation, 143
  procedures for performing, 462
Color vision
  progressive loss of, 425-426
Colorectal cancer (CRC)
  causing anorectal bleeding, 330, 331-332b
  and constipation, 118-119, 118-119b
  screening for, 116b, 321b
  symptoms associated with, 321-322, 330, 331-332b
Common cold, 127-128, 131-132b
Comorbid insomnia, 352, 354-355b
Complete blood counts (CBCs); *See* each chapter's laboratory
      and diagnostic studies sections
Complete heart block
  causing syncope, 367
Complicated urethritis
  causing penile discharge, 301, 302b
Computed tomography (CT scans); *See* chapter "Laboratory
      and Diagnostic Studies" sections
  definition and procedures for performing, 454-455, 463
Concentration lapses
  with depression, 102
  with psychological disorders, 30
Conditioned insomnia, 349, 353-354, 354-355b
Condyloma acuminata, 330, 331-332b, 407-408, 408-410b

Confusion
  abrupt and short-lived
      indicating transient ischemic attack (TIA), 99
  caused by head trauma, 99
  cognitive losses with, 100
  cranial nerve factors, 104
  definition of, 98
  differential diagnoses associated with
      delirium, 105-106, 109-110b
      dementia, 107, 109-110b
      depression, 107, 109-110b
  hallucinations, 99
  health conditions that might cause, 100, 101b
  key questions of family or close contact, 98-101
      alcohol or drug use, 98
      onset, duration and characteristics of, 98-99
      suicidal thoughts, 98
  laboratory and diagnostic studies, 104-105
  medications that can cause, 100
  neurological exams, 103-104
  physical examination to analyze
      level of consciousness assessment, 102
      mental status examination, 102-103
  proprioception and cerebellar function tests, 104
  symptoms of, 99
  tremors and gait disturbances, 99
  and urinary incontinence, 375, 375b, 381
Confusion Assessment Method (CAM), 103
Congenital aganglionic megacolon, 113-114, 115, 117-118, 118-119b
Congenital coronary anomalies, 92, 95b
Congenital diseases
  and amenorrhea, 51
  of eyes, 432, 433-434b
  of heart, 367
Congenital TORCH infections, 426, 432, 433-434b
Congestive heart failure
  as pulmonary embolus risk factor, 160-161
Conjunctiva
  anatomical illustration of, 335f
  conditions causing red eye
      allergic conjunctivitis, 342, 343-344b
      bacterial conjunctivitis, 341, 343-344b
      chemical conjunctivitis, 342, 343-344b
      N. gonorrhoeae conjunctivitis, 342, 343-344b
      subconjunctival hemorrhage, 342, 343-344b
      viral conjunctivitis, 341-342, 343-344b
  inspection of, 339
Constipation
  abdominal x-ray illustrating, 459-460, 460f
  and anal fissures, 324
  and anorectal disorders, 324-325
  chronic verus acute, 111
  defining, 111
  diagnostic reasoning/key history questions, 111-115
      age of onset, 112
      alternating with diarrhea, 113
      bleeding, 112, 114
      bowel habits, 113
      breakfast habits, 113
      in children, 113-114
      cow's milk use, 113-114
      crying with defecation, 114
      delayed passage of meconium stool, 114
      dietary patterns or changes, 112-113, 114
      enema, laxative and suppository use, 113

Constipation *(Continued)*
    fecal soiling of underpants, 114
    genetic history of, 114-115
    medications, 113
    onset and duration, 112
    pain, 114
    recent and chronic illnesses, 112
    red flags, 111-112
    with sedentary lifestyles, 113
    stool color, size, consistency and frequency, 111-112, 113-114
    toilet training, 114
    urge to defecate, 113-114
    urinary tract problems, 114-115
    vomiting, 114
    weight loss (unintentional), 112
  differential diagnoses of
    anorectal lesions, 118, 118-119b
    colorectal cancer, 118-119, 118-119b
    congenital aganglionic megacolon, 115, 118, 118-119b
    drug-induced constipation, 118, 118-119b
    fecal impaction, 117, 118-119b
    functional constipation, 117, 118-119b
    Hirschsprung disease, 118, 118-119b
    idiopathic slow transit, 117-118, 118-119b
    irritable bowel syndrome (IBS), 117, 118-119b
    simple constipation, 117, 118-119b
    tumors, 118-119, 118-119b
  with female and child urinary dysfunction, 388
  functional causes of, 111, 117
  laboratory and diagnostic studies, 115-117
  painful, 114-115
  physical examination procedures, 115
  urinary incontinence due to, 381, 382-383b
Contact dermatitis, 315, 316-320b
Continuous-loop monitoring
  for syncope evaluation, 370
Contraceptive use
  and amenorrhea, 47
Conversion charts
  metric system, 465t
  temperature, 466
Coordination
  and imbalance with vertigo, 149-150
  testing in older adults, 104
Core body temperature
  and fever, 194
Core needle biopsy, 69
Cornea
  anatomical illustration of, 335f
  cloudy with glaucoma, 343
  conditions causing red eye
    corneal abrasion, 342, 343-344b
    herpetic infections, 342-343, 343-344b
    keratitis, 342, 343-344b
  inspection with red eye, 339
  testing corneal light reflex, 429
Corneal abrasion, 342, 343-344b
Corneal light reflex, 429
Coronary artery disease (CAD)
  and dyspnea, 161-162
  and palpitations, 288, 294-295b
  risk factors for, 82-83
Cortical defecation control, 111
Cost/benefit analysis
  and clinical decision-making, 5

Costochondritis, 78, 79-80b, 93, 95b
Costophrenic angle
  as seen on chest x-rays, 452, 454, 452f, 454f, 455b
Cough
  defining and categorizing, 120
  description and reflexes associated with, 120
  diagnostic reasoning/key questions
    asthma history, 120-121
    characteristics and nature of, 122-123
    choking episode history, 122
    chronic health problems, 124
    duration categories, 120
    eating or GERD issues and, 123
    environmental irritant exposure, 123-124
    exercise-related, 123
    family history, 123
    fever accompanying, 121
    foreign body, 121
    headache accompanying, 121-122
    immunocompromise issues, 124
    life-threatening conditions, 120
    nasal congestion accompanying, 121
    occupation/hobbies of patient, 122
    season and allergies, 123
    severity and progression of, 122
    shortness of breath, 120
    smoking/smoke exposure, 124
    sputum characteristics, 121-122
    timing of, 122
    tuberculosis, 124
  and fever with red eye, 338
  history of and dyspnea, 160
  and hoarseness, 237-238
  laboratory and diagnostic studies, 126-127
  physical examination procedures, 124-126
  recent onset differential diagnoses
    acute bronchitis, 129, 131-132b
    acute laryngotracheobronchitis, 129, 131-132b
    bacterial pneumonia, 128, 131-132b
    Bordetella pertussis infection, 128, 131-132b
    bronchiolitis, 129, 131-132b
    chlamydial pneumonia, 129, 131-132b
    chronic obstructive pulmonary disease (COPD), 128, 131-132b
    common cold, 127-128, 131-132b
    croup, 129, 131-132b
    Mycoplasma pneumoniae, 128, 131-132b
    nasopharyngitis, 127-128, 131-132b
    pertussis, 128, 131-132b
    viral upper respiratory infections, 128, 131-132b
    whooping cough, 128, 131-132b
  and sore throat, 357
  and sputum production, 84, 121-122
  and stress incontinence, 380
  subacute and chronic differential diagnoses
    allergic rhinitis, 130, 132-133b
    angiotensin-converting enzyme inhibitor-induced, 130, 132-133b
    asthma, 129, 132-133b
    bronchogenic carcinoma, 130, 132-133b
    chronic bronchitis, 130, 132-133b
    chronic sinusitis, 130, 132-133b
    cystic fibrosis, 130, 132-133b
    foreign body aspiration, 130, 132-133b
    gastroesophageal reflux disease (GERD), 129-130, 132-133b
    postnasal drainage syndrome, 129, 132-133b

Cough *(Continued)*
  psychogenic origin, 131, 132-133b
  smoking-related, 131, 132-133b
  tuberculosis, 130-131, 132-133b
  and syncope, 371, 372b
Cough tests
  during urinary incontinence evaluation, 378
Cover/uncover eye tests, 429
Cow's milk
  and constipation, 113-114
  or soy protein hypersensitivity
    causing diarrhea, 138
Crackles, 87, 167
Cranial nerves
  and confusion, 104
  cranial pain mechanisms and pathways, 221, 222f
  and earaches, 180
  function assessment in hoarseness evaluation, 239
  and headaches, 227-228
  referred pain symptoms and earaches, 182, 182-183b
Craniopharyngiomas, 432, 433-434b
Cranium auscultation
  during headache evaluation, 227
C-reactive protein (CRP)
  tests during limb pain evaluation, 253
Crohn disease, 444, 445-446b
Croup, 129, 131-132b, 169, 171-172b, 237, 240, 241-242b
Cruciate ligament test, 258, 261t
Cullen sign, 16
Cultures; *See also* "Laboratory and diagnostic studies"
    sections
  for anorectal disorder diagnosis, 327
  bacterial for skin rash/lesion evaluation, 313
  and gram stains in red eye cases, 340-341
  and sensitivity tests
    for penile discharge evaluation, 299-300
    testing male genitourinary system, 214-215
  for sexually transmitted diseases (STDs), 19
C-urea breath test, 20
Cushing syndrome
  as possible amenorrhea cause, 57, 58-59t
  and weight gain (unintentional), 444, 445-446b
Cyanosis
  appearance of with dyspnea, 166
Cyclic mastalgia, 74, 78, 79-80b
Cystic fibrosis
  and coughing, 130, 132-133b
  and diarrhea, 139
  and weight loss (unintentional), 438, 444, 445-446b
Cystitis
  description and diagnosis of male, 208, 217, 219-220b
  urinary problems due to, 391-392, 392b, 394b
Cystoscopy and contrast radiography
  for urinary incontinence evaluation, 380
Cysts
  breast, 70, 72-73b
  ovarian, 24, 25-29b
  skin, 304-305t, 307f
Cytological smear, 69, 76-78

D

Dacryocystitis, 341, 343-344b
Databases
  supporting evidence-based practice (EBP), 4-5, 5b

Day care
  diarrhea risks, 137
  and earaches, 175
  and parasites, 15
  skin rashes and lesions, 310
Daytime wetting
  by children, 374
Deep eye pain
  with glaucoma, 343
Deep tendon reflexes (DTRs) tests
  during ALBP examination, 273-274
  in confused patients, 104
  in constipation cases, 115t
  during headache evaluation, 228
Deep vein thrombosis (DVT), 160-161
Defecation; *See also* bowel movements
  constipation (*See* constipation)
  crying in children, 114
  five areas of problems in, 111
  pain relieved by, 14
  painful, 114-115
  precipitating syncope, 367
Degenerative eye diseases, 425-426
Dehydration
  and diarrhea, 135
  and fever, 195-196
  status assessment, 139-140, 140t
  causing stool hardening, 112
Dehydroepiandrosterone sulfate, 56
Delayed puberty
  as possible cause of amenorrhea, 57, 58-59t
Delayed sleep phase syndrome, 352, 354-355b
Delirium
  cognitive losses with, 100, 102
  confusion indicating possible, 98
  definition of, 98
  distinguishing characteristics of, 105-106, 106t,
    109-110b
  fluctuating symptoms with, 99
  hallucinations, 99
  possible causes of, 98
  and wake cycle sleep disturbance, 99
Dementia
  agnosia, 104
  causes of, 99b
  cognitive losses with, 100, 102
  common presentations of, 107b
  definition of, 98
  distinguishing characteristics of, 106t, 107, 109-110b
  gradual onset of, 99
  phases of Alzheimer-type, 107b
  reflex abnormalities with, 104
  and urinary incontinence, 375, 375b, 381
  and weight loss (unintentional), 443-444, 445-446b
Densities
  of chest x-rays, 448t
Dental problems
  examining during nasal evaluation, 283
  headaches caused by, 227, 229-230, 232-233b
  causing referred pain earaches, 174
Depression
  as clue to psychological disorders, 30
  cognitive losses with, 102
  diagnostic questions, 33-34, 34b
  and fatigue, 187, 189-190, 191-192b

Depression *(Continued)*
  medications that can cause, 31, 32b
  in older adults
    causing confusion, 98
    distinguishing characteristics of, 106t, 107, 109-110b
    Geriatric Depression Scale, 103, 103f
  SIG E CAPS depression mnemonic, 34b
  sleep problems due to, 346, 348
  symptoms of, 34
  and urinary incontinence, 375, 375b, 381
  and weight loss/gain (unintentional), 443, 445-446b
Deprivation amblyopia, 426
Dermal cysts
  spinal, 271
Dermatological conditions; *See also* skin rashes and lesions
  descriptive terminology regarding lesions, 306t
  lesion types, 304-305t
  morphological criteria, 304-305t, 306t, 307f, 308, 308f
  origins and mechanisms of, 303
Detrusor muscle
  and urinary incontinence, 374, 376
Developmental enuresis, 376-377, 382, 382-383b
Diabetes insipidus
  causing urinary incontinence, 381, 382-383b
Diabetes mellitus
  and anorectal disorders, 326
  and earaches, 176
  and female and child urinary dysfunction, 388
  causing urinary incontinence, 381, 382-383b
  and weight loss (unintentional), 437-438, 443, 445-446b
Diabetic retinopathy, 426, 432, 433-434b
Diagnostic and Statistical Manual of Mental Disorders IV,
  text revision (DSM-IV-TR), 35
Diagnostic imaging
  abdominal x-rays (*See* abdominal x-rays)
  chest x-rays (*See* chest x-rays)
  image and organ/tissue density, 447, 455-456t
  radiolucent and radiopaque, 447, 455-456t
  tissue density, 447, 455-456t
Diagnostic process
  COLDSPA mnemonic, 2-4
  experts *versus* novice proficiency in, 3-4
  OLDCARTS mnemonic, 3
  in primary care context, 2-3
  symptom analysis, 2-4
Diagnostic reasoning; *See also* individual chapters
  definition of, 2
  experts *versus* novice proficiency in, 3-4
  goals of, 2
  key history and information-gathering questions (*See* "Diagnostic
    reasoning: focused history" sections)
  physical exam process (*See* "Diagnostic reasoning: focused
    physical examination" sections)
  process of, 2-3
Diamond culture, 417
DIAPERS urinary incontinence mnemonic, 375b
Diaphragm
  normal vs abnormal x-ray findings, 463-464b
  as seen on chest x-rays, 451, 453, 454f, 455b
Diaphragm contraceptive device
  and female urinary dysfunction, 387
Diarrhea
  acute *versus* chronic in children, 135-136
  alternating with constipation, 113

Diarrhea *(Continued)*
  and anorectal disorders, 324
  bacteria and parasites causing, 143-145, 146-147b
  and blood in stool, 13-15, 136
  diagnostic reasoning/key history questions
    acute *versus* chronic adult, 135
    acute *versus* chronic in children, 135-136
    animal contact infections, 137
    antibiotics and other medications, 138
    blood in stools, 136
    celiac sprue, 139
    color of stools, 136
    cow's milk/soy protein hypersensitivity, 138
    cystic fibrosis, 139
    day care risks, 137
    dehydration risks, 135
    dietary habits, 138
    distal colon symptoms, 135
    excessive high-carbohydrate fluids, 138
    fever, 137
    food poisoning, 137, 139
    gastrointestinal surgery, 138
    gluten enteropathy, 139
    immunocompromised patients, 138
    inflammatory bowel disease family history, 139
    lactose intolerance, 138
    pain occurrence, location, and severity, 136-137
    proximal colon symptoms, 134-135
    recent travel, 137-138
    sexual activities, 138
    sleep disruptions with persistent, 137
    starvation stools, 139
    stool frequency, intervals, volume and consistency, 134
    tears and dehydration, 135
    thirst and dehydration, 135
    vomiting, 137
    wet diapers and dehydration, 135
  differential diagnoses of acute
    antibiotic-induced, 144, 146-147b
    Bacillus aureus food poisoning, 143, 146-147b
    C. difficile, 144, 146-147b
    Clostridium perfringens, 143, 146-147b
    Entamoeba histolytica, 144, 146-147b
    Enterotoxic *E. coli,* 143-144, 146-147b
    food poisoning, 143, 146-147b
    hemolytic uremic syndrome, 144, 146-147b
    hemorrhagic disease of newborns, 144, 146-147b
    necrotizing enterocolitis, 144, 146-147b
    pseudomembranous colitis, 144, 146-147b
    Salmonella, 143, 146-147b
    Shigella, 143, 146-147b
    Staphylococcus food poisoning, 143, 146-147b
    Vibrio cholerae, 143, 146-147b
    viral gastroenteritis, 143, 146-147b
  differential diagnoses of chronic
    carbohydrate malabsorption, 145, 147-148b
    Celiac sprue, 145, 147-148b
    Crohn disease, 145, 147-148b
    Cryptosporidium and Isospora belli, 145, 147-148b
    diabetic enteropathy, 145, 147-148b
    drug-induced, 145, 147-148b
    fat malabsorption, 145, 147-148b
    Giardia parasite, 145, 147-148b
    HIV enteropathy, 145, 147-148b
    irritable bowel syndrome (IBS), 144, 147-148b

Diarrhea *(Continued)*
   Isospora belli and *Cryptosporidium,* 145, 147-148b
   lactose intolerance, 145, 147-148b
   medication-induced, 145, 147-148b
   postgastrectomy dumping syndrome, 145, 147-148b
   protein hypersensitivity, 145, 147-148b
   toddler's diarrhea, 145, 147-148b
   ulcerative colitis, 144, 147-148b
  exudative, 134
  laboratory and diagnostic studies, 141-143
  lactose intolerance, 134
  origins and incidence of, 134
  osmotic or malabsorptive, 134
  pain occurrence, location, and severity, 136-137
  parasites and bacteria causing, 143-145, 146-147b
  physical examination procedures, 139-141
   abdomen contour and bowel sounds, 140-141
   digital rectal examination, 141
   hydration status assessment, 139-140, 140t
   urine output/specific gravity, 140, 140t
  secretory, 134
  traveler's diarrhea, 134
Diascopy
  for skin rash/lesion evaluation, 312
Diet
  and constipation, 112-113, 114
  and diarrhea, 138
  and fatigue, 184-185, 189
  causing headaches, 224, 231, 232-233b
  and weight loss/gain (unintentional), 436, 438
Diet pills
  causing sleep disruption, 348
Dietary fiber
  and constipation, 111, 117
  and fecal incontinence, 113
  affecting stool consistency, 111-112
Dietary habits
  and constipation, 111, 112-113, 114
  and weight, 435-436, 436b, 438-439, 440t, 444, 445-446b
Diethylstilbestrol (DES) exposure, 402
DIG FAST bipolar assessment, 34-35, 35b
Digital rectal examination (DRE)
  in abdominal pain evaluation, 18
  in anorectal evaluation, 326-327
  in constipation evaluation, 115
  correlated with PSA, 216
  in diarrhea evaluation, 141
  digital rectal prostate exam, 213
  in male genitourinary evaluation, 213
  in urinary incontinence evaluation, 378
Digital rectal prostate exam
  in male genitourinary evaluation, 213
Digitalis
  as pulmonary embolus risk factor, 161
Dilation and curettage (D&C), 405
Disability
  with acute low back pain (ALBP), 267, 277, 277-279b
Diskitis
  causing acute low back pain (ALBP), 275, 277-279b
Dissection of aortic aneurysm, 22, 25-29b
Disseminated systemic urethral infection, 297
Distal colon
  symptoms with diarrhea, 135
Distal interphalangeal (DIP) joints
  osteoarthritis in, 250, 250f

Diuretics
  causing urinary incontinence, 375, 375t, 381, 382-383b
Diurnal enuresis, 374
Diverticular disease
  causing lower abdominal pain, 24, 25-29b
Diverticulitis
  and blood in stool, 13-15
Diving
  and earaches, 175-176
  nasal symptoms due to, 282
Dix-Hallpike maneuvers, 153, 153b
Dizziness
  central differential diagnoses of
   brainstem dysfunction, 155
   cerebellar dysfunction, 155
   migraine headaches, 155
   multiple sclerosis, 155
  with chest pain, 84
  in children, 149
  diagnostic reasoning/key patient questions
   activity, 150
   anxiety, 150
   cholesteatoma, 152
   double vision, facial numbness and hemiparesis, 150
   duration of episodes, 151
   head trauma history, 152
   headaches, 150
   hearing loss and tinnitus, 151
   medical and cardiovascular history, 150
   medications, 151
   middle ear infections, 151
   onset, 151
   recent or recurrent illnesses, 151
   sensations, 149-150
   timing, 151
   vestibular neuronitis, 151
  with earaches, 177
  with headaches, 225
  laboratory and diagnostic studies, 154-155
  other differential diagnoses
   salt retention with ototoxic drugs, 156
   trauma, 156
  peripheral differential diagnoses of
   acoustic neuroma, 156
   benign paroxysmal positional vertigo (BPPV), 155-156
   benign paroxysmal vertigo (BPV) of childhood, 155
   cholesteatoma, 156
   labyrinthitis, 155-156
   Meniere disease, 155
   otitis, 156
   perilymph fistula, 156
   sinusitis, 156
   vestibular neuronitis, 155
  physical examination procedures, 152-154
   Bárány maneuvers, 153
   Dix-Hallpike maneuvers, 153, 153b
   ear exam, 152
   gait tests, 153-154
   positional maneuvers, 153
   provocation maneuvers, 152-153
   rapid alternating movement (RAM) tests, 154
   Rinne (AC:BC) test, 152
   Valsalva maneuver, 152
   Weber test, 152

Dizziness *(Continued)*
  versus syncope, 366, 367-368
  systemic differential diagnoses of
    cardiac dysrhythmias, 156
    cardiovascular causes, 156
    neurosyphilis, 156
    orthostatic hypotension, 156
    psychogenic causes, 156
    syphilis, 156
    vertigo, 149-158
DNA probes/testing
  for infectious organisms
    during abdominal pain evaluation, 19
    to evaluate male genitourinary system, 215
    in female/child urinary problem evaluation, 391
    in penile discharge evaluation, 300
    for urinary incontinence evaluation, 379
    in vaginal discharge cases, 417
Domestic violence
  indications of, 31f, 32, 40, 42-45b
  key questions to detect, 31f, 32
Doppler blood flow test
  for penile discharge evaluation, 300
Doppler Flow studies
  of male genitourinary system, 217
Doppler ultrasonography
  for syncope evaluation, 370
Double vision
  and red eye, 337
  with vertigo, 150
Drawer sign, 258, 261t
Dribbling
  assessing in urinary incontinence patients, 377
  with overflow small-volume incontinence, 380-381
  as primary male symptom of overflow incontinence, 376
  stream and hesitancy evaluation, 209, 210t
Drooling
  with sore throats, 356
Drug abuse
  causing acute fatigue, 190, 191-192b
  assessing during HEEADSSS interview, 34-35, 36t
  and fatigue, 185
  history and penile discharge issues, 296
  or alcohol causing confusion, 98
  causing palpitations, 293, 294-295b
  RAFFT adolescent questionnaire, 34b
Drug withdrawal
  causing headaches, 231, 232-233b
Drug-induced constipation, 118, 118-119b
Drug-induced syncope, 368, 371, 372b
Drugs; *See* medications
Dry cough
  versus moist, 125
Duct ectasia, 71, 72-73b
Ductography, 69
D-Xylose absorption test
  to evaluate diarrhea, 142
Dyscrasias
  causing vaginal bleeding
    leukemia, 408, 408-410b
    von Willebrand disease, 408, 408-410b
Dysfunctional uterine bleeding (DUB), 396, 398
Dysmenorrhea
  in absence of menses, 53
  causing lower abdominal pain, 24, 25-29b

Dyspareunia
  assessing in urinary incontinence patients, 375
  and endometriosis, 398
  introital and deep vaginal, 415
  and pain with vaginal discharge, 415
  with sexual activity, 13
Dyspepsia
  causing upper abdominal pain, 25, 25-29b
Dyspnea
  and breast pain, 76
  with coughs, 120
  description and sensations of, 159
  diagnostic reasoning/key patient questions
    acute *versus* progressive onset of, 159
    aggravating or precipitating factors, 161-162
    allergen possibilities, 160, 162
    anaphylaxis, 160
    anxiety, 161
    asthma history, 160
    confinement, surgery or fractures, 161
    cough accompanying, 160
    eczema or atopic dermatitis history, 163
    farm residence/chemical exposure, 163
    foreign body aspiration, 160
    honey ingestion, 163
    hyperventilation, 162, 165
    immunization history, 163
    leg trauma, 161
    medications taken, 161-162
    neuromuscular conditions, 162-163
    obesity, 163
    occupational hazards, 163
    oral contraceptives/estrogen, 161
    preexisting conditions or diseases, 161-162
    pulmonary embolus considerations, 160-161
    relieving factors, 162
    smoking, 163
    trauma or pneumothorax, 160
  emergent differential diagnoses
    acute epiglottis, 169, 171-172b
    anaphylaxis, 169, 171-172b
    bacterial tracheitis, 169, 171-172b
    botulism, 170, 171-172b
    croup, 169, 171-172b
    foreign body aspiration, 169, 171-172b
    pneumothorax, 169, 171-172b
    pulmonary embolus, 169, 171-172b
    status asthmaticus, 169, 171-172b
  laboratory and diagnostic studies, 168-169
  nonemergent differential diagnoses
    anemia, 170, 172-173b
    asthma, 170-171, 172-173b
    chronic obstructive pulmonary disease (COPD), 170, 172-173b
    heart failure, 170, 172-173b
    hyperventilation syndrome, 171, 172-173b
    laryngomalacia, 171, 172-173b
    pneumonia, 171, 172-173b
    poor physical conditioning, 170, 172-173b
    vascular ring, 171, 172-173b
  and palpitations, 288
  physical examination procedures, 163-168
  with sore throats, 356
  and syncope, 367
  three causes of, 165

Dysthymia, 41, 42-45b
Dysuria
  symptoms and origins of, 386-387

E

Earache, 174-183
  definition of, 174
  diagnostic reasoning/focused history questions
    age, 174
    airplane travel, 175-176
    barotrauma, 175-176
    bottle propping, 175
    cerumen impaction, 177
    cleft palate, 176
    day care attendance, 175
    diabetes mellitus, 176
    discharge, 176-177
    diving, 175-176
    dizziness or ringing in ear, 177
    drainage, 176-177
    ear trauma, 177
    family history, 174-175
    fever, 174
    foreign bodies, 177
    head trauma, 177
    hearing loss in adults and children, 177
    insect bites, 177
    itching, 176-177
    loud noises, 177
    pain location, 176
    pain onset, timing and duration, 176
    pain quality, severity and quantity, 176
    previous infections, 174
    psoriasis, 176
    seborrheic dermatitis, 176
    smoke exposure, 175
    swimming, 175
    upper respiratory infections, 174
  differential diagnoses of
    acute otitis media (AOM), 181, 182-183b
    barotrauma, 181-182, 182-183b
    cerumen impaction, 181, 182-183b
    cervical lymphadenitis, 182, 182-183b
    cervical nerve referred pain, 182, 182-183b
    cholesteatoma, 181, 182-183b
    cranial nerve referred pain, 182, 182-183b
    external otitis, 181, 182-183b
    foreign bodies, 181, 182-183b
    mastoiditis, 181, 182-183b
    otitis media with effusion, 181, 182-183b
    temporomandibular joint disorder, 182, 182-183b
    trauma or tympanic membrane perforation, 182, 182-183b
  laboratory and diagnostic studies of, 180-181
  physical examination procedures
    ear canals and external ear inspection, 177-180
    pneumatic otoscopy, 179
    tympanic membrane examination, 175b, 178-180
  referred pain, 174
Eardrum
  anatomic diagram of, 175f
  cholesteatoma behind, 178-179
Ears; See also earaches
  anatomic diagram of, 175f
  exam during dizziness and vertigo evaluation, 152

Ears (Continued)
  exam during earache evaluation, 177-180
  exam during headache evaluation, 227
  as indicator of psychological or substance abuse disorders, 39
  infections, 204, 206-207b
  symptoms and fever, 196, 204, 206-207b
  trauma, 177
Eating; See also diet
  assessing during HEEADSSS interview, 34-35, 36t
  GERD issues and coughing, 123
Eating disorders
  anorexia nervosa, 54, 57, 58-59t, 439, 443, 445-446b
  bulimia, 54, 57, 58-59t
  screening during amenorrhea evaluation, 54
Eating habits
  and weight, 435-436, 436b, 438-439, 440t, 444,
    445-446b
  and weight gain (unintentional), 439, 440t
  and weight loss (unintentional), 436, 438
Ecchymosis, 16
Echocardiography
  for chest pain evaluation, 89
  definition and procedures, 455
  for dyspnea evaluation, 168
  of palpitations, 292
  for syncope evaluation, 370
Economic status
  and weight loss/gain (unintentional), 444, 445-446b
Ectodermal dysplasia, 199
Ectopic pregnancy
  abdominal pain from, 9, 14, 21, 25-29b
  indications of, 397, 397b, 403
  pelvic exams to rule out, 17
  causing vaginal bleeding, 406, 408-410b
Ectropion
  and entropion, 338, 341, 343-344b
Eczema
  characteristics, associations and diagnosis of,
    316-320b
  definition and mechanisms of, 315
  history of and dyspnea, 163
Edema
  and fluid buildup in joint capsules, 251-252
  with limb injuries, 251-252
  in middle ear, 174
Education
  assessing during HEEADSSS interview, 34-35, 36t
Elbow
  anatomical diagram of, 248f
  diagnostic pain questions, 245
  patient locating pain in, 245, 250
  tennis elbow test, 256, 261t
  trauma or overuse injuries
    lateral humeral epicondylitis, 256, 262-265b
    nursemaid's elbow, 256, 262-265b
    olecranon bursitis, 255-256, 262-265b
    subluxation of radial head, 256, 262-265b
    tennis elbow, 256, 262-265b
Electrocardiography (ECGs)
  during abdominal pain evaluation, 20
  to analyze confusional states, 105
  during chest pain evaluation, 89
  for dyspnea evaluation, 168
  of palpitations, 291
  for syncope evaluation, 369

Electroencephalography (EEGs)
to analyze confusional states, 105
during dizziness and vertigo evaluation, 154
for syncope evaluation, 370
Electronystagmography (ENG)
during dizziness and vertigo evaluation, 154
Electrophysiology studies (EPSs), 370
Employment
assessing during HEEADSSS interview, 34-35, 36t
Endocrine system
disorders
associated with confusional states, 101b
and weight gain (unintentional), 439-440, 444,
445-446b
and weight loss (unintentional), 438, 443, 445-446b
Endocrinopathies
hyperprolactinemia, 407, 408-410b
polycystic ovary syndrome, 407, 408-410b
thyroid dysfunction, 407, 408-410b
Endometrial biopsy
during amenorrhea evaluation, 56
in vaginal bleeding cases, 405
Endometrial cancer
causing vaginal bleeding, 406, 408-410b
warnings and risk factors, 400, 400b
Endometrial cycle
and ovarian cycle correlation, 46, 48t
Endometriosis
and amenorrhea, 53
and deep vaginal dyspareunia, 415
pain, 14
Endometritis, 407, 408-410b
Endoscopy
during chest pain evaluation, 91
definition and procedures for performing, 463
to evaluate diarrhea, 143
Enemas
and constipation, 113
Energy; *See also* calories/activity levels
changes with thyroid dysfunction, 51-52
deficits with psychological disorders, 30, 34, 34b
and fatigue, 184
Enophthalmos, 427
Entamoeba histolytica, 144, 146-147b
Enterotoxic *E. coli*
causing diarrhea, 143-144, 146-147b
Enterovirus
fever characteristics with, 205, 206-207b
Entropion
and ectropion, 338, 341, 343-344b
Enuresis; *See also* urinary incontinence
from nonorganic causes
primary enuresis, 382
secondary (developmental) enuresis, 382
sickle cell anemia, 382
small bladder, 382
from organic causes
genitourinary causes, 381
neurological causes, 381-382
Environment
assessing during HEEADSSS interview, 34-35, 36t
hazards and fatigue, 186
and hoarseness, 237
irritant exposure and coughing, 123-124
Enzyme-linked immunosorbent assay (ELISA), 189, 253

Epididymitis
description and diagnosis of male, 218,
219-220b
causing penile discharge, 298, 301, 302b
Epigastric pain
structures associated with, 12t
Epiglottis
function and illustration of, 235, 236f
and sore throat, 356, 361-362, 364-365b
Epiglottitis, 237
Episcleritis, 342, 343-344b
Epstein-Barr virus (EBV), 189, 191, 191-192b
Epworth Sleepiness Scale, 346, 347b
Erythema
in dark-skinned patients, 311
Erythema chronicum migrans (ECM)
with Lyme disease, 310
Erythema infectiosum
definition and mechanisms of, 313
fever and rash eruption periods, 196, 310
Erythema multiforme, 315, 316-320b
Erythema nodosum
and travel to Southeast Asia, 310
Erythrocyte sedimentation rate (ESR)
during chest pain evaluation, 91
for fatigue cases, 188-189
for headache evaluation, 228
tests during limb pain evaluation, 252
Escherichia coli
causing adult female and child urinary problems, 385
causing chronic bacterial prostatitis, 208, 217-218,
219-220b
causing diarrhea, 143-144, 146-147b
Esophageal pH
during chest pain evaluation, 91
during cough evaluation, 127
Esophageal probe
during cough evaluation, 127
Esophagitis
causing chest pain, 93, 95b
pain factors with, 12
causing upper abdominal pain, 24-25, 25-29b
Estrogen
deficiency and amenorrhea, 53
drugs that may increase levels of, 52, 52b
as pulmonary embolus risk factor, 160-161
that produce nipple discharge, 64, 64b
causing vaginal bleeding, 400-401
Estrogen progesterone challenge test, 56
Estrogen therapy, 400-401
Eustachian tube
anatomic diagram of, 175f
blockage with otitis media with effusion, 181
failure in air travelers and divers, 175-176
Evidence-based practice (EBP)
clinical diagnosis of appendicitis, 21b
definition of, 4-5
prostate cancer screening, 216, 216b
Ewing sarcoma
back pain due to, 267
Exanthema, 205, 206-207b
Excessive high-carbohydrate fluids
causing diarrhea, 138
Excisional biopsy, 69, 313
Excoriation, 304-305t, 307f

Exercise
amenorrhea induced by, 57, 58-59t
assessing during HEEADSSS interview, 34-35, 36t
and calorie balance, 435, 436b, 437b, 439, 440t
coughing due to, 123
hematuria, 386
intolerance with dyspnea, 161-162
nipple discharge induced by, 65
precipitating syncope, 367
recent and chest pain, 84
and sleep problems, 348
syncope with, 367
training intensity and amenorrhea, 51
Exercise myocardial perfusion imaging, 89
Exercise stress tests, 370
Exophthalmos, 426
Expectations
clarifying with patients, 4
Experience
importance of practical nursing, 4
Experts
versus novice clinicians, 3-4
External auditory canal
anatomic diagram of, 175f
External genitals
examination of female, 415-416
palpation and percussion
during male genitourinary evaluation, 213
External otitis
symptoms and earaches from, 181, 182-183b
Extraocular movement tests, 340, 429-430
Extremities; *See also* limb pain
examination of
during chest pain evaluation, 89
during cough evaluation, 126
during dyspnea evaluation, 166
during headache evaluation, 228
during palpitations evaluation, 291
during syncope evaluation, 369
sensations and jerking
causing sleep problems, 346, 346
Exudative diarrhea, 134
Eye tests
alternating cover/uncover eye tests, 429
Amsler grid, 429, 429f
cover/uncover eye tests, 429
extraocular movements test, 429-430
of older adults, 104
ophthalmoscopic examination, 430
pupillary response tests, 430
Eyelids
assessment of, 428-429
conditions causing red eye
blepharitis, 341, 343-344b
chalazion, 341, 343-344b
entropion and ectropion, 341, 343-344b
hordeolum, 341, 343-344b
inspection/eversion, 338-339
palpation during red eye evaluation, 340
Eyes; *See also* vision; vision loss
anatomical illustration of, 335f
assessing during fatigue evaluation, 187
cataracts, 431, 433-434b
chemical or thermal trauma to, 425
congenital infections, 432, 433-434b

Eyes *(Continued)*
discharge characteristics, 337
disorders of
allergic conjunctivitis, 342, 343-344b
bacterial conjunctivitis, 341, 343-344b
blepharitis, 341, 343-344b
chalazion, 341, 343-344b
chemical conjunctivitis, 342, 343-344b
corneal abrasion, 342, 343-344b
dacryocystitis, 341, 343-344b
entropion and ectropion, 341, 343-344b
episcleritis, 342, 343-344b
glaucoma, 343, 343-344b
herpetic infections, 342-343, 343-344b
hordeolum, 341, 343-344b
hyphema, 342, 343-344b
iritis, 343, 343-344b
keratitis, 342, 343-344b
N. gonorrhoeae conjunctivitis, 342, 343-344b
orbital cellulitis, 343, 343-344b
periorbital cellulitis, 343, 343-344b
scleritis, 342, 343-344b
subconjunctival hemorrhage, 342, 343-344b
viral conjunctivitis, 341-342, 343-344b
enophthalmos, 427
exophthalmos, 426
as indicator of psychological or substance abuse disorders, 39
inflammation with red eye, 338
normal movements and development, 427, 427b
ophthalmoscopic examinations, 430
pain
with glaucoma, 343
versus nonpainful red eye, 336, 336b
with vision loss, 424-425
ptosis, 427
red eye (*See* red eye)
squinting, 426
swelling, redness and fever, 334, 337
testing (*See* eye tests)
trauma to, 425, 431, 433-434b

F
FABER test
during ALBP examination, 272, 272f
Facial disorders
causing referred pain earaches, 174
Facial fullness
and pressure symptoms, 284
Facial numbness
with vertigo, 150
Factitious fever
characteristics with, 205, 206-207b
Failure to thrive, 130, 437
Fainting; *See also* syncope
with chest pain, 84
in family history, 369
with lightheadedness, 149-150
Falls
spinal fractures, 267-268, 274, 277-279b
False vocal cords, 235, 236f
Familial adenomatous polyposis (FAP), 325-326
Family history; *See* individual conditions
Farm residence/chemical exposure
and dyspnea, 163

Farsightedness, 431
Fasting blood glucose tests, 189, 441
Fat necrosis
  and breast lumps, 70, 72-73b
Fatigue
  acute *versus* chronic, 184
  classification of, 184
  defining, 184
  diagnostic reasoning/key patient questions
    activities of daily living, 185
    alcohol and drug use, 185
    anxiety and depression, 187
    appetite, 185
    bleeding, 186
    body fluids exposure, 185
    diseases associated with, 185
    and fever, 186
    joint tenderness, 185-186
    lifestyle habits, 185
    Lyme disease exposure, 186
    medications, 185
    menopause, 185
    menstrual period, 185-186
    and night sweats or hot flashes, 185
    occupational and environmental hazards,
      186
    onset, severity and pattern, 186
    psychological origins of, 186-187
    school performance, 187
    sleep patterns, 184-185
    stress, 186-187
    urination increases, 185
    weakness *versus* fatigue, 184
    weight loss, 185
  and Epstein-Barr virus (EBV), 189, 191,
      191-192b
  laboratory and diagnostic studies, 188-189
  organic causes of acute
    alcoholism or drug abuse, 190, 191-192b
    anemia, 190, 191-192b
    Graves disease, 190, 191-192b
    hyperthyroidism, 190, 191-192b
    hypothyroidism, 190, 191-192b
    myxedema, 190, 191-192b
  organic causes of chronic
    cancer, 191, 191-192b
    chronic fatigue syndrome, 191, 191-
      192b
    fibromyalgia, 191, 191-192b
    heart failure, 190-191, 191-192b
    hepatitis, 191, 191-192b
    medications, 190, 191-192b
    mononucleosis, 191, 191-192b
    sleep apnea, 190, 191-192b
  physical examination procedures, 187-188
  physiological differential diagnoses
    nutritional deficiencies, 189, 191-192b
    sleep and rest deficits, 189, 191-192b
  physiological *versus* psychological, 184
  psychological causes of, 30
    anxiety, 190, 191-192b
    depression, 189-190, 191-192b
Faun's beard, 271
Febrile seizures, 195-196
Fecal and gastrointestinal tests, 442
Fecal fat test, 141-142

Fecal immunochemical test (FIT)
  for anorectal disorder diagnosis, 321b, 327-328
  for colorectal cancer detection, 321b, 327-328
  for constipation evaluation, 116
  to evaluate diarrhea, 141
Fecal immunochemical test (iFOBT)
  during abdominal pain evaluation, 19-20
  during constipation evaluation, 116
Fecal impaction
  and constipation, 117, 118-119b
  and urinary incontinence, 375-376, 381, 382-383b
Fecal incontinence, 113, 324
Fecal leukocytes, 141
Fecal occult blood test (FOBT)
  during abdominal pain evaluation, 19
  during constipation evaluation, 115-116
  to evaluate diarrhea, 141
  during rectal pain evaluation, 327
Fecal soiling
  from anorectal disorders, 324
Fecal/stool DNA
  for anorectal disorder diagnosis, 327
Females
  Tanner stages of sexual maturity in girls, 49, 50-51, 50f
Ferritin level tests
  for fatigue cases, 188
  with sleep problems, 351
Fever
  with abdominal pain, 16
  accompanying coughs, 121
  with acute low back pain (ALBP), 267
  with breast lumps, 63
  caused by defective heat loss mechanism, 194
  with chest pain, 84
  and chills
    in females and children, 385
    in males, 208
  definition of, 194
  diagnostic reasoning/key patient history questions
    aches, 196
    alkaloid atropine plant exposure, 198
    animal exposure, 198
    behavior changes in children, 197
    camping or outdoor activities, 197
    cat-scratch disease, 198
    chronic diseases, 196-197
    duration and height of, 195
    ear, nose and throat symptoms, 196
    food poisoning, 198
    gastrointestinal symptoms, 196
    genitourinary tract symptoms, 196
    Haemophilus influenzae, 195
    head trauma or headaches, 195
    heat exposure or heatstroke, 199
    hyperthermia in hot environments, 199
    immunizations, 197-198
    infants, 195
    infection exposure, 195-196, 197
    joint pain, 196
    lethargy, 195
    location of symptoms, 196
    medications, 197
    meningococcal disease exposure, 195
    narrowing diagnostic focus with, 196
    obesity, 199
    occurrence and patterns of, 194-195

Fever *(Continued)*
   otitis media, 195
   overdressing, 199
   respiratory symptoms, 196
   sexual activity, 197
   skin rashes, 196
   stiff necks, 195
   surgery, 197
   temperature measurement, 194-195
   travel, 184b, 197
   tuberculosis or hepatitis exposure, 197
   vomiting, 195
  with diarrhea, 137
  differential diagnoses of
   bone infections, 205, 206-207b
   ear infections, 204, 206-207b
   enterovirus, 205, 206-207b
   exanthema, 205, 206-207b
   factitious fever, 205, 206-207b
   gastroenteritis, 204, 206-207b
   Kawasaki disease, 205, 206-207b
   meningitis, 204-205, 206-207b
   occult bacteremia, 205-206, 206-207b
   osteomyelitis, 205, 206-207b
   otitis media, 204, 206-207b
   pelvic inflammatory disease (PID), 204, 206-207b
   periodic or unidentifiable in children, 199, 206,
    206-207b
   pharyngitis, 204, 206-207b
   prostatitis, 204, 206-207b
   roseola infantum, 205, 206-207b
   sinusitis, 204, 206-207b
   upper respiratory infections (URIs), 204, 206-207b
   urinary tract infections (UTIs), 204, 206-207b
   viral infections, 204, 206-207b
  with earaches, 174
  and fatigue, 186
  with female and child urinary dysfunction, 385
  associated with head trauma, 99
  heat production over heat loss, 194
  hypothalamus regulation of, 194
  laboratory and diagnostic studies, 202-204
  with penile discharge, 297-298
  physical examination procedures, 199-202
  with seizures in infants, 202
  skin rashes and lesions with, 308-311
  with sore throat, 357
  causing stool hardening, 112
  three categories of childhood, 195
  three types of, 194
Fever of unknown origin (FUO), 194
Fiber
  and constipation, 111, 117
  and fecal incontinence, 113
  affecting stool consistency, 111-112
Fibroadenoma
  of breasts, 70, 72-73b
Fibrocystic breast changes, 71, 72-73b
Fibroids
  and deep vaginal dyspareunia, 415
  causing vaginal bleeding, 406, 408-410b
Fibromyalgia
  causing chest pain, 85
  causing chronic fatigue, 191, 191-192b
  definition and limb pain with, 259, 262-265b
Fibromyositis, 253-254, 262-265b

Fibrositis, 253-254, 262-265b
Fifth disease, 313
Fine-needle aspiration (FNA), 69, 76-78
Finger fractures, 256, 262-265b
Finkelstein test, 261t
First metatarsophalangeal (MTP) joints
  osteoarthritis in, 250
Fissures
  anal, 111, 115, 324, 328-329, 331-332b
  description and examples of skin, 304-305t, 307f
  as seen on chest x-rays, 454, 454f, 455b
Flank pain
  and female/child urinary system, 386, 389, 391-393
  and male genitourinary system, 211-212
  with penile discharge, 297-298
  structures associated with, 12t
  and tenderness, 14, 17
Flash of light
  and red eye, 337
  with vision loss, 425
Flea bites, 311
Flexible fiberoptic laryngoscopy, 239
Flexible sigmoidoscopy
  and colonoscopy
   for anorectal disorder diagnosis, 327
   for colon cancer screening, 116b, 117
   during constipation evaluation, 116b, 117
   to evaluate diarrhea, 143
Flip-flopping palpitations, 289
Floaters, 337, 425
Fluid intake
  assessing in urinary incontinence patients, 376-377
  and female and child urinary dysfunction, 388
Fluids
  buildup in joint capsules, 251-252
  buildup in middle ear, 174
  normal vs abnormal x-ray findings, 463-464b
Fluorescein staining
  for red eye evaluation, 340
Fluorescent treponemal antibody absorption test (FTA-ABS), 300
Fluttering palpitations, 289
Follicle-stimulating hormones (FSHs), 55, 404, 418
Follicular eruption skin lesions
  acne vulgaris, 313
  rosacea, 313
Folliculitis, 313, 316-320b
Fontanel, 140, 140t
Food poisoning
  diarrhea caused by, 137, 139, 143, 146-147b
  fever caused by, 198
Food-borne infections, 137, 139
Foods
  association with chest pain, 85
  causing female and child urinary dysfunction, 388
  causing headaches, 224, 231, 232-233b
  relieving pain, 12-13
Foot
  plantar fasciitis, 258-259, 262-265b
Foreign bodies
  child urinary symptoms due to, 387
  description and vaginal discharge with, 419, 421b
  in ears, 177, 181, 182-183b
  inspecting oral cavity for, 166
  sensations in eyes, 336
  vaginal bleeding and discharge due to, 399, 408, 408-410b,
   415

Foreign body aspiration
  and coughing, 121, 130, 132-133b
  and dyspnea, 160, 169, 171-172b
Formula-fed infants
  and weight loss (unintentional), 436
Foucher sign, 258, 261t
Fractures
  diagnostic reasoning/key questions, 244
  history of and dyspnea, 161
  spinal, 267-268, 274, 277-279b
Free air
  on abdominal x-ray, 461-462, 462f, 463-464b
Frontal sinuses
  percussion/palpation of, 284
Functional bladder neck obstruction
  assessing in urinary incontinence patients, 377
Functional constipation, 117, 118-119b
Functional dyspepsia
  causing upper abdominal pain, 25, 25-29b
Functional pain
  versus organic, 15, 15t
Fungal infection skin lesions
  candidiasis, 314-315
  pityriasis versicolor, 315
  tinea, 315
Furuncle
  characteristics, associations and diagnosis of,
      316-320b
  definition and mechanisms of, 313

G

Gait
  abnormalities and limb pain, 249-250
  assessment of
    during ALBP examination, 271
    during dizziness and vertigo evaluation, 153-154
    during headache evaluation, 226, 228
    during urinary incontinence evaluation, 378
  circumduction, 249
  of confused patients, 104
  disturbances in older adults, 99
  as indicator of psychological or substance abuse disorder,
      39
Gait tests
  during dizziness and vertigo evaluation, 153-154
Galactorrhea
  and amenorrhea, 52
  medications that promote, 58, 58-59t
  patient history of, 52
  pituitary, genetic or medical causes of, 65
Gallstones
  causing acute low back pain (ALBP), 276, 277-279b
Ganglion, 256, 262-265b
Gardner syndrome, 325-326
Gardnerella vaginalis
  DNA probe and saline prep testing for, 19
Gas patterns
  in abdominal x-rays, 459f, 460, 461f
Gas stoppage symptoms, 13-15
Gastric air bubbles
  normal vs abnormal x-ray findings, 463-464b
  as seen on chest x-rays, 452, 455b
Gastritis
  causing upper abdominal pain, 25, 25-29b

Gastroenteritis
  fever characteristics with, 204, 206-207b
  causing upper abdominal pain, 25, 25-29b
Gastroesophageal reflux disease (GERD)
  and coughing, 123, 126-127, 129-130, 132-133b
  and hoarseness, 238, 240, 241-242b
  causing sleep problems, 347, 352
  causing upper abdominal pain, 24-25, 25-29b
Gastroesophageal reflux in infants
  and weight loss (unintentional), 444, 445-446b
Gastrointestinal system
  bleeding, 323
  and chest pain, 85
  considering during abdominal pain evaluation, 14
  surgery causing diarrhea, 138
  symptoms accompanying fever, 196
General appearance
  observation of (*See* chapter "Diagnostic reasoning/focused physical
      examination" sections)
Generalized anxiety disorder
  causing palpitations, 293, 294-295b
  symptoms of, 41, 42-45b
Generalized pain
  structures associated with, 12t
Genital/prostate examination
  for men
    during abdominal pain evaluation, 17
Genital warts, 407-408, 408-410b
  itching and lesions with, 420, 421b
Genitals
  female
    examination of, 415-416
    itching and lesions
      genital warts, 420, 421b
      herpes simplex, 420, 421b
      molluscum contagiosum, 420, 421b
      syphilis, 420, 421b
  male
    exam during male genitourinary evaluation, 213
    exam during urinary incontinence evaluation, 378
Genitourinary system
  and abdominal pain, 14
  male (*See* male genitourinary system)
  and urinary incontinence, 377, 381
Genitourinary tract symptoms
  accompanying fever, 196
Geriatric Depression Scale, 103, 103f
Giant cell arteritis
  causing headaches, 230, 232-233b
Giardia antigen test
  to evaluate diarrhea, 142
Glans penis
  inflammation/redness with penile discharge, 297, 299
  inspecting during male genitourinary evaluation, 213
  Tanner stage development illustration, 77f
Glaucoma
  definition and vision loss from, 431-432, 432b, 433-434b
  halos with acute, 337
  intraocular pressure measurement, 341
  causing red eye, 343, 343-344b
Glenohumeral joint instability, 255, 262-265b
Global cognitive loss
  with delirium, 100, 102-103
Glottis
  function and illustration of, 235, 236f

Glucose and ketones
  for female/child urinary problem evaluation, 390
Gluten enteropathy
  causing diarrhea, 139
Glycosuria, 299
Glycosylated hemoglobin test, 441-442
Goals
  clarifying with patients, 4
Gonococcal infections
  penile discharge with, 296
  Thayer-Martin culture to detect, 417
  vaginal discharge with, 420, 421b
Gonococcal pharyngitis, 363, 364-365b
Gonococcal urethritis
  causing penile discharge, 296, 300-301, 302b
Gout, 255, 262-265b
Gram stains
  during abdominal pain evaluation, 19
  of male genitourinary system, 214-215
  for penile discharge evaluation, 300
  red eye, 340-341
Gram-negative bacteria
  causing urinary tract infections, 385
Graves disease, 190, 191-192b
Grey Turner sign, 16
Grief
  normal *versus* psychological, 39-40, 42-45b
  as risk factor for confusional states, 101
Groin
  palpation during abdominal pain evaluation, 17
  patient locating pain in, 250
Group A β-hemolytic streptococcus (GABHS) infections
  ASO titer to detect, 361
  groups at risk for, 362t
  sore throat indications of, 356-357, 358
"Growing pains," 247
Growth and development
  and amenorrhea, 54
Growth parameters
  during headache evaluation, 226
Gulf War veterans
  fatigue symptoms in, 186
Gynecological problems
  and amenorrhea, 53
Gynecomastia
  and breast pain in men, 74

H

Habitual constipation
  causing lower abdominal pain, 24, 25-29b
Haemophilus influenzae
  and fever, 195
  causing hoarseness, 239-240
Hair
  inspection of
    during fatigue evaluation, 187
    during skin rash/lesion evaluation, 312
  and skin changes with thyroid dysfunction,
    51, 54
Hallucinations
  with confusion, 99
Halos, 337
Hand-foot-and-mouth disease
  skin rashes and lesions, 314, 316-320b

Head and neck examination
  during amenorrhea evaluation, 54
  during cough evaluation, 125
  during fever evaluation, 201
  during headache evaluation, 228
  during hoarseness evaluation, 238-239
  during nasal evaluation, 283
  during palpitations evaluation, 291
Head trauma
  causing confused state, 99
  and earaches, 177
  and fever, 195
  history and vertigo, 152
  loss of vision following, 425
Headaches
  accompanying coughs, 121-122
  acute, subacute, or chronic, 221
  cerebrovascular origins of secondary
    brain abscesses, 231, 232-233b
    hydrocephalus, 231, 232-233b
    intracerebral hemorrhage, 231, 232-233b
    intracranial tumors, 231, 232-233b
    pseudotumor cerebri, 231, 232-233b
    subdural hematoma, 231, 232-233b
  defining and classifying, 221, 223b
  diagnostic reasoning/key focused questions
    age at onset, 225
    alleviating factors, 225
    aura and prodrome, 224
    carbon dioxide or toxin exposure, 226
    chronic disease accompanying, 223-224
    current health, 226
    dizziness with, 225
    duration of, 224
    family history of, 226
    frequency, 224
    lifestyle habits, 225
    life-threatening assessment, 221-222
    medications taken, 225
    nausea and vomiting, 225
    onset and severity, 222-223
    pain characteristics, 224
    pain location, 224
    pattern and duration of, 224-225
    photophobia, 225
    prior history of, 225
    symptoms accompanying, 223
    trauma history, 223
    triggers and aggravating factors, 224, 226
    vision changes, 225
  and fever, 195
  goals for evaluating and treating, 221
  associated with head trauma, 99
  infectious origins of secondary
    dental problems, 229-230, 232-233b
    meningitis, 230, 232-233b
    otitis media, 230, 232-233b
    pharyngitis, 230, 232-233b
    sinusitis, 229, 232-233b
  laboratory and diagnostic studies, 228-229
  mechanisms and pathways, 221, 222f
  metabolic origins of secondary
    carbon monoxide poisoning, 230-231,
      232-233b
    dietary ingestion, 231, 232-233b

Headaches *(Continued)*
　　drug withdrawal, 231, 232-233b
　　severe hypoglycemia, 231, 232-233b
　　neurogenic origins of secondary
　　　cervical spine disorders, 222f, 230, 232-233b
　　　giant cell arteritis, 230, 232-233b
　　　optic neuritis, 230, 232-233b
　　　temporal arteritis, 230, 232-233b
　　　trigeminal neuralgia, 230, 232-233b
　　physical examination procedures, 226-228
　　skin rashes and lesions with, 310
　　skull radiographs to evaluate, 229
　　and syncope, 367
　　types of primary
　　　benign exertional headaches, 229, 232-233b
　　　cluster headaches, 229, 232-233b
　　　migraine with aura, 229, 232-233b
　　　migraine without aura, 229, 232-233b
　　　mixed headaches, 229, 232-233b
　　　tension-type headaches (TTHs), 229, 232-233b
　　and vertigo, 150
Health assessments; *See* assessments
Hearing acuity tests
　　during dizziness and vertigo evaluation, 152
　　during earache evaluation, 179
Hearing loss
　　and earaches, 177
　　and hoarseness evaluation, 238-239
　　testing in older adults, 104
　　and tinnitus and vertigo, 151-152
Heart
　　exam during syncope evaluation, 369
　　palpitations (*See* palpitations)
　　as seen on chest x-rays, 452, 454, 453f, 454f, 455b
Heart disease
　　causing syncope, 367, 370-371, 372b
Heart failure
　　causing chronic fatigue, 190-191, 191-192b
　　and dyspnea, 161-162, 170, 172-173b
Heart sound auscultation
　　during chest pain evaluation, 88
　　during cough evaluation, 126
　　during dyspnea evaluation, 168
Heartburn; *See also* gastroesophageal reflux disease (GERD)
　　and esophagitis, 14, 24-25
Heat stroke
　　fever from, 199
Heberden (DIP) joint nodes, 250, 250f
HEEAD adolescent assessment method, 34-35, 34b, 36t
Hematuria
　　with female and child urinary dysfunction, 385-386
　　and male genitourinary disorders, 209
　　with penile discharge, 297
Hemiparesis
　　with vertigo, 150
Hemoglobin and hematocrit level tests, 168
Hemolytic uremic syndrome, 144, 146-147b
Hemorrhagic disease of newborns
　　causing diarrhea, 144, 146-147b
Hemorrhoids
　　causing anorectal bleeding, 323, 330, 330t, 331-332b
　　classification of internal, 330t
　　pain with, 324
Henoch-Schönlein purpura
　　abdominal pain from, 16, 23, 25-29b

Hepatic function tests
　　for fatigue cases, 189
Hepatitis
　　causing chronic fatigue, 191, 191-192b
　　exposure and fever, 197
　　fatigue symptoms with, 185
Hereditary nonpolyposis colon cancer, 325-326
Hernia
　　causing lower abdominal pain, 24, 25-29b
　　palpation during abdominal pain evaluation, 17
Herniated disk
　　causing acute low back pain (ALBP), 275, 277-279b
Herpangina, 363, 364-365b
Herpes simplex virus (HSV)
　　anorectal infections with, 322-323
　　herpes virus antigen detection test, 327
　　itching and lesions, 420, 421b
　　causing red eye, 342-343, 343-344b
　　skin burning preceding rash, 310
　　skin rashes and lesions, 310, 314, 316-320b
　　causing sore throat, 363, 364-365b
　　causing urethritis, 385
Herpes virus antigen detection test, 327
Herpes zoster
　　and breast pain, 79, 79-80b
　　and chest pain, 93-94, 95b
　　causing red eye, 343
　　skin rashes and lesions, 314, 316-320b
Hesitancy
　　with overflow small-volume incontinence, 380-381
Heuristics
　　in diagnostic reasoning process, 3
Hilar area
　　as seen on chest x-rays, 452, 456b
Hip
　　and leg injuries or disorders
　　　iliopsoas tendinitis, 257, 262-265b
　　　Legg-Calvé-Perthes disease, 256-257, 262-265b
　　　proximal fibula fracture, 257, 257f, 262-265b
　　　slipped capital femoral epiphysis, 256, 262-265b
　　　stress fracture, 257, 262-265b
　　　transient synovitis of hip, 256, 262-265b
Hip mobility test
　　during ALBP examination, 273
Hips
　　Ortolani sign for congenital dislocation, 251, 251f
　　osteoarthritis in, 250
　　patient locating pain in, 250
Hirschsprung disease, 113-114, 117-118, 118-119b
HIV encephalopathy
　　signs of, 104
Hoarseness
　　definition of, 235
　　diagnostic reasoning/key history questions
　　　alcohol consumption, 237
　　　allergies, 237
　　　asthma, 237
　　　duration, 235
　　　exposure, 237
　　　gastroesophageal reflux disease (GERD), 238
　　　immunizations, 237
　　　neurological disease, 238
　　　onset, 236
　　　pain, 237
　　　progression, 235-236

Hoarseness *(Continued)*
    recurrence, 235
    smoking, 237
    surgical history, 236
    associated symptoms, 237-238
    timing, 237
    trauma, 236
    upper respiratory infections, 237
    voice habits, 237
  differential diagnoses of common causes of
    acute epiglottis, 239-240, 241-242b
    acute laryngeal edema, 240, 241-242b
    acute laryngitis, 239, 241-242b
    chronic laryngitis, 240, 241-242b
    croup, 240, 241-242b
    gastroesophageal reflux disease (GERD), 240, 241-242b
    hypothyroidism, 240, 241-242b
    laryngeal cancer, 240, 241-242b
    laryngeal papillomas, 241, 241-242b
    laryngotracheobronchitis, 240, 241-242b
    neoplasm, 240, 241-242b
    psychogenic hoarseness, 241, 241-242b
    trauma, 240, 241-242b
    vocal cord paralysis, 240, 241-242b
    vocal cord polyps, 240, 241-242b
  laboratory and diagnostic studies, 239
  physical examination procedures, 238-239
  with sore throat, 358
Holistic medicine
  diagnostic reasoning, 5
Home environment
  assessing during HEEADSSS interview, 34-35, 36t
Homonymous hemianopsia, 424f
Honey ingestion
  and dyspnea, 163
Hordeolum
  causing red eye, 341, 343-344b
Hormone therapy
  causing female and child urinary dysfunction, 387-388
  and vaginal bleeding, 400-401
Hormones
  and weight gain (unintentional), 439
Hot flashes
  and fatigue, 185
Hot or red breast, 75
Human chorionic gonadotropin (β-hCG) test
  to test for pregnancy, 76
  in vaginal bleeding cases, 403-404
Human immunodeficiency virus (HIV)
  and coughs, 124
  fatigue symptoms with, 185
  and fever, 197
  questions during anorectal evaluation, 322-323, 324
  as risk factor for confusional states, 101
  tests to diagnose, 189, 202
  and weight loss (unintentional), 444, 445-446b
Human leukocyte antigen
  for penile discharge evaluation, 300
Human papilloma virus (HPV)
  acetic acid test to detect, 418
Hydration status
  assessing
    in diarrhea cases, 139-140, 140t
    during syncope evaluation, 369

Hydrocephalus
  and headaches, 231, 232-233b
Hygiene
  anorectal disorders from poor, 325-326
  evaluating in penile discharge cases, 297
  sleep, 348, 352, 354-355b
  vaginal discharge due to poor, 414-415
Hygiene products
  and douching causing vaginitis, 414-415
  causing female and child urinary dysfunction, 388, 393, 394b
Hypercoagulability, 160-161
Hypernatremia, 198
Hyperopia, 431
Hyperprolactinemia
  and amenorrhea, 52, 52b
  causing breast lumps, 71, 72-73b
  causing vaginal bleeding, 407, 408-410b
Hypertension
  and coronary artery disease (CAD), 82-83
Hyperthermia
  causing fever, 198
  in hot environments and fever, 199
Hyperthyroidism
  and abnormal menstrual bleeding, 407
  and acute fatigue, 190, 191-192b
  and fever, 198
  and palpitations, 293-294, 294-295b
  and skin and hair changes, 51, 54
  and weight loss (unintentional), 443, 445-446b
Hyperventilation
  and chest pain, 87
  and dyspnea, 162, 165
  and syncope, 368
  test during dizziness/vertigo evaluation, 152
Hyperventilation syndrome
  and dyspnea, 171, 172-173b
Hyphema
  causing red eye, 334-335, 342, 343-344b
Hypnotics
  causing urinary incontinence, 375, 375t, 381, 382-383b
Hypoglycemia, 231, 232-233b
Hypomenorrhea
  description of, 396
Hypopharyngeal cyst, 235
Hypothalamic set point
  antipyretics to lower, 194
Hypothalamic-pituitary-ovarian (HPO) axis
  imbalances
    and amenorrhea, 52
    and menses changes, 396
Hypotheses
  criteria for testing, 3
  formulating and testing diagnostic, 3
Hypothyroidism
  causing abnormal menstrual bleeding, 407
  causing acute fatigue, 190, 191-192b
  and hoarseness, 240, 241-242b
  causing skin and hair changes, 51, 54
  and weight gain (unintentional), 444, 445-446b
Hypoxia, 124
Hysterectomy
  and vaginal bleeding, 400, 405
Hysterical syncope, 367

I

Itching
  skin rashes and lesions with, 309, 310b
Ideal body weight, 439, 440t
Idiopathic slow transit
  and constipation, 117-118, 118-119b
Ileus
  abdominal pain from, 23, 25-29b
Iliopsoas tendinitis, 257, 262-265b
Images
  abdominal x-ray, 457-464
  chest x-ray, 448-450, 449f, 450f, 451f, 452f,
    454f
Imbalance
  sensations of, 149-150
Immigrant patients/sexual partners
  questions and penile discharge, 298
Immunizations
  and fever, 197-198
  history of
    and dyspnea, 163
    and hoarseness, 237
  skin rashes and lesions due to, 311
  and sore throats, 358
Immunochemical FOBT (iFOBT)
  for anorectal disorder diagnosis, 327-328
  during constipation evaluation, 116
  to evaluate diarrhea, 141
Immunocompromised patients; *See also* human immunodeficiency
    virus (HIV)
  anorectal disorders in, 322-323
  coughs in, 124
  diarrhea in, 138
  and female and child urinary dysfunction, 386
  and male genitourinary evaluation, 208
Immunological skin lesions
  allergic dermatitis, 315
  contact dermatitis, 315
  eczema, 315
  psoriasis, 315
  seborrheic dermatitis, 315
Imperforate hymen
  and amenorrhea, 57, 58-59t
Impetigo
  characteristics, associations and diagnosis of,
    316-320b
  contacting methods, 310
  definition and mechanisms of, 313
  itching of, 310b
Incarcerated hernia
  abdominal pain from, 23, 25-29b
Incontinence
  fecal (*See* fecal incontinence)
  urinary (*See* urinary incontinence)
Indirect hemagglutinin assay (IHA), 142
Infants
  anorectal disorders in, 323
  bowel movement frequency in, 111
  constipation and congenital hypothyroidism, 112
  earache behaviors in, 178
  eye tests and screens, 427-428, 428t
  fever in, 184b, 195, 199
  irritable with urinary dysfunction, 386
  retinopathy of prematurity, 431
  sleep problems in, 345, 346-347, 348-350

Infections
  with acute low back pain (ALBP), 267
  DNA probe testing, 19
  exposure and fever, 195
  exposure days and symptom onset
    with penile discharge, 296
  associated with headaches, 223
    dental problems, 229-230, 232-233b
    meningitis, 230, 232-233b
    otitis media, 230, 232-233b
    pharyngitis, 230, 232-233b
    sinusitis, 229, 232-233b
  history and fever, 197
  and penile discharge, 296
  revealed by white blood cell counts, 18
  stages with penile discharge, 297
  tests to detect anorectal, 327-328
Infectious diseases
  conditions associated with confusional states,
    101b
  causing skin rashes and lesions
    carbuncle, 313
    folliculitis, 313
    furuncle, 313
    impetigo, 313
Infectious rhinitis
  nasal symptoms with, 285, 287b
Infertility
  and amenorrhea, 52-53
Inflammatory bowel disease
  and blood in stool, 13-15
  family history of, 139
Inflammatory breast cancer
  causing breast lumps, 71, 72-73b
Inflammatory skin lesions
  allergic dermatitis, 315
  contact dermatitis, 315
  eczema, 315
  psoriasis, 315
  seborrheic dermatitis, 315
Information gathering
  in diagnostic reasoning process (*See* "Diagnostic reasoning: focused
    history" sections)
Injuries; *See* trauma
Inner ear
  anatomic diagram of, 175f
  disruption causing peripheral vertigo, 149
Insect bites
  and earaches, 177
  itching of, 310b
  skin rashes and lesions, 314, 316-320b
Insomnia; *See also* sleep problems
  comorbid, 352, 354-355b
  description of, 349
Inspiratory stridor
  with sore throats, 356
Insufflation tests
  on eardrum, 179
Insulin
  and diabetes, 437-438
Intact uterus
  and vaginal bleeding, 400
Interstitial cystitis
  urinary problems due to, 393, 394b
Intestinal parasites, 15

Intracerebral hemorrhage
   and headaches, 222-223, 231, 232-233b
Intracranial tumors
   and headaches, 231, 232-233b
Intraductal papilloma, 71, 72-73b
Intraocular inflammation
   indications of, 428-429
Intraocular pressure measurement
   and glaucoma, 341, 431-432, 432b, 433-434b
   during red eye evaluation, 341
Intraotic manipulation
   during earache evaluation, 179-180
Intrauterine devices (IUDs), 398-399
Intussusception
   abdominal pain from, 23, 25-29b
   causing anorectal bleeding, 331, 331-332b
Iris
   anatomical illustration of, 335f
   characteristics and functions of, 339-340
   inspection with red eye, 339-340
   iritis, 343, 343-344b
Iritis, 343, 343-344b
Irritable bowel syndrome (IBS)
   and constipation, 117, 118-119b
   and gas entrapment, 14
   causing lower abdominal pain, 8, 23-24, 25-29b
   ribbonlike stools with, 113
Ischemia
   abdominal pain from, 8
Ischemic chest pain
   versus nonischemic, 82t
Ischemic heart disease
   and chest pain, 81
   as pulmonary embolus risk factor, 160-161
Itching
   anorectal, 324
   and earaches, 176-177
   with pain and bleeding in anorectal area, 321-333
   skin rashes and lesion, 309
   and tearing with red eye, 338

J

Joint aspiration
   tests during limb pain evaluation, 253
Joint capsules
   edema, 251-252
Joint disease
   versus musculoskeletal disorders, 245
Joints
   inflammation differential diagnoses
      gout, 255, 262-265b
      juvenile rheumatoid arthritis, 254, 262-265b
      osteoarthritis, 254, 262-265b
      rheumatoid arthritis, 254, 262-265b
      septic arthritis, 254-255, 262-265b
   pain and fever, 196
   stiffness or locking, 246
   tenderness
      and fatigue, 185-186
Jugular venous pressure (JVP)
   assessing during palpitations evaluation, 291
Juvenile polyps
   causing anorectal bleeding, 331, 331-332b
Juvenile rheumatoid arthritis, 254, 262-265b

K

Karyotyping, 56, 78
Kawasaki disease
   fever characteristics with, 205, 206-207b
   and heart conditions, 85
   skin rashes and fever, 310
   and syncope, 368
Keratitis
   causing red eye, 342, 343-344b
Kernig sign, 202, 204-205
Ketones
   testing in urinary dysfunction cases, 390
Kidney stones
   causing urinary tract infections, 385
Kidneys
   anatomic diagram and x-ray view of, 458f, 459,
      459f
   dysfunction of (*See* male genitourinary problems; urinary
      dysfunction)
   neoplasm and infections of, 208
   normal vs abnormal x-ray findings, 463-464b
   tumors, 219, 219-220b
   urinary incontinence (*See* urinary incontinence)
Klinefelter syndrome, 74, 76, 79, 79-80b
Knees
   anatomical diagram of, 249f
   osteoarthritis in, 250
   pain questions to patients, 245-248, 250
   tests to assess
      Bulge sign, 261t
      collateral ligament test, 258, 261t
      cruciate ligament test, 258, 261t
      drawer sign, 258, 261t
      Foucher sign, 258, 261t
      Lachman test, 258, 261t
      McMurray maneuver, 258, 261t
   trauma or injuries
      anterior cruciate ligament tear, 258, 262-265b
      Baker cyst, 258, 262-265b
      chondromalacia patellae, 257, 262-265b
      medial collateral ligament sprain, 258, 262-265b
      medial meniscus tear, 258, 262-265b
      Osgood-Schlatter disease, 258, 262-265b
      patellar tendinitis, 257, 262-265b
      popliteal cyst, 258, 262-265b
Kyphoscoliosis, 164

L

Labyrinthitis, 155-156
Lachman test, 258, 261t
Lacrimal puncta, 340
Lacrimal sac
   dacryocystitis, 341, 343-344b
Lactation
   and breast lumps, 63
   and mastitis, 71, 72-73b, 78
   and nipple discharge, 64
Lactose intolerance
   causing diarrhea, 134, 138
   causing lower abdominal pain, 24, 25-29b
Language
   as clue to psychological or substance abuse disorders, 30,
      39
   problems indicating dementia, 104, 107, 107b

Large bowel
 normal vs abnormal indications in x-rays, 463-464b
 obstruction
  abdominal x-ray illustrating, 460f
Laryngeal cancer, 237, 240, 241-242b
Laryngeal diphtheria, 237
Laryngeal edema, 240, 241-242b
Laryngeal papillomas
 as possible cause of hoarseness, 235-236, 241, 241-242b
Laryngitis
 and hoarseness, 237, 239-240, 241-242b
Laryngomalacia
 and dyspnea, 171, 172-173b
Laryngotracheobronchitis, 129, 131-132b, 237, 240, 241-242b
Larynx
 definition and illustration of, 235, 236f
 examination in hoarseness evaluation, 238-239
Lateral humeral epicondylitis, 256, 262-265b
Lateralization test
 during dizziness and vertigo evaluation, 152
Lavage
 of cerumen obstructions, 177-178
Laxatives
 and constipation, 113
Leakage
 assessing in urinary incontinence patients, 377
Left lateral abdominal x-rays, 462
Left lower quadrant pain
 structures associated with, 12t
Left nasal hemianopsia, 424f
Left upper quadrant pain
 structures associated with, 12t
Legg-Calvé-Perthes disease, 256-257, 262-265b
Legs; *See also* limb pain
 and hip injuries or disorders
  iliopsoas tendinitis, 257, 262-265b
  Legg-Calvé-Perthes disease, 256-257, 262-265b
  proximal fibula fracture, 257, 257f, 262-265b
  slipped capital femoral epiphysis, 256, 262-265b
  stress fracture, 257, 262-265b
  transient synovitis of hip, 256, 262-265b
 Iliopsoas test, 257, 261t
 patient locating pain in, 250
 trauma history and dyspnea, 161
Leiomyomas
 causing vaginal bleeding, 406, 408-410b
Lens
 anatomical illustration of, 335f
 characteristics and functions of, 339-340
 inspection of eye, 339-340
Leprosy, 310
Lethargy
 and fatigue, 186
 and fever, 195
Leukemia
 causing vaginal bleeding, 408, 408-410b
Leukocyte count
 in fatigue cases, 188-189
 inflammation or infections indicated by, 18
 and male genitourinary problems, 214-215
Leukocyte esterase, 390
Leukocytosis, 18
Leukoencephalopathy
 associated with confusional states, 101b
Leukokoria, 428-429

Level of consciousness
 assessing during dyspnea evaluation, 164
 with dementia, depression and delirium, 99, 102
 with head trauma, 99
 with syncope, 366
Lice, 310, 418
Lichen planus
 itching of, 310b
Lichenification, 304-305t, 307f
Lifestyle
 and constipation, 112-113
 and fatigue, 185
 headaches due to, 225
 sleep problems due to, 348, 352, 354-355b
Ligaments
 elbow, 248f
 knees
  anterior cruciate ligament tear, 258, 262-265b
  medial collateral ligament sprain, 258, 262-265b
 shoulder, 248f
Lightheadedness
 with chest pain, 84
 defining *versus* dizziness, 149-150
 with palpitations, 288
Limb pain
 ankle or foot trauma or injury
  Achilles tendinitis, 258, 262-265b
  ankle sprain, 258, 262-265b
  medial tibial stress syndrome, 258, 262-265b
  plantar fasciitis, 258-259, 262-265b
  shin splints, 258, 262-265b
 diagnostic reasoning/key patient questions
  activities affected by, 246
  acute *versus* chronic, 246
  ankle pain questions, 245-248
  assistive devices, 245
  compensation activities or actions, 245
  elbow pain questions, 245
  fever, 243-244
  fractures, 244
  immediate treatment injuries, 243
  joint stiffness or locking, 246
  knee pain questions, 245-248
  limping, 247
  location of, 244
  lower extremity pain, 245-248
  Lyme disease, 247-248, 250-251
  mixed conditions, 248
  musculoskeletal *versus* joint disease, 245
  night pain, 247
  overuse injuries, 244-245
  pain description by patient, 245
  severity of, 244
  shoulder pain questions, 245
  sprains, 244
  strains, 244
  swelling, 246
  systemic diseases causing, 247
  upper extremity pain, 245
  wrist pain questions, 245
 elbow trauma or overuse injuries
  lateral humeral epicondylitis, 256, 262-265b
  nursemaid's elbow, 256, 262-265b
  olecranon bursitis, 255-256, 262-265b

Limb pain *(Continued)*
  subluxation of radial head, 256, 262-265b
  tennis elbow, 256, 262-265b
  hip and leg injuries or disorders
    iliopsoas tendinitis, 257, 262-265b
    Legg-Calvé-Perthes disease, 256-257, 262-265b
    proximal fibula fracture, 257, 257f, 262-265b
    slipped capital femoral epiphysis, 256, 262-265b
    stress fracture, 257, 262-265b
    transient synovitis of hip, 256, 262-265b
  joint inflammation differential diagnoses
    gout, 255, 262-265b
    juvenile rheumatoid arthritis, 254, 262-265b
    osteoarthritis, 254, 262-265b
    rheumatoid arthritis, 254, 262-265b
    septic arthritis, 254-255, 262-265b
  knee trauma or injury
    anterior cruciate ligament tear, 258, 262-265b
    Baker cyst, 258, 262-265b
    chondromalacia patellae, 257, 262-265b
    medial collateral ligament sprain, 258,
      262-265b
    medial meniscus tear, 258, 262-265b
    Osgood-Schlatter disease, 258, 262-265b
    patellar tendinitis, 257, 262-265b
    popliteal cyst, 258, 262-265b
  laboratory and diagnostic studies, 252-253
  musculoskeletal, systemic or joint origins of, 243
  musculoskeletal inflammation differential diagnoses
    bursitis, 253, 262-265b
    fibromyositis, 253-254, 262-265b
    fibrositis, 253-254, 262-265b
    myofascitis, 253-254, 262-265b
    osteomyelitis, 254, 262-265b
    tendinitis, 253, 262-265b
    tenosynovitis, 253, 262-265b
  myalgia or muscle conditions causing
    fibromyalgia, 259, 262-265b
    psychogenic, 259, 262-265b
    viral infections, 259, 262-265b
  nerve entrapment causes of
    carpal tunnel syndrome, 260, 261t, 262-265b
    neuritis, 260, 262-265b
    peroneal nerve compression, 260, 262-265b
    tarsal tunnel syndrome, 260, 262-265b
    thoracic outlet syndrome, 260, 262-265b
  physical examination procedures, 248-252, 248f
  shoulder trauma or overuse injuries
    acromioclavicular joint injuries, 255, 262-265b
    bicipital tendinitis, 255, 262-265b
    dislocation, 255, 262-265b
    glenohumeral joint instability, 255, 262-265b
    rotator cuff tear, 255, 262-265b
  systemic disorders causing
    acute leukemia, 259, 262-265b
    Lyme arthritis, 259-260, 262-265b
    neuroblastomas, 260, 262-265b
    osteogenic sarcoma, 260, 262-265b
    sickle cell disease, 259, 262-265b
    systemic lupus erythematosus, 259,
      262-265b
  wrist or hand injuries
    finger fractures, 256, 262-265b
    ganglion, 256, 262-265b
    wrist fractures, 256, 262-265b

Limping; *See also* gait
  assessment of, 247
  and gait tests, 249-250
Lipoma
  breast, 70, 72-73b
Liver
  anatomic diagram and x-ray view of, 458f, 459,
    459f
  normal vs abnormal x-ray findings, 463-464b
Lobar pneumonia
  asymmetrical chest movement with, 165b
Localized infections
  and fever, 195-196
Localized pain
  structures associated with, 12t
Localized skin lesions
  description and examples of skin, 304-305t, 307f
Loss of consciousness
  with syncope, 366
Loud noises
  and earaches, 177
Low back pain; *See* acute low back pain (ALBP)
  from male genitourinary problems, 211-212
  vaginal bleeding with, 397
Lower abdominal pain
  structures associated with, 12t
Lumbar puncture
  to analyze confusional states, 105
  for headache evaluation, 228
  for meningitis diagnosis, 203-204
Lung disease
  as pulmonary embolus risk factor, 160-161
Lung evaluation
  during dyspnea evaluation, 167
Lungs
  abnormal sounds, 87-88
  and chest pain, 83-84
  chest x-ray image of, 453-454, 454f,
    455-456b
  examination of
    during fatigue evaluation, 187-188
    during nasal evaluation, 284
    during syncope evaluation, 369
  tumors
    causing chest pain, 94, 95b
Luteinizing hormones (LH), 55-56, 404
Lyme arthritis, 259-260, 262-265b
Lyme disease
  confusional states associated with, 101b
  and fatigue, 186
  and fever, 197
  and limb pain, 247-248, 250-251
  and syncope, 369
  transmission and skin symptoms of, 310
Lyme titer enzyme-linked immunosorbent assay serology
    (ELISA)
  tests during limb pain evaluation, 253
Lymph nodes
  palpation
    during amenorrhea evaluation, 54
    during breast lump evaluation, 66, 67f
    during diarrhea evaluation, 141
    during fever evaluation, 201
    during hoarseness evaluation, 239
    during skin rash/lesion evaluation, 312

M

Macula
    anatomical illustration of, 335f
Macular degeneration
    definition and blindness, 432, 433-434b
    painless vision loss with, 425
Macular skin eruptions
    Erythema infectiosum, 313
    fifth disease, 313
    measles, 314
    pityriasis, 314
    roseola, 314
    rubella, 314
    rubeola, 314
    scarlet fever, 314
    slapped cheek disease, 313
Macules
    description and examples of skin, 304-305t, 307f
Magnetic resonance imaging (MRIs)
    during abdominal pain evaluation, 20
    to analyze confusional states, 105
    for breast evaluation, 69
    for chest pain evaluation, 90
    definition and procedures, 455
    during dizziness and vertigo evaluation, 154
Major depressive disorder
    definition and symptoms of, 41, 42-45b
Malabsorption
    and weight loss (unintentional), 443, 445-446b
Malabsorptive diarrhea, 134
Male acute mastitis, 71, 72-73b
Male breast cancer, 71-73, 72-73b
Male external genitals
    palpation and percussion
        during male genitourinary evaluation, 213
Male genitourinary system
    cystitis, 208
    definition and components of, 215
    diagnostic reasoning/key history questions
        age, 211-212
        American Urological Association Symptom Index, 209, 210t
        anuria, 209
        bed-confined patients, 212
        bicycle riding, 212
        family history, 211
        fever and chills, 208
        hematuria, 209
        immunocompromised patients, 208
        low back, flank, or abdominal pain, 211-212
        nephrotoxic drug use, 212
        nocturia, 211
        other previous urinary problems, 211
        pain, 209, 212
        penile discharge with frequency, urgency and dysuria, 211
        perianal aching, 211
        polyuria, 211
        recent sexually transmitted infections (STIs), 212
        recent urinary catheters or instrumentation, 212
        sexually active/unprotected sex, 212
        suprapubic discomfort, 211
        timing, 209
        toxin exposure, 212
        turbidity with foul odor, 214
        urinary incontinence, 211
        urine hesitancy, stream and dribbling, 209, 210t

Male genitourinary system *(Continued)*
    differential diagnoses
        acute bacterial prostatitis, 217, 219-220b
        asymptomatic inflammatory prostatitis, 218, 219-220b
        benign prostatic hyperplasia, 218, 219-220b
        bladder or kidney tumors, 219, 219-220b
        chronic bacterial prostatitis, 217-218, 219-220b
        chronic pelvic pain syndrome, 218, 219-220b
        chronic prostatitis, 218, 219-220b
        cystitis, 217, 219-220b
        epididymitis, 218, 219-220b
        kidney or bladder tumors, 219, 219-220b
        orchitis, 218, 219-220b
        perineal compression syndrome, 219, 219-220b
        prostate cancer, 218, 219-220b
        pyelonephritis, 217, 219-220b
        testicular torsion, 218, 219-220b
        tumors of bladder or kidney, 219, 219-220b
        urethritis, 217, 219-220b
        urolithiasis, 217, 219-220b
    laboratory and diagnostic studies, 213-217
    overview of, 208
    physical examination procedures, 212-213
    urinary tract conditions and diseases of, 215
        chronic bacterial prostatitis, 208
        cystitis, 208
        dysuria, 208
        kidney problems, 208
        neoplasm, 208
        sexually transmitted diseases, 208
        trauma, 208
        urinary flow problems, 208
Males
    Tanner stage development illustration, 77f
Malrotation
    abdominal pain from, 23, 25-29b
Mammary duct ectasia, 78, 79-80b
Mammograms
    to evaluate breast lumps, 68-69
    to evaluate breast pain, 76
    questions regarding past, 75
Mania
    definition of, 34-35, 35b, 41-45, 42-45b
    medications that can cause, 31, 32b
    symptoms of, 35b
Mantoux test
    for fatigue cases, 189
Marfan syndrome, 81, 85
Mastalgia; *See* breast pain
Mastitis
    and breast pain, 78, 79-80b
    description of, 71, 72-73b, 78
    and lactation-related breast lumps, 63
Mastoid bone
    illustration of, 175f
    mastoiditis, 181
    radiography of, 181
Mastoid process radiography
    to evaluate earaches, 181
Mastoiditis
    symptoms and earaches from, 181, 182-183b
Maternal blood ingestion, 330, 331-332b
Maturation index
    during amenorrhea evaluation, 56-57

Maxillary sinuses
    percussion/palpation of, 284
Maxillary sinusitis
    nasal symptoms with, 281
McMurray maneuver, 258, 261t
Meares-Stamey 4-glass test
    of male prostatitis, 214-215, 214b
Measles
    definition and skin eruptions, 314, 316-320b
    fever and rash eruption periods, 196
Meckel diverticulum
    causing anorectal bleeding, 331, 331-332b
Meconium stool
    delayed passage and constipation, 114
Medial collateral ligament sprain, 258, 262-265b
Medial meniscus tear, 258, 262-265b
Medial tibial stress syndrome, 258, 262-265b
Mediastinum
    as seen on chest x-rays, 452, 455b
Medications; *See also* drug abuse
    and abdominal pain, 15
    and acute low back pain (ALBP), 269
    and alcohol use, 346-347
    and amenorrhea, 52, 52b, 58, 58-59t
    causing breast pain, 75
    causing chronic fatigue, 190, 191-192b
    causing constipation, 113, 118
    and difficulty staying asleep, 346
    and fatigue, 185
    and fever, 197
    causing headaches, 225
    history and dyspnea, 161-162
    affecting mental state, 100
    causing mood disorders, 31, 32b
    nasal symptoms due to, 283
    causing nipple discharge, 64, 64b
    causing palpitations, 289-290, 293, 294-295b
    skin rashes and lesions from, 310-311
    causing sleep problems, 346-347, 352, 354-355b
    causing sore throats, 358
    and syncope, 368, 371, 372b
    causing urinary incontinence, 375, 375t, 381,
        382-383b
    vaginal bleeding caused by, 401
    vaginal discharge caused by, 413
    and vertigo, 151
    and weight gain (unintentional), 439-440
    and weight loss (unintentional), 438-439
Medscape, 5b
Melena, 323
Memory
    losses with delirium, 100, 107, 107b
    losses with dementia, 102
Meniere disease
    causing peripheral vertigo, 155
Meninges
    inflammation and fever, 202
Meningismus, 228
Meningitis
    fever characteristics with, 204-205, 206-207b
    headaches caused by, 226, 230, 232-233b
Meningococcal disease exposure
    and fever, 195
Menometrorrhagia, 396
Menopausal syndrome, 400

Menopause
    age at, 400
    and breast pain, 74
    and fatigue, 185
    mammary duct ectasia, 78
    sleep problems with, 353, 354-355b
    symptoms of, 400
    vaginal bleeding during, 400
    vaginal bleeding following, 398, 400
    and weight gain (unintentional), 439
Menorrhagia
    definition of, 398
Menses
    average duration of, 396
    heaviness with HPO axis imbalances, 396,
        398
    irregular, 398
Menstrual cycles
    diagram of interrelationships throughout, 47f, 48t
    history questions regarding, 47, 47f, 51
    normal *versus* abnormal, 396
    oligomenorrhea and polymenorrhea, 396
    relationship to breast pain, 74
    stages of, 48t
    vaginal bleeding with irregular, 399-400
Menstrual cyclic mastalgia, 78, 79-80b
Menstrual periods
    average duration of, 396
    and fatigue, 185-186
    irregular, 398
    missed and breast pain, 75
Menstruation
    onset and amenorrhea, 47
Mental function
    affective changes, 38-39
    confusion (*See* confusion)
    losses with delirium, 100
    and syncope, 371, 372b
    and urinary incontinence, 375-376, 378-379, 381,
        382-383b
Mental status assessments
    components of, 102-103
    Confusion Assessment Method (CAM), 103
    during cough evaluation, 124
    during fever evaluation, 202
    Geriatric Depression Scale, 103, 103f
    during palpitations evaluation, 291
    in urinary incontinence patients, 375-376, 378-379, 381,
        382-383b
Merkel diverticulum
    technetium 99m scan to identify, 328
Mesenteric adenitis, 22, 25-29b
Metabolic system
    and confusional states, 101b
    and fatigue, 184
Metric system
    conversion charts, 465t
Micturition; *See* urination
Middle ear
    anatomic diagram of, 175f
    earaches, 174-183
    evaluation with pneumatic otoscopy, 180f
    fluid buildup in, 174
    infections causing vertigo, 151
    tympanograms, 180f

Migraine headaches
  and aura, 229, 232-233b
  causing central vertigo, 155
  and dizziness, 150
  pain location and characteristics, 224
  and syncope, 367-368, 371, 372b
  transient loss of vision with, 425
Migraine with aura
  description and pain associated with, 229, 232-233b
Migraine without aura
  description and pain associated with, 229, 232-233b
Mini Mental State Examination (MMSE), 102-103, 102f
Miscarriages
  causing vaginal bleeding, 405, 408-410b
Mitral regurgitation, 93, 95b
Mitral valve prolapse, 93, 95b
Mixed headaches
  description and pain associated with, 229, 232-233b
Mixed incontinence
  definition of, 374
  causing urinary incontinence, 381, 382-383b
Mobility
  with acute low back pain (ALBP), 271
  affected by limb pain, 246
  testing in older adults, 104
  and urinary incontinence, 375-376, 378, 381, 382-383b
Modified Diamond culture, 417
Molluscum contagiosum
  itching and lesions, 420, 421b
Mononucleosis
  causing chronic fatigue, 191, 191-192b
  skin rashes and other symptoms with, 310
  causing sore throats, 358, 362-363, 364-365b
Monospot
  for fatigue cases, 189
Mood disorders
  secondary to physiological conditions, 31
  types and symptoms of, 41-45, 42-45b
Motile trichomonads, 412f
Motor system
  assessing during headache evaluation, 228
Mouth
  anatomical structures of, 359, 360f
  disorders
    causing referred pain earaches, 174
  as indicator of psychological or substance abuse disorders, 39
  inspection
    during fatigue evaluation, 187
    during headache evaluation, 227
    during nasal evaluation, 283
    during skin rash/lesion evaluation, 312
Movements
  problems with acute low back pain (ALBP), 271
  testing in older adults, 104
  causing vertigo, 150
Mucous membranes
  examining in diarrhea cases, 139-140, 140t
  inspection during male genitourinary evaluation, 212
Multi-infarct dementia
  versus Alzheimer-type, 109t
Multiple sclerosis
  causing central vertigo, 155
Muscle strength tests
  during ALBP examination, 273
  during limb pain evaluation, 252, 252t

Muscles
  aches
    and fatigue, 186
  disorders of
    fibromyalgia, 259, 262-265b
    psychogenic, 259, 262-265b
    viral infections, 259, 262-265b
  inflammation causing chest pain, 85
  weakness
    and fatigue, 184
Musculoskeletal disorders
  versus joint disease, 245
Musculoskeletal system; See also limb pain
  evaluation of
    in abdominal pain cases, 14
    during fatigue evaluation, 188
    during fever evaluation, 201-202
    in urinary incontinence cases, 378
  inflammation
    bursitis, 253, 262-265b
    fibromyositis, 253-254, 262-265b
    fibrositis, 253-254, 262-265b
    myofascitis, 253-254, 262-265b
    osteomyelitis, 254, 262-265b
    tendinitis, 253, 262-265b
    tenosynovitis, 253, 262-265b
  strains
    causing acute low back pain (ALBP), 275, 277-279b
Myasthenia gravis
  hoarseness due to, 238
Mycoplasma pneumoniae, 128, 131-132b
Myocardial infarction (MI)
  and abdominal pain, 22, 25-29b
  and chest pain, 81, 91, 95b
  causing dyspnea, 161-162
  causing syncope, 367
Myocardial ischemia
  and chest pain, 81
Myocarditis, 92, 95b
Myofascitis, 253-254, 262-265b
Myomas
  causing vaginal bleeding, 406, 408-410b
Myopia, 431
Myringitis, 178-179
Myxedema, 190, 191-192b

N

Narcolepsy, 346-347, 352, 354-355b
Narcotics
  causing urinary incontinence, 375, 375t, 381,
    382-383b
Nasal cavity
  amplifying voice sounds, 235
Nasal congestion
  accompanying coughs, 121
Nasal discharge
  color and odor, 284
Nasal endoscopy, 285
Nasal mucosa
  and turbinate inspection, 284
Nasal obstruction
  conditions causing, 280
  symptoms with, 286, 287b
Nasal polyposis, 286, 287b

Nasal polyps
  causing nasal obstruction, 280
  nasal symptoms with, 286, 287b
  or masses evaluation, 284
Nasal smears
  during nasal evaluation, 284-285, 285t
  for pertussis, 127
Nasal spray
  nasal symptoms due to, 282
Nasal symptoms, 280-287
  conditions which aggravate, 280
  diagnostic reasoning/key questions, 283
    acute sinusitis, 281
    acute symptoms, 281-282
    allergic rhinitis with seasonal, 280-281
    chronic symptoms, 281-282
    cocaine use, 283
    diving and swimming, 282
    duration and history of symptoms, 280
    exposure to viral infections, 282
    maxillary sinusitis, 281
    medication use, 283
    nasal spray use, 282
    pain location, 281
    pregnancy, 282
    seasonal occurrence, 280-281
    smoking history, 282
    systemic disorders causing, 283
    trauma history, 282
    unilateral or bilateral, 282
    viral or bacterial, 282
  differential diagnoses
    acute sinusitis, 286, 287b
    allergic rhinitis, 285-286, 287b
    chronic sinusitis, 286, 287b
    infectious rhinitis, 285, 287b
    nasal obstruction, 286, 287b
    nasal polyposis, 286, 287b
    nonallergic rhinitis, 286, 287b
    osteomyelitis of frontal bone, 287, 287b
    rhinitis medicamentosa, 286, 287b
    sinus obstruction, 286, 287b
  laboratory and diagnostic studies, 284-285
  overview of, 280
  paranasal sinus anatomy, 280, 281f
  physical examination procedures, 283
Nasopharyngeal cancer, 174
Nasopharyngitis, 127-128, 131-132b
National Guideline Clearinghouse websource, 5b
Nausea and vomiting
  accompanying headaches, 225
  with female and child urinary dysfunction, 385
  associated with head trauma, 99
  with peripheral vertigo, 150
  as prodromal symptom of syncope, 366
Nearsightedness, 431
Necrotizing enterocolitis
  causing diarrhea, 144, 146-147b
  presenting symptoms and seriousness of, 331, 331-332b
Neisseria gonorrhoeae
  conjunctivitis, 342, 343-344b
  description and vaginal discharge with, 420, 421b
  DNA probe to test for, 19, 215, 417
  as gram-positive organism, 327
  incubation period of, 296

Neisseria gonorrhoeae (Continued)
  causing pelvic inflammatory disease (PID), 407
  causing penile discharge, 300, 302b
  causing urethritis, 300-301, 385
Neonatal discharge, 71, 72-73b
Neoplasms; *See also* cancer
  bladder or kidney, 219, 219-220b
  confusion from, 98
  and constipation, 118-119, 118-119b
  description and examples of skin, 304-305t, 307f
  genitourinary system, 208
  pituitary adenoma, 52, 58-59t, 58-59
  as possible cause of hoarseness, 240, 241-242b
  spinal cord, 271
Nephrocalcinosis, 460, 461f
Nephrotoxic drug use
  and male genitourinary evaluation, 212
Nerve entrapment
  causing limb pain
    carpal tunnel syndrome, 260, 261t, 262-265b
    neuritis, 260, 262-265b
    peroneal nerve compression, 260, 262-265b
    tarsal tunnel syndrome, 260, 262-265b
    thoracic outlet syndrome, 260, 262-265b
Nerve root compression
  tests to assess, 271-274
Neuritis, 260, 262-265b
Neuroblastomas, 260, 262-265b, 268-269
Neurocardiogenic syncope
  arrhythmias, 371, 372b
  breath-holding, 372b
  carotid sinus hypersensitivity, 371, 372b
  cough syncope, 371, 372b
  situational syncope, 371, 372b
  vasovagal syncope, 371, 372b
Neurofibromatosis
  and vision loss, 425-426
Neurogenic bladder, 380-381
Neurological and reflex tests
  during limb pain evaluation, 252
Neurological system
  conditions associated with confusional states, 101b
  examination
    during dizziness and vertigo evaluation, 153-154
    during fatigue evaluation, 188
    during fever evaluation, 202
    and hoarseness, 238
    during nasal evaluation, 284
    and syncope evaluation, 369
    during urinary incontinence evaluation, 378
    in urinary incontinence patients, 381-382
  and migraine headaches, 371, 372b
  seizures
    and syncope, 371, 372b
Neurosyphilis, 156
Neutrophils
  definition of, 18
Newborns
  anorectal disorders in, 323
  bloody vaginal discharge in, 407, 408-410b
  congenital hydronephrosis, 385
  dysplastic kidney, 385
  eye tests and screens, 427-428, 428t
  nipple discharge in, 65
  retinopathy of prematurity, 431

Newborns *(Continued)*
  sleep problems in, 352-353, 354-355b
  vision loss risks in, 426
Nicotine
  causing sleep disruption, 348
Night itching
  and vaginal discharge, 413, 413f
Night pain
  acute low back, 270
  in limbs, 247
Night sweats
  or hot flashes, 185
Night terrors or nightmares, 349, 353, 354-355b
Nighttime wetting, 374
Nipple discharge
  and breast lumps, 62
  breast pain with, 75
  conditions causing, 71, 72-73b
  drugs that produce, 64, 64b
  from exercise or sexual stimulation, 65
  galactorrhea, 65
    and amenorrhea, 52
    medications that promote, 58, 58-59t
    patient history of, 52
    pituitary, genetic or medical causes of, 65
  microscopy of, 69
  in newborns, 65
  nipple well, 68
  versus normal, 64
  postmenopausal, 65
  pregnancy and lactation-related, 64
  and prolactin levels, 63
  single *versus* multi-duct, 65
  spontaneous *versus* expressed, 65
  timing and duration of, 64
Nipple stimulation
  and amenorrhea, 52, 58, 58-59t
Nipple well, 68
Nipples
  sore or cracked, 63
Nitrite strips
  for female/child urinary problem evaluation, 390
Nocturia, 208, 211
Nocturnal enuresis, 377
Nocturnal wetting, 374
Nodules
  description and examples of skin, 304-305t, 307f
Nonallergic rhinitis
  nasal symptoms with, 286, 287b
Non-contrast-enhanced helical CT, 20
Noncyclic mastalgia, 78, 79-80b
Nongonococcal urethritis
  causing penile discharge, 296, 301, 302b
Non–rapid eye movement (NREM) sleep
  stages of, 345
Nonsuppurative otitis
  definition of, 174
Nose; *See also* nasal symptoms
  assessing during fatigue evaluation, 187
  assessing during headache evaluation, 227
  as indicator of psychological or substance abuse disorders, 39
  inspection during dyspnea evaluation, 166
  symptoms and fever, 196
Novices
  versus expert clinicians, 3-4

Nuchal rigidity, 202, 204-205
Nucleic acid amplification tests (NAATs), 215, 417
Numbness
  facial, 150
  or tingling with acute low back pain (ALBP), 267, 271
Nursemaid's elbow, 256, 262-265b
Nutritional deficiency
  assessing during amenorrhea evaluation, 54
  and fatigue, 184, 189, 191-192b
  and weight loss (unintentional), 436, 443, 445-446b
Nystagmus
  definition of, 152-153, 153t
  diagnosing, 429
  in infants, 423
  vision, 423

O

Obesity
  activity and weight recommendations, 436b, 437b
  and amenorrhea, 51, 54
  body mass index (BMI) chart, 467f
  and coronary artery disease (CAD), 82-83
  and dyspnea, 163
  and heat stroke/fever, 199
  and obstructive sleep apnea (OSA), 351, 351b, 354-355b
  and polycystic ovary syndrome (POS), 398-399
  and vaginal bleeding, 402
Obstipation
  defining, 111
  symptoms of, 10, 23
Obstructive sleep apnea hypopnea syndrome (OSAHS), 351, 351b, 354-355b
Obstructive sleep apnea (OSA)
  definition of, 346
  description and causes of, 351, 351b, 354-355b
Occult bacteremia
  fever characteristics with, 205-206, 206-207b
Occupational and environmental hazards
  and acute low back pain (ALBP), 267, 277, 277-279b
  and coughing, 122
  and dyspnea, 163
  and fatigue, 186
Office cystometrography
  for urinary incontinence evaluation, 379
OLDCARTS mnemonic
  in diagnostic process, 3
Older adults
  activity and weight recommendations for, 436b, 437b
  alcohol withdrawal in, 104
  balance testing in, 104
  cataracts in, 431
  confusion in, 98-110
  Geriatric Depression Scale, 103, 103f
  glaucoma in, 431-432
  hearing loss in, 104
  sleep problems in, 345, 349, 353, 354-355b
  syncope in, 366b
  urinary incontinence occurrence in, 375
  vision testing in, 104
Olecranon bursitis, 255-256, 262-265b
Oliguria, 385-386
Online Journal of Clinical Innovations, 5b

Ophthalmoscopy
  during headache evaluation, 227
  procedures of, 430
  in red eye evaluation, 340
  to test vision, 430
Optic chiasm
  illustration of, 424f
Optic disc
  anatomical illustration of, 335f
Optic gliomas, 425-426, 432
Optic nerve
  anatomical illustration of, 335f
  glioma, 425-426, 432, 433-434b
  illustration of, 424f
Optic neuritis
  description of, 431, 433-434b
  causing headaches, 230, 232-233b
Optic tract
  illustration of, 424f
Oral cavity
  amplifying voice sounds, 235
  inspection during dyspnea evaluation, 166
Oral contraceptives
  discontinuing and heavy bleeding, 399
  history and dyspnea, 161
Oral thrush, 415
Orbital cellulitis, 334, 343, 343-344b
Orbits
  assessment of, 338, 428-429
  disorders causing red eye
    orbital cellulitis, 343, 343-344b
    periorbital cellulitis, 343, 343-344b
  infections, 334
  trauma to, 425
Orchitis
  description and diagnosis of male, 218, 219-220b
  causing penile discharge, 301, 302b
Organ systems
  abdominal anatomic diagram of, 458f
  and abdominal pain, 14-15
Organic pain
  versus functional, 15, 15t
Orientation losses
  with dementia, 102
Orthostasis
  and syncope, 368
Orthostatic hypotension
  with pneumonia or status asthmaticus, 165-166
  and syncope, 371, 372b
  causing vertigo, 149-150, 156
Ortolani signs
  for congenital hip dislocation test, 251, 251f
Osgood-Schlatter disease, 258, 262-265b
Osmotic diarrhea, 134
Osteoarthritis
  definition and deformities caused by, 250, 250f
  diagnosis of, 250f
  and limb pain, 254, 262-265b
Osteoblastoma
  causing acute low back pain (ALBP), 275, 277-279b
Osteogenic sarcoma, 260, 262-265b
Osteoid osteoma, 275, 277-279b
Osteomyelitis
  causing acute low back pain (ALBP), 275, 277-279b
  fever characteristics with, 205, 206-207b

Osteomyelitis *(Continued)*
  of frontal bone, 287, 287b
  and limb pain, 254, 262-265b
Osteoporosis
  causing acute low back pain (ALBP), 276, 277-279b
Otitis
  causing peripheral vertigo, 156
Otitis media
  definition of, 174
  fever with, 195, 204, 206-207b
  headaches caused by, 230, 232-233b
  symptoms and earaches from, 181, 182-183b
Otoscopy
  to examine ear canals, 178
  during hoarseness evaluation, 238-239
  pneumatic, 179, 180f
Oucher Pain Scale
  for children, 10, 11f
Outdoor activities
  and fever, 197
  and Lyme disease (*See* Lyme disease)
  and parasites, 15
  skin rashes and lesions, 310-311
Ova/parasite stool test
  for anorectal disorder diagnosis, 328
  to evaluate diarrhea, 142
Ovarian cycles
  and endometrial cycle correlation, 46, 48t
Ovarian cysts
  causing lower abdominal pain, 24, 25-29b
Ovarian toxicity
  drugs that may cause, 52, 52b
Overflow incontinence
  in children, 113
  definition of, 374
  medications that can cause, 375t
  symptoms and causes of, 380-381, 382-383b
Overuse injuries, 244-245, 275, 277-279b
Overweight; *See* obesity
Oximetry
  transcutaneous pulse, 168

P
Pain
  abdominal, 8 (*See* abdominal pain)
  acute low back pain (ALBP), 269-271
  anorectal disorder, 324
  Apley rule, 10
  breast (*See* breast pain)
  chest (*See* chest pain)
  children's Oucher Pain Scale, 10, 11f
  constipation, 114
  cranial mechanisms and pathways, 222f
  diagnostic analysis of, 2-3
  and difficulty staying asleep, 346
  ear, 176, 176 (*See also* earache)
  with eye motion, 334
  with female and child urinary dysfunction, 385-386
  with glaucoma, 343
  headache, 224
  with hematuria, 386
  with hoarseness, 237
  itching and bleeding in anorectal area, 321-333
  location and structures, 10-11, 12t

Pain *(Continued)*
  male genitourinary system, 209, 212
  migraine headache, 224, 367
  nasal location of, 281
  organic *versus* functional, 15, 15t
  with penile discharge, 297-298
  precipitating syncope, 367
  radiation of, 11-12
  with red eye, 336, 336b, 338
  referred
    with acute low back pain (ALBP), 270-271
    definition of, 8, 9b
    earache, 174
  associated with skin rashes/lesions, 310
  causing sleep problems, 346-347
  with vaginal discharge, 415
  with vision loss, 424-425
Pallor
  of skin with dyspnea, 166
Palpitations
  and chest pain, 84
  in children, 288
  definition of heart, 288
  diagnostic reasoning/key history questions
    angina pectoris, 288
    arrhythmia information, 290b
    cardiac surgery, 289
    chest pain, 288
    coronary artery disease (CAD) history, 288
    description of, 289
    dyspnea, 288
    flip-flopping, fluttering or pounding, 289
    genetic disorders, 290
    illness, 290
    lightheadedness, 288
    medications taken, 289-290
    occurrence of, 289
    panic, stress, or anxiety disorders, 289
    risks associated with, 288
    stimulants used, 290
    sudden cardiac death family history, 289
    syncope, 288
  differential diagnoses
    alcohol or drug abuse, 293, 294-295b
    anemia, 293, 294-295b
    cardiac arrhythmias, 292, 292b, 294-295b
    drugs and medications, 293, 294-295b
    generalized anxiety disorder, 293, 294-295b
    hyperthyroidism, 293-294, 294-295b
    nonarrhythmic causes, 293, 293b, 294-295b
    panic disorders, 293, 294-295b
    pheochromocytoma, 293, 294-295b
    psychological causes, 292-293, 294-295b
    stimulant use, 293, 294-295b
  evidence-based practice (EBP)
    arrhythmia predictions, 290b
  laboratory and diagnostic studies, 291-292
  overview of causes, 288
  physical examination procedures, 290-291
  and syncope, 367
Panic attacks/disorders
  definition of, 34, 41, 42-45b
  and fatigue, 190
  history and chest pain evaluation, 86
  causing palpitations, 289, 293, 294-295b
  and syncope, 368

Pap test, 401, 442
Papules
  description and examples of skin, 304-305t, 307f
Papulosquamous eruptions
  in children, 308f
Paranasal sinuses; *See also* nasal symptoms
  anatomy of, 280, 281f
Parasite/ova stool test
  for anorectal disorder diagnosis, 328
  to evaluate diarrhea, 142
Parasites; *See also* pinworms
  abdominal pain from, 15
  causing anorectal itching, 325, 330, 331-332b
  and diarrhea, 142
  intestinal, 15
  scotch tape test, 328
Parietal pain, 10
Parkinson disease, 238, 238t
Parotitis
  causing referred pain earaches, 174
Paroxysmal nocturnal dyspnea (PND), 347
Parsimony
  as hypothesis testing characteristic, 3
Partial thromboplastin time (PTT), 404
Passive range-of-motion tests
  during limb pain evaluation, 252
Past-pointing test
  during dizziness and vertigo evaluation, 154
Patches
  skin, 304-305t, 307f
Patellar tendinitis, 257, 262-265b
Pediatrics; *See* children
Pediculosis
  contacting methods, 310
  itching of, 310b
Pelvic examinations
  during amenorrhea evaluation, 55
  to evaluate urinary dysfunction, 389
  process of, 402-403
  during urinary incontinence evaluation, 378
  for vaginal bleeding evaluation, 402-403
  for women with abdominal pain, 17
Pelvic inflammatory disease (PID)
  abdominal pain from, 8, 22-23, 25-29b
  causing acute low back pain (ALBP), 277, 277-279b
  and deep vaginal dyspareunia, 415
  description and causes of, 407, 408-410b
  fever characteristics with, 196-197, 204, 206-207b
  vaginal discharge with, 420, 421b
Penile discharge
  color, consistency and amount, 296-297
  diagnostic reasoning/key history questions
    abdominal pain, 297-298
    acute pain, 297-298
    alcohol or drug abuse history, 296
    discharge color, consistency and amount, 296-297
    disseminated systemic urethral infection, 297
    exposure days and symptom onset, 296
    fever, 297-298
    flank pain, 297-298
    glans penis inflammation/redness, 297
    hematuria, 297
    hygiene practices, 297
    immigrant patient/partner, 298
    recent STI treatment, 298
    recent travel, 298

Penile discharge *(Continued)*
    Reiter syndrome symptoms, 297
    scrotal or testicular pain, 297-298
    sexual practices and partners, 296
    stage of infection, 297
    substance abuse history, 296
    symptom onset and description, 296-297, 298
    unprotected sex, 296
    urethritis questions, 297
    urinary frequency, urgency and other symptoms, 297
    urinary tract pain, 297-298
  differential diagnoses of
    balanitis, 301, 302b
    C. trachomatis, 300, 302b
    Chlamydia infections, 301, 302b
    complicated urethritis, 301, 302b
    epididymitis, 301, 302b
    gonococcal urethritis, 300-301, 302b
    N. gonorrhoeae, 300, 302b
    nongonococcal urethritis, 301, 302b
    orchitis, 301, 302b
    prostatitis, 301, 302b
    Reiter syndrome, 301, 302b
    urethritis, 300, 302b
  DNA probe testing, 19
  evaluation with frequency, urgency and dysuria, 211
  laboratory and diagnostic studies, 299-300
  overview of causes and infections, 296
  physical examination procedures, 298-299
Penis
  inspecting during male genitourinary evaluation, 213
  inspection during penile discharge evaluation, 297, 299
  Tanner stage development illustration, 77f
Peptic ulcers
  causing chest pain, 94, 95b
  perforation, 21, 25-29b
  causing upper abdominal pain, 25, 25-29b
Perianal aching, 211
Perianal pruritus
  vaginal discharge with, 413, 413f, 418
Perianal streptococcal cellulitis, 329, 331-332b
Pericarditis, 92, 95b
Perilymph fistula, 156
Perimenopause
  vaginal bleeding during, 406, 408-410b
Perineal compression syndrome
  description and diagnosis of male, 219, 219-220b
Perineal electromyelography, 379
Periodic leg movement
  sleep problems due to, 351, 354-355b
Periorbital cellulitis, 334, 343, 343-344b
Peripheral blood smear
  to evaluate diarrhea, 142
Peripheral perfusion, 140, 140t
Peripheral pulse test
  during abdominal pain evaluation, 18
Peripheral vertigo
  definition of, 149
  and nystagmus, 152-153, 153t
Perirectal area
  abscesses, 322-323, 328-329, 331-332b
  inspection of, 326
Perirectal fistula, 328-329, 331-332b
Peristaltic reflex, 111
Peritoneal pain
  abdominal, 10

Peritoneum
  inflammation and abdominal pain, 8
Peritonitis
  acute abdominal pain from, 8-9, 22, 25-29b
  features and mnemonic, 9b
Peritonsillar abscesses, 356, 362, 364-365b
Periumbilical pain
  structures associated with, 12t
Peroneal nerve compression, 260, 262-265b
Persistent hyperplastic primary vitreous (PHPV) retinal detachment, 428-429
Pertussis, 127-128, 131-132b
Pets; *See* animal exposure
Phalen test, 260, 261t
Pharyngitis
  fever characteristics with, 204, 206-207b
  headaches caused by, 230, 232-233b
  causing referred pain earaches, 174
  sore throat *(See* sore throat)
  with ulcers
    and aphthous stomatitis, 363, 364-365b
    and candidiasis, 363, 364-365b
    and canker sores, 363, 364-365b
    and herpangina, 363, 364-365b
    and herpes simplex virus (HSV), 363, 364-365b
    and Vincent angina, 363, 364-365b
  without ulcers
    and epiglottis, 361-362, 364-365b
    and gonococcal pharyngitis, 363, 364-365b
    and inflammation, 363, 364-365b
    and mononucleosis, 362-363, 364-365b
    and peritonsillar abscess, 362, 364-365b
    and retropharyngeal abscess, 362, 364-365b
    and streptococcal pharyngitis, 362, 362t, 364-365b
    and viral pharyngitis, 362, 364-365b
Pharynx; *See also* pharyngitis
  amplifying voice sounds, 235
Pheochromocytoma, 293, 294-295b
Photophobia
  with eye pain and vision loss, 424-425
  with glaucoma, 343
  with headaches, 225-226
  and red eye, 337
Physical activities; *See* activities; activity levels; exercise
Pilonidal disease, 329, 331-332b
Pinworms
  causing anorectal itching, 325, 330, 331-332b
  assessing in urinary incontinence patients, 377
  scotch tape test, 328
  vaginal discharge with, 413, 413f, 418
Pituitary adenoma, 52, 58-59t, 58-59
Pityriasis
  definition and skin eruptions, 314, 316-320b
Pityriasis rosea
  itching of, 310b
Pityriasis versicolor, 315, 316-320b
Placenta abruptio, 406, 408-410b
Placenta previa, 405, 408-410b
Plantar fasciitis, 258-259, 262-265b
Plaque
  description and examples of skin, 304-305t, 307f
Pleura
  as seen on chest x-rays, 452, 454, 454f, 455b
Pleural effusion
  asymmetrical chest movement with, 165b
Pleural friction rub, 167

Pleuritis, 93, 95b, 276-277, 277-279b
Pleurodynia, 94, 95b
Pneumatic otoscopy, 179, 180f
Pneumonia
    abdominal pain from, 23, 25-29b
    chest pain with, 81-82
    definition and diagnosis of, 93, 95b
    and dyspnea, 171, 172-173b
Pneumoperitoneum, 460, 461f
Pneumothorax
    chest pain with, 81-82
    definition and diagnosis of, 92, 95b
    and dyspnea, 160, 169, 171-172b
Polycystic ovary syndrome (PCOS)
    causing amenorrhea, 57, 58-59t
    chronic bleeding with, 398-399, 407, 408-410b
Polymenorrhea, 396
Polymyositis, 85
Polypharmacy
    as risk factor for confusional states, 101
Polyuria, 211
Popliteal cyst, 258, 262-265b
Positional maneuvers
    during dizziness and vertigo evaluation, 153
Positional nystagmus test
    during dizziness and vertigo evaluation, 152-153
Positron emission tomography (PET scan)
    to analyze confusional states, 105
    definition and procedures, 455
Postmenopausal women
    breast lumps in, 62
    stress incontinence in, 380
    vaginal bleeding in, 398, 400
Postnasal drainage syndrome, 129, 132-133b
Postnasal drip, 235
Poststreptococcal glomerulonephritis, 393, 394b
Postural strains
    causing acute low back pain (ALBP), 275, 277-279b
Posture
    assessing during dyspnea evaluation, 163-164
Postvoid residual volume measurement, 378-379
Potassium hydroxide test (KOH)
    during abdominal pain evaluation, 19
    for skin rash/lesion evaluation, 312
Practitioners
    expert *versus* novice, 3-4
Preauricular nodes, 340
Precordial catch syndrome, 94, 95b
Pregnancy
    activity and weight recommendations for, 436b, 437b
    and amenorrhea, 46, 55, 57
    and anorectal disorders, 326
    breast pain with, 75, 78, 79-80b
    and lactation-related nipple discharge, 64
    nasal symptoms with, 282
    tests to determine, 18
    and vaginal bleeding, 396-397, 405, 408-410b
    weeks of gestation, 397
Premenarche
    and vaginal discharge, 413
Premenstrual symptoms
    with amenorrhea, 53
Prenatal systemic lupus erythematosus (SLE)
    and syncope, 369
Prepubertal bleeding, 399

Primary care
    diagnostic process in, 2-3
Primary enuresis
    versus secondary in children, 376-377
    symptoms and causes of, 382
Primary nonorganic enuresis, 374, 377, 382
Proctalgia fugax, 324, 329, 331-332b
Proctitis/proctocolitis, 322-323, 324, 329, 331-332b
Progesterone level tests, 56-57, 404
Progressive degenerative eye diseases, 425-426
Prolactin levels
    drugs that may increase, 52, 52b
    and nipple discharge, 63, 69
    testing in amenorrhea evaluation, 55
Proprioception tests
    in confusion cases, 104
Proptosis, 343
Prostate
    extension into rectum scale, 213
Prostate cancer
    description and diagnosis of male, 218, 219-220b
    screening with prostate-specific antigen, 216, 216b
Prostate-specific antigen (PSA)
    for cancer screening, 216, 216b
Prostatitis
    acute bacterial, 217, 219-220b
    chronic bacterial, 208, 217-218, 219-220b
    fever characteristics with, 204, 206-207b
    NIH classification, 214-215, 215b
    causing penile discharge, 301, 302b
    ruling out in men, 17
Protein strips
    for female/child urinary problem evaluation, 390
Proteinuria, 299
Prothrombin time (PT)
    during chest pain evaluation, 90
    tests during vaginal bleeding evaluation, 404
Provocation maneuvers
    during dizziness and vertigo evaluation, 152-153
Provocative stress tests
    during urinary incontinence evaluation, 378
Proximal fibula fracture, 257, 257f, 262-265b
Proximal interphalangeal (PIP) joints
    osteoarthritis in, 250, 250f
Pruritus ani, 325, 329-330, 331-332b
Pseudomembranous colitis, 144, 146-147b
Pseudotumor cerebri, 231, 232-233b
Psoriasis
    characteristics, associations and diagnosis of, 316-320b
    definition and mechanisms of, 315
    itching of, 310b
    and sebum overproduction, 176
Psychogenic disorders
    and coughing, 94, 95b, 131, 132-133b
    and hoarseness, 241, 241-242b
    of muscles, 259, 262-265b
    and vertigo, 150, 156
Psychogenic dizziness, 150
Psychogenic syncope, 368
Psychological disorders
    and acute low back pain (ALBP), 267, 277, 277-279b
    diagnostic reasoning/key questions, 30-39, 31f
        in adolescents, 34-35, 34b
        anxiety, 34
        BATHE model, 32-34

Psychological disorders *(Continued)*
    bipolar, 34-35, 35b
    depression, 33-34, 34b
    DIG FAST bipolar assessment, 34-35, 35b
    and domestic violence detection, 31f, 32
    evaluation diagram, 31f
    HEEAD adolescent assessment method, 34-35, 34b, 36t
    and substance abuse, 33, 33b, 34b
    suicide risk questions, 35
  differential diagnoses
    anxiety disorders, 34, 41, 42-45b
    autism spectrum disorder, 40, 40b, 42-45b
    bipolar disorder, 34-35, 35b, 41-45, 42-45b
    domestic violence, 31f, 32, 40, 42-45b
    dysthymia, 41, 42-45b
    generalized anxiety disorder, 41, 42-45b
    major depressive disorder, 41, 42-45b
    mania, 34-35, 35b, 41-45, 42-45b
    mood disorders, 41-45, 42-45b
    normal grief, 40, 42-45b
    normal stress, 39-40, 42-45b
    panic disorder, 41, 42-45b
    social anxiety disorder, 41, 42-45b
    social phobia, 41, 42-45b
    substance abuse, 33, 33b, 34b, 40, 42-45b
  and fatigue, 184, 186-187
  hysterical syncope, 371, 372b
  causing palpitations, 292-293, 294-295b
  physical exam clues, 35-39
  THINC MED mnemonic, 31, 32b
Psychosocial problems
  HEEAD method to analyze, 34-35, 34b, 36t
  questions to determine, 30
  and weight loss/gain (unintentional), 436-437, 444,
    445-446b
Psychotropic drugs
  causing vertigo, 151
Ptosis, 427, 428-429
Pubertal development stages, 47, 49, 49f, 50f
Pulmonary angiography
  during chest pain evaluation, 90
  for dyspnea evaluation, 168-169
Pulmonary embolus
  and chest pain, 81, 91-92, 95b
  and dyspnea, 160-161, 169, 171-172b
  causing syncope, 367
Pulmonary hypertension, 160-161
Pulmonary vasculature
  as seen on chest x-rays, 452, 455b
Punch biopsy
  for skin rash/lesion evaluation, 313
Pupillary response tests, 430
Pupils
  anatomical illustration of, 335f
  assessment of, 428-429
  characteristics and functions of, 339-340
  inspection with red eye, 339-340
  pupillary response tests, 430
Pustules, 304-305t, 307f
Pyelonephritis
  abdominal pain from, 22, 25-29b, 385-386
  causing acute low back pain (ALBP), 276, 277-279b
  description and diagnosis of male, 208, 217,
    219-220b
  urinary problems due to, 385-386, 393, 394b

Q
Qualitative urine/serum human chorionic gonadotropin tests (hCG),
    18, 403
Quantitative serum human chorionic gonadotropin (hCG) test, 18, 403

R
Radiography; *See also* abdominal x-rays; chest x-rays
  for abdominal pain evaluation, 20
  for chest pain evaluation, 90
  to evaluate causes of hoarseness, 239
  during limb pain evaluation, 253
RAFFT adolescent questionnaire, 34b
Range-of-motion (ROM) tests
  during ALBP examination, 272
  in limb pain cases, 252
Rapid alternating movement (RAM) tests
  during dizziness and vertigo evaluation, 154
  in older adults, 104
Rapid eye movement (REM) sleep, 345
Rapid influenza testing
  during cough evaluation, 127
Rashes; *See* skin rashes and lesions
Rectal bleeding
  versus vaginal bleeding, 401
Rectocele, 115
Rectum
  anal soreness, 321
  anatomy of, 321-322, 322f
  bleeding differential diagnoses
    allergic colitis, 330-331, 331-332b
    bowel inflammation, 331, 331-332b
    colorectal cancer, 330, 331-332b
    condyloma acuminata, 330, 331-332b
    hemorrhoids, 330, 330t, 331-332b
    intussusception, 331, 331-332b
    juvenile polyps, 331, 331-332b
    maternal blood ingestion, 330, 331-332b
    Meckel diverticulum, 331, 331-332b
    necrotizing enterocolitis, 331, 331-332b
  diagnostic reasoning/key history questions
    anorectal bleeding, 322
    bleeding disorders, 322
    bowel movement straining and habits,
      325
    constipation, 324-325
    diabetes mellitus, 326
    diarrhea, 324
    family history, 326
    fecal soiling, 324
    hygiene, 325-326
    immunocompromised patients, 322-323
    itching, 324
    masses, 324
    pain, 324
    pregnancy and childbirth, 326
    regarding newborns, infants and children, 323
    sexual abuse determination, 325
    sexual activities/practices, 324, 324b
    symptom analysis, 323
    tenesmus, 324
  itching differential diagnoses
    pinworms, 325, 330, 331-332b
    pruritus ani, 325, 329-330, 331-332b
  laboratory and diagnostic studies, 327-328

Rectum *(Continued)*
  pain, itching and bleeding, 321-333
  pain differential diagnoses, 328-329, 331-332b
    anal fissure, 328-329, 331-332b
    perianal streptococcal cellulitis, 329, 331-332b
    perirectal abscess, 328-329, 331-332b
    perirectal fistula, 328-329, 331-332b
    pilonidal disease, 329, 331-332b
    proctalgia fugax, 329, 331-332b
    proctitis/proctocolitis, 329, 331-332b
  physical examination procedures, 326-327
    anoscopy, 327
    digital rectal examination, 326-327
    perirectal area inspection, 326
  sphincter contraction tenesmus, 321
  sphincter tone assessment, 274
  tears and fissures, 321
Recurrent abdominal pain (RAP), 8-9, 25-29, 25-29b
Red blood cell (RBC) analysis, 391
Red eye
  anterior chamber causes of
    hyphema, 342, 343-344b
  conjunctiva causes of
    allergic conjunctivitis, 342, 343-344b
    bacterial conjunctivitis, 341, 343-344b
    chemical conjunctivitis, 342, 343-344b
    N. gonorrhoeae conjunctivitis, 342, 343-344b
    subconjunctival hemorrhage, 342, 343-344b
    viral conjunctivitis, 341-342, 343-344b
  corneal causes of
    corneal abrasion, 342, 343-344b
    herpetic infections, 342-343, 343-344b
    keratitis, 342, 343-344b
  diagnostic reasoning/key questions, 335
    blurring, 336
    chemicals, 334
    discharge characteristics, 337
    double vision, 337
    flashing lights, 337
    floaters, 337
    halos, 337
    itching and tearing, 338
    onset and recurrence of, 335-336
    orbital infections, 334
    pain location and severity, 336, 336b, 338
    pain with eye motion, 334
    painful *versus* nonpainful causes, 336, 336b
    photophobia, 337
    sinus infections, 334-335, 338
    swelling, redness and fever, 334, 337
    tears, 337-338
    trauma, 334-335
    with vision loss, 336, 336b
  erythematous swelling, 338
  eyelid causes of
    blepharitis, 341, 343-344b
    chalazion, 341, 343-344b
    entropion and ectropion, 341, 343-344b
    hordeolum, 341, 343-344b
  glaucoma causing, 343, 343-344b
  inflammation inspection, 338
  intraocular pressure measurement, 341
  laboratory and diagnostic studies, 340-341
  lacrimal sac causes of
    dacryocystitis, 341, 343-344b

Red eye *(Continued)*
  orbit causes of
    orbital cellulitis, 343, 343-344b
    periorbital cellulitis, 343, 343-344b
  physical examination procedures, 338-340
  sclera causes of
    episcleritis, 342, 343-344b
    scleritis, 342, 343-344b
  uveal tract causes of
    iritis, 343, 343-344b
Referral pain
  with acute low back pain (ALBP), 270-271
  definition of, 8, 9b
  earache, 174
Reflexes
  testing
    during limb pain evaluation, 252
    in older adults, 104
    during palpitations evaluation, 291
Refractive amblyopia, 426
Refractive errors, 430-431, 433-434b
Reiter syndrome, 297, 301, 302b
Relieving factors
  aiding diagnoses, 12-13, 14
Renal insufficiency, 208
Reproductive life cycle
  and age affecting vaginal bleeding, 397-398
Respiration rate
  during cough evaluation, 125
  during dyspnea evaluation, 164, 165b
  measuring during chest pain evaluation, 86-87
  and pattern during chest pain evaluation, 86-87
Respiration rhythm and depth
  during dyspnea evaluation, 164, 165b
Respiratory epithelium
  and nasal drainage, 280
Respiratory system
  considering during abdominal pain evaluation, 15
  examination during hoarseness evaluation, 238
  and fever, 196
Rest deficits
  causing fatigue, 189, 191-192b
Restless legs syndrome
  sleep problems due to, 351, 354-355b
Restlessness
  as clue to psychological disorders, 30
Restrictive pulmonary disease
  features of, 164
Retina
  anatomical illustration of, 335f
Retinal artery occlusion, 423-424, 424f
Retinal detachment
  definition and vision loss, 432, 433-434b
  flash of light symptoms, 423, 425
Retinoblastomas
  definition and symptoms of, 431, 433-434b
  indications of, 428-429
Retinopathy of prematurity, 431, 433-434b
Retropharyngeal abscesses, 362, 364-365b
Retrosternal area
  as seen on chest x-rays, 454, 454f, 455b
Rheumatoid arthritis (RA)
  description and symptoms of, 254, 262-265b
  diagnostic criteria for, 254b

Rheumatoid factor (RF)
tests during limb pain evaluation, 253
Rhinitis medicamentosa, 286, 287b
Rhinoplasty, 236
Rhinorrhea, 357
Rhonchi
assessing during dyspnea evaluation, 167
Ribs and intracostal spaces
as seen on chest x-rays, 451, 451f, 455b
Rigidity
causes of, 104
Rinne test, 152, 179
Rocky Mountain spotted fever
fever and rash eruption periods, 196-197, 200-201
transmission and skin symptoms of, 310
Rosacea, 313, 316-320b
Roseola, 314, 316-320b
Roseola infantum
fever characteristics with, 205, 206-207b
rash eruption periods, 196
Rotator cuff
patient locating pain in, 250
tears, 255, 262-265b
tests, 255, 261t
Rubella, 196, 314, 316-320b
Rubeola, 314, 316-320b
"Rule-in" and "rule-out" strategies, 4
"Rules of thumb"
in diagnostic reasoning process, 3
Ruptured abdominal aortic aneurysm, 9

S

Safety
assessing risks during HEEADSSS interview, 34-35, 36t
Saline prep test, 19
Salmonella, 143, 146-147b
Salpingitis, 22-23, 25-29b
Salt retention with ototoxic drugs
causing dizziness, 156
Savagery
assessing risks during HEEADSSS interview, 34-35, 36t
Scabies, 308f, 310, 310b, 418
Scapulae
as seen on chest x-rays, 451, 455b
Scarlet fever, 196, 310, 314, 316-320b, 360
Scheuermann disease, 276, 277-279b
Sciatica
causing acute low back pain (ALBP), 267, 275,
277-279b
pain characteristics with, 269, 270-271, 277-279b
Sclera
anatomical illustration of, 335f
episcleritis, 342, 343-344b
inspection with red eye, 339
scleritis, 342, 343-344b
Scoliosis, 88
Scotch tape test, 328, 418
Scrotum
inspecting during male genitourinary evaluation, 213
pain and penile discharge, 297-298, 299
Tanner stage development illustration, 77f
Seasonal allergies
and coughs, 123
nasal symptoms with, 280-281

Seborrheic dermatitis
characteristics, associations and diagnosis of, 316-320b
definition and mechanisms of, 315
description and location in children, 308f
Sebum
overproduction and earaches, 176
Secondary amenorrhea
definition of, 46
Secondary (developmental) enuresis
versus primary in children, 376-377, 382, 382-383b
symptoms of, 382
Secondary nonorganic enuresis, 374, 377, 382, 382-383b
Secretory diarrhea, 134
Secretory otitis, 174
Sedatives
causing urinary incontinence, 375, 375t, 381, 382-383b
Sedentary lifestyles
and constipation, 113
and weight problems (*See* activity levels; obesity)
Segmented urine collection
for male genitourinary evaluation, 214-215
Seizures
in height of fever, 195-196
as prodromal symptom of syncope, 366, 371, 372b
versus syncope, 367
Sensory impairments
function test during ALBP exam, 273
in older adults, 104
Septic arthritis, 254-255, 262-265b
Septic joints, 248
Septum deviation, 280
Serology test for syphilis, 105, 155, 300, 328, 417-418
Serous otitis media, 174
Serum B_{12} and folate tests, 105
Serum electrolytes
and depression, 39
tests during constipation evaluation, 116
Serum estradiol levels, 404
Serum estrogen receptor modulators, 161
Serum follicle-stimulating hormones (FSHs) level tests, 55, 404
Serum luteinizing hormones (LHs) level tests, 55-56, 404
Serum thyroid-stimulating hormones (TSHs) tests, 55, 116, 442
Severe acute respiratory syndrome (SARS), 197, 198b
Sexual abuse
assessing during HEEADSSS interview, 34-35, 36t
determination of, 325
Sexual activities/practices/partners
and anorectal disorders, 324, 324b
assessing during HEEADSSS interview, 34-35, 36t
and diarrhea, 138
and disease exposure through body fluids, 185
dyspareunia pain with, 13, 375, 398, 415
causing female urinary dysfunction, 387
and fever, 197
history and male genitourinary evaluation, 212
pain during, 13
and partner history, 296
and penile discharge problems, 296, 298, 302b
vaginal discharge due to, 412, 414
Sexual maturity assessment, 49f, 50f, 54
Sexually transmitted infections (STIs)
evaluating recent male, 212, 298
causing female urinary dysfunction, 388
and penile discharge, 298
ruling out in women and men, 17

Sexually transmitted infections *(Continued)*
  and urethritis in males, 296
  causing urinary tract infections in men, 208
  vaginal bleeding with, 397, 399
  vaginal discharge with, 412-413, 414
Shaken baby syndrome, 425
Sheehan syndrome, 58, 58-59t
Shigella, 143, 146-147b
Shin splints, 258, 262-265b
Shingles
  causing breast pain, 79, 79-80b
  causing chest pain, 93-94, 95b
  skin rashes and lesions, 314, 316-320b
Shortness of breath; *See* dyspnea
Shoulder
  anatomical diagram of, 248f
  diagnostic reasoning/key questions, 245
  patient locating pain in, 250
  tests to assess, 261t
  trauma or overuse injuries
    acromioclavicular joint injuries, 255, 262-265b
    bicipital tendinitis, 255, 262-265b
    dislocation, 255, 262-265b
    glenohumeral joint instability, 255, 262-265b
    rotator cuff tear, 255, 261t, 262-265b
Sickle cell anemia
  urinary incontinence due to, 377, 382
Sickle cell disease (SCD), 85, 259, 262-265b
SIG E CAPS depression mnemonic, 34b
Sigmoidoscopy
  for abdominal pain evaluation, 20
  procedures for performing, 463
Simple constipation, 24, 25-29b, 117, 118-119b
Sinus aspiration, 285
Sinus headaches, 224-225
Sinus infections, 334-335, 338
Sinus obstruction
  nasal symptoms with, 286, 287b
Sinuses; *See also* nasal symptoms
  amplifying voice sounds, 235
  unilateral or bilateral symptoms in, 282
Sinusitis
  fever characteristics with, 204, 206-207b
  headaches caused by, 224-225, 229, 232-233b
  causing hoarseness, 235
  causing peripheral vertigo, 156
Situational stress, 32-33
Situational syncope, 368, 371, 372b
Sjögren syndrome, 238, 336
Skin; *See also* skin rashes and lesions
  and hair changes with thyroid dysfunction, 51, 54
  as indicator of psychological or substance abuse disorders, 39
  inspection of
    during ALBP examination, 271
    during amenorrhea evaluation, 51, 54
    during breast examination, 76
    during breast lump evaluation, 66
    during chest pain evaluation, 87
    during cough evaluation, 126
    during dyspnea evaluation, 166
    during fatigue evaluation, 187
    during limb pain evaluation, 250-251, 250f
    during male genitourinary evaluation, 212
    in sore throat cases, 360

Skin *(Continued)*
  pigmentation issues with, 304-305t
  types and examples of lesions, 304-305t, 307f
Skin rashes and lesions
  acute *versus* chronic, 309b
  allergic reactions
    erythema multiforme, 315, 316-320b
    urticaria, 315, 316-320b
  descriptive dermatological terminology, 306t
  diagnostic reasoning/focused history questions
    acute *versus* chronic, 308, 309b
    allergic reactions, 308
    burning, 310
    drug reactions, 310
    evolution stage of lesion, 309, 309b
    family history, 311
    fever, 308-311
    headache with, 310
    immunizations, 311
    initial presentation of, 309
    itching, 309, 310b
    living situation/day care, 310
    medications, 311
    mucosal involvement and fever, 308
    onset and duration, 308, 309b
    outdoor or leisure exposure to, 310-311
    pain associated with, 310
    pets and flea bites, 311
    sore throat, 310
    spread and movement of, 309
    travel, 310
    triggers, 311
    viral infections, 310
  with fever, 196, 200-201
  follicular eruption differential diagnoses
    acne vulgaris, 313, 316-320b
    rosacea, 313, 316-320b
  fungal infection differential diagnoses
    candidiasis, 314-315, 316-320b
    pityriasis versicolor, 315, 316-320b
    tinea, 315, 316-320b
  illustration of types of, 307f
  immunological and inflammatory differential diagnoses
    allergic dermatitis, 315, 316-320b
    contact dermatitis, 315, 316-320b
    eczema, 315, 316-320b
    psoriasis, 315, 316-320b
    seborrheic dermatitis, 315, 316-320b
  infectious eruption differential diagnoses
    carbuncle, 313, 316-320b
    folliculitis, 313, 316-320b
    furuncle, 313, 316-320b
    impetigo, 313, 316-320b
  laboratory and diagnostic studies, 312-313
  with Lyme disease, 247, 310-311
  macular/papular eruption differential diagnoses
    Erythema infectiosum, 313, 316-320b
    fifth disease, 313, 316-320b
    measles, 314, 316-320b
    pityriasis, 314, 316-320b
    roseola, 314, 316-320b
    rubella, 314, 316-320b
    rubeola, 314, 316-320b
    scarlet fever, 314, 316-320b
    slapped cheek disease, 313, 316-320b

Skin rashes and lesions *(Continued)*
  mechanisms and evaluation criteria, 303, 304-305t, 316-320b
  neoplastic eruption differential diagnoses, 316, 316-320b
    basal cell carcinoma, 316, 316-320b
    malignant melanoma, 315-316, 316-320b
    squamous cell carcinoma, 316, 316-320b
  overview of, 303, 316-320b
  physical examination procedures, 311-312
  shape and border characteristics of, 314, 316-320b
  vesicular and bullous differential diagnoses
    chickenpox, 314, 316-320b
    hand-foot-and-mouth disease, 314, 316-320b
    herpes simplex virus (HSV), 314, 316-320b
    herpes zoster, 314, 316-320b
    insect bites, 314, 316-320b
    shingles, 314, 316-320b
    varicella zoster, 314, 316-320b
Skin scraping, 312
Skull
  examining during headache evaluation, 226
Slapped cheek disease, 313, 316-320b
Sleep; *See also* sleep problems
  assessing during HEEADSSS interview, 34-35, 36t
  bedtime routines and environment, 348
Sleep apnea
  causing chronic fatigue, 190, 191-192b
Sleep diaries, 350
Sleep enuresis, 374
Sleep problems, 345-355
  in adolescents, 349, 353, 354-355b
  age-related, 349, 352-353, 354-355b
  anxiety, 346, 348
  awakening with or awakening from chest pain, 84
  bedtime routines and environment, 348-349
  in children and infants, 345, 348-349, 352-353, 354-355b
  chronic obstructive pulmonary disease (COPD), 347, 352
  consequences of chronic, 345
  daytime sleepiness and dozing, 346-347
  defining nature and degree of, 345-346
  delayed sleep phase syndrome, 352, 354-355b
  with depression, 346, 348
  difficulty falling asleep, 346
  difficulty staying asleep, 346
  duration of, 346
  Epworth Sleepiness Scale, 346, 347b
  exercise factors, 348
  and fatigue, 184-185, 189, 191-192b
  gastroesophageal reflux (GERD) disease, 347, 352
  hygiene, 352, 354-355b
  illnesses, 347, 352, 354-355b
  insomnia, 349
    comorbid, 352, 354-355b
    conditioned, 349, 353-354, 354-355b
  laboratory and diagnostic studies, 350-351
    actigraphy, 350
    ferritin levels, 351
    sleep diaries, 350
    sleep studies, 350
  lifestyle issues, 348, 352, 354-355b
  limb sensations and jerking, 346, 346
  medications and alcohol use, 346-347, 352, 354-355b
  in menopausal women, 353, 354-355b
  narcolepsy, 352, 354-355b
  in newborns, 352-353, 354-355b
  nightmares and night terrors, 349, 353, 354-355b

Sleep problems *(Continued)*
  obstructive sleep apnea hypopnea syndrome (OSAHS), 351, 351b, 354-355b
  obstructive sleep apnea (OSA), 346, 351, 351b, 354-355b
  in older adults, 345, 349, 353, 354-355b
  and pain, 346-347
  paroxysmal nocturnal dyspnea (PND), 347
  periodic leg movement, 351, 354-355b
  persistent diarrhea, 137
  physical examination procedures, 350
  poor sleep hygiene, 352, 354-355b
  processes regulating
    circadian rhythm, 345
    physiological need, 345
  with psychological disorders, 30, 34b
  restless legs syndrome, 351, 354-355b
  sleep refusal, 353, 354-355b
  snoring, 346
  somnambulism, 350, 354, 354-355b
  stages of
    non–rapid eye movement (NREM) sleep, 345
    rapid eye movement (REM) sleep, 345
  statistics and types of, 345
  stimulant consumption, 348
  trained night crier or feeder, 353-354, 354-355b
  and travel, 348-349
  and wake cycle disturbance
    with delirium, 99
Sleep studies, 350
Slipped capital femoral epiphysis, 256, 262-265b
Small intestine
  anatomic diagram and x-ray view of, 458f, 459-460, 461f
  normal vs abnormal x-ray findings, 463-464b
  obstruction abdominal x-ray of, 461f
  series, 462
Small-volume incontinence, 380-381
Smell test
  during nasal evaluation, 283
Smoke exposure
  and coughing, 124
  and earaches, 175
Smoking
  assessing during HEEADSSS interview, 34-35, 36t
  cessation and weight gain, 439
  and coronary artery disease (CAD), 82-83
  coughs, 124, 131, 132-133b
  and dyspnea, 163
  and hoarseness, 236-237
  nasal symptoms with, 282
  as pulmonary embolus risk factor, 160-161
Sneezing
  and sore throats, 358
  stress incontinence from, 380
Snellen tests, 427-428
Snoring
  and sleep problems, 346
Social anxiety disorder
  definition of, 41, 42-45b
Social isolation
  and weight loss (unintentional), 444, 445-446b
Social phobia, 41, 42-45b
Social skills
  as clue to psychological disorders, 30
Social support
  assessing during HEEADSSS interview, 34-35, 36t

Soft tissue
as seen on chest x-rays, 450, 455b
Somatic pain, 10
Somnambulism, 350, 354, 354-355b
Sore throat
β-hemolytic streptococcus (GABHS) infections,
356-357, 358, 362t
causes and origins of, 356
classifying with/without pharyngeal ulcers, 356
diagnostic reasoning/key questions
in adolescents, 358
age, 358
conjunctivitis, 357
cough and rhinorrhea, 357
drooling, dyspnea, and inspiratory stridor, 356
emergency signals, 356
epiglottis and acute epiglottis, 356
exposure, onset and severity, 357-358
fever, 357
hoarseness, 358
immunizations, 358
medications, 358
mononucleosis, 358
peritonsillar abscesses, 356
sexual behaviors, 358
sneezing, 358
symptoms, 357-358
drooling, dyspnea, and inspiratory stridor, 356
emergency signals, 356
exposure, onset and severity, 357-358
laboratory and diagnostic studies, 361
pharyngitis with ulcers causing
aphthous stomatitis, 363, 364-365b
candidiasis, 363, 364-365b
canker sores, 363, 364-365b
herpangina, 363, 364-365b
herpes simplex virus (HSV), 363, 364-365b
Vincent angina, 363, 364-365b
pharyngitis without ulcers causing
epiglottis, 361-362, 364-365b
gonococcal pharyngitis, 363, 364-365b
inflammation, 363, 364-365b
mononucleosis, 362-363, 364-365b
peritonsillar abscess, 362, 364-365b
retropharyngeal abscess, 362, 364-365b
streptococcal pharyngitis, 362, 362t, 364-365b
viral pharyngitis, 362, 364-365b
physical examination procedures, 358-361
skin rashes and lesions with, 310
Soy protein hypersensitivity, 138
Specific gravity test
for female/child urinary problem evaluation, 389-390
for urinary incontinence evaluation, 379
Speech
as indicator of psychological or substance abuse disorders, 39
Sphincter
anal
anal fissures and tears, 321, 328-329, 331-332b
contraction tenesmus, 321
relaxation and defecation problems, 111
weakness
and urinary incontinence, 374
Sphincter-detrusor dyssynergia, 374
Spinal arc, 111
Spinal cord tumors, 271

Spinal metastasis
causing acute low back pain (ALBP), 275, 277-279b
Spinal stenosis, 276, 277-279b
Spine
fractures, 267-268, 274, 277-279b
normal vs abnormal x-ray findings, 463-464b
osteoarthritis in, 250
palpation in children, 378
scoliosis evaluation, 88
Spirometry
for dyspnea evaluation, 168
Spleen
anatomic diagram and x-ray view of, 458f, 459, 459f
normal vs abnormal x-ray findings, 463-464b
Spondylolisthesis, 270, 275, 277-279b
Spontaneous abortions
causing vaginal bleeding, 397, 405, 408-410b
Sports; *See* exercise
Sprains
ankle, 258, 262-265b
and limb pain, 244
Sputum
for acid-fast bacilli (AFB), 203
characteristics and coughs, 121-122
and chest pain, 84
for culture and sensitivity tests, 127, 203
for gram staining, 203
Squinting, 426
Stable angina, 92, 95b
Staphylococcus infections
food poisoning, 143, 146-147b
and red eye, 335, 341-342
Starvation stools, 139
Status asthmaticus
and dyspnea, 169, 171-172b
Stein-Leventhal syndrome, 398-399
Stereotactic or needle localization biopsy, 69
Stereotyping
cautioning against diagnostic, 3
Stethoscopes, 126
Stiff necks
and fever, 195
Stimulant use
causing palpitations, 293, 294-295b
causing sleep problems, 348
Stomach
anatomic diagram and x-ray view of, 458f, 459, 459f
gas pattern x-ray images, 459f, 460, 461f
Stool antigen test, 20
Stool culture and sensitivity test, 142, 203
Stool leukocyte test, 203
Stool sample for ova and parasites, 203
Stools
analyzing during abdominal pain assessment, 13-15
black, 112
blood in with diarrhea, 136
color of, 114, 136
and constipation, 111
delayed passage and constipation, 114
fecal immunochemical test (iFOBT), 19-20, 115-116
fecal occult blood test (FOBT), 19, 115-116
frequency, volume and consistency, 111, 134
intervals, 134
with irritable bowel syndrome (IBS), 113
loose bloody, 323

Stools *(Continued)*
  melena, 323
  in newborns, infants and children, 323
  "normal" frequency, 111
  pH to evaluate diarrhea, 142
  size and caliber, 113
  stool antigen test, 20
Strabismic amblyopia, 426
Strabismus, 430, 433-434b
Straight leg raising (SLR) test
  during ALBP examination, 272-273
Strains
  description of, 244
Streptococcal infections
  causing female and child urinary dysfunction, 389
  and red eye, 335, 341-342
  sore throat
    β-hemolytic streptococcus (GABHS) infections, 356-357, 358,
      362t
Streptococcal pharyngitis, 362, 362t, 364-365b
Stress
  and acute low back pain (ALBP), 267, 277, 277-279b
  and fatigue, 186-187
  normal *versus* psychological or situational, 39-40, 42-45b
  palpitations, 289
  precipitating syncope, 367
  causing vertigo, 150
Stress fractures, 257, 262-265b
Stress incontinence
  definition of, 374
  medications that can cause, 375t
  symptoms and causes of, 380, 382-383b
  Valsalva maneuver to test for, 378
Stress tests
  during chest pain evaluation, 89
  for syncope evaluation, 370
Stridor
  assessing during dyspnea evaluation, 165
Stroke
  as pulmonary embolus risk factor, 160-161
  and transient ischemic attacks (TIAs), 367-368
Styes, 341, 343-344b
Subarachnoid hemorrhage (SAH)
  acute and sudden headache with, 221, 222-223
Subconjunctival hemorrhage, 342, 343-344b
Subdural hematoma
  confusion from, 98
  and headaches, 231, 232-233b
Subjective judgments
  in hypothesis formation, 3
Subluxation of radial head, 256, 262-265b
Substance abuse; *See also* alcohol abuse; drug abuse
  CAGE questionnaire, 33, 33b
  categories of substances, 40
  as clue to psychological disorders, 30
  diagnostic questions and symptoms of, 33, 33b, 34b
  history and penile discharge issues, 296
  RAFFT adolescent questionnaire, 34b
Sudden death family history, 369
Suicide
  assessing risk during HEEADSSS interview, 34-35,
    36t
  risk questions, 35, 98
Suppositories
  and constipation, 113

Suprapubic discomfort
  with female and child urinary dysfunction, 387
  history and male genitourinary evaluation, 211
Supraventricular tachycardia
  and syncope, 367
Surgery
  associated with abdominal pain, 15
  and dyspnea, 161
  and hoarseness, 236
  recent and fever, 197
Sweat chloride test, 127, 442
Sweating
  as prodromal symptom of syncope, 366
Swelling
  with limb injuries, 246, 251-252
Swimming
  and earaches, 175
  nasal symptoms due to, 282
Syncope
  cardiac differential diagnoses
    arrhythmias, 370-371, 372b
    organic heart disease, 370-371, 372b
  definition of, 366, 366b
  diagnostic reasoning/key history questions
    after sudden head rotation, 368
    chest pain or shortness of breath, 367
    event and post-event characteristics, 367
    with exercise, 367
    fainting in family history, 369
    frequency of, 368
    headaches, 367
    health problems, 368
    heart disease/congenital heart problem history, 367
    Kawasaki disease history, 368
    loss of consciousness, 366
    Lyme disease, 369
    medications, 368
    migraine headaches, 367-368
    orthostasis, 368
    palpitations, 367
    pre-event characteristics, 367
    prenatal systemic lupus erythematosus (SLE), 369
    prodromal symptoms, 366
    psychogenic syncope, 368
    situational or vasovagal, 368
    sudden death family history, 369
    vertigo, dizziness and visual symptoms, 367-368
    witness information, 367
  evidence-based practice (EBP) for diagnosis of, 366b
  laboratory and diagnostic studies, 369-370
  with lightheadedness, 149-150
  loss of consciousness with, 366
  medication-related differential diagnoses
    drug-induced, 371, 372b
    prescribed medications, 371, 372b
  neurocardiogenic differential diagnoses
    arrhythmias, 371, 372b
    breath-holding, 372b
    carotid sinus hypersensitivity, 371, 372b
    cough syncope, 371, 372b
    situational syncope, 371, 372b
    vasovagal syncope, 371, 372b
  neurological differential diagnoses
    migraine headaches, 371, 372b
    seizures, 371, 372b

Syncope *(Continued)*
in older adults, 366b
orthostatic hypotension, 371, 372b
with palpitations, 288
physical examination procedures, 369
psychiatric differential diagnoses
hysterical reactions, 371, 372b
mental disorders, 371, 372b
psychiatric evaluations, 366b
types of, 366
unknown causes of, 371, 372b
without warning, 367
Syphilis, 156, 420, 421b
Systemic lupus erythematosus, 85, 259, 262-265b

T
T-ACE prenatal alcohol-use questionnaire, 33b
Tachycardia
description of, 165, 165b
Tamoxifen
vaginal bleeding due to, 401
Tanner stages
illustration of boy, 77f
of sexual maturity in girls, 49, 50-51, 50f
Tarsal tunnel syndrome, 260, 262-265b
T-cells
production and fever, 194
Technetium 99m scan
for anorectal disorder diagnosis, 328
Teeth
inspection during nasal evaluation, 283
causing referred pain earaches, 174
Temperature
charting during amenorrhea evaluation, 56
during dyspnea evaluation, 165-166
examining in diarrhea cases, 140
hypothalamus regulation of, 194
measurement for fever evaluation, 194-195, 200
Temporal arteritis
causing headaches, 230, 232-233b
Temporomandibular joint (TMJ)
and earaches, 174, 182, 182-183b
pain with headaches, 221, 224, 227
Tendinitis, 253, 262-265b
Tenesmus
and anorectal disorders, 324
with ulcerative colitis in children, 323
Tennis elbow, 256, 261t, 262-265b
Tenosynovitis, 253, 262-265b
Tension pain, 8
Tension-type headaches (TTHs)
pain location and characteristics, 224, 229, 232-233b
pattern and duration of, 224-225
Testes
pain and penile discharge evaluation, 297-298, 299
Tanner stage development illustration, 77f
Testicular torsion, 218, 219-220b
Thermal trauma
vision loss from, 425, 432, 433-434b
Thermometers
for accurate fever gauging, 194-195
THINC MED
mnemonic for evaluating psychological/physiologic conditions, 31, 32b

Thirst
assessing in urinary incontinence patients, 376
and dehydration with diarrhea, 135
Thoracic outlet syndrome, 260, 262-265b
Thoracic spine
as seen on chest x-rays, 451, 455b
Threatened abortion, 405, 408-410b
Throat
assessing during fatigue evaluation, 187
assessing during headache evaluation, 227
symptoms and fever, 196
Thrombus
dislodging and pulmonary embolus, 160-161
formation factors, 160-161
Thyroid function tests
to analyze confusional states, 105
and breast evaluation, 69
during constipation evaluation, 116
and depression, 39
Thyroid gland
and amenorrhea, 51, 54, 57, 58-59t
and hoarseness, 239
and palpitations, 291
and vaginal bleeding, 407, 408-410b
Thyroidectomy
causing hoarseness, 236
Thyroid-stimulating hormones (TSHs)
and depression, 39
for fatigue cases, 189
tests, 55, 116, 442
Tietze syndrome, 78, 79-80b, 93, 95b
Tilt-table testing
for syncope evaluation, 370
Tinea
characteristics, associations and diagnosis of, 316-320b
definition and mechanisms of, 315
infections, 311
itching of, 310b
Tinel sign, 260, 261t
Tinnitus, 151
Tiredness
in adolescents, 184
and fatigue, 184
Toddlers
sleep refusal, 353, 354-355b
Toilet training
and stool withholding, 114
Tolerance
alcohol, 33b
Tones and guarding percussion, 16
Tonsillectomy, 236
TORCH infections, 426, 432, 433-434b
Total blindness, 424f
Total iron-binding capacity (TIBC)
for fatigue cases, 188
Total serum protein test, 442
Toxicology screening
for drugs and alcohol, 39, 105
for syncope evaluation, 370
Toxins
exposure and male genitourinary problems, 212
causing headaches, 226

Toxocara canis, 428-429
Trachea
    and chest palpation during chest pain evaluation, 87
    location of, 236f
    as seen on chest x-rays, 450, 455b
Trained night crier or feeder, 353-354, 354-355b
Transcranial Doppler ultrasonography, 370
Transcutaneous pulse oximetry
    for dyspnea evaluation, 168
Transient ischemic attacks (TIAs)
    cerebral perfusion and syncope, 367-368
    confusion indicating possible, 99
Transient synovitis of hip, 256, 262-265b
Transient vision loss, 425
Transillumination of sinuses
    during nasal evaluation, 284
Trauma
    and acute low back pain (ALBP), 268
    causing dizziness, 156
    earaches due to, 182, 182-183b
    to eyes, 425, 431, 433-434b
    causing female and child urinary dysfunction, 387
    history of
        and dyspnea, 160
        and headaches, 223
        and hoarseness, 236
    nasal symptoms due to, 282
    as possible cause of hoarseness, 236, 240, 241-242b
    as pulmonary embolus risk factor, 160-161
    causing red eye, 334-335
    to urinary tract, 208
    causing urinary tract infections, 385
    causing vision loss, 425
Travel
    recent
        and fever, 184b, 197
        and penile discharge, 298
        and skin rashes and lesions, 310
    sleep problems due to, 348-349
    traveler's diarrhea, 134, 137-138
Treatment plans
    development from diagnostic reasoning, 5
Tremors
    causes of, 99, 104
Treponema pallidum-specific tests, 300
Trichomonas
    in men, 296
Trichomonas vaginalis
    diamond culture to identify, 417
    DNA probe and saline prep testing for, 19, 215, 417
Trichomoniasis
    description and vaginal discharge with, 418b, 419, 421b
    microscopic illustration of, 412f
    tests to detect, 412f, 417
    vaginal bleeding and discharge due to, 399
Trigeminal autonomic cephalalgias, 221
Trigeminal neuralgia
    causing headaches, 230, 232-233b
True vocal folds, 235, 236f
Tuberculin skin tests
    during cough evaluation, 127
    for fatigue cases, 189
Tuberculosis
    causing breast lumps, 70, 72-73b
    and coughing, 124, 130-131, 132-133b
    exposure and fever, 197

Tuberculosis *(Continued)*
    and travel, 310
    and weight loss (unintentional), 438, 444, 445-446b
Tubular, red cell and hyaline casts, 391
Tumbling E chart, 427-428
Tumors
    bladder or kidney, 219, 219-220b
    and constipation, 118-119, 118-119b
    description and examples of skin, 304-305t, 307f
    pituitary adenoma, 52, 58-59t, 58-59
    spinal cord, 271
Tuning fork test, 179
Turbidity with foul odor
    with male genitourinary conditions, 214
Turbinate, 284
Turner syndrome, 51, 54, 57, 58-59t
Tympanic membrane
    anatomic diagram of, 175f
    examination in red eye cases, 340
    illustration of usual landmarks, 179f
    perforation symptoms, 182
Tympanometry, 180-181, 180f
Tzanck smear
    for skin rash/lesion evaluation, 312
    of vaginal discharge, 417

U
Ulcerative colitis
    bloody diarrhea, cramping and tenesmus with, 323
Ultrasonography
    definition and procedures for performing, 463
    to evaluate breasts, 68, 76
    for female/child urinary problem evaluation, 391
    for urinary incontinence evaluation, 380
    vaginal/lower abdomen, 404-405
Uncomplicated urinary tract infections (UTIs), 391-392, 392b, 394b
Unilateral breast lumps
    versus bilateral, 61
Unprotected sex; *See* sexual activities/practices
Upper respiratory infections (URIs)
    and earaches, 174
    fever characteristics with, 204, 206-207b
    and hoarseness, 237
Ureaplasma urealyticum, 296
Ureterolithiasis, 14, 22, 25-29b
Urethra
    obstruction, 375-376
    recent treatment and penile discharge, 298
Urethral meatus
    inspecting
        during male genitourinary evaluation, 213
        during penile discharge evaluation, 299
Urethritis
    description and diagnosis of male, 217, 219-220b
    in males and sexually transmitted infections (STIs), 296
    causing penile discharge, 297, 300, 302b
    urinary problems due to, 392
Urge incontinence
    definition of, 374
    medications that can cause, 375t
    symptoms and causes of, 380, 382-383b
Urge to defecate
    and constipation, 113-114

Urge to urinate
  with female and child urinary dysfunction, 388
Urgency
  as primary male symptom of urinary incontinence, 376
Urinalysis
  for abdominal pain evaluation, 19
  in constipation evaluation, 116
  in dizziness and vertigo evaluation, 154-155
  in fatigue cases, 188
  for female/child urinary problem evaluation, 390-391
  for male genitourinary evaluation, 214
  for penile discharge evaluation, 299
  testing in confused older adults, 105
  for urinary incontinence evaluation, 379
Urinary bleeding
  versus vaginal bleeding, 401
Urinary catheters, 212
Urinary dysfunction (female adult and children)
  diagnostic reasoning/key questions
    acute pain, 385-386
    bleeding without urination, 386
    constipation, 388
    diabetes mellitus, 388
    diaphragm use, 387
    excessive urination, 388
    exercise-related hematuria, 386
    family history, 388
    fever and chills, 385
    fluid intake, 388
    foods, caffeine or alcohol use, 388
    foreign objects, 387
    hematuria, 386
    hormone therapy, 387-388
    hygiene products or bubble baths, 388, 393, 394b
    immunocompromised patients, 386
    irritable infants, 386
    nausea and vomiting, 385
    pain with hematuria, 386
    previous urinary problems, 388
    primary symptoms, 386-387
    recent instrumentation, 388
    risk factors, 388
    sexual activity, 387
    sexually transmitted infections (STIs), 388
    streptococcal infections, 389
    suprapubic discomfort, 387
    trauma, 387
    urge to urinate, 388
    urinary incontinence, 387
    vaginal discharge, 387-388
    vaginitis, 388
  differential diagnoses
    atrophic vaginitis, 392-393, 394b
    bacterial cystitis, 391-392, 392b, 394b
    chemical irritation, 393, 394b
    cystitis, 391-392, 392b, 394b
    interstitial cystitis, 393, 394b
    poststreptococcal glomerulonephritis, 393, 394b
    pyelonephritis, 393, 394b
    uncomplicated urinary tract infections (UTIs), 391-392, 392b, 394b
    urethritis, 392
    urinary tract infections (UTIs), 391-392, 392b, 394b
    urolithiasis, 393, 394b
    vulvovaginitis, 392-393, 394b

Urinary dysfunction *(Continued)*
  laboratory and diagnostic studies, 389-391
  physical examination procedures, 389
Urinary flow; *See* urine flow
Urinary frequency
  with penile discharge, 297
Urinary incontinence
  anatomical causes of
    overflow incontinence, 380-381, 382-383b
    stress incontinence, 380, 382-383b
    urge incontinence, 380, 382-383b
  categorizing, 374
  caused by reversible factors
    constipation and fecal impaction, 381, 382-383b
    diabetes insipidus, 381, 382-383b
    diabetes mellitus, 381, 382-383b
    medications, 381, 382-383b
    mental or mobility function, 381, 382-383b
    mixed incontinence, 381, 382-383b
    urinary tract infections, 381, 382-383b
    vaginitis, 381, 382-383b
  definition of, 374
  diagnostic reasoning/key questions
    abnormal daytime voiding, 377
    atrophic vaginitis, 375
    bowel function, 375-376
    chronic health problems and, 375-376
    dribbling or chronic leakage, 377
    dyspareunia, 375
    family history of, 377
    fecal impaction, 375-376
    fluid intake, 376-377
    functional bladder neck obstruction, 377
    gender and birth order, 377
    genitourinary system questions, 377
    medications, 375, 375t
    mental status, 375-376
    and mobility, 375-376
    nervous system issues, 377
    nocturnal enuresis, 377
    pinworms, 377
    presenting primary symptoms, 376
    primary *versus* secondary enuresis in children, 376-377
    reversible factors and questions, 374-375, 375b
    sickle cell disease, 377
    thirst, 376
    urethra obstruction, 375-376
    urinary tract infections, 375
    urine lost per episode, 376
    vaginal dryness, 375
    voiding frequency and stream characteristics, 376
    weight loss or gain, 376
  DIAPERS mnemonic, 375b
  enuresis from nonorganic causes
    primary enuresis, 382
    secondary (developmental) enuresis, 382
    sickle cell anemia, 382
    small bladder, 382
  enuresis from organic causes
    genitourinary causes, 381
    neurological causes, 381-382
  with female and child urinary dysfunction, 387
  laboratory and diagnostic studies, 379-380
  with male genitourinary conditions, 211
  overview of, 375

Urinary incontinence *(Continued)*
  physical examination procedures, 378-379
  types of, 374, 380b
Urinary stones
  in men, 208
  pain, bleeding and infection with, 385
Urinary tract
  and constipation, 114-115
  pain with penile discharge, 297-298
  problems and vaginal discharge, 415
  problems in males (*See* male genitourinary system)
  urinary incontinence, 374-384
Urinary tract infections (UTIs); *See also* male genitourinary system;
      urinary dysfunction (females and children)
  abdominal pain from, 14, 22, 25-29b
  causes of, 208
  fever characteristics with, 204, 206-207b
  causing urinary incontinence, 375, 381, 382-383b
  urinary problems due to, 391-392, 392b, 394b
Urinary urgency
  with penile discharge, 297
Urination
  American Urological Association Symptom Index, 210t
  assessing volume lost in UI patients, 376
  differential diagnoses relating to problems with, 380-382, 382-383b
  increases and fatigue, 185
  precipitating syncope, 367
  urinary incontinence (*See* urinary incontinence)
Urine
  American Urological Association Symptom Index, 210t
  discoloration with urinary dysfunction, 386, 389, 390-391
  lost per episode, 376
  odor with urinary tract infections, 381
  postvoid residual volume, 378-379
  testing of, 389-391
Urine culture and sensitivity
  for abdominal pain evaluation, 19
  for female/child urinary problem evaluation, 391
  during fever evaluation, 202
  for urinary incontinence evaluation, 379
Urine cytology, 379
Urine dipstick
  for female/child urinary problem evaluation, 389-390
  for male genitourinary evaluation, 214
  for penile discharge evaluation, 299
Urine flow
  American Urological Association Symptom Index, 210t
  observation of voiding, 213
  problems in men, 209, 208 (*See also* male genitourinary system)
  studies, 215
Urine hesitancy
  stream and dribbling evaluation, 209, 210t
Urodynamic testing, 379, 379b
Uroflowmetry
  for male genitourinary evaluation, 215
  during urinary incontinence evaluation, 379
Urolithiasis
  description and diagnosis of male, 217, 219-220b
  urinary problems due to, 393, 394b
Urticaria
  definition and causes of, 315
  itching of, 310b
US Preventive Services Task Force, 5b
Uterine cancer
  causing vaginal bleeding, 406, 408-410b

Uterine fibroids
  causing lower abdominal pain, 24, 25-29b
Uterine prolapse, 398
Uterus
  amenorrhea, 53
  anatomic diagram and x-ray view of, 458f, 459
  normal vs abnormal x-ray findings, 463-464b
Uveal tract, 343, 343-344b
Uveitis, 272, 432, 433-434b

V
Vagina
  bleeding (*See* vaginal bleeding)
  passage of tissue from, 397
Vaginal bleeding; *See also* menopause; menstrual cycle
  anovulatory cycle systemic causes of, 406-407,
      408-410b
    in newborns, 407, 408-410b
    perimenarche, 406-407, 408-410b
    perimenopause, 406, 408-410b
  blood dyscrasias causing
    leukemia, 408, 408-410b
    von Willebrand disease, 408, 408-410b
  diagnostic reasoning/key history questions
    acute *versus* chronic, 398-399
    age and reproductive life cycle, 397-398
    age at menarche, 400
    amounts of, 396
    anticoagulant use, 396
    birth control method, 399
    bleeding or clotting disorders, 396, 401-402
    blood dyscrasias, 401-402
    diethylstilbestrol (DES) exposure, 402
    discharge accompanying, 399
    ectopic pregnancy, 397, 397b, 403
    endometrial cancer warnings and risk factors, 400, 400b
    hormone therapy, 400-401
    hysterectomy, 400
    intact uterus, 400
    irregular masses causing, 398
    with irregular menstrual cycles, 399-400
    last Pap test, 401
    lesions and lumps, 401
    with low back or abdominal pain, 397
    and maternal age, 397
    medications that might cause, 401
    menopausal symptoms, 400
    pediatric or prepubertal, 399
    postmenopausal, 398, 400
    and pregnancy, 396-397
    recent childbirth, 397
    sexually transmitted infections (STIs), 397, 399
    spontaneous abortions, 397
    symptom analysis, 398
    tamoxifen and other medication use, 401
    urinary or rectal bleeding *versus*, 401
    vaginal discharge, 401
  endocrinopathy systemic causes of
    hyperprolactinemia, 407, 408-410b
    polycystic ovary syndrome, 407, 408-410b
    thyroid dysfunction, 407, 408-410b
  heavy and acute menses, 397-398
  laboratory and diagnostic studies, 403-405
  medications causing, 408, 408-410b

Vaginal bleeding *(Continued)*
  normal *versus* excessive, 396, 398
  organic causes of
    adenomyosis, 406, 408-410b
    ectopic pregnancy, 406, 408-410b
    endometrial cancer, 406, 408-410b
    fibroids, 406, 408-410b
    leiomyomas, 406, 408-410b
    miscarriage, 405, 408-410b
    myomas, 406, 408-410b
    placenta abruptio, 406, 408-410b
    placenta previa, 405, 408-410b
    pregnancy, 405, 408-410b
    spontaneous abortion, 405, 408-410b
    threatened abortion, 405, 408-410b
    uterine cancer, 406, 408-410b
  physical examination procedures, 402-403
  vaginal infections causing
    atrophic vaginitis, 407, 408-410b
    condylomata acuminata, 407-408, 408-410b
    endometritis, 407, 408-410b
    foreign bodies, 408, 408-410b
    genital warts, 407-408, 408-410b
    pelvic inflammatory disease, 407, 408-410b
Vaginal cultures
  for female urinary problem evaluation, 391
  fungal or Sabouraud agar culture, 417
  for urinary incontinence evaluation, 379
Vaginal discharge
  accompanying vaginal bleeding, 399, 401
  characteristics of, 402-403, 411-412
  chronic vulvovaginitis, 414
  clinical diagnosis of vaginitis, 418b
  diagnostic reasoning/key history questions
    activities that cause infections, 413
    chronic vulvovaginitis, 414
    dyspareunia and pain, 415
    foreign bodies, 415
    and hygiene, 414-415
    medications or chemotherapy, 413
    and night itching, 413, 413f
    odor and color characteristics, 411-412, 412f
    pain issues, 415
    perianal pruritus, 413, 413f, 418
    pinworms, 413, 413f, 418
    premenarche, 413
    recent illnesses or infections, 413-414
    sexual activities/practices, 412, 414
    sexually transmitted infection history, 412-413, 414
    symptom occurrence and chronology, 413-414
    urinary tract symptoms accompanying, 415
  DNA probes, 417
  with female urinary dysfunction, 387-388
  with itching and lesions
    genital warts, 420, 421b
    herpes simplex, 420, 421b
    molluscum contagiosum, 420, 421b
    syphilis, 420, 421b
  laboratory and diagnostic studies, 416-418
  physical examination procedures, 415-416
    external and internal genital exam, 415-416
    vaginal-rectal exam, 416
  types of
    allergic vaginitis, 419, 421b
    atrophic vaginitis, 419, 421b

Vaginal discharge *(Continued)*
    bacterial vaginosis, 419, 421b
    Candida vulvovaginitis, 419, 421b
    Chlamydia infections, 419-420, 421b
    Chlamydia trachomatis, 420, 421b
    foreign bodies, 419, 421b
    gonorrhea infections, 420, 421b
    N. gonorrhoeae, 420, 421b
    pelvic inflammatory disease (PID), 420, 421b
    physiological discharge, 419, 421b
    trichomoniasis, 419, 421b
Vaginal infections
    atrophic vaginitis, 407, 408-410b
    condylomata acuminata, 407-408, 408-410b
    endometritis, 407, 408-410b
    foreign bodies, 408, 408-410b
    genital warts, 407-408, 408-410b
    pelvic inflammatory disease, 407, 408-410b
Vaginal-rectal exam, 416
Vaginitis; *See* vaginal discharge
Vaginosis
    symptoms and diagnosis of, 418b
    vaginal bleeding and discharge due to, 399
Valsalva maneuver
    during dizziness and vertigo evaluation, 152
    during urinary incontinence evaluation, 378
Valvular heart disease
    causing dyspnea, 161-162
Varicella, 196
Vasovagal syncope, 368, 371, 372b
Venereal Disease Research Laboratory (VDRL), 300, 328
Ventilation/perfusion lung scan, 89-90
Ventilatory system
    dysfunction causing dyspnea, 165
Ventricular tachycardias
    and syncope, 367
Vertebral bodies
    as seen on chest x-rays, 453, 454f, 455b
Vertigo
    adult and children sensations of, 149-150
    dizziness and visual symptoms, 367-368
    origins of, 149
    as prodromal symptom of syncope, 366
    versus syncope, 366, 367-368
Vesicles, 304-305t, 307f
Vesicoureteral reflux (VUR), 385
Vestibular nerves
    anatomic diagram of, 175f
Vestibular neuronitis
    causing peripheral vertigo, 151, 155
Vibrio cholerae, 143, 146-147b
Vincent angina, 363, 364-365b
Violence
    assessing risks during HEEADSSS interview, 34-35, 36t
Viral conjunctivitis
    causing red eye, 341-342, 343-344b
Viral gastroenteritis, 143, 146-147b
Viral infections
    fever characteristics with, 196, 204, 206-207b
    affecting muscles, 259, 262-265b
    nasal symptoms with, 282
    skin rashes and lesions due to, 310
    upper respiratory, 128, 131-132b, 196
Viral pharyngitis, 362, 364-365b

Vision
blurring of, 423
changes
and headaches, 225
evaluating in dizziness or vertigo cases, 152
focus abilities, 423
normal development and eye movements, 427b
nystagmus, 423
ophthalmoscopic examinations, 430
Snellen or Tumbling E chart to test, 427-428
squinting, 426
testing in older adults, 104
total absence of, 423
visual fields illustration, 339, 424f
visual fixation, 423
Vision loss
with aging, 427
versus blurry vision, 336
causes of
amblyopia, 426, 430, 433-434b
astigmatism, 431, 433-434b
cataracts, 431, 433-434b
central retinal artery occlusion, 431, 433-434b
chemical or thermal trauma, 432, 433-434b
congenital infections, 432, 433-434b
craniopharyngioma, 432, 433-434b
deprivation amblyopia, 426
diabetic retinopathy, 426, 432, 433-434b
eye trauma, 425
glaucoma, 431-432, 432b, 433-434b
head trauma, 425
injuries, 431, 433-434b
macular degeneration, 432, 433-434b
optic nerve glioma, 432, 433-434b
optic neuritis, 431, 433-434b
refractive amblyopia, 426
refractive errors, 430-431, 433-434b
retinal detachment, 432, 433-434b
retinoblastomas, 431, 433-434b
retinopathy of prematurity, 431, 433-434b
strabismic amblyopia, 426
strabismus, 430, 433-434b
TORCH infections, 426, 432, 433-434b
uveitis, 432, 433-434b
chemical or thermal trauma causing, 425
degrees of, 423
and delayed development, 427, 427b
eye pain with, 424-425
family history of, 426
flash of light with, 425
laboratory and diagnostic tests, 425
neonatal risks, 426
onset of, 423-424
pattern of, 427
physical examination procedures, 427-430
progressive degenerative, 425-426
with red eye, 336, 336b
transient, 425
Visual acuity
progressive loss of, 425-426
routine testing and glaucoma screening, 432b
Snellen or Tumbling E chart to test, 427-428
testing in red eye cases, 338

Visual fields
assessing, 429
illustration of, 424f
testing in red eye cases, 338
Visuospatial problems, 102
Vital signs; *See* specific conditions
Vitamin deficiency
associated with confusional states, 101b
Vitreous hemorrhage, 425, 428-429
Vocal cord paralysis, 240, 241-242b
Vocal cord polyps, 240, 241-242b
Vocal cords
and hoarseness, 235-242
Vocal folds
function and illustration of, 235, 236f
Vocal fremitus, 167
Voice
changes and dyspnea, 165, 167
definition of, 235
habits and hoarseness, 237
overuse causing hoarseness, 235-236
quality, pitch and volume, 235, 238, 238t
Voiding
abnormal daytime, 377
differential diagnoses relating to problems with, 380-382, 382-383b
frequency in urinary incontinence patients, 376
observation
in male genitourinary evaluation, 213
during urinary incontinence evaluation, 378-379
stream characteristics, 376
Voiding cystourethrography (VCUG), 379
Vomiting
and abdominal pain, 13
causes of, 13
with constipation, 114
with diarrhea, 137
with fever, 195-196
Vomitus
appearance of, 13
Von Willebrand disease
causing vaginal bleeding, 408, 408-410b
Vulvovaginitis
urinary problems due to, 392-393, 394b
vaginal bleeding and discharge due to, 399

W
Weakness
versus fatigue, 184
Web sources
supporting evidence-based practice (EBP), 4-5, 5b
Weber test
during dizziness and vertigo evaluation, 152
for hearing acuity, 179
WebMD, 5b
Weight; *See also* weight gain; weight loss
activity levels for maintaining healthy, 437b
and amenorrhea, 51, 53-54
assessing during HEEADSSS interview, 34-35, 36t
and body mass index (BMI), 435
body mass index (BMI) chart, 467f
calorie intake and activity levels, 435, 436b, 437b, 440t
changes with aging, 100, 435
examining in diarrhea cases, 140
of infants and children, 435

Weight *(Continued)*
  key recommendations for maintaining healthy, 436b
  loss or gain in urinary incontinence patients, 376
  measuring, 435
  and vaginal bleeding, 402
Weight gain (unintentional)
  diagnostic reasoning/key questions
    aging-related, 439
    alcohol use, 439
    calories and activity level table, 439, 440t
    eating patterns and activity levels, 439, 440t
    endocrine assessment, 439-440
    medications, 439-440
    menopause and hormones, 439
    smoking, 439
  differential diagnoses
    aging, 444, 445-446b
    anxiety, 443, 445-446b
    cognitive impairment, 443, 445-446b
    Cushing syndrome, 444, 445-446b
    depression, 443, 445-446b
    endocrine disorders, 444, 445-446b
    hypothyroidism, 444, 445-446b
    imbalance in calorie/activity levels, 444, 445-446b
  lab tests to assess
    basal metabolic rate (BMR) test, 442, 443b
    complete blood count (CBC) with indices and differential, 441
    sweat chloride test, 442
    thyroid-stimulating hormone (TSH) test, 442
  physical examination procedures, 440-442
Weight loss (unintentional)
  and abdominal pain, 15
  and constipation, 112
  defining, 435
  diagnostic reasoning/key questions
    acute or chronic conditions, 437
    age, 435
    anorexia, 439
    appetite, 436, 438
    breastfeeding, 436
    cancer screening, 438
    concerns regarding ideal weight, 439
    cystic fibrosis, 438
    diabetes, 437-438
    eating habits/diet changes, 436, 438
    endocrine disorders, 438
    failure to thrive, 437
    family history, 438
    formula-fed infants, 436
    indications of, 435
    medication history, 438-439
    nutritional adequacy, 436
    physical activity, 436, 437b, 438
    psychosocial factors, 436-437
    tuberculosis, 438
  diagnostic reasoning/physical examination, 440-442
  differential diagnoses of
    Addison disease, 443, 445-446b
    alcohol use, 444, 445-446b
    anorexia nervosa, 443, 445-446b
    cancer, 442-443, 445-446b

Weight loss *(Continued)*
    Crohn disease, 444, 445-446b
    cystic fibrosis, 444, 445-446b
    dementia, 443-444, 445-446b
    depression, 443, 445-446b
    diabetes mellitus, 443, 445-446b
    economic status, 444, 445-446b
    endocrine disorders, 443, 445-446b
    gastroesophageal reflux in infants, 444, 445-446b
    HIV/AIDS, 444, 445-446b
    hyperthyroidism, 443, 445-446b
    malabsorption, 443, 445-446b
    nutritional deficiency, 443, 445-446b
    psychosocial factors, 444, 445-446b
    social isolation, 444, 445-446b
    tuberculosis, 444, 445-446b
  and fatigue, 185
  laboratory and diagnostic studies
    basal metabolic rate (BMR) test, 442, 443b
    complete blood count (CBC) with indices and differential, 441
    fasting blood glucose test, 441
    sweat chloride test, 442
    thyroid-stimulating hormone (TSH) test, 442
West Nile virus (WNV)
  characteristics and dangers of, 197, 198b
Wet diapers
  and dehydration with diarrhea, 135
Wet mount tests
  to evaluate diarrhea, 142
  for female/child urinary problem evaluation, 391
Wheals, 304-305t, 307f
Wheezing, 87-88, 165, 167
Whisper test
  for hearing acuity, 179
White blood cell (WBC) count
  for fatigue cases, 188-189
  for female/child urinary problem evaluation, 391
  inflammation or infections indicated by, 18
Whooping cough, 128, 131-132b
Witch's milk, 71, 72-73b
Wood's light
  for skin rash/lesion evaluation, 312
Wrist
  diagnostic reasoning/key pain questions, 245
  Finkelstein test, 261t
  fractures, 256, 262-265b
  Phalen test, 260, 261t
  Tinel sign, 260, 261t

X

X-rays; *See* abdominal x-rays; chest x-rays; radiography

Y

Yale Observation Scale Predictive Model
  for quantifying fever and illness in children, 199, 200t
Yawning
  as prodromal symptom of syncope, 366
Yergason test, 255, 261t